SEVENTH EDITION

Critical Care Handbook of the Massachusetts General Hospital

SEVENTH EDITION

Critical Care Handbook of the Massachusetts General Hospital

SENIOR EDITOR

Edward A. Bittner, MD, PhD, MSEd
Associate Professor
Department of Anesthesia
Harvard Medical School
Program Director, Critical Care Anesthesiology Fellowship
Department of Anesthesia, Critical Care and Pain Medicine
Massachusetts General Hospital
Boston, Massachusetts

ASSOCIATE EDITORS

Lorenzo Berra, MD
Reginald Jenney Associate Professor
Department of Anesthesia, Critical Care and Pain Medicine
Harvard Medical School
Staff Anesthesiologist and Critical Care Physician
Medical Director, Respiratory Care
Department of Anesthesia, Critical Care and Pain Medicine
Massachusetts General Hospital
Boston, Massachusetts

Peter J. Fagenholz, MD
Associate Professor
Harvard Medical School
Department of Surgery
Massachusetts General Hospital
Boston, Massachusetts

Jean Kwo, MD
Assistant Professor
Department of Anaesthesia
Harvard Medical School
Staff Anesthesiologist and Critical Care Physician
Medical Director, Surgical Intensive Care Unit
Department of Anesthesia, Critical Care and Pain Medicine
Massachusetts General Hospital
Boston, Massachusetts

Jarone Lee, MD
Associate Professor
Surgery and Emergency Medicine
Harvard Medical School
Vice Chief, Critical Care
Department of Trauma, Emergency Surgery, Surgical Critical Care
Massachusetts General Hospital
Boston, Massachusetts

Abraham Sonny, MD
Assistant Professor
Department of Anesthesia
Harvard Medical School
Cardiac Anesthesiologist and Critical Care Physician
Department of Anesthesia, Critical Care and Pain Medicine
Massachusetts General Hospital
Boston, Massachusetts

Wolters Kluwer

Philadelphia • Baltimore • New York • London
Buenos Aires • Hong Kong • Sydney • Tokyo

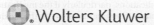

Senior Acquisitions Editor: Keith Donnellan
Senior Development Editor: Ashley Fischer
Editorial Coordinator: Sunmerrilika Baskar
Marketing Manager: Kirsten Watrud
Production Project Manager: Bridgett Dougherty
Design Coordinator: Stephen Druding
Manufacturing Coordinator: Beth Welsh
Prepress Vendor: S4Carlisle Publishing Services

Seventh Edition

9 8 7 6 5 4 3 2 1

Printed in the United States of America

Library of Congress Cataloging-in-Publication Data

ISBN-13: 978-1-975183-79-0

ISBN-10: 1-975183-79-7

Library of Congress Control Number: 2023904026

---

shop.lww.com

MPP0223

To our patients, teachers, and trainees—
past, present, and future.

CONTRIBUTORS

Chiaka O. V. Akarichi, MD
Assistant Professor
Department of Surgery
University of Texas Southwestern Medical School
Associate Medical Director of Parkland Burn Center
Department of Surgery
Parkland Hospital
Dallas, Texas

Katherine H. Albutt, MD, MPH
Assistant Professor
Department of Surgery
Harvard Medical School
Attending Surgeon
Departments of Trauma, Emergency Surgery, and Surgical Critical Care
Massachusetts General Hospital
Boston, Massachusetts

Clíodhna Ashe, BA, BDentSc, BMBS
Fellow in Critical Care Medicine
Department of Anesthesia, Critical Care and Pain Medicine
Massachusetts General Hospital
Boston, Massachusetts

Aranya Bagchi, MBBS
Assistant Professor of Anesthesia
Department of Anesthesia, Critical Care and Pain Medicine
Harvard Medical School
Staff Anesthesiologist and Intensivist
Heart Center ICU, Corrigan Minehan Heart Center and Department of Anesthesia, Critical Care and Pain Medicine
Massachusetts General Hospital
Boston, Massachusetts

Lisa M. Bebell, MD
Associate Professor
Harvard Medical School
Associate Physician
Division of Infectious Diseases
Department of Medicine
Massachusetts General Hospital
Boston, Massachusetts

William J. Benedetto, MD
Assistant Professor
Department of Anesthesia, Critical Care and Pain Medicine
Harvard Medical School
Massachusetts General Hospital
Boston, Massachusetts

Lorenzo Berra, MD
Reginald Jenney Associate Professor
Department of Anesthesia, Critical Care and Pain Medicine
Harvard Medical School
Staff Anesthesiologist and Critical Care Physician
Medical Director, Respiratory Care
Department of Anesthesia, Critical Care and Pain Medicine
Massachusetts General Hospital
Boston, Massachusetts

Edward A. Bittner, MD, PhD, MSEd
Associate Professor
Department of Anesthesia
Harvard Medical School
Program Director, Critical Care Anesthesiology Fellowship
Department of Anesthesia, Critical Care and Pain Medicine
Massachusetts General Hospital
Boston, Massachusetts

Sharon E. Brackett, RN, BSN
Registered Nurse
Surgical Intensive Care Unit
Massachusetts General Hospital
Boston, Massachusetts

Diana Barragan Bradford, MD
Staff Anesthesiologist and Critical Care Intensivist
Instructor, Harvard Medical School
Department of Anesthesia, Critical Care and Pain Medicine
Massachusetts General Hospital
Boston, Massachusetts

Benjamin R. M. Brush, MD
Assistant Professor
Department of Neurology
New York University
Attending Physician
Department of Neurology
NYU Langone Health Tisch Hospital
New York, New York

Ryan W. Carroll, MD, MPH
Assistant Professor
Department of Pediatrics
Harvard Medical School
Attending Faculty
Division of Pediatric Critical Care Medicine
Massachusetts General Hospital
Boston, Massachusetts

Marvin G. Chang, MD, PhD
Assistant Professor
Department of Anesthesia, Critical Care and Pain Medicine
Harvard Medical School
Associate Program Director, Critical Care Medicine Fellowship
Director, Perioperative Transthoracic Echocardiography
(Point of Care Ultrasound)
Department of Anesthesia, Critical Care and Pain Medicine
Massachusetts General Hospital
Boston, Massachusetts

Hovig V. Chitilian, MD
Anesthesiologist
Department of Anesthesia, Critical Care and Pain Medicine
Massachusetts General Hospital
Boston, Massachusetts

Devan Cote, MD
Instructor in Anesthesia
Harvard Medical School
Anesthesiologist
Department of Anesthesia, Critical Care and Pain Medicine
Massachusetts General Hospital
Boston, Massachusetts

Jerome Crowley, MD, MPH
Clinical Instructor
Department of Anesthesia, Critical Care and Pain Medicine
Harvard Medical School
ECMO Director
Heart Center ICU
Massachusetts General Hospital
Boston, Massachusetts

Brian M. Cummings, MD
Assistant Professor
Department of Pediatrics
Harvard Medical School
Pediatric Intensive Care
Department of Pediatrics
Massachusetts General Hospital
Boston, Massachusetts

Roberta Ribeiro De Santis Santiago, MD, PhD, RRT
Instructor in Anesthesia
Department of Anesthesia, Critical Care and Pain Medicine
Harvard Medical School
Research Staff
Department of Anesthesia, Critical Care and Pain Medicine
Massachusetts General Hospital
Boston, Massachusetts

Paige McLean Diaz, MD
Gastroenterology Fellow
Department of Medicine
Massachusetts General Hospital
Boston, Massachusetts

Ander Dorken-Gallastegi, MD
Post-Doctoral Research Fellow
Department of Surgery
Harvard Medical School
Post-Doctoral Research Fellow
Division of Trauma, Emergency Surgery, and Surgical Critical Care
Massachusetts General Hospital
Boston, Massachusetts

David M. Dudzinski, MD
Assistant Professor
Cardiology and Critical Care
Harvard Medical School
Director, Cardiac Intensive Care Unit
Department of Cardiology, Cardiac Intensive Care, Echocardiography
Massachusetts General Hospital
Boston, Massachusetts

Walter (Sunny) Dzik, MD
Associate Professor
Department of Pathology
Harvard Medical School
Consulting Hematologist
Department of Medicine
Massachusetts General Hospital
Boston, Massachusetts

Michael G. Fitzsimons, MD
Associate Professor
Department of Anesthesia, Critical Care and Pain Medicine
Harvard Medical School
Director, Division of Cardiac Anesthesia
Department of Anesthesia, Critical Care and Pain Medicine
Massachusetts General Hospital
Boston, Massachusetts

Rachel C. Frank, MD
Fellow
Division of Cardiology
Department of Medicine
Harvard Medical School
Fellow
Division of Cardiology
Department of Medicine
Massachusetts General Hospital
Boston, Massachusetts

Manolo Rubio Garcia, MD
Interventional Cardiology, Vascular Medicine and Endovascular Intervention Specialist
Interventional Cardiology
Cardiovascular Institute of San Diego
Chula Vista, California

Ed George, MD, PhD
Assistant Professor
Department of Anesthesiology
Harvard Medical School
Director of Disaster Planning and Resource Management Perioperative Services
Department of Anesthesia and Critical Care
Massachusetts General Hospital
Boston, Massachusetts

Lauren E. Gibson, MD
Clinical Fellow
Department of Anesthesia, Critical Care and Pain Medicine
Massachusetts General Hospital
Boston, Massachusetts

Dusan Hanidziar, MD, PhD
Instructor in Anesthesia
Harvard Medical School
Anesthesiologist and Intensivist
Department of Anesthesia, Critical Care and Pain Medicine
Massachusetts General Hospital
Boston, Massachusetts

Bryan D. Hayes, PharmD
Associate Professor
Division of Medical Toxicology, Department of Emergency Medicine
Attending Pharmacist
Department of Pharmacy
Massachusetts General Hospital
Boston, Massachusetts

Dean R. Hess, PhD, RRT
Lecturer
Respiratory Care, College of Professional Studies
Northeastern University
Respiratory Care Services
Massachusetts General Hospital
Boston, Massachusetts

Ronald E. Hirschberg, MD
Assistant Professor
Director, Physical Medicine and Rehabilitation Consultation Service
Department of Physical Medicine and Rehabilitation
Massachusetts General Hospital
Boston, Massachusetts

Ryan J. Horvath, MD, PhD
Instructor in Anesthesia
Department of Anesthesia, Critical Care and Pain Medicine
Harvard Medical School
Post Anesthesia Care Unit (PACU) Director
Staff Anesthesiologist and Critical Care Intensivist
Department of Anesthesia, Critical Care and Pain Medicine
Massachusetts General Hospital
Boston, Massachusetts

Joanne C. Huang, PharmD, BCIDP
Infectious Diseases Clinical Pharmacist
Department of Pharmacy
Massachusetts General Hospital
Boston, Massachusetts

Paul S. Jansson, MD, MS
Instructor
Departments of Surgery and Emergency Medicine
Harvard Medical School
Emergency and Critical Care Physician
Departments of Surgery and Emergency Medicine
Mass General Brigham
Boston, Massachusetts

Kristin Kennedy, DO
Clinical Fellow
Harvard Medical School
Surgical Critical Care Fellow
Department of Surgery
Massachusetts General Hospital
Boston, Massachusetts

Emmett Alexander Kistler, MD
Fellow
Harvard Medical School
Division of Pulmonary and Critical Care Medicine
Massachusetts General Hospital
Boston, Massachusetts

Alexander S. Kuo, MS, MD
Assistant Professor
Department of Anesthesia, Critical Care and Pain Medicine
Massachusetts General Hospital
Assistant Professor
Department of Anesthesia, Critical Care and Pain Medicine
Harvard Medical School
Boston, Massachusetts

Carolyn J. La Vita, MHA, RRT
Director
Department of Respiratory Care
Massachusetts General Hospital
Boston, Massachusetts

Yvonne Lai, MD
Assistant Professor
Harvard Medical School
Associate Program Director, Anesthesiology Residency
Department of Anesthesiology, Critical Care and Pain Medicine
Massachusetts General Hospital
Boston, Massachusetts

Sameer Lakha, MD
Assistant Professor
Anesthesiology, Perioperative and Pain Medicine
Institute for Critical Care Medicine
Icahn School of Medicine at Mount Sinai
The Mount Sinai Hospital
New York, New York

Benjamin Levi, MD
Associate Professor
Division Chair for General Surgery
Department of Surgery
University of Texas Southwestern Medical Center
Dallas, Texas

Ying Hui Low, MD, FASA, FASE
Staff Physician
Department of Anesthesiology
Massachusetts General Hospital
Boston, Massachusetts

Shu Yang Lu, MD
Clinical Instructor
Department of Anesthesia, Critical Care and Pain Medicine
Harvard Medical School
Department of Anesthesia, Critical Care and Pain Medicine
Massachusetts General Hospital
Boston, Massachusetts

Robert S. Makar, MD, PhD
Associate Professor
Department of Pathology
Harvard Medical School
Director, Blood Transfusion Service
Department of Pathology
Massachusetts General Hospital
Boston, Massachusetts

Christopher J. Mariani, MD, PhD
Fellow
Department of Anesthesia, Critical Care and Pain Medicine
Harvard Medical School
Massachusetts General Hospital
Boston, Massachusetts

Laurie O. Mark, MD
Attending Anesthesiologist and Critical Care Physician
Department of Anesthesiology
Jesse Brown VA Medical Center
Chicago, Illinois

Lukas H. Matern, MD
Chief Resident
Department of Anesthesia, Critical Care and Pain Medicine
Massachusetts General Hospital
Boston, Massachusetts

April E. Mendoza, MD, MPH
Assistant Professor
Department of Surgery
Massachusetts General Hospital
Boston, Massachusetts

Ilan Mizrahi, MD
Instructor
Department of Anesthesia
Harvard Medical School
Anesthetist
Department of Anesthesia, Critical Care and Pain Medicine
Massachusetts General Hospital
Boston, Massachusetts

Catherine E. Naber, MD
Clinical Instructor in Pediatrics
Harvard Medical School
Pediatric Intensivist
Massachusetts General Hospital
Boston, Massachusetts

Emily E. Naoum, MD
Instructor in Anesthesia
Harvard Medical School
Clinical Instructor
Program Director, Obstetric Anesthesia Fellowship
Department of Anesthesia, Critical Care and Pain Medicine
Massachusetts General Hospital
Boston, Massachusetts

Michael O'Brien, PharmD
Emergency Medicine Clinical Pharmacist
Department of Pharmacy
Massachusetts General Hospital
Boston, Massachusetts

Peter O. Ochieng, MD
Instructor in Anesthesia
Department of Anesthesia, Critical Care and Pain Medicine
Harvard Medical School
Staff Anesthesiologist
Department of Anesthesia, Critical Care and Pain Medicine
Massachusetts General Hospital
Boston, Massachusetts

Jonathan J. Parks, MD, FACS
Clinical Instructor in Surgery
Department of Surgery
Harvard Medical School
Instructor in Surgery
Department of Surgery
Massachusetts General Hospital
Boston, Massachusetts

Kristin Parlman, PT, DPT, NCS
Physical Therapy Clinical Specialist
Department of Physical Therapy
Massachusetts General Hospital
Boston, Massachusetts

Sylvia Ranjeva, MD, PhD
Resident Physician
Department of Anesthesia, Critical Care and Pain Medicine
Massachusetts General Hospital
Boston, Massachusetts

Benjamin Christian Renne, MD
Instructor
Harvard Medical School
Critical Care Attending Physician
Division of Trauma, Emergency Surgery, and Surgical Critical Care
Massachusetts General Hospital
Boston, Massachusetts

Josanna Rodriguez-Lopez, MD
Assistant Professor
Department of Medicine
Harvard Medical School
Assistant Physician
Division of Pulmonary and Critical Care
Department of Medicine
Massachusetts General Hospital
Boston, Massachusetts

Katarina J. Ruscic, MD, PhD
Instructor in Anesthesia
Department of Anesthesia, Critical Care and Pain Medicine
Harvard Medical School
Director of Anesthesia for Plastic, Reconstructive and Breast Oncology Surgery
Department of Anesthesia, Critical Care and Pain Medicine
Massachusetts General Hospital
Boston, Massachusetts

Daniel Saddawi-Konefka, MD, MBA
Assistant Professor
Harvard Medical School
Program Director, Anesthesiology Residency
Department of Anesthesia, Critical Care and Pain Medicine
Massachusetts General Hospital
Boston, Massachusetts

Kyan C. Safavi, MD, MBA
Assistant Professor
Department of Anesthesia
Harvard Medical School
Anesthesiologist and Critical Care Physician
Department of Anesthesia, Critical Care and Pain Medicine
Massachusetts General Hospital
Boston, Massachusetts

Noelle N. Saillant, MD, FACS
Assistant Professor
Department of Surgery
Boston University School of Medicine
Surgeon
Department of Surgery
Trauma, Acute Care and Surgical Critical Care
Boston Medical Center
Boston, Massachusetts

Takashi Sakano, MD
Instructor
Department of Anesthesia, Critical Care and Pain Medicine
Harvard Medical School
Anesthesiologist
Department of Anesthesia, Critical Care and Pain Medicine
Massachusetts General Hospital
Boston, Massachusetts

Esperance A. K. Schaefer, MD, MPH
Instructor
Department of Medicine
Harvard Medical School
Assistant in Medicine
Gastroenterology Unit, Department of Medicine
Massachusetts General Hospital
Boston, Massachusetts

Kenneth Shelton, MD
Assistant Professor
Harvard Medical School
Chief of the Critical Care Division
Department of Anesthesiology, Critical Care and Pain Medicine
Massachusetts General Hospital
Boston, Massachusetts

Robert Sheridan, MD
Professor of Surgery
Harvard Medical School
Chief of Staff
Department of Surgery
Shriners Hospital for Children
Boston, Massachusetts

Robert D. Sinyard, III, MD, MBA
Post-doctoral Research Fellow
Ariadne Labs
Harvard TH Chan School of Public Health
Surgical Resident
Department of Surgery
Massachusetts General Hospital
Boston, Massachusetts

Jamie L. Sparling, MD
Instructor of Anesthesia
Department of Anesthesia
Harvard Medical School
Staff Anesthesiologist and Intensivist
Department of Anesthesia, Critical Care and Pain Medicine
Massachusetts General Hospital
Boston, Massachusetts

Zachary P. Sullivan, MD, MS
Fellow, Critical Care Medicine
Department of Anesthesiology, Perioperative and Pain Medicine
Stanford University
Stanford, California
Resident-Anesthesiology
Department of Anesthesiology, Critical Care and Pain Medicine
Massachusetts General Hospital
Boston, Massachusetts

Gina H. Sun, MD
Resident Physician
Department of Anesthesia, Critical Care and Pain Medicine
Massachusetts General Hospital
Boston, Massachusetts

Alan J. Sutton, MD
Staff Physiatrist
Department of Physical Medicine & Rehabilitation
Encompass Health Rehabilitation Hospital of Braintree
Braintree, Massachusetts

Lauren A. Sweetser, MD, MA
Clinical and Research Fellow
Department of Pediatric Critical Care
Harvard Medical School
Clinical and Research Fellow
Department of Pediatric Critical Care
Massachusetts General Hospital for Children
Boston, Massachusetts

Parsia Vagefi, MD, FACS
Professor of Surgery
Executive Vice Chair of Strategy and Finance
Chief, Division of Surgical Transplantation
Ernest Poulos, M.D. Distinguished Chair in Surgery
UT Southwestern Medical Center
Dallas, Texas

Karen Waak, PT, DPT, CCS
Physical Therapy Clinical Specialist
Department of Physical Therapy
Massachusetts General Hospital
Boston, Massachusetts

Elisa C. Walsh, MD
Instructor
Department of Anesthesia
Harvard Medical School
Staff Anesthesiologist and Intensivist
Department of Anesthesia, Critical Care and Pain Medicine
Massachusetts General Hospital
Boston, Massachusetts

Alison S. Witkin, MD
Assistant Professor of Medicine
Department of Medicine
Harvard Medical School
Assistant in Medicine
Department of Medicine
Massachusetts General Hospital
Boston, Massachusetts

Victor W. Wong, MD
Staff Surgeon
Plastic and Reconstructive Surgery
The Permanente Medical Group
Santa Rosa, California

Amanda S. Xi, MD, MSE
Instructor
Harvard Medical School
Director of Pre-Procedure Evaluation and Procedural Sedation
Department of Anesthesia, Critical Care, and Pain Medicine
Massachusetts General Hospital
Boston, Massachusetts

Michael J. Young, MD, MPhil
Associate Director, MGH NeuroRecovery Clinic
Center for Neurotechnology and NeuroRecovery (CNTR)
Division of Neurocritical Care, Department of Neurology
Massachusetts General Hospital and Harvard Medical School
Boston, Massachusetts

Adil Yunis, MD
Physician
Department of Cardiovascular Medicine
Massachusetts General Hospital
Boston, Massachusetts

Sahar F. Zafar, MD, MSc
Neurointensivist
Department of Neurology
Massachusetts General Hospital
Boston, Massachusetts

Hilary L. Zetlen, MD, MPH
Fellow
Division of Pulmonary and Critical Care
Massachusetts General Hospital
Boston, Massachusetts

PREFACE

The Critical Care Handbook of the Massachusetts General Hospital, Seventh Edition is designed to be a concise, didactic, and practical guide for health care providers caring for patients with life-threatening illness and injuries. Care for the critically ill patient is broad in scope and practice. It can take place in a variety of settings including prehospital situations, the emergency department, hospital ward, operating room, and intensive care unit. The critical care provider needs to be knowledgeable not only about a broad range of medical and surgical conditions causing critical illness but also with the technological procedures and devices used in support of organ system dysfunction. To that end, this handbook includes basic principles of diagnosis and management of the critically ill patient including fundamental physiology, monitoring, diagnostic and therapeutic procedures, as well as more advanced knowledge of specific patient conditions and treatments. The handbook also includes chapters devoted to many of the complicated ethical and social issues encountered in critical care practice such as end-of-life decision-making, the economics of care, quality improvement, and understanding of the ongoing challenges faced by survivors of critical illness. While endeavoring to maintain the structure and style of successful prior editions, the handbook chapters have been updated to reflect the rapid changes in critical care management. In addition, new sections and chapters have been added to describe recent innovations in thought and practice. As with prior editions, the handbook reflects the current clinical practice at the Massachusetts General Hospital that is the foundation of our critical care training programs.

I am indebted to a number of people who were essential in the publication of the Seventh Edition of *The Critical Care Handbook of the Massachusetts General Hospital*. First, I wish to gratefully acknowledge the past editors and contributors to the previous editions of this handbook. They established the solid foundation upon which our clinical practice and this current edition are based. My coeditors of this edition deserve special acknowledgment for their dedication and diligent editing efforts despite the unrelenting demands of post-COVID-19 health care practice. The professional staff at Wolters Kluwer including Keith Donnellan, Ashley Fischer, and Sunmerrilika Baskar have been indispensable throughout the planning and organizing stages of this book, and by providing "gentle reminders" to submit our chapters on time. Finally, I am grateful to my wife Karen and sons Daniel and Andrew for their ongoing love and support.

Edward A. Bittner, MD, PhD, MSEd

CONTENTS

1 Hemodynamic Monitoring

Christopher J. Mariani and Daniel Saddawi-Konefka

I. HEMODYNAMIC MONITORING

Hemodynamic monitoring is one of the cornerstones of patient evaluation in the intensive care unit (ICU) and provides diagnostic and prognostic value. The choice of monitoring depends on the diagnostic needs of the patient and the risk-benefit balance of monitor placement and maintenance and complications associated with its use. This chapter outlines an approach to the assessment of hemodynamics and perfusion in patients who are critically ill and the technical principles of commonly used monitoring methods.

A. Perfusion: *The goal of hemodynamic monitoring is to ensure adequate tissue perfusion* for gas, nutrient, and waste exchange, with the goal of decreasing morbidity and mortality. It is difficult to link optimization of a single hemodynamic parameter to an improvement in morbidity and mortality. For this reason, intensivists should not rely solely on any one physical monitor or parameter but should evaluate multiple potential signs of adequate perfusion such as mental status, urine output, or laboratory findings (eg, central venous oxygen saturation, base deficit, and lactate).

B. Optimizing Perfusion: *Hemodynamic monitors are not therapeutic.* Hemodynamic data, however, can be used to guide therapy. Optimizing perfusion may require fluid administration, diuresis, administration of pharmacologic agents (eg, vasoconstrictors, inotropic agents), or interventions (eg, intra-aortic balloon pumps, ventricular assist devices, extracorporeal membrane oxygenation). With this in mind, any monitor must be used dynamically to ensure that employed therapies are optimizing perfusion over time.

1. Fluid challenge: Much discussion around optimization of hemodynamics revolves around fluid status. The "fluid challenge" is a time-honored test to aid in determining whether fluid administration could be beneficial. With a fluid challenge test, intravenous (IV) fluid is rapidly administered while hemodynamics are monitored to determine whether the administration improves hemodynamic parameters (and thereby be of benefit to the patient). Although the fluid challenge is not standardized, it most commonly involves the rapid administration of 500 mL of fluid, with a positive test defined as an increase in cardiac output (CO) greater than 10% to 15%. A "passive leg raise" test can be used to provide similar information. To perform this test, a clinician passively elevates a supine patient's legs. Blood moves to the central veins from the elevated limbs, providing an "autotransfusion" of approximately 150 to 300 mL. An improvement in stroke volume suggests fluid responsiveness, whereas deterioration in hemodynamics can be quickly reversed by lowering the legs. A passive leg raise test may also be performed using pulse pressure as a surrogate for stroke volume. The sensitivity and specificity of a passive leg raise are reduced when changes in pulse pressure are measured in place of stroke volume.

II. ARTERIAL BLOOD PRESSURE MONITORING

A. General Principles

1. Blood pressure describes the pressure exerted by circulating blood within the blood vessels. Because this pressure drives flow, it is used as a surrogate measure of blood flow and, in turn, organ perfusion (Figure 1.1). This simplified view has limitations and notably poor correlation with CO in some situations, such as emergency resuscitation of the patient with hypovolemia who is critically ill. Nonetheless, arterial blood pressure monitoring as a target for perfusion is used in almost all critical care settings.
2. Under normal circumstances, tissue perfusion is maintained across a range of pressures by autoregulation, which describes the intrinsic capacity of vascular beds to maintain flow by adjusting local vascular resistance. However, pathologic conditions common in the ICU such as chronic hypertension, trauma, and sepsis may impair autoregulation, resulting in blood flow that may depend directly on perfusion pressure.
3. The "gold standard" for blood pressure measurement is aortic root pressure, which is representative of the pressures received by the major organs (eg, heart, brain, kidneys). As the pressure wave travels distally from the aorta, the measured mean pressure decreases while the measured pulse pressure (systolic pressure minus diastolic pressure) is increased owing to pulse wave reflection from the high-resistant distal arterioles. In addition to being amplified, as one progresses distally, the arterial waveform is slightly delayed (Figure 1.2).

B. Noninvasive Blood Pressure Monitoring: Various techniques can be used to measure blood pressure noninvasively, including manual palpation, determination

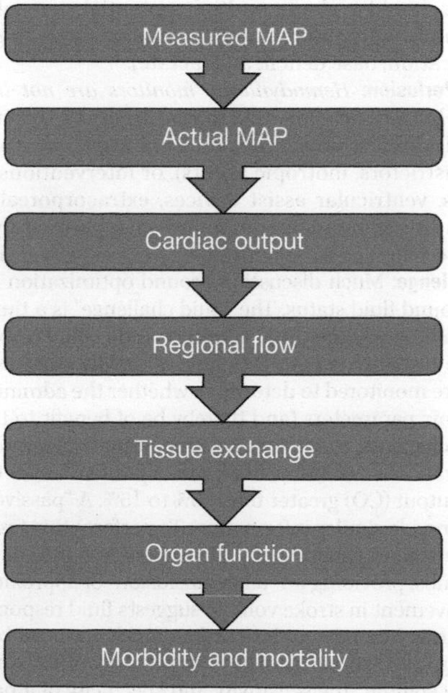

FIGURE 1.1 The assumptions when extrapolating mean arterial pressure (MAP) to a morbidity and mortality benefit.

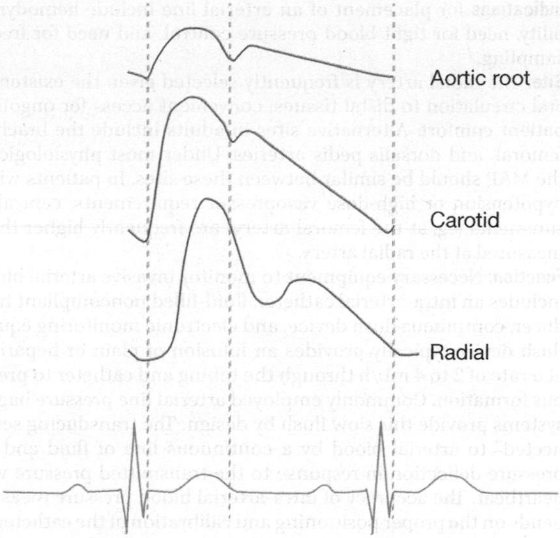

FIGURE 1.2 Arterial waveforms as one travels distally along the arterial tree.

of Korotkoff sounds with a sphygmomanometer and stethoscope or Doppler ultrasound, and automated oscillometric methods, which are most common in the ICU.

1. **Function:** The oscillometric method uses a pneumatic cuff with an electric pressure sensor, most commonly over the brachial artery. The cuff is inflated to high pressure and then slowly deflated. Arterial pulsations are recorded as oscillations. The pressure that produces the greatest oscillation recording is closely associated with mean arterial pressure (MAP). Systolic and diastolic pressures are then **calculated**, often using proprietary algorithms.
2. **Technique:** Accurate noninvasive blood pressure measurement requires appropriate cuff sizing and placement. Most blood pressure cuffs display reference lines for an acceptable arm length, and the cuffs should be sized as recommended in relationship to arm circumference. Cuffs that are too small may overestimate blood pressure, whereas cuffs that are too large may underestimate blood pressure.
3. **Limitations and risks**
   - **a.** The pressure measured by a noninvasive cuff is the pressure at the cuff site. When an extremity pressure is measured to estimate coronary perfusion, either the extremity should be placed at the level of the heart or the extremity level relative to the heart should be accounted for (eg, a pressure measured at a site 10 cm below the heart will be 10 cm H_2O or ~7.4 mm Hg greater than the pressure at the heart).
   - **b.** Tissues, including vessels and nerves, can be damaged by cyclical compression of pneumatic cuffs with frequent cycling. As such, automatic methods may not be appropriate in rapidly changing situations. They may also be less accurate with extremes of blood pressure or in patients with dysrhythmias.

C. Invasive Arterial Blood Pressure Monitoring provides beat-to-beat pressure transduction and allows for convenient blood sampling.

1. **Indications** for placement of an arterial line include hemodynamic instability, need for tight blood pressure control, and need for frequent blood sampling.
2. **Site:** The radial artery is frequently selected given the existence of collateral circulation to distal tissues, convenient access for ongoing care, and patient comfort. Alternative sites in adults include the brachial, axillary, femoral, and dorsalis pedis arteries. Under most physiologic conditions, the MAP should be similar between these sites. In patients with profound hypotension or high-dose vasopressor requirements, central MAP measurements (eg, at the femoral artery) are frequently higher than the MAP measured at the radial artery.
3. **Function:** Necessary equipment to monitor invasive arterial blood pressure includes an intra-arterial catheter, fluid-filled noncompliant tubing, transducer, continuous flush device, and electronic monitoring equipment. The flush device typically provides an infusion of plain or heparinized saline at a rate of 2 to 4 mL/h through the tubing and catheter to prevent thrombus formation. Commonly employed arterial line pressure bag/transducer systems provide this slow flush by design. The transducing sensor is "connected" to arterial blood by a continuous line of fluid and measures a pressure deflection in response to the transmitted pressure wave of each heartbeat. The accuracy of intra-arterial blood pressure measurement depends on the proper positioning and calibration of the catheter-transducer monitoring system.
   a. **Positioning:** The arterial pressure reflects the pressure at the level of the transducer, not the pressure at the level of the cannulation site. This is because of the fluid-filled tubing between the patient and transducer, which maintains energy by exchanging potential energy for pressure (Bernoulli's equation). For example, if the transducer is lowered, the fluid in the tubing exerts an additional pressure on the transducer and the measured pressure will be higher. Therefore, the arterial transducer should be placed at the level of interest. For example, positioning at the fourth intercostal space on the midaxillary line ("the phlebostatic axis") corresponds to the level of the aortic root, and positioning at the external acoustic meatus corresponds to the level of the circle of Willis.
   b. **Static calibration** zeros the system to atmospheric pressure. The transducer is opened to air and the recorded pressure (the atmospheric pressure) is set to zero.
   c. **Dynamic response** is important to account for because it affects the pressure readings in ways that are unrelated to the actual pressure wave at the cannulation site (eg, the reading may appear flattened [damped] or stretched [underdamped]). Dynamic response occurs as a result of the natural frequency of the arterial line system as well as the damping coefficient. The natural frequency is the frequency at which a pressure pulse oscillates within the system. The damping coefficient is a measure of how quickly an oscillating waveform decays in the system. These two characteristics of an arterial line system can be illustrated using a fast flush (also known as a square wave) test. In this test, the transducer and tubing system is transiently flushed with fluid at 300 mm Hg. Following the flush, the arterial pressure trace will exhibit a series of oscillations before returning to baseline. The frequency of these oscillations (calculated by dividing the monitor speed by the wavelength of the oscillating waves) represents the natural frequency of the system. The damping coefficient is related to the amplitude ratio of successive oscillations (eg, the height of the first oscillation relative to the second oscillation). To have an adequate dynamic response, and thereby accurately measure arterial blood pressure, the correct combinations of natural frequencies

and damping coefficients are required. When a system has an inadequate dynamic response, over- or underdamping will be observed. Generally, return of the pressure signal to baseline after one to two oscillations following a fast flush test is indicative of a system with an adequate dynamic response.

1. Overdampened systems will underestimate systolic pressure and overestimate diastolic pressure (because the waveforms will tend to collapse around the MAP). Overdamped systems will return to baseline following a fast flush after one or less oscillations. Overdampening may be caused by air bubbles, clots, kinking of the catheter or tubing, or loose connections.
2. Underdampened systems will overestimate the systolic blood pressure and underestimate the diastolic pressure. Underdampened systems will have greater than two oscillations following the fast flush before returning to the baseline. Underdamping may be caused by excessive tubing length, stiff tubing, or tachycardia.
3. In both over- and underdampened systems, the measured mean pressure will still be accurate.

4. **Complications:** Arterial cannulation is relatively safe. Risks depend on the site of cannulation. For radial cannulation, reported serious risks include permanent ischemic damage (0.09%), local infection and sepsis (0.72% and 0.13%, respectively), and pseudoaneurysm (0.09%). Fastidious attention to the adequacy of distal perfusion is important. Thrombotic sequelae are associated with larger catheters, smaller arterial size, administration of vasopressors, duration of cannulation, and multiple arterial cannulation attempts. With regard to infectious risk, the aseptic technique was not standardized in the studies that yielded the aforementioned percentage of risk and longer duration of cannulation increased risk. Less serious risks include temporary occlusion (19.7%) and hematoma (14.4%). Axillary and femoral sites have been associated with higher risks of infection. Brachial cannulation has been associated with median nerve injury (0.2%-1.4%). However, in a center with standardized use of brachial catheters for cardiac surgery, no nerve injuries were reported following 21 000 brachial artery catheterizations, suggesting that previous risk of nerve injury may overestimate complications in centers where this approach is standard.
5. **Respiratory variation:** Increased intrathoracic pressure decreases preload, arterial pressure, and pulse pressure. This effect is marked in patients with hypovolemia who are more susceptible to increased intrathoracic pressures. Variation of more than 10% to 12% in systolic pressure or pulse pressure is suggestive of fluid responsiveness. Importantly, this has been validated in patients with regular cardiac rhythm and breathing pattern, and it is dependent on the ventilatory pressure delivered.
6. **Arterial waveform analysis** has been used to gauge stroke volume and is discussed later in this chapter.

D. **Discrepancies Between Noninvasive and Invasive Arterial Blood Pressure Measurements** exist, with noninvasive measurements tending to yield higher measurements during hypotension and lower measurements during hypertension. These discrepancies persist even with appropriate cuff sizing in patients who are critically ill. Retrospective data suggest that the higher noninvasive systolic blood pressures during hypotension are overestimates of perfusion because the incidence of acute kidney injury and mortality is higher with noninvasive versus invasive systolic blood pressures. There was no difference in acute kidney injury or mortality when mean pressures were compared, which suggests that mean pressures should be targeted when the patient who is hypotensive and critically ill is treated with a noninvasive cuff.

III. CENTRAL VENOUS PRESSURE MONITORING

A. Indications for placement of a central venous catheter (CVC) include administration of certain medications, concentrated vasopressors, or total parenteral nutrition (TPN); need for dialysis; need for long-term medication administration such as chemotherapy or IV antibiotics; need for IV access in patients with difficult peripheral access; need for sampling central venous blood; or need for central venous pressure (CVP) hemodynamic data to guide management efforts.

B. Site: Common central venous cannulation sites are the internal jugular, subclavian, and femoral veins. The ideal site of cannulation varies with the characteristics of the patient and the indications for insertion. For example, the subclavian site is relatively contraindicated in patients with coagulopathies because it is not directly compressible, and the femoral vein may be ideal in emergency situations because of ease of cannulation. Table 1.1 summarizes the advantages and disadvantages of the most commonly used sites for venous access.

C. CVP Waveform: CVP provides an estimate of right ventricular preload and should be measured with the transducer positioned at the phlebostatic axis. The CVP tracing contains three positive deflections (Figure 1.3). The *a* wave corresponds to atrial contraction and correlates with the P wave on the electrocardiogram (ECG). The *c* wave corresponds to ventricular contraction (and bulging of the tricuspid valve into the right atrium) and correlates with the end of the QRS complex on the ECG. The *v* wave corresponds to atrial filling against a closed tricuspid valve and occurs with the end of the T wave on ECG. The *x* descent after the *c* wave is thought to be due to the downward displacement of the atrium during ventricular systole and the *y* descent by the tricuspid valve opening during diastole.

1. **Abnormal waveforms:** Arrhythmias and valvular abnormalities can result in different central venous waveform morphologies. For example, the loss of atrial contraction that occurs with atrial fibrillation results in the loss of *a* waves on CVP tracings. Large *a* waves ("cannon *a* waves") may occur when the atrium contracts against a closed valve, as occurs during atrioventricular dissociation or ventricular pacing. Abnormally large *v* waves that begin immediately after the QRS complex and often incorporate the *c* wave are associated with tricuspid regurgitation. Abnormally large *v* waves may also be observed during right ventricular failure or ischemia, constrictive pericarditis, or cardiac tamponade due to the volume and/or pressure overload seen by the right atrium. Tricuspid stenosis is a diastolic defect in atrial emptying and can result in an attenuated *y* descent with a prominent *a* wave.

TABLE 1.1 Risks and Benefits of Different Central Line Access Approaches

Site	Infection risk	Bleeding risk	Thrombotic risk	Patient comfort	Comments
Internal jugular	++	+	++	++	Compressible, low pneumothorax risk
Subclavian	+	+++	+	+++	Higher risk of pneumothorax, difficult to compress in case of bleeding
Femoral	+++	+	+++	+	Often easiest place in an emergency, high infection rate
PICC	+	–	++	+++	Good for long-term access, low flow rate

PICC, peripherally inserted central catheter.
-, insignificant; +, to a less extent; ++, to a moderate extent; +++, to a substantial extent.

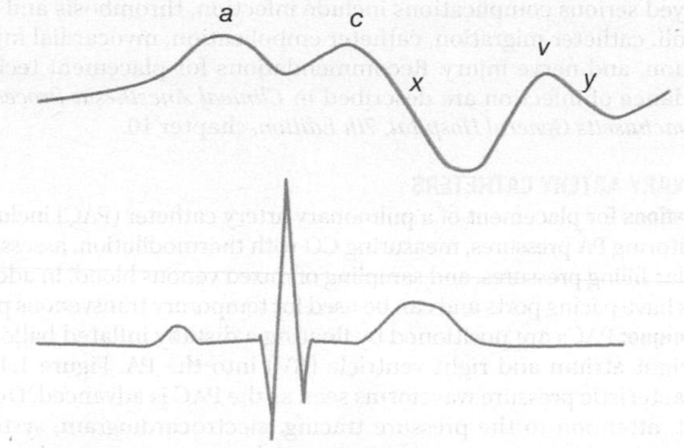

FIGURE 1.3 The central venous pressure (CVP) waveform.

D. Interpretation of CVP

1. **Measurement:** CVP, when measured as a surrogate for end-diastolic filling, should be measured at the valley just before the *c* wave (ie, at the end of the diastole, just before ventricular contraction). Because CVP changes with respiration (owing to changes in intrathoracic pressure), it should be measured at end expiration, when the lung is closest to functional residual capacity and confounding intrathoracic pressure influences are minimized.
2. **Utility and controversy:** CVP has been used clinically to assess fluid status for decades. The physiologic determinants of CVP include patient position, the circulating volume status, interactions between systemic and pulmonary circulations, alterations in rhythm or valvular function (see **Section III.C.1**), and the dynamic changes in the respiratory system over the breathing cycle. Not surprisingly, the accurate interpretation of CVP can be difficult and a number of studies have challenged its use. Systematic review has suggested poor correlation of CVP with circulating blood volume as well as poor correlation of CVP (or trend in CVP) with fluid responsiveness.
3. **Clinical confounders:** When used clinically, CVP measurements are used to estimate end-diastolic volume, given in the following relationship:

$$V_{RV} = C_{RV} \cdot (\mathrm{CVP} - P_{extracardiac})$$

where V_{RV} is end-diastolic volume, C_{RV} is compliance of the right ventricle, CVP approximates the pressure inside the ventricle, and $P_{extracardiac}$ is extracardiac pressure. Given this relationship, the general categories of physiologic perturbation that alter the direct relation between CVP and volume are as follows:

a. **Abnormal cardiac compliance**, as in concentric hypertrophy
b. **Altered extracardiac pressure**, as with high positive end-expiratory pressure (PEEP), abdominal compartment syndrome, or tamponade, for example
c. **Valvular abnormalities**, as with tricuspid insufficiency or stenosis (where CVP will no longer approximate right ventricular pressures)
d. **Ventricular interdependence**

E. Complications: Central venous cannulation complications vary depending on the selected anatomic site (see Table 1.1) and operator experience. Serious immediate complications include catheter malposition, pneumo- or hemothorax, arterial puncture, bleeding, air or wire embolism, arrhythmia, and thoracic duct injury (with left subclavian or left internal jugular approach).

Delayed serious complications include infection, thrombosis and pulmonary emboli, catheter migration, catheter embolization, myocardial injury or perforation, and nerve injury. Recommendations for placement technique and avoidance of infection are described in *Clinical Anesthesia Procedures of the Massachusetts General Hospital, 7th Edition*, chapter 10.

IV. PULMONARY ARTERY CATHETERS

A. Indications for placement of a pulmonary artery catheter (PAC) include need for monitoring PA pressures, measuring CO with thermodilution, assessing left ventricular filling pressures, and sampling of mixed venous blood. In addition, some PACs have pacing ports and can be used for temporary transvenous pacing.

B. Technique: PACs are positioned by floating a distally inflated balloon through the right atrium and right ventricle (RV) into the PA. Figure 1.4 shows the characteristic pressure waveforms seen as the PAC is advanced. During placement, attention to the pressure tracing, electrocardiogram, systemic blood pressure, and oxygen saturation is essential to ensure proper placement of the catheter and to minimize known complications.

1. Fluoroscopic guidance may be useful in certain situations, such as in the presence of a recently placed permanent pacemaker (generally within 6 weeks), the need for selective PAC placement (eg, following pneumonectomy), and the presence of significant structural or physiologic abnormalities (eg, severe RV dilation, large intracardiac shunts, or severe pulmonary hypertension).

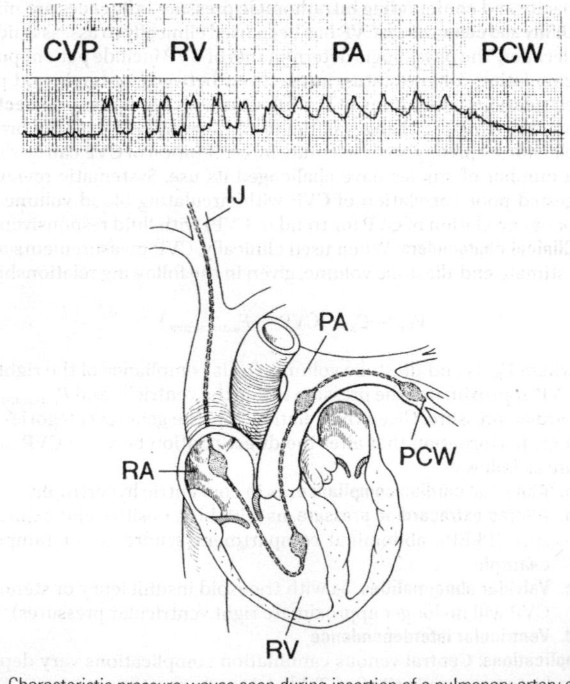

FIGURE 1.4 Characteristic pressure waves seen during insertion of a pulmonary artery catheter. CVP, central venous pressure; IJ, internal jugular; PA, pulmonary artery; PCW, pulmonary capillary wedge; RA, right atrium; RV, right ventricle.

C. Waveforms During Placement: The right atrial pressure waveform is the same as the CVP waveform previously described. The pressure waveform in the RV has a systolic upstroke (in phase with the systemic arterial upstroke) with low diastolic pressures that increase during diastole, owing to ventricular filling. The PA pressure waveform will also be in phase with systemic pressures during systole but will differ from the RV tracing as the pressure decreases during diastole. Often, the diastolic pressure will increase when the balloon enters the PA, but the better marker of this advancement is the transition to a downward slope during diastole. The pulmonary artery occlusion pressure (PAOP) or wedge pressure waveform will resemble the CVP trace with *a, c,* and *v* waves, although these are often difficult to distinguish clinically.

D. Physiologic Data

1. Thermodilution CO

a. Method: A rapid bolus of cold saline is injected proximal to the right heart and temperature is monitored at the distal tip of the PAC. With higher CO, more blood is mixed with the cold fluid bolus and the temperature recorded over time will be attenuated, as described by the modified Stewart-Hamilton equation:

$$CO = \frac{(T_{body} - T_{injectate}) \times V \times K}{AUC}$$

where CO is cardiac output, T_{body} is the temperature of the body, $T_{injectate}$ is the temperature of the saline bolus, V is the volume of the bolus, K reflects properties of the catheter system, and AUC is the area under the curve of temperature change.

b. Reliability: Averaging of serial measurements is recommended for each CO determination because the calculated CO may vary by as much as 10% without a change in clinical condition. It is important to minimize variations in the rate and volume of injection, which also introduce error. Colder solutions (ie, increased $T_{body} - T_{injectate}$) decrease error, although attention should be paid to potential tachy- or bradyarrhythmias. Tricuspid regurgitation may affect calculations as a result of recirculated blood between the right atrium and RV. Intracardiac shunt can likewise introduce error.

2. Pulmonary artery occlusion pressure: Occluding the PA recreates a static fluid column between the distal tip of the catheter and the left atrium, allowing for equilibration of pressures between the two sites. In this manner, PAOP approximates left atrial pressure, a surrogate for left ventricular end-diastolic volume. For an accurate measure of PAOP, the proper atrial trace, similar to the "*a-c-v*" trace of the CVP waveform, should be visualized. As highlighted in the discussion of CVP measurements, volume is only one parameter that influences the PAOP measurements. Other variables include cardiac compliance, intrathoracic pressures, valvular lesions, ventricular interdependence, and so forth.

3. Mixed venous oxygen saturation ($S\bar{v}O_2$): As CO increases, tissue oxygen demand is met with less per-unit oxygen extraction and $S\bar{v}O_2$ increases. This is a loose correlation because $S\bar{v}O_2$ also depends on hemoglobin concentration and oxygen consumption, as outlined by the Fick equation:

$$CO = \frac{\dot{V}O_2}{(SaO_2 - S\bar{v}O_2) \cdot hgb \cdot 1.34 \cdot 10}$$

where CO is cardiac output in liters per minute, $\dot{V}O_2$ is oxygen consumption in millimeters per minute, SaO_2 and $S\bar{v}O_2$ are arterial and mixed venous oxygen saturation, and hgb is hemoglobin in grams per deciliter.

$S\bar{v}O_2$ correlates with CO, and a low $S\bar{v}O_2$ suggests low CO (assuming adequate oxygen extraction by the tissues and an adequate hemoglobin). $Sc\bar{v}O_2$, an oxygen saturation drawn from a non-PA central line, can act as a surrogate for $S\bar{v}O_2$. It is typically higher than the $S\bar{v}O_2$ is by about 5% because it does not include the oxygen-depleted blood from the heart itself (returned to the right atrium from the coronary sinus), although the exact difference between $Sc\bar{v}O_2$ and $S\bar{v}O_2$ is not predictable.

E. **Complications:** In addition to complications associated with central venous access, PAC placement is associated with an increased risk of arrhythmia including right heart block (especially in patients with recent myocardial infarction [MI] or pericarditis) and PA rupture. PA rupture risk is increased with pulmonary hypertension, advanced age, mitral valve disease, hypothermia, and anticoagulant therapy. It requires emergent thoracotomy. Catheter-related complications, including knotting or balloon rupture with subsequent air or balloon fragment emboli, have also been reported.

F. **Relative Contraindications** to PA placement include left heart block (because a superimposed right heart block would lead to a complete block), presence of a transvenous pacer or recently placed pacemaker or implantable cardioverter-defibrillator (ICD) leads, tricuspid or pulmonary stenosis or prosthetic tricuspid or pulmonary valves (given the associated difficulty in passing the catheter and balloon), and patient predisposition for arrhythmia, coagulopathy, or severe pulmonary hypertension. Need for magnetic resonance imaging (MRI) is also a contraindication because most PA lines contain ferromagnetic material.

G. **Controversy Over PACs:** Although hemodynamic data derived from PACs enhance understanding of cardiopulmonary physiology, the risk-to-benefit profile has been questioned. Since the mid-1990s, several large outcome studies assessing the benefit of PACs have been conducted without clear evidence of mortality benefit. Moreover, PAC-guided therapy has been associated with more complications than has CVC-guided therapy. Although these results are not sufficiently convincing to completely discourage the use of PACs, they underscore the importance of using PACs only when the benefit of management guidance derived from PA data is strongly believed to outweigh the associated risks.

V. ALTERNATIVES TO BLOOD PRESSURE MONITORING

Numerous alternative hemodynamic monitors have been developed to assess either cardiovascular function or tissue perfusion.

A. **Transthoracic Ultrasound:** The use of ultrasound for hemodynamic assessment of cardiac function and fluid status has been growing in critical care and is discussed further in **Chapter 3**.

B. **Continuous Esophageal Doppler:** Blood velocity in the descending aorta can be measured with a transesophageal Doppler ultrasound. The average velocity over one heartbeat is multiplied by the cross-sectional area of the aorta (either estimated on the basis of patient data or measured by the probe) to calculate stroke volume. Stroke volume is multiplied by heart rate (HR) to obtain CO. Notably, because this is only the flow in the descending aorta, a certain percentage (typically around 30%) is added to estimate total CO. Modern probes are roughly the size of nasogastric tubes, much smaller than are ordinary transesophageal echocardiography probes, and can provide "corrected flow time" and stroke volume variation in addition to CO, which can be used to gauge fluid responsiveness.

1. **Advantages:** Esophageal Doppler monitoring allows for continuous measurement with minimal risk of infection, is simple to use with a short setup time, and has a low incidence of iatrogenic complications.

2. **Disadvantages:** Esophageal Doppler monitoring can only be performed in intubated patients, requires frequent repositioning if the patient is moved, is operator dependent, and is not widely available.

C. Partial CO_2 Rebreathing Method: The partial CO_2 rebreathing method is based on the Fick principle:

$$CO = \frac{\dot{V}O_2}{CaO_2 - C\bar{v}O_2}$$

where CO is cardiac output, CaO_2 is the arterial blood oxygen content of oxygen, $C\bar{v}O_2$ is the venous blood oxygen content, and $\dot{V}O_2$ is oxygen consumption.

Clinical measurement of $\dot{V}O_2$ is challenging, so this technique is based on a restatement of the Fick equation for carbon dioxide elimination rather than for oxygen consumption:

$$CO = \frac{\dot{V}O_2}{C\bar{v}CO_2 - CaCO_2}$$

Using an intermittent partial rebreathing circuit, the change in CO_2 production and end-tidal CO_2 concentration in response to a brief, sudden change in minute ventilation is measured. The changes in end-tidal CO_2 are used to calculate CO.

1. **Advantages:** This method is low risk, noninvasive, and can be performed every few minutes. The partial rebreathing CO_2 CO method has also shown reasonably good agreement with gold standard thermodilution in clinical trials in some settings.
2. **Disadvantages:** As currently designed, this method requires tracheal intubation for measurement of exhaled gases. Measurements can be affected by changing patterns of ventilation and intrapulmonary shunting. Furthermore, this technique has a relatively long response time.

D. Transpulmonary Thermodilution and Transpulmonary Indicator Dilution: With these techniques, the same principles for PAC thermodilution are employed but only a CVC and an arterial line are required. A bolus of either cold saline (with the PiCCO device) or lithium chloride (with the LiDCO device) is injected into the central line and the dilution over time in a peripheral artery is used to derive the CO. These are commonly used in conjunction with pulse contour analysis (see **Section V.E**) to provide continuous assessment of CO.

1. **Advantages:** Both of these methods have been shown to correlate reasonably well with PAC thermodilution. Transpulmonary thermodilution has the added benefit of providing an assessment of extravascular lung water and intrathoracic blood volume.
2. **Disadvantages:** Both methods require repetitive blood draws, and calibration may be affected by neuromuscular blocking agents. Notably, the PiCCO system typically requires the placement of an axillary or femoral arterial catheter.

E. Pulse Contour Analysis: This modality for measuring CO relies on the principle that stroke volume and CO can be gauged from characteristics of the arterial waveform, using calculations that are based on estimates of compliance of the arterial tree. Commercially available devices require calibration, typically against thermodilution or indicator dilution methods.

1. **Advantages:** Pulse contour analysis devices are continuous and employ catheters (CVCs and arterial lines) that are commonly employed in patients in the ICU.
2. **Disadvantages:** This technique requires patients who are mechanically ventilated and has shown reduced accuracy in patients who are hemodynamically labile or on vasoactive medications. The altered arterial waveform of patients with aortic insufficiency may also decrease the accuracy of this technique.

F. Impedance Cardiography (Also Known as Electrical Impedance Plethysmography): With impedance cardiography, a high-frequency, low-magnitude current is applied to the chest, and impedance is measured. As the aorta fills with blood with each heartbeat, impedance decreases, and this change is used to determine stroke volume and CO. Advances in phased-array and signal processing technologies have improved impedance cardiography, largely overcoming artifact due to electrode placement, HR and rhythm disturbances, and differences in body habitus, although its use is still fairly limited in the ICU. Both electrical velocimetry and bioreactance employ similar principles. Electrical velocimetry relates the velocity of blood flow in the aorta to determine CO, whereas bioreactance uses changes in electrical current frequency (rather than in impedance) to measure changes in blood flow during the cardiac cycle.

1. **Advantages:** This method is noninvasive and continuous.
2. **Disadvantages:** Impedance cardiography is more time consuming to set up and its usefulness is limited, with noisy environments, extravascular fluid accumulation, or arrhythmias.

G. Tissue Perfusion Monitors: Most hemodynamic monitors are surrogates for adequate perfusion, whereas a few aim to assess perfusion at the tissue level. Notably, these only assess tissue perfusion in the tissues where they are measured. Gastric tonometry measures gastric CO_2, which decreases with low perfusion states. Tissue oxygenation (StO_2) measures the percentage of oxygenated hemoglobin at the microcirculation/tissue level. Although there are many tissue perfusion monitors, most of these are still used primarily for research and not for clinical applications at this time.

Selected Readings

Bartels K, Esper S, Thiele R. Blood pressure monitoring for the anesthesiologist: a practical review. *Anesth Analg.* 2016;122(6):1866-1879.

Cavallaro F, Sandroni C, Marano C, et al. Diagnostic accuracy of passive leg raising for prediction of fluid responsiveness in adults: systematic review and meta-analysis of clinical studies. *Intensive Care Med.* 2010;36(9):1475-1483.

Galluccio ST, Finnis ME, Chapman MJ. Femoral-radial arterial pressure gradients in critically ill patients. *Crit Care Resusc.* 2009;11(1):34-38.

Gardner RM. Direct blood pressure measurement—dynamic response requirements. *Anesthesiology.* 1981;54(3):227-236.

Kaufmann T, Cox EGM, Wiersema R, et al. Non-invasive oscillometric versus invasive arterial blood pressure measurements in critically ill patients: a post hoc analysis of a prospective observational study. *Crit Care.* 2020;57:118-123.

Kaur B, Kaur S, Yaddanapudi LN, et al. Comparison between invasive and noninvasive blood pressure measurements in critically ill patients receiving inotropes. *Blood Press Monit.* 2019;24(1):24-29.

Kim WY, Jun JH, Huh JW, et al. Radial to femoral arterial blood pressure differences in septic shock patients receiving high-dose norepinephrine therapy. *Shock.* 2013;40(6):527-531.

Kobe J, Mishra N, Arya VK, et al. Cardiac output monitoring: technology and choice. *Ann Card Anaesth.* 2019;22(1):6-17.

Messina A, Longhini F, Coppo C, et al. Use of the fluid challenge in critically ill adult patients: a systematic review. *Anesth Analg.* 2017;125(5):1532-1543.

Monnet X, Rienzo M, Osman D. Passive leg raise predicts fluid responsiveness in the critically ill. *Crit Care Med.* 2006;34(5):1402-1407.

Riley LE, Chen GJ, Latham HE. Comparison of noninvasive blood pressure monitoring with invasive arterial pressure monitoring in medical ICU patients with septic shock. *Blood Press Monit.* 2017;22(4):202-207.

Saugel B, Kouz K, Mediert A, et al. How to measure blood pressure using an arterial catheter: a systematic 5-step approach. *Crit Care.* 2020;24(1):172.

Singh A, Bahadorani B, Wakefield BJ, et al. Brachial arterial pressure monitoring during cardiac surgery rarely causes complications. *Anesthesiology.* 2017;126(6):1065-1076.

2 Respiratory Monitoring

Catherine E. Naber and Ryan W. Carroll

INTRODUCTION

Intensive care units (ICUs) provide high-resolution and high-frequency surveillance for patients who are critically ill to capture disease trajectory in real time. This intensive monitoring enables clinicians to alter, add, or remove interventions to match the progression of disease, thereby reducing mortality, morbidity, and length of stay.

Intensive monitoring in the ICU promotes a culture of safety and provides the data needed to develop thresholds for initiating, escalating, deescalating, and ceasing treatment. Whether by invasive or noninvasive means, this monitoring aims to accurately capture disease progression.

Respiratory monitoring, invasive and noninvasive, and subsequent treatment are the mainstays of critical care; it is what separates the subspecialty from all others.

This chapter discusses the core aspects of respiratory monitoring in the ICU setting and how to troubleshoot a shift in a patient's respiratory trajectory.

I. BASIC CONCEPTS: The chief focus of respiratory monitoring is on the delivery and removal (exchange) of gases, oxygen (O_2), and carbon dioxide (CO_2), respectively.

A. Hypoxia is the condition of inadequate oxygen. Hypoxia can occur in the whole body (generalized hypoxia) or regionally (tissue hypoxia).

1. Reasons for **hypoxia** include the following:
   - **a. Hypoxemia**
   - **b. Ischemia:** a deficiency in oxygen supply due to insufficient blood flow
   - **c. Histotoxic:** inability of cells to use oxygen despite appropriate delivery (eg, cyanide toxicity)
   - **d. Anemia**
   - **e. Inhibition of the function of hemoglobin** such as in carbon monoxide poisoning or elevated methemoglobinemia

B. Hypoxemia is low partial pressure of O_2 in the arterial blood **(Pao_2)** resulting in a reduction of oxygen in the arterial blood. The Pao_2 should always be interpreted in relation to the level of supplemental oxygen or **$F{\rm IO}_2$** (fraction of inspired oxygen).

- **a.** For example, a Pao_2 of 95 mm Hg breathing 100% oxygen is quite different from a Pao_2 of 95 mm Hg breathing air (21% oxygen).
- **b.** The relationship between Pao_2 and $F{\rm IO}_2$ is often captured in the Pao_2/$F{\rm IO}_2$ (P/F) ratio and is used to determine severity of lung injury, specifically acute respiratory distress syndrome (ARDS). A low P/F ratio reflects poor oxygen exchange, for example.

1. Causes of hypoxemia include the following:

- **a.** Pulmonary diseases or conditions resulting in increased passage of deoxygenated blood from the right side of the heart to the left without participating in gas exchange
  1. Increased shunt ($\dot{Q}S/\dot{Q}T$)
  2. Ventilation-perfusion ($\dot{V}/\dot{Q}$) mismatch
  3. A low mixed venous Po_2 (eg, decreased cardiac output) will magnify the effect of shunt on Pao_2.

- **b.** Hypoventilation
- **c.** Diffusion defect
- **d.** PaO_2 is also decreased with decreased inspired oxygen (eg, at high altitude).

C. Anoxia: complete deprivation of oxygen

D. Hyperoxemia (increased PaO_2) may occur when breathing supplemental oxygen. The PaO_2 also increases with hyperventilation.

E. Ventilation/CO_2 removal: Arterial partial pressure of CO_2 ($PaCO_2$) is the balance between carbon dioxide production ($\dot{V}CO_2$) and alveolar ventilation ($\dot{V}A$).

$$PaCO_2 = K \times \dot{V}CO_2/VA$$

where K is a constant.

F. Dead space: Portions of the airways that do not participate in gas exchange. Physiologic dead space (VDphys) is considered the TOTAL dead space and is the sum of the anatomic dead space (VDana) and the alveolar dead space (VDalv).

$$VDphys = VDana + VDalv$$

1. Anatomic dead space comprises airways known to be devoid of gas exchange mechanisms—areas without alveoli (ie, trachea, bronchi).
   - **a.** Anatomic dead space in an adult is usually considered 150 mL (and in children or small adults, ~2 mL/kg).
2. Alveolar dead space is ventilated alveoli that lack concomitant perfusion, essentially leading to ventilation (gas flow) with reduced CO_2 removal.
   - **a.** This occurs whenever the pulmonary vasculature blood flow is lower than the level of gas exchange in the corresponding alveolar space. The extreme of dead space ventilation is cardiac arrest (all V and no Q); but a pulmonary embolism (PE) is the pathophysiology more commonly encountered.
3. Note: Be mindful of added dead space from inappropriate additions to the airway circuit, which manifests greater relative impact in patients with smaller lung volumes (eg, pediatric, patients with severe kyphoscoliosis and achondroplasia).
4. **Dead space**, total ($\dot{V}_{DS}/\dot{V}_T$) can also be calculated from the **Bohr equation by calculating** the discrepancy between arterial blood gas (ABG)-based $PaCO_2$ and end-tidal CO_2 ($ETCO_2$), which measures the ratio of dead space to total ventilation:

$$V_{DS}/V_T = (PaCO_2 - ETCO_2)/PaCO_2$$

where V_{DS} is the volume of dead space and V_T is the total tidal volume.

   - **a.** The normal VDS/V_T is 0.3 to 0.4, so 30% to 40% of the total tidal volume.

G. Minute ventilation:

Minute ventilation (liters per minute, LPM) = Tidal volume (V_T, in mL or L) × respiratory rate (breaths per minute)

1. **Minute ventilation (LPM)** can also be framed as the sum of physiologic dead-space minute ventilation + alveolar minute ventilation.
   - **a.** Multiplying the respiratory rate (RR) by the dead-space volume determined by the Bohr equation results in the minute ventilation of the respective volume.
     1. For example, a physiologic dead space (or V_{DS}) of 200 mL (0.33 of a total V_T of 600 mL) at an RR of 14 = 2.8 LPM of dead-space minute

ventilation; and conversely, the alveolar minute ventilation of the same patient receiving 600 mL V_T results from subtracting the dead-space volume from the total (600 mL − 200 mL = 400 mL) × RR of 14 = alveolar minute ventilation of 5.6 LPM. The total minute ventilation, as displayed on the ventilator, would be 8.4 LPM.

II. METHODS OF MONITORING GAS EXCHANGE

A. Arterial Blood Gas (ABG)

1. ABG analysis is considered the standard assessment of pulmonary gas exchange. ABGs provide the following values:
   a. Arterial partial pressure of oxygen (PaO_2)
      1. Normal PaO_2 is 90 to 100 mm Hg breathing room air at sea level.
   b. Arterial partial pressure of carbon dioxide ($PaCO_2$)
      1. Normal $PaCO_2$ is 35 to 45 mm Hg.
   c. pH
   d. Base excess
   e. Blood oxygen saturation (or saturation level of oxyhemoglobin, SaO_2), which can help verify pulse oximetry
   f. HCO_3^- (bicarbonate)
      1. A calculated value using pH and $PaCO_2$ through the Henderson-Hasselbalch equation

$$pH = 6.1 + \log [HCO_3^- / (0.03 \times PaCO_2)]$$

   g. ABG testing can also report dyshemoglobin subtypes such as the following:
      1. **Carboxyhemoglobin** (COHb): reflects carbon monoxide inhalation. Endogenous COHb levels are 1% to 2% and can be elevated in cigarette smokers and people living in polluted environments. Because carboxyhemoglobin does not transport oxygen, the SaO_2 is proportionally reduced by the COHb level.
      2. **Methemoglobin** (metHb): The iron in the hemoglobin molecule can be oxidized to the ferric form in the presence of a number of oxidizing agents, the most notable of which are nitrates. Because methemoglobin (metHb) does not transport oxygen, the SaO_2 is also proportionally reduced by the metHb level.
      3. **Fetal hemoglobin** (HbF): has a higher affinity for oxygen than does adult hemoglobin and is involved in transportation of oxygen from the mother's bloodstream to the fetus. Levels remain high in an infant until around 4 months of age, nearing 1% by 6 months of age.

B. Peripheral venous blood gas (VBG): reflects PCO_2 and PO_2 at the local tissue level

1. **Arterial PO_2 (PaO_2) versus venous PO_2 (PvO_2)**
   a. PvO_2 is affected by oxygen delivery and oxygen consumption at the tissue level, whereas PaO_2 is affected by lung function. Thus, PvO_2 should not be used as a surrogate for PaO_2.
2. **Venous pH versus arterial pH**
   a. Venous pH is typically lower than arterial pH.
3. **Venous PCO_2 ($PvCO_2$) versus arterial $PaCO_2$**
   a. Venous $\mathbf{PCO_2}$ is typically higher than arterial.
4. Hemodynamic instability affects the difference between arterial and venous pH and PCO_2.
   a. During cardiac arrest, for example, it has been shown that $PvCO_2$ can be very high even when $PaCO_2$ is low, a consequence of low cardiac output in the context of equivalent CO_2 production.

C. Mixed venous or central venous blood gas: preferred when using venous blood to assess acid-base status

1. Drawn from blood in the pulmonary artery that stems from blood flowing from the superior and inferior vena cavae and the coronary sinus.
2. Mixed venous oxygen (Pvo_2 and Svo_2) provides an indication of global tissue oxygen extraction.
   a. Normal partial pressure of mixed venous oxygen (Pvo_2) is 35 to 45 mm Hg.
   b. Normal mixed venous oxygen saturation (Svo_2) is 65% to 75%.
   c. Factors affecting mixed venous oxygen level can be illustrated by the following equation, a rearrangement of the **Fick equation**:

$$Svo_2 = Sao_2 - [Vo_2 / (CO \times Hb \times 1.36)]$$

   where Svo_2 is the mixed venous oxygen saturation; Sao_2, arterial oxygen saturation; Vo_2, oxygen consumption; CO, cardiac output; and Hb is hemoglobin.
3. Svo_2 **is decreased** if the following apply:
   a. Oxygen consumption is increased in the absence of increased delivery, such as in hyperthermia or pain.
   b. Cardiac output is decreased, such as in hypovolemia or shock.
   c. The patient is anemic.
   d. Oxygen saturation is decreased.
4. Svo_2 **is elevated** under conditions of increased oxygen delivery:
   a. Increased inspired oxygen concentration
   b. Conditions of decreased oxygen utilization
      1. Hypothermia
      2. Sepsis
      3. Extreme vasodilation

D. Minimization of errors in blood gas sample collection

1. Care must be taken to avoid sample contamination with air because the Po_2 and Pco_2 of room air at sea level are approximately 155 and 0 mm Hg, respectively.
2. Care should also be taken to avoid contamination of the sample with saline from the sample line or venous blood.
3. Leukocyte larceny (spurious hypoxemia, pseudohypoxemia). The Pao_2 in samples drawn from subjects with very high leukocyte counts can decrease rapidly. Immediate chilling and analysis are necessary.

E. Laboratory analysis of blood gases

1. Blood gases and pH are measured at 37 °C. Using empiric equations, the blood gas analyzer can adjust the measured values to the patient's body temperature. This feature is important to consider in the context of targeted hypothermia after cardiac arrest and focal cerebral ischemia.
2. Once the results of blood gases are available, they are often used to adjust the patient's acid-base status through ventilation or medications. Two strategies for management exist.
   a. **α-stat** ("alpha-stat") management is the acid-base adjustment method in which blood gas measurements (pH, $Paco_2$) obtained at 37 °C from the blood gas machine are directly used to reach the targets ($Paco_2 = 40$ mm Hg, pH = 7.4). Using empiric equations, the blood gas analyzer can adjust the measured values to the patient's body temperature.
      1. Most ICUs utilize the α-stat strategy. The choice of ventilation strategy is becoming increasingly important with the use of targeted hypothermia as a therapeutic tool. Because of increased gas solubility during hypothermia, the α-stat strategy results in relative

hyperventilation (and, therefore, relative cerebral vasoconstriction and reduced cerebral blood flow).

b. pH-stat management is an alternative method in which measurements obtained at 37 °C are corrected to the patient's actual body temperature before use to achieve those same numerical targets. It may be necessary to enquire with your laboratory to determine whether the laboratory is reporting temperature-compensated values (ie, that may facilitate the use of the pH-stat strategy).

c. There are different conditions under which each of these methods can be more or less advantageous.

F. Pulse oximetry: Pulse oximetry has become a standard of care in the ICU. It is useful for titrating supplemental oxygen in patients with hypoxemia receiving noninvasive and invasive respiratory support. It displays the Spo_2, or pulse oxygen saturation

a. An Spo_2 of 92%, or more, reliably predicts a Pao_2 of 60 mm Hg or higher. Spo_2 should be periodically confirmed by blood gas analysis of Sao_2.

1. Principles of operation (Figure 2.1)

a. The commonly used pulse oximeter emits two wavelengths of light (infrared at 940 and red at 660 nm) from light-emitting diodes through a pulsating vascular bed to a photodetector.

b. The ratio of absorption of red and infrared lights is used to determine the fraction of oxygenated hemoglobin (oxyhemoglobin).

c. A variety of probes are available in disposable or reusable designs and include digital probes (finger or toe), ear probes, and nasal probes.

2. Accuracy

a. Pulse oximeters use empiric calibration curves developed from studies of healthy volunteers. They are typically accurate within ±2% for Spo_2 readings as low as 70%. Thus, their accuracy may be reduced in the clinical setting (see Limitations in **Section II.F.6**).

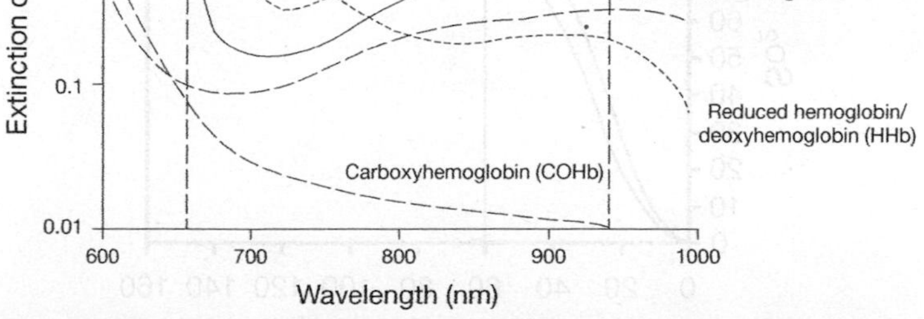

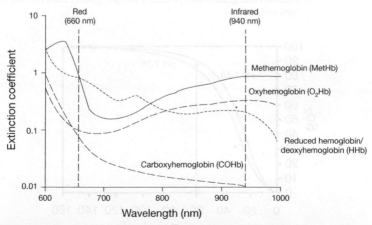

FIGURE 2.1 Red and infrared wavelengths used in pulse oximetry and corresponding types of hemoglobin: oxyhemoglobin (O_2Hb), reduced hemoglobin (sometimes labeled "deoxyhemoglobin," HHb), methemoglobin (MetHb), and carboxyhemoglobin (COHb). Note where the lines of each hemoglobin subtype intersect with the corresponding red and infrared wavelength cutoffs. (Reprinted from Jubran A. Pulse oximetry. *Crit Care.* 2015;19(1):272. doi:10.1186/s13054-015-0984-8, with permission from Springer.)

  b. As illustrated by the oxyhemoglobin dissociation curve (Figure 2.2), if the pulse oximeter displays an oxygen saturation (Spo_2) of 95%, the true saturation could be as low as 93% or as high as 97%. This range of Spo_2 translates to a Pao_2 range from as low as about 60 mm Hg to greater than 150 mm Hg.

3. What do traditional pulse oximeters detect?

  a. Oxyhemoglobin and deoxyhemoglobin

4. What can multiple-wavelength pulse oximetry and co-oximetry detect?

  a. COHb, metHb, and total hemoglobin, in addition to Spo_2.

5. Additional monitoring features of pulse oximetry

  a. Respiratory variation in the plethysmographic waveform

    1. Photoplethysmography of peripheral perfusion is displayed by some pulse oximeters. The beat-to-beat plethysmogram displayed on the pulse oximeter reflects beat-to-beat changes in local blood volume. The cyclic changes in the blood pressure and plethysmographic waveform baseline can be caused by changes in intrathoracic pressure relative to the intravascular volume (likened to pulsus paradoxus).

  b. Perfusion index (PI) is a measurement displayed on many pulse oximeters. It is the ratio of the pulsatile blood flow to the nonpulsatile and thus represents a noninvasive measure of peripheral perfusion.

  c. Plethysmographic variability index (PVI) is a measure of the dynamic changes in the PI that occur during the respiratory cycle. The lower the number, the lesser the variability.

    1. PVI may be increased in patients with severe airflow obstruction and/or in patients who are hypovolemic. It has been proposed as a predictor of fluid responsiveness in patients who are mechanically ventilated, although individual variability in waveform amplitude can be a limitation (Figure 2.3).

6. Limitations of pulse oximetry

  a. Dyshemoglobinemia: Carboxyhemoglobinemia and **methemoglobinemia** (Figure 2.1) result in significant inaccuracy in dual-wavelength pulse oximeters. Multiple-wavelength pulse oximeters address these issues by measuring COHb% and metHb%.

    1. Carboxyhemoglobinemia produces an Spo_2 greater than the true oxygen saturation.

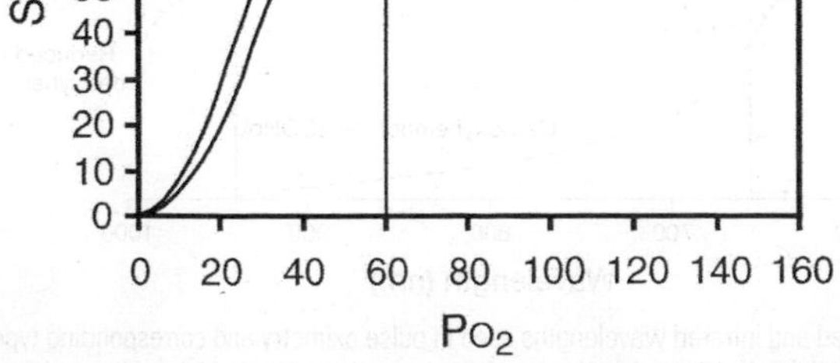

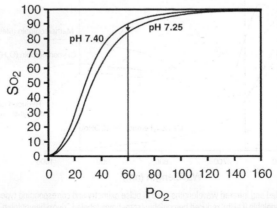

FIGURE 2.2 Oxyhemoglobin dissociation curve. Note that small changes in oxygen saturation relate to large changes in partial pressure of oxygen (PO_2) when the saturation is greater than 90%. Also note that the saturation can change without a change in PO_2 if there is a shift in the oxyhemoglobin dissociation curve.

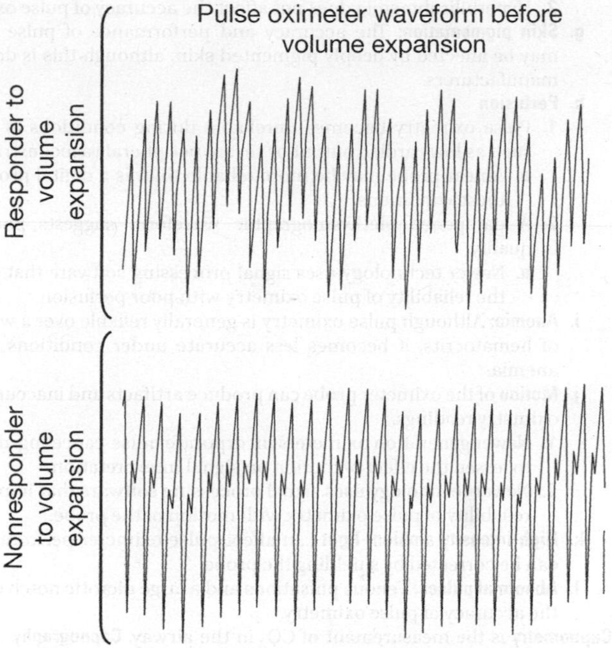

FIGURE 2.3 Pulse oximeter waveform from a patient who responded to volume expansion and from another who did not respond to volume expansion. (Reprinted from Cannesson M, Desebbe O, Rosamel P, et al. Pleth variability index to monitor the respiratory variations in the pulse oximeter plethysmographic waveform amplitude and predict fluid responsiveness in the operating theatre. *Br J Anaesth.* 2008;101:200-206, with permission from Elsevier.)

2. Methemoglobinemia causes the Spo_2 to reduce commensurate with the rise in metHb but hovers around 85% when metHb levels rise beyond 15%.
3. HbF does not affect the accuracy of pulse oximeters.

b. Spo_2 (oxygen saturation) versus Po_2: Because of the shape of the oxyhemoglobin dissociation curve, pulse oximetry is a poor indicator of hyperoxemia. It is also an insensitive indicator of hypoventilation. If the patient is breathing supplemental oxygen, significant hypoventilation can occur without desaturation measured by pulse oximetry.

c. Ventilation versus oxygenation: Pulse oximetry provides no clinical information related to $Paco_2$ and acid-base balance.

d. Differences between devices and probes: Calibration curves vary from manufacturer to manufacturer. The output of the light-emitting diodes of pulse oximeters varies from probe to probe.

e. The penumbra effect occurs when the pulse oximeter probe does not fit correctly and light from the light-emitting diodes escapes the photodetector. It leads to an Spo_2 reading that is erroneously lower than the actual value.

f. Endogenous and exogenous dyes and pigments

1. Intravascular dyes (eg, methylene blue) and nail polish can also affect the accuracy of pulse oximetry.
   a. Although this issue may be less problematic in newer generations of pulse oximeters, it is nonetheless prudent to remove nail polish before applying the pulse oximetry probe.

2. Hyperbilirubinemia does not affect the accuracy of pulse oximetry.

g. **Skin pigmentation:** The accuracy and performance of pulse oximetry may be affected by deeply pigmented skin, although this is debated by manufacturers.

h. **Perfusion**
   1. Pulse oximetry becomes unreliable during conditions of low flow such as low cardiac output or severe peripheral vasoconstriction.
      a. An ear probe may be more reliable than is a digital probe under these conditions.
   2. A dampened plethysmographic waveform suggests poor signal quality.
      a. Newer technology uses signal processing software that improves the reliability of pulse oximetry with poor perfusion.

i. **Anemia:** Although pulse oximetry is generally reliable over a wide range of hematocrits, it becomes less accurate under conditions of severe anemia.

j. **Motion** of the oximeter probe can produce artifacts and inaccurate pulse oximetry readings.
   1. Newer generation oximeters incorporate noise-canceling algorithms to lessen the effect of motion on signal interpretation.
   2. Newer technology uses signal processing software that improves the reliability of pulse oximetry with motion of the probe.

k. **High-intensity ambient light** can affect pulse oximeter performance and can be corrected by shielding the probe.

l. **Abnormal pulses:** Venous pulsations and a large dicrotic notch can affect the accuracy of pulse oximetry.

G. **Capnometry** is the measurement of CO_2 in the airway. **Capnography** is the display of a CO_2 waveform called the **capnogram** (Figure 2.4).
   1. The PCO_2 measured at end exhalation is called the **end-tidal PCO_2 ($ETCO_2$)**.
      a. The $ETCO_2$ represents alveolar PCO_2. It is a function of the rate at which CO_2 is added to the alveoli and the rate at which CO_2 is cleared from the alveoli. Thus, the $ETCO_2$ is a function of the ($\dot{V}/\dot{Q}$).
      b. With a normal and homogeneously distributed ($\dot{V}/\dot{Q}$), the $ETCO_2$ approximates the $PaCO_2$.

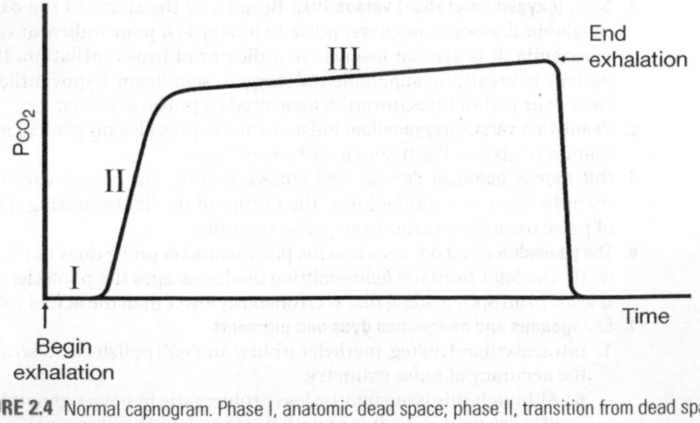

FIGURE 2.4 Normal capnogram. Phase I, anatomic dead space; phase II, transition from dead space to alveolar gas; phase III, alveolar plateau.

c. With a high $\dot{V}/\dot{Q}$ ratio (dead-space effect), the $ETCO_2$ is lower than the $PaCO_2$.

d. With a low $\dot{V}/\dot{Q}$ ratio (shunt effect), the $ETCO_2$ approximates the mixed venous PCO_2.

e. Changes in $ETCO_2$ can be due to changes in CO_2 production, CO_2 delivery to the lungs, or changes in the magnitude and distribution of the alveolar ventilation.

2. Types of capnometers

a. Quantitative capnometers measure CO_2 using the principles of infrared spectroscopy, Raman spectroscopy, or mass spectroscopy.

b. Nonquantitative capnometers indicate CO_2 by a color change of an indicator material, based on a shift in pH.

c. Mainstream capnometer chambers are placed directly into the airway circuit.

d. Sidestream capnometers aspirate gas from the airway circuit through tubing to a measurement chamber in the capnometer.

3. Uses of capnometers

a. $ETCO_2$ monitoring to confirm tracheal intubation is generally regarded as the standard of care for clinically confirming the correct placement of the endotracheal tube. Low-cost, disposable devices that produce a color change in the presence of CO_2 are commercially available.

b. Capnometers can aid in the detection of increases in dead space, prompting corrective interventions. This early dead-space detection is useful during resuscitation.

1. Be mindful of added dead space from inappropriate additions to the airway circuit.

c. Capnometers can indicate obstructive respiratory mechanics via waveform changes.

1. Waveform: normal (Figure 2.4) and abnormal, as seen in a patient with obstructive lung disease when the waveform changes from box/plateau to saw-toothed (Figure 2.5).

4. Volumetric capnometry, also called volume-based capnometry, displays exhaled CO_2 as a function of exhaled tidal volume (Figure 2.6). Note that the

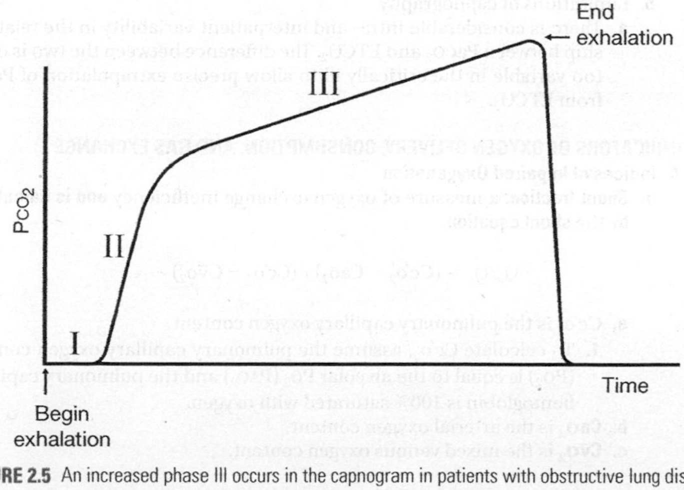

FIGURE 2.5 An increased phase III occurs in the capnogram in patients with obstructive lung disease.

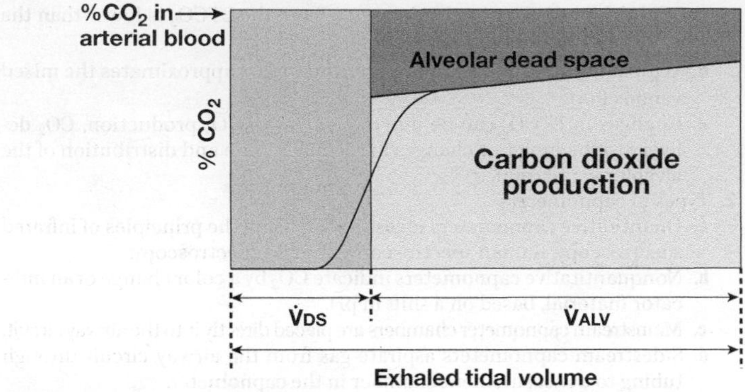

FIGURE 2.6 The volume-based capnogram. Note that the area under the curve represents carbon dioxide elimination, which equals carbon dioxide production during steady-state conditions.

area under the volume-based capnogram is the volume of CO_2 exhaled. Assuming steady-state conditions, this represents **carbon dioxide production** ($\dot{V}CO_2$). Because $\dot{V}CO_2$ is determined by metabolic rate, it can be used to estimate **resting energy expenditure** (REE):

$$REE = CO_2\ (L/min) \times 5.25\ kcal/L \times 1440\ min/d$$

a. Using volume-based capnometry and a partial-rebreathing circuit, **pulmonary capillary blood flow** can be measured by applying a modification of the Fick equation using a capnography tool called the NICO (noninvasive cardiac output monitor; Figure 2.7). With corrections for intrapulmonary shunt, this allows noninvasive estimation of cardiac output. There is significant variability in the clinical application of this method.

5. Limitations of capnography

a. There is considerable intra- and interpatient variability in the relationship between $PaCO_2$ and $ETCO_2$. The difference between the two is often too variable in the critically ill to allow precise extrapolation of $PaCO_2$ from $ETCO_2$.

III. INDICATORS OF OXYGEN DELIVERY, CONSUMPTION, AND GAS EXCHANGE

A. Indices of Impaired Oxygenation

1. Shunt fraction: a measure of oxygen exchange inefficiency **and is calculated by** the **shunt equation:**

$$\dot{Q}_s/\dot{Q}_t = (Cc'O_2 - CaO_2)\ /\ (Cc'O_2 - C\bar{v}O_2)$$

a. $Cc'O_2$ is the pulmonary capillary oxygen content.

1. To calculate $Cc'O_2$, assume the pulmonary capillary oxygen content (PO_2) is equal to the alveolar PO_2 (PAO_2) and the pulmonary capillary hemoglobin is 100% saturated with oxygen.

b. $\mathbf{CaO_2}$ is the arterial oxygen content.

c. $\mathbf{C\bar{v}O_2}$ is the mixed venous oxygen content.

$$C\bar{v}O_2 = (1.34 \times Hb \times HbO2) + (0.003 \times PaO_2)$$

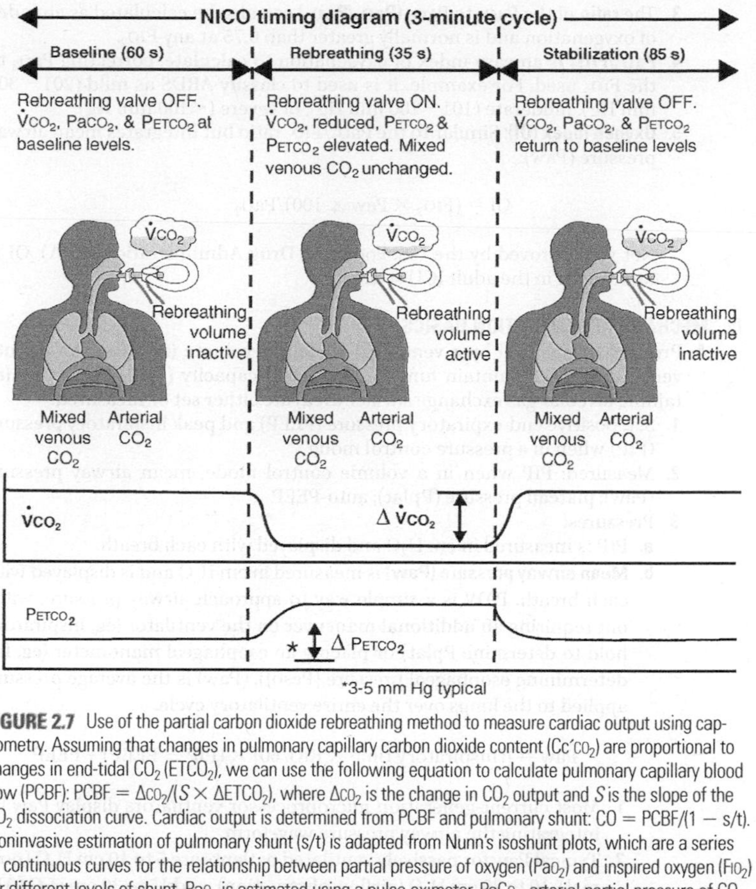

FIGURE 2.7 Use of the partial carbon dioxide rebreathing method to measure cardiac output using capnometry. Assuming that changes in pulmonary capillary carbon dioxide content ($Cc'CO_2$) are proportional to changes in end-tidal CO_2 ($ETCO_2$), we can use the following equation to calculate pulmonary capillary blood flow (PCBF): PCBF = $\Delta CO_2/(S \times \Delta ETCO_2)$, where ΔCO_2 is the change in CO_2 output and *S* is the slope of the CO_2 dissociation curve. Cardiac output is determined from PCBF and pulmonary shunt: CO = PCBF/(1 − s/t). Noninvasive estimation of pulmonary shunt (s/t) is adapted from Nunn's isoshunt plots, which are a series of continuous curves for the relationship between partial pressure of oxygen (PaO_2) and inspired oxygen (FIO_2) for different levels of shunt. PaO_2 is estimated using a pulse oximeter. $PaCO_2$, arterial partial pressure of CO_2. (Non invasive cardiac output (NICO) timing diagram courtesy of Novametrix, Wallingford, CT.)

d. If measured when the patient is breathing 100% oxygen, the $\dot{Q}_S/\dot{Q}_T$ represents shunt (ie, blood that flows from the right heart to the left heart without passing functional alveoli). If measured at FIO_2 less than 1.0, the $\dot{Q}_S/\dot{Q}_T$ represents shunt and $\dot{V}/\dot{Q}$ mismatch (ie, venous admixture).

2. An increased $P(A-a)O_2$ gradient is another measure of oxygen exchange inefficiency. The $P(A-a)O_2$ is normally 10 mm Hg or less breathing room air and 50 mm Hg or less breathing 100% oxygen. The alveolar partial pressure of oxygen, PAO_2, is calculated from the alveolar gas equation:

$$PAO_2 = [FIO_2 \times (P_B - PH_2O)] - [PaCO_2/R]$$

where PB is the barometric pressure, PH_2O the water vapor pressure, and R the respiratory quotient. For calculation of PAO_2, an R of 0.8 is commonly used.

a. An increased difference the **$P(A-a)O_2$ gradient** can be caused by

1. Shunt

2. $\dot{V}/\dot{Q}$ mismatch

3. Diffusion defect

3. The **ratio** of the Pa_{O_2} to PA_{O_2} (**Pa_{O_2}/PA_{O_2}**) can also be calculated as an index of oxygenation and is normally greater than 0.75 at any F_{IO_2}.
4. **Pa_{O_2}/F_{IO_2}** is an easy index of oxygenation to calculate, correcting Pa_{O_2} to the F_{IO_2} used. For example, it is used to classify ARDS as mild (201 − 300 mm Hg), moderate (101 − 200 mm Hg), or severe (<100 mm Hg).
5. **Oxygen index (OI):** Similar to the Pa_{O_2}/F_{IO_2} ratio but integrates mean airway pressure (Paw):

$$OI = (F_{IO_2} \times Paw \times 100)/Pa_{O_2}$$

Not yet approved by the U.S. Food and Drug Administration (FDA), OI is rarely used in the adult ICU setting.

IV. MECHANICAL VENTILATION BASICS

A. Pressures generated by a ventilator to deliver volume (and thereby minute ventilation) and maintain functional residual capacity (FRC; thereby maintaining alveolar gas exchange surface area) are either set or measured.

1. Set: positive end-expiratory pressure (PEEP) and peak inspiratory pressure (PIP) when in a pressure control mode
2. Measured: PIP when in a volume control mode; mean airway pressure (Paw); plateau pressure (Pplat); auto-PEEP
3. Pressures:
   - **a.** PIP is measured in cm H_2O and displayed with each breath.
   - **b.** **Mean airway pressure (Paw)** is measured in cm H_2O and is displayed with each breath. PAW is a simple way to approach airway pressure, without requiring an additional maneuver on the ventilator (eg, inspiratory hold to determine Pplat) or placing an esophageal manometer (eg, for determining esophageal pressure [Peso]). ($\bar{P}aw$) is the average pressure applied to the lungs over the entire ventilatory cycle.

$$\bar{P}aw = [(\text{Inspiratory time} \times RR)/60] \times (PIP - PEEP) + PEEP$$

   1. Most current-generation microprocessor ventilators display $\bar{P}aw$ by integrating the airway pressure waveform.
   2. Typical $\bar{P}aw$ for passively ventilated patients are 5 to 10 cm H_2O (normal), 10 to 20 cm H_2O (airflow obstruction), and 15 to 30 cm H_2O (ALI [acute lung injury] or ARDS).
   3. Factors affecting $\bar{P}aw$ are as follows:
      - **a.** PIP (an increase in PIP increases airway pressure)
      - **b.** PEEP (an increase in PEEP increases airway pressure)
      - **c.** I:E ratio (inspiratory-to-expiratory ratio: the longer the inspiratory time, the higher the $\bar{P}aw$)
      - **d.** Inspiratory pressure waveform (a rectangular inspiratory pressure waveform produces a higher Paw than does a triangular inspiratory pressure waveform)
   - **c.** **Plateau pressure (Pplat):** Pplat is the pressure manifest in the distal airways/alveoli after the inspiratory pressure has been given time to equilibrate.
   1. **Measurement:** measured during an inspiratory hold maneuver on the ventilator, lasting 0.5 to 2.0 seconds.
      - **a.** During the breath-hold, pressure equilibrates throughout the system so that the pressure measured at the proximal airway approximates the alveolar pressure (Figure 2.8).

b. Note, the ventilator must be in a volume control mode and the patient must be fully synchronous with the ventilator and cannot trigger breaths (achieved by an escalation in sedation and/or use of neuromuscular blockade [NMB]).

2. An increased Pplat indicates a greater risk of alveolar overdistension during mechanical ventilation. Many authorities recommend that Pplat be maintained at 30 cm H_2O or less in patients with acute respiratory failure. This assumes that chest wall compliance is normal. A higher Pplat may be necessary if chest wall compliance is decreased (eg, abdominal distension).

d. Auto-PEEP (aka intrinsic PEEP) is measured by an expiratory hold maneuver. As the inspiratory pressure equilibrates in the airways, the resulting stable pressure reading at expiration is the amount of back pressure generated by the lungs during exhalation. This pressure reading is termed auto-PEEP. Patients with obstructive lung disease may generate large auto-PEEP. Again, the patient must be fully synchronous with the ventilator and able to accommodate the maneuver. An expiratory hold maneuver can be performed in a pressure or volume control mode.

V. LUNG MECHANICS: Lung mechanics directly influence the level of mechanical ventilation support needed to adequately exchange gas

A. Compliance: the amount of volume (tidal volume, V_T, in mL) generated for every unit of pressure delivered (cmH_2O). Normal compliance is 100 mL/cm H_2O and on a ventilator, usually 50 to 100 mL/cmH_2O, the reduction likely caused by supine or semirecumbent position and microatelectasis. For example, a patient who is ventilated but has normal compliance can demonstrate a **driving pressure (Pplat – PEEP)** of 10 cmH_2O and a V_T of 500 to 1000 mL. A decrease in compliance will result in reduced V_T, requiring an escalation in driving pressure. Two types of compliance measured are static compliance and dynamic compliance.

1. Static compliance is a measurement performed in conditions of no flow or, more likely, a very low flow (quasi-static condition) achieved by the

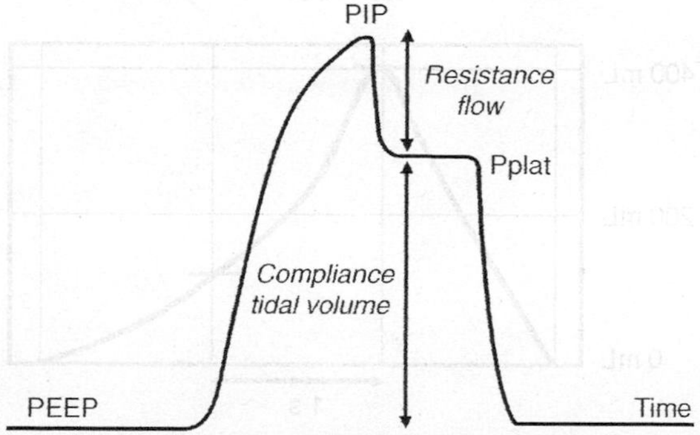

FIGURE 2.8 Peak alveolar pressure (Pplat) is determined by applying an end-inspiratory breath-hold. The peak inspiratory pressure (PIP)-Pplat difference is determined by resistance and end-inspiratory flow, and the Pplat-positive end-expiratory pressure (PEEP) difference is determined by compliance and tidal volume.

end-inspiratory hold maneuver (or pause). It is influenced by the compliance of the lungs and the chest wall.

$$C_{STAT} = V_T/(Pplat - PEEP).$$

a. Static compliance is more frequently used in the ICU because it specifically reflects compliance of the lung tissue (and chest wall).

2. Dynamic compliance is measured during active inspiration and during gas flow.

$$C_{DYN} = V_T/(PIP - PEEP)$$

As with static compliance, dynamic compliance is influenced by lung and chest wall compliance, with the additional component of airway resistance.

a. Dynamic compliance is not as commonly used to guide therapeutic decisions in the ICU but can be used to better identify a component of airway resistance.

B. Airway Resistance (R_{AW}) is determined by the driving pressure and the flow.

1. Ohm's law of V = IR, rearranged: R = V/I, wherein V is the delta pressure (driving pressure) and I is flow (LPM).

$$R_{AW} = (PIP - Pplat)/flow\ (60\ L/min\ or\ 1\ L/s).$$

a. Normal, therefore, is 10 to 15 cm H_2O/L/s at a flow of 60 LPM (1 L/s) in a patient who is ventilated (for comparison, in a patient who is healthy, spontaneously breathing, and nonintubated, airway resistance is 2-3 cm H_2O/L/s).

2. Inspiratory airway resistance can be estimated during volume ventilation from the PIP − Pplat difference and the end-inspiratory flow:

$$R_I = (PIP \times Pplat)/rR_I = (PIP \times Pplat)/I$$

where I is the end-inspiratory flow.

a. A simple way to measure this is to deliver a constant inspiratory flow of 60 L/min (1 L/s) through the ventilator, and, thus, the inspiratory airway resistance is the PIP − Pplat difference.

3. Expiratory resistance can be estimated from the time constant (τ) of the lung (Figure 2.9):

$$RE = \tau/C$$

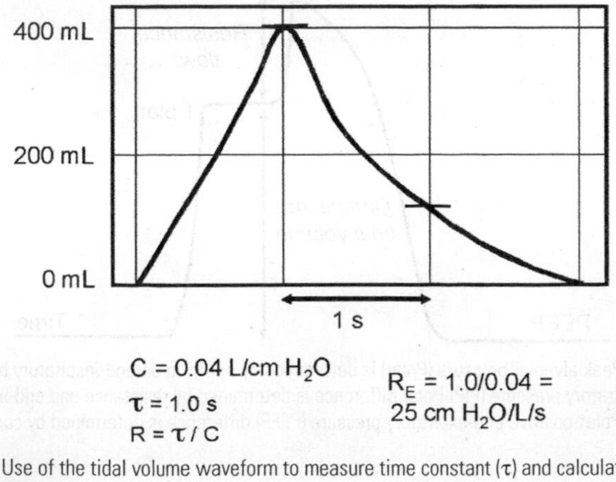

FIGURE 2.9 Use of the tidal volume waveform to measure time constant (τ) and calculate expiratory airway resistance.

4. **Common causes** of increased airway resistance are bronchospasm, secretions, small endotracheal tube (ETT), and thoracic mass.
   a. For patients who are intubated and mechanically ventilated, as mentioned earlier, airway resistance should be less than 10 cm H_2O/L/s at a flow of 1 L/s. Expiratory airway resistance is typically greater than inspiratory airway resistance.

VI. MEASUREMENT OF LUNG MECHANICS

A. It is important to understand that compliance of the respiratory system is influenced by the combination of lung compliance and chest wall compliance. Esophageal balloon manometry is used to estimate pleural pressure (Ppl). Transpulmonary pressure is the difference between Pplat and **esophageal pressure (Peso)**. Transpulmonary pressure, or the change in pleural pressure, can be used to estimate the contributions made by the lung and the chest wall to the total compliance of the respiratory system.

1. **Esophageal pressure (Peso) measured by esophageal balloon manometry**
   a. Esophageal pressure changes reflect changes in pleural pressure, but the absolute esophageal pressure does not reflect absolute pleural pressure (Figure 2.10).
   b. The change in esophageal pressure (ΔPeso) during passive inflation of the lungs can be used to calculate chest wall compliance (Ccw).
      1. Ccw = VT/ΔPeso
   c. Changes in esophageal pressure, relative to changes in alveolar pressure, can be used to calculate transpulmonary pressure (an indirect estimate of lung stress).
      1. Transpulmonary pressure (difference between Pplat and Peso) is targeted at $<$27 cm H_2O.
   d. Esophageal pressure monitoring can provide data that allow for more precise setting of tidal volume (and Pplat) in patients with reduced chest wall compliance (eg, those who are obese).
   e. Although esophageal pressure has been used to target the appropriate setting for PEEP, its clinical application is debated. The concept is that patients with a higher Peso require more PEEP to counterbalance the alveolar collapsing effect of the higher pleural pressure. Currently, our practice is to measure esophageal pressure for patients who are hypoxemic and weigh more than 120 kg.
   f. **Chest wall compliance** is calculated from changes in esophageal pressure (pleural pressure) during passive inflation. It is normally 200 mL/cm H_2O and can be **decreased** because of abdominal distension, chest wall edema, chest wall burns, and thoracic deformities (eg, kyphoscoliosis), and, more dynamically, a patient asynchronous with the ventilator (ie, "bucking the vent"). Chest compliance is **increased** with flail chest, open chest or abdomen, and NMB.
   g. **Lung compliance** is calculated from changes in transpulmonary pressure. **Transpulmonary pressure** is the difference between alveolar pressure (Pplat) and pleural pressure (esophageal). Normal lung compliance is 100 mL/cm H_2O.
      1. Lung compliance is **reduced** by pulmonary edema, ARDS, pneumothorax, pneumonia/infiltrate, atelectasis, and interstitial lung disease (ILD).
         a. When compliance is decreased, a larger transpulmonary pressure is required to deliver a given tidal volume into the lungs. Thus, a decreased compliance will result in the need for a higher Pplat and PIP. To avoid dangerous levels of airway pressure, lower tidal volumes are used to ventilate the lungs of patients with decreased compliance. Determining the source of the decreased compliance is critical to appropriate management and optimization of

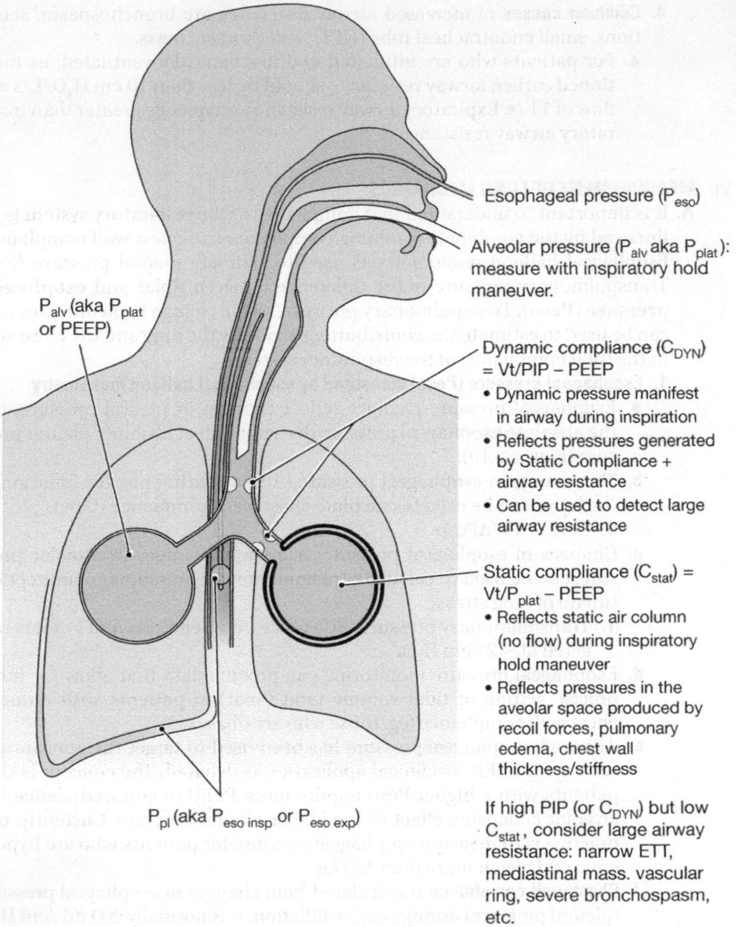
Esophageal pressure (P_{eso})
Alveolar pressure (P_{alv} aka P_{plat}): measure with inspiratory hold maneuver.
P_{alv} (aka P_{plat} or PEEP)
Dynamic compliance (C_{DYN}) = Vt/PIP – PEEP
• Dynamic pressure manifest in airway during inspiration
• Reflects pressures generated by Static Compliance + airway resistance
• Can be used to detect large airway resistance
Static compliance (C_{stat}) = Vt/P_{plat} – PEEP
• Reflects static air column (no flow) during inspiratory hold maneuver
• Reflects pressures in the aveolar space produced by recoil forces, pulmonary edema, chest wall thickness/stiffness
If high PIP (or C_{DYN}) but low C_{stat}, consider large airway resistance: narrow ETT, mediastinal mass. vascular ring, severe bronchospasm, etc.
P_{pl} (aka $P_{eso\ insp}$ or $P_{eso\ exp}$)

C_{cw} = Vt/ $P_{eso\ insp}$ – $P_{eso\ exp}$

C_{lung} = Vt/ End-inspiration transpulmonary pressure – End-expiratory transpulmonary pressure

Where:

End-inspiratory transpulmonary pressure = P_{plat}– $P_{eso\ insp}$ (used for estimating overdistention)

End-expiratory transpulmonary pressure = PEEP– $P_{eso\ exp}$ (used for optimizing PEEP)

Summarized: Compliance Lung only = Vt/(P_{plat}– $P_{eso\ ins}$)– (PEEP– $P_{eso\ exp}$)

FIGURE 2.10 Approaches to determining transpulmonary pressure, chest wall versus lung compliance, and dynamic and static compliance. Of note, certain elements are used as surrogates for other elements. For example: Plateau pressure (Pplat) is a proxy of alveolar pressure (Palv) on inspiration, and the relationship is identified by "aka" in this figure. C_{CW}, chest wall compliance; C_{lung}, lung compliance; P_{pl}, pleural pressure; P_{plat}, plateau pressure; P_{alv}, alveolar pressure; Peso, esophageal pressure; C_{DYN}, dynamic compliance; C_{stat}, static compliance; V_t = tidal volume; V = volume; PIP = peak inspiratory pressure; PEEP = positive end-expiratory pressure; Insp = inspiratory; Exp = expiratory.

invasive respiratory support. Decreased lung compliance also increases the work of breathing, decreasing the likelihood of successful weaning from the ventilator (Figure 2.10).

2. Lung compliance is **increased** by emphysematous changes.

2. **Measurement:** Esophageal pressure is measured by placing a thin-walled balloon containing a small volume of air (<1 mL) into the distal third of the esophagus. The measurement and display of esophageal pressure are facilitated by commercially available systems.
3. **Clinical implications**
   a. Esophageal pressure monitoring provides additional data that can optimize PIP, Pplat, or driving pressure to maintain a tidal volume adequate for effective ventilation while minimizing barotrauma.
   b. Changes in esophageal pressure can be used to assess respiratory effort and the work of breathing during spontaneous breathing and patient-triggered modes of ventilation; to assess chest wall compliance during full ventilatory support; and to assess auto-PEEP during spontaneous breathing and patient-triggered modes of ventilation.
   c. If exhalation is passive, the change in esophageal (ie, Ppl) pressure required to reverse flow at the proximal airway (ie, trigger the ventilator) reflects the amount of auto-PEEP. Negative esophageal pressure changes that produce no flow in the airway indicate failed trigger efforts —in other words, the patient's inspiratory efforts are insufficient to overcome the level of auto-PEEP and trigger the ventilator. Clinically, this is recognized as a patient RR (observed by inspecting chest wall movement) that is greater than the triggered rate on the ventilator.

B. **Gastric Pressure** is sometimes measured to determine whether it influences respiratory system compliance and/or reduces FRC.

1. **Measurement:** Gastric pressure is measured by a balloon-tipped catheter similar to that used to measure esophageal pressure. It reflects changes in intra-abdominal pressure. An alternative for measuring gastric pressure is measuring **bladder pressure.**
2. **Clinical implications:** During a spontaneous inspiratory effort, gastric pressure normally increases because of contraction of the diaphragm. A decrease in gastric pressure with spontaneous inspiratory effort is consistent with diaphragmatic paralysis (Figure 2.11). A high baseline gastric pressure reflects elevated intra-abdominal pressure, which may affect chest wall compliance and lung function.

C. **Electrical Impedance Tomography (EIT)** is an imaging technique in which the conductivity is inferred from surface electrical measurements. EIT adhesive electrodes are applied to the skin and an electric current, typically a few milliamperes of alternating current at a frequency of 10 to 100 kHz, is applied across two or more electrodes. The resulting electrical potentials are measured and the process is repeated for different configurations of applied current. The lungs become less conductive as the alveoli become filled with air and more conductive when alveoli become airless (collapsed, edematous, or consolidated). EIT helps identify areas of poor $\dot{V}/\dot{Q}$ matching and can help highlight problematic quadrants (eg, ventral left and right and dorsal left and right; Figure 2.12).

VII. MEASUREMENTS TAKEN FROM A SPONTANEOUSLY BREATHING PATIENT ON A VENTILATOR

A. **Occlusion Pressure ($P_{0.1}$, sometimes denoted as "P-one-hundred")** is the negative airway pressure generated 100 ms after the onset of inhalation against an occluded airway.

1. $P_{0.1}$ is an index of ventilatory drive. It can be measured manually and/or automatically on some ventilators.

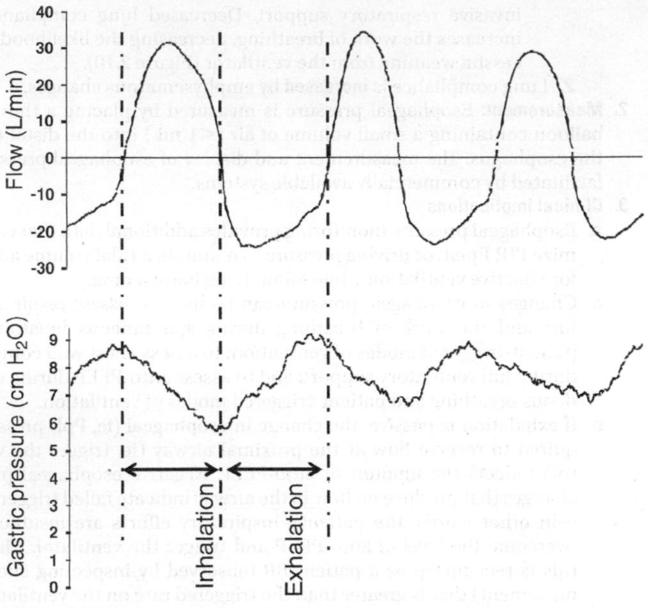

FIGURE 2.11 Gastric pressure measurement in a patient with diaphragm paralysis. Note that the gastric pressure decreases during the inspiratory phase.

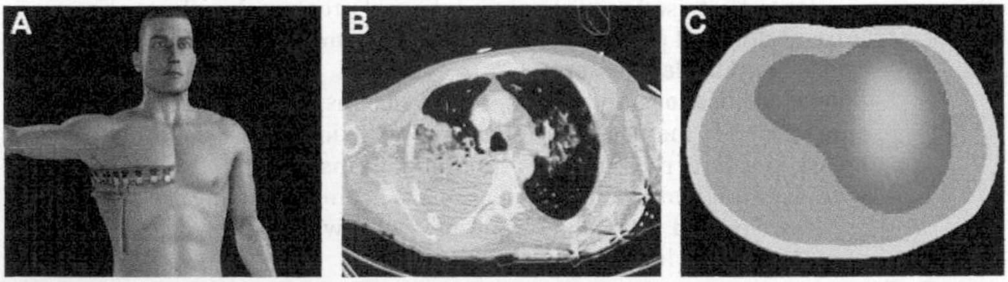

FIGURE 2.12 Electric impedance tomography (EIT). **A:** A belt of EIT electrodes is placed around the chest, between the fifth and sixth intercostal space. **B:** A computed tomography (CT) scan of a chest with pneumonia in the right lower lobe. **C:** The EIT readout of the same chest in "B," demonstrating an area of nonventilation, correlating with the CT findings. (Courtesy of Timpel.)

2. Normal $P_{0.1}$ is 3 to 4 cm H_2O.
3. A $P_{0.1}$ greater than 6 cm H_2O has been associated with weaning failure.

B. **Maximum Inspiratory Pressure (PImax or MIP),** the most negative pressure generated during a maximal inspiratory effort against an occluded airway
1. PImax is an index of the strength of the inspiratory muscles.
2. The off-ventilator manual measurement technique uses a one-way valve, allowing exhalation, but not inhalation, and an occlusion for approximately 15 to 20 seconds, provided no arrhythmias or desaturations occur. Some ventilators perform this measurement electronically by occluding both inspiratory and expiratory valves.
3. Normal PImax is less than or equal to 100 cm H_2O (varies with sex and age).
4. Although PImax equal to or greater than 30 cm H_2O has been associated with weaning failure; its predictive value is poor.

C. Maximum expiratory pressure (PEmax or MEP), the most positive pressure generated during a maximal inspiratory effort against an occluded airway

1. PEmax is an index of the strength of the expiratory muscles.

D. Asynchrony with ventilatory support has been correlated with worse outcomes. Asynchrony is recognized by observing the flow and volume curves on the ventilator in conjunction with patient effort. Minimizing asynchrony requires several approaches: increasing sedation, NMB, a change in flow trigger or mode of assisted ventilation, or neurally adjusted ventilatory assist (NAVA).

1. NAVA is a ventilation mode that delivers ventilatory support synchronized with and proportional to the electrical activity of the patient's diaphragm (EAdi). EAdi is measured using esophageal electrodes positioned at the level of the diaphragm and provides a measure of respiratory drive. The ratio of tidal volume (Vt) to EAdi can be used as a measure of a patient's neuroventilatory efficiency.

E. Spontaneous breathing trial and/or spontaneous awake trial (see **Chapter 24**)

VIII. WORK OF BREATHING

A. The Campbell Diagram (Figure 2.13) is used to determine the work of breathing. This diagram includes the effects of chest wall compliance, lung compliance, and airway resistance on the work of breathing. Work of breathing is increased with decreased chest wall compliance, decreased lung compliance, or increased airway resistance.

1. Clinical implications: Work of breathing requires special equipment and an esophageal balloon to quantify, and, for this reason, it is not frequently measured. Moreover, it is not clear that measuring work of breathing improves patient outcome. It may be useful for quantifying patient effort

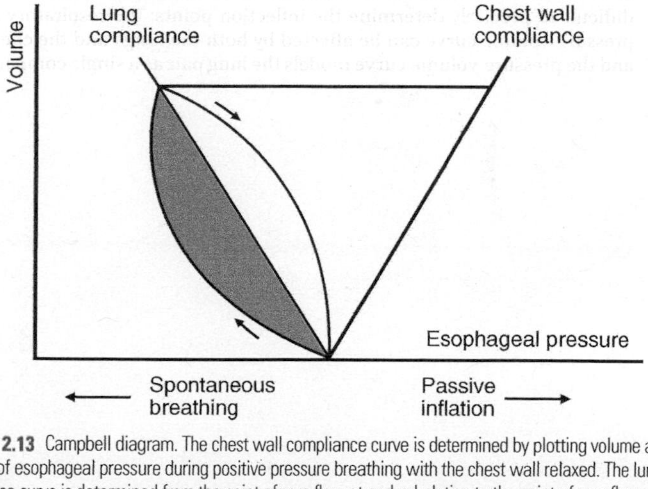

FIGURE 2.13 Campbell diagram. The chest wall compliance curve is determined by plotting volume as a function of esophageal pressure during positive pressure breathing with the chest wall relaxed. The lung compliance curve is determined from the point of zero flow at end exhalation to the point of zero flow at end inhalation during spontaneous breathing. Because of airway resistance, the esophageal pressure is more negative than that predicted from the lung compliance curve. The areas indicated on the curve represent elastic work of breathing and resistive work of breathing. Note that a decreased chest wall compliance will shift the compliance curve to the right, thus increasing the elastic work of breathing. A decrease in lung compliance shifts the curve to the left, also increasing the work of breathing. An increased airway resistance causes a more negative esophageal pressure during spontaneous breathing, increasing the resistive work of breathing.

during mechanical ventilation but this can often be achieved by simply observing the respiratory variation on a central venous pressure tracing. Large inspiratory efforts produce large negative deflections of the central venous pressure trace during inspiratory efforts. Increasing the level of ventilatory assistance should reduce these negative deflections.

B. There are emerging technologies aimed at measuring the work of breathing or a change in respiratory effort (ie, tidal volume), noninvasively.

IX. STATIC PRESSURE-VOLUME CURVES measure the pressure-volume relationship of the respiratory system.

A. Measurement

1. The manual method with a super syringe is relatively simple but requires disconnecting the patient from the ventilator to perform the maneuver.
2. Alternatively, a pressure-volume curve can be measured automatically in select ventilators without disconnecting the patient from the ventilator.
3. The multiple occlusion method involves repeated end-inspiratory breath occlusions at different lung volumes, and the constant flow technique measures the change in airway opening pressure with a constant slow flow (≤10 L/min).
4. The optimal technique is unknown.

B. Lower and Upper Inflection Points can be determined from the pressure-volume curve. Some authors have suggested that the level of PEEP should be set above the lower inflection point to avoid alveolar collapse and that Pplat should be set below the upper inflection point to avoid alveolar overdistension. However, the clinical benefits of this approach are unclear, and setting the ventilator using the pressure-volume curve is not currently recommended because there are important limitations to the clinical use of pressure-volume curves. Accurate measurements require heavy sedation (and, often, NMB); it is unclear whether the inflation or deflation curve should be assessed; it can be difficult to precisely determine the inflection points; the respiratory system pressure-volume curve can be affected by both the lungs and the chest wall; and the pressure-volume curve models the lung pair as a single compartment.

3 Use of Ultrasound in Critical Illness

Lauren E. Gibson and Marvin G. Chang

Critical care ultrasonography (CCUS, or point-of-care ultrasound) has become an increasingly valuable skill in the diagnosis and management of patients who are critically ill presenting in a variety of clinical scenarios (Table 3.1). Widespread adoption has been facilitated by advances in ultrasound technology because modern devices have become increasingly portable, less expensive, and yet capable of high-quality imaging. Conceptually, CCUS functions as an extension of the physical examination. It is immediately available at the bedside, is noninvasive, and in skilled hands provides a wealth of information that can be used to rapidly narrow differential diagnoses and to initiate or modify treatment. CCUS is not intended to replace other more comprehensive forms of diagnostic imaging. Rather, the **real-time acquisition and interpretation** of images that are then **interpreted in the context of the physiology** of a patient who is acutely unstable is the hallmark of CCUS. Of the very broad range of techniques that comprise CCUS, this chapter focuses primarily on the use of ultrasound to evaluate cardiorespiratory status.

I. ULTRASOUND BASICS

A. An ultrasound image is produced from the emission of sound waves and the interaction of these sound waves with various tissue interfaces that are then reflected and detected by a transducer. The **wavelength** of a sound wave is the distance between two repetitive points along a single cycle, whereas the **frequency** of a wave is the number of repetitions per second. The wavelength and frequency of the sound wave determine the **spatial resolution.** The shorter the wavelength, and thus the higher the frequency, the better the spatial resolution. High-frequency waves provide excellent near-field resolution but poor tissue penetration because they are subject to attenuation with increasing tissue depth. Conversely, low-frequency waves offer improved tissue penetration, allowing visualization of deeper structures, but poor spatial resolution. Thus, higher frequency probes (~5-10 MHz) are used for visualization of relatively superficial vascular structures and lower frequency probes (~2-5 MHz) for imaging deeper tissues such as the heart and abdomen. The three main probe types used are the linear probe, the curvilinear probe, and the phased-array probe.

B. Spatial resolution differs from temporal resolution. Spatial resolution relates to the ability to determine the location of a structure in space. **Temporal resolution** relates to the ability to determine the position of a structure at a particular instant in time. Temporal resolution is determined by the **pulse repetition frequency (PRF).** The higher the PRF, the higher the temporal resolution. A higher PRF increases the number of frames per second. This becomes important when assessing a fast-moving structure such as the heart. The temporal resolution can be improved by decreasing the sector width or imaging depth.

C. **Doppler ultrasonography** is of great value in the assessment and quantification of blood flow through the heart. Doppler techniques are divided into pulsed-wave Doppler (PWD), continuous-wave Doppler (CWD), and color Doppler. **PWD** is used to measure flow velocities at a single defined location, such as at a point (defined by the sampling volume) in the left ventricular

TABLE 3.1 Suggested Uses for Point-of-Care Ultrasound in the Critical Care Setting

Clinical scenario	Potential uses of ultrasound
Newly admitted patient	Supplement physical exam by assessing cardiac function, confirming bilateral lung sliding and presence or absence of B-lines, determining the presence of ascites
	Procedural guidance for line placements
	Confirm positioning of existing lines, tubes, and drains
New-onset hypotension	Assess left ventricular systolic function to diagnose cardiogenic shock
	Check for regional wall motion abnormalities to assist in diagnosing acute coronary syndrome or stress cardiomyopathy
	Assess right ventricular systolic function to check for hemodynamically significant pulmonary embolism
	Check for major valvular stenosis or regurgitation
	Determine presence of pericardial effusion and/or tamponade
	Measure LVOT VTI to diagnose hyperdynamic function, possible distributive shock
	Assess IVC size and collapsibility to determine hypovolemic shock
New-onset hypoxemia	Confirm endotracheal tube positioning by transtracheal ultrasound
	Assess lung sliding and check for pneumothorax
	Determine presence or absence of B-lines and consolidations
	Perform bubble study to determine presence of intracardiac or intrapulmonary shunting
	Check for pleural effusions
	Procedural guidance for drainage of large pleural effusion
Titrating ventilation settings	Monitor for changes in B-lines with titration of PEEP
	Assess cardiopulmonary interactions with changes in mechanical ventilation
	Monitor progression or improvement of ARDS
Determining readiness for extubation	Check for resolution of B-lines, consolidations
	Assess cardiac filling pressures to determine the need for further diuresis
	Measure diaphragmatic excursion during spontaneous breathing efforts
Optimize patient volume status	Measure LVOT VTI before and after a fluid challenge or passive leg raise to determine fluid responsiveness
	Measure cardiac filling pressures to help determine the need for fluid vs diuresis
	Measure respiratory variation in LVOT or carotid VTI
	Assess IVC size and collapsibility
Cardiac arrest	Check for reversible etiologies such as large pericardial effusion or tension pneumothorax
	Monitor for return of spontaneous cardiac activity
	Perform carotid artery pulse checks
	Confirm cardiac standstill upon cessation of resuscitation
Evaluation of trauma patient	FAST exam to check for hemoperitoneum, pericardial effusion, and free fluid in the pelvis
	Assess for pneumothorax
	Procedural guidance for pericardiocentesis

TABLE 3.1 Suggested Uses for Point-of-Care Ultrasound in the Critical Care Setting (*continued*)

Clinical scenario	Potential uses of ultrasound
	Measure optic nerve sheath diameter as an indicator of intracranial pressure if head trauma is suspected
	Assess gastric size and emptying to determine the need for rapid sequence intubation if patient requires general anesthesia
Patient with suspected DVT	Check vein compressibility to determine presence of thrombus in deep veins
	Assess right ventricular systolic function to check for hemodynamically significant pulmonary embolism
Patient requiring mechanical circulatory support	Confirm correct cannula or device positioning
	Monitor for thrombus formation
	Assess cardiac function upon weaning of support

ARDS, acute respiratory distress syndrome; DVT, deep venous thrombosis; FAST, focused assessment with sonography for trauma; IVC, inferior vena cava; LVOT, left ventricular outflow tract; PEEP, positive end-expiratory pressure; VTI, velocity time integral.

outflow tract (LVOT). However, the maximum velocities that it can accurately measure is limited, beyond which PWD is susceptible to a form of sampling error called **aliasing. CWD**, on the other hand, is not limited by aliasing and can be used to measure very high flow velocities (such as those from a stenotic aortic valve). However, the trade-off is **range ambiguity**, that is, CWD cannot identify the precise location of the maximum velocity—it simply measures the maximum velocity anywhere in the path of the ultrasound beam. **Color Doppler** is a form of pulsed Doppler (and thus subject to aliasing) that measures flow at multiple sampling volumes on a two-dimensional (2D) grid rather than along a single line. One important caveat to the use of these techniques is that they are all **angle dependent**. In other words, they are accurate when the angle of the transducer beam is less than **20°** to the direction of blood flow. Consequently, Doppler measurements may underestimate true flows or provide inconsistent values on serial examination.

D. **M-mode** or motion mode is another useful ultrasonography tool that displays a view of all structures along a single vertical line over time. Because M-mode is confined to a single scan line, it provides the highest temporal resolution. This is useful for accurately measuring distances, such as the diameter of the inferior vena cava (IVC) or the size of a pericardial effusion, determining presence and absence of lung sliding, and for tracking the path of structures, such as valve opening (see Figures 3.1F and 3.2D).

E. Cardiac ultrasound, or echocardiography, can be performed by a **transthoracic echocardiographic (TTE)** or **transesophageal echocardiographic (TEE)** approach, depending on patient factors and the specific clinical question. TTE offers the advantages of being noninvasive, presenting no risk to the patient, and can be rapidly deployed. TTE imaging may be limited in situations such as increased patient body habitus, recent sternotomy, or the presence of dressings or drains. TEE overcomes many of these limitations related to image acquisition and can offer better image resolution, making it the preferred technique for detailed examination of valvular morphology such as for diagnosing endocarditis or assessing the position and function of implanted valves, for determining the presence of left atrial thrombus, for guiding placement of cannulas such as for extracorporeal membrane oxygenation (ECMO), and guiding resuscitation during cardiac arrest. However, TEE is invasive, often requires sedation, and, although rare, poses risk of damage to the oropharynx or esophagus during probe placement and manipulation. Because of its accessibility, faster deployment, and absent risk profile, TTE should be the initial approach for patients in the intensive care unit (ICU), whereas TEE is reserved for specific indications or in patients in whom TTE images proved inadequate by a skilled operator. The remainder of this chapter focuses on the use of TTE.

II. BASIC VERSUS ADVANCED CRITICAL CARE ECHOCARDIOGRAPHY

A. Basic Critical Care Echocardiography: Critical care echocardiography (CCE) is divided into basic and advanced levels. At the basic level, the intensivist performs a **"goal-directed" examination** that is designed to answer a specific binary question, such as the following:

1. Is there severe LV systolic dysfunction? (Based on gross inspection of LV contractility)
2. Is there marked right ventricular (RV) dilation? (Based on the comparison of LV to RV size)
3. Is there a severe valvular abnormality? (Based on color Doppler assessment)
4. Is there a significant pericardial effusion? (Based on the assessment of pericardial space, assessing for tamponade physiology)
5. Is the patient likely to be volume responsive? (Based on IVC size and variability)

Basic CCE can be performed rapidly and assists the intensivist in determining the cause of hemodynamic instability and guiding management in the acute setting. The scope of basic CCE has been defined by several governing bodies and is the focus of this chapter. A basic CCE exam comprises five standard 2D views that allow qualitative assessment as well as simple quantitative measures such as diameters of the IVC and pericardial effusions using M-mode. Although there are structured training programs, basic CCE competency does not require formal certification and proficiency can be achieved with brief (2- to 3-hour) didactics and hands-on training. Practitioners should have an awareness of their own limitations when it comes to performing echocardiography, and assistance from more experienced sonographers should be freely sought to resolve equivocal findings.

B. Standard Views for Basic Critical Care Echocardiography: A basic CCE exam consists of five standard 2D views that are obtained in each patient (see Figure 3.1). The views are obtained in the following order: (i) parasternal long-axis (PLAX), (ii) parasternal short-axis (PSAX) at the level of the mid-papillary muscle, (iii) apical four chamber (A4C), (iv) subcostal four chamber (SC4C), and (v) subcostal IVC. This sequence may be modified depending on the clinical situation—for example, in a patient receiving chest compressions, it is often most practical to begin with the subcostal four-chamber view to assess the adequacy of compressions and/or the presence of spontaneous cardiac activity while minimizing interruption of resuscitative efforts.

C. Advanced Critical Care Echocardiography: Advanced CCE allows the intensivist to perform a more comprehensive evaluation of a patient's underlying pathophysiology, in a capability similar to that of a formal exam performed by a cardiologist. This includes additional 2D views and more advanced quantitative measures such as PWD and CWD to characterize valvular lesions, estimate stroke volume and cardiac output, assess RV and LV filling pressures, and evaluate diastolic function. Further training is required to achieve proficiency in advanced CCE, with the option of receiving formal certification.

III. LUNG ULTRASOUND

A. For many years, the air-filled lungs were thought to be impossible to view in a meaningful way with ultrasound. However, by taking advantage of ultrasound artifacts produced by the air-filled lung interface with fluid and/or

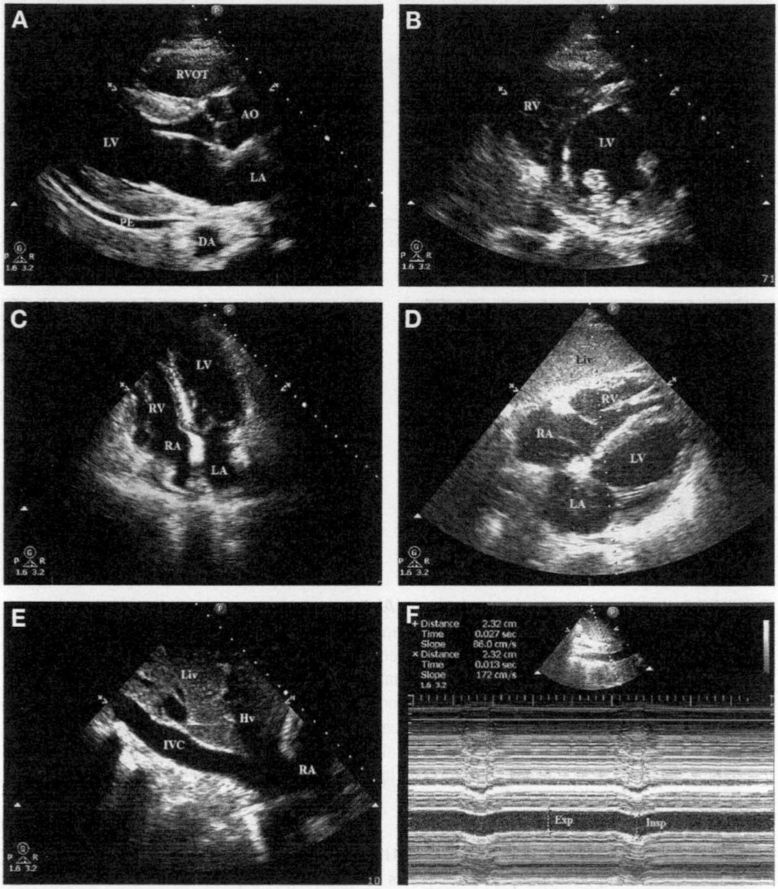

FIGURE 3.1 Transthoracic echocardiograms showing the basic views needed for a goal-directed echocardiographic examination in the intensive care unit (ICU). Salient anatomic features are noted on the figures. **(A)** Parasternal long-axis view in diastole (mitral valve wide open; aortic valve closed). Note the small posterior pericardial effusion (PE). **(B)** Parasternal short-axis view. **(C)** Apical four-chamber view. **(D)** Subcostal four-chamber view. **(E)** Visualization of the inferior vena cava (IVC). **(F)** M-mode interrogation of the IVC—no change in diameter between inspiration and expiration. AO, ascending aorta; DA, descending thoracic aorta; Exp, expiration; Hv, hepatic vein; Insp, inspiration; LA, left atrium; Liv, liver; LV, left ventricle; RA, right atrium; RV, right ventricle; RVOT, right ventricular outflow tract. (Images Courtesy of Aranya Bagchi, MBBS.)

surrounding tissue, useful information can be obtained. In fact, ultrasound has a higher sensitivity and specificity than do auscultation and plain film radiographs for the detection of pleural effusion, consolidation, and pneumothorax.

B. The Normal Lung Exam

1. The lung exam is best performed with either the linear or phased-array probe in 2D mode (see Figure 3.2). The operator should scan the chest in each of the four quadrants on both the left and right sides of a supine

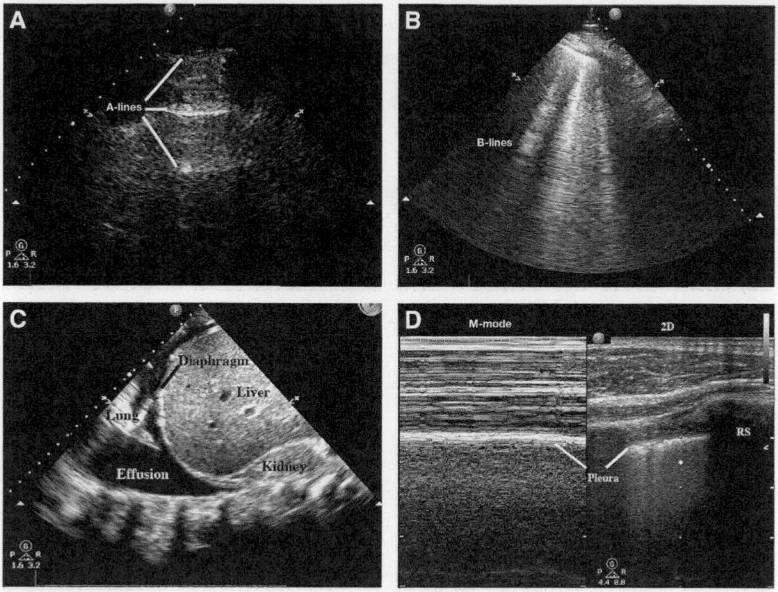

FIGURE 3.2 Ultrasound examination of the lung: **(A)** A-lines, which are consistent with normal aeration of the lung field under examination. **(B)** Multiple B-lines seen in this sector, suggesting excess interstitial fluid. Note that A-lines are not visible because they are effaced by B-lines. **(C)** An uncomplicated pleural effusion. It is important to use the anatomic landmarks (in this case, liver and diaphragm below and a portion of atelectatic lung above) to confirm that the fluid being visualized is pleural fluid and not ascites. **(D)** M-mode interrogation of the pleural surface to show the "seashore sign" that is caused by the movement of the parietal and visceral pleura over each other. The two-dimensional (2D) image being scanned by M-mode is shown to the right. RS, rib shadow. (Images Courtesy of Aranya Bagchi, MBBS.)

patient. The anterior border of the scanning area is defined by the parasternal line, the posterior border is defined by the posterior axillary line, and the midpoint of the scanning area is defined by the anterior axillary line. In the normal lung, the windows between each rib should reveal a hyperechoic pleural line sliding along the chest wall with each inspiration and expiration.

2. Placing the M-mode across the pleural line produces a characteristic "**seashore sign**" wherein a linear, laminar pattern appears in the tissue superficial to the hyperechoic pleural line and a granular, "sandy" pattern appears in the tissues deep to the pleural line (Figure 3.2D). This visualization of lung sliding is produced by the movement of the parietal pleura over the visceral pleura with inspiration and expiration. The "sandy" pattern vanishes in the absence of lung sliding, indicating the presence of a pneumothorax (see subsequent text).
3. **A-lines** are horizontal reverberation artifacts produced by the hyperechoic pleural line that repeat at regular intervals from the superficial to the deep portion of the ultrasound image. These are present in the normal lung because of the presence of the air-filled lung, although patients with severe asthma/emphysema may have a more pronounced A-line pattern (Figure 3.2A).

4. **B-lines** are vertical, discrete, laser-like reverberation artifacts that arise from the pleural line and extend to the bottom of the image without fading. B-lines move synchronously with the pleural line during inspiration and expiration. These indicate the presence of fluid in the lung, and a few B-lines (typically <3 per ultrasound field) are normal in the dependent portions of the healthy lung. However, multiple B-lines in a lung field represent increased interstitial fluid. Patients with cardiogenic and noncardiogenic pulmonary edema will have an extensive B-line profile over their anterior lungs (Figure 3.2B). B-lines efface normal A-lines.

IV. ULTRASOUND UTILITY IN CRITICAL CARE MEDICINE

A. **Assessing Undifferentiated Shock:** Acute hypotension can be caused by distributive shock such as due to sepsis, hypovolemic shock, cardiogenic shock due to LV or RV dysfunction or to severe valvular disease, or obstructive shock such as due to pericardial tamponade, pulmonary embolism, or tension pneumothorax. Each of these can be confirmed or excluded using basic CCE, allowing the clinician to then determine the most appropriate treatment. **Any finding should be confirmed in at least two orthogonal views** to reduce the risk of misinterpretation such as due to ultrasound artifact or misidentification of structures.

1. **Distributive shock:** The characteristic features of distributive shock are low vascular tone, due to impaired endothelial function, and high cardiac output. CCE will often reveal hyperdynamic LV function even in patients with underlying cardiac dysfunction, resulting from the low afterload state. Cardiac output can be assessed by placing the PWD across the LVOT and measuring the velocity time integral (VTI) or stroke distance. When measuring VTI, it is important to align the PWD cursor along the direction of blood flow to avoid underestimation. Stroke volume can be calculated by multiplying the stroke distance by the cross-sectional area of the LVOT, estimated from the diameter of the LVOT in the PLAX view. However, in point-of-care settings, we recommend using the stroke distance (ie, LVOT VTI) as a proxy for stroke volume because this excludes errors derived from the estimation of the LVOT cross-sectional area. An LVOT VTI 18 to 22 cm indicates normal cardiac output, and an LVOT VTI greater than 22 cm indicates a hyperdynamic cardiac output consistent with distributive/septic shock, whereas an LVOT VTI less than 18 cm is consistent with hypovolemic, obstructive, and cardiogenic shock. Patients in distributive shock are often volume responsive because of a decrease in stressed blood volume from vasodilation and CCE can be instrumental in guiding fluid resuscitation in these patients, as described here.
2. **Hypovolemic shock:** Assessment of intravascular volume status can be challenging in the patients who are critically ill. Hypovolemic shock is diagnosed depending on low cardiac output that improves with fluid administration. Although CCE can be extremely useful in detecting significant hypovolemia, it is important to use multiple methods to assess volume status because each method has drawbacks. Echocardiographic signs of hypovolemia include end-systolic ventricular effacement (also known as "kissing papillary muscles") in the PLAX and PSAX views, which can also be seen in patients with hyperdynamic cardiac function such as in vasodilatory and septic shock. An IVC that is less than 2 cm in diameter and that collapses by at least 50% with inspiration or with a quick "sniff" in patients who are not intubated and spontaneously breathing (IVC distensibility >18% in patients who are intubated) suggests volume responsiveness. IVC size and collapsibility can be easily quantified using the M-mode, with the cursor placed across the IVC approximately 3 cm before the right atrial

junction. IVC assessment for volume responsiveness may be of limited use in patients with RV failure, pulmonary hypertension, or severe tricuspid regurgitation. Volume responsiveness can be more reliably determined in patients who are both intubated and spontaneously breathing by assessing for an LVOT VTI increase of more than 12% with a fluid challenge or passive leg raise. Furthermore, respirophasic variation (>12%) in the stroke volume is also an indicator of hypovolemia or fluid responsiveness in a patient who is mechanically ventilated. Keep in mind that for adequate assessment, the patient must be in sinus rhythm and receiving tidal volumes of at least 8 mL/kg. Stroke volume variation can be estimated by the variation in the LVOT VTI.

In addition to these echocardiographic findings, the lung ultrasound exam (see **Section III.B**) can also be a useful adjunct because patients with less than 3 B-lines in bilateral lung windows are likely to tolerate additional volume, whereas those with three or more B-lines in bilateral lung windows are unable to tolerate additional volume (suggesting increased interstitial fluid; see Figure 3.2B). In a patient with hypovolemia with a recent history of trauma, hemorrhagic shock should be presumed and a **focused assessment with sonography for trauma** (FAST) exam should be performed to help identify the source of bleeding (see **Section V.A**). It is important to note that the FAST exam is unable to reliably evaluate for retroperitoneal hemorrhage.

3. **Cardiogenic shock:** The presence of cardiogenic shock can be suggested depending on certain physical exam findings such as cool extremities, jugular venous distension, and/or crackles, and can be confirmed using basic CCE. These patients will have low cardiac output (LVOT VTI <18 cm) and elevated cardiac filling pressures that can be assessed using diastology. Furthermore, more than 3 B-lines is generally seen bilaterally on lung ultrasound, which is consistent with cardiogenic pulmonary edema. CCE exam will demonstrate grossly abnormal LV and/or RV function, as discussed subsequently.
   a. **LV function** should be assessed in the PLAX, PSAX, A4C, and SC4C views. Is the left ventricle dilated or hypertrophied? What is the global function of the left ventricle (hyperdynamic, normal, mildly depressed, or severely depressed)? More experienced echocardiographers can perform more quantitative measures of LV systolic function, such as E-point septal separation and mitral annular plane systolic excursion (MAPSE), and diastolic function using PWD to measure mitral inflow velocities. The PSAX view is unique in that it allows the assessment of regional wall motion abnormalities (WMAs) in each of the major coronary arterial territories, which can be helpful in determining whether there is major cardiac dysfunction that is likely ischemic in origin. However, detecting more subtle WMAs requires expertise and is typically beyond the scope of a basic exam. Regional ballooning of the left ventricle may suggest Takotsubo or stress cardiomyopathy that is not due to obstructive coronary disease or plaque rupture. Severe valvular disease, such as acute regurgitation from a ruptured papillary muscle or aortic dissection, can also cause cardiogenic shock and acute respiratory failure, and can be identified using color Doppler across each of the valves. Furthermore, the identification of significant valvular disease may be beneficial for hemodynamic optimization.
   b. **RV function** should be assessed in the A4C, PSAX, and SC4C views. Dilatation of the right ventricle may be visible in the PLAX view but cannot be adequately assessed in this view. Basic assessment includes the size of the right ventricle on A4C or SC4C views. If the right ventricle is as large

or larger than the left ventricle in the basal diameter, it is considered dilated. The interventricular septum should be assessed in the PSAX view and will appear flattened (known as the "D sign") during diastole in the setting of RV volume overload or flattened during systole in the setting of RV pressure overload. Assessment of the right ventricle is especially important in patients with acute respiratory distress syndrome or in those receiving mechanical ventilation at high inspiratory pressures because these patients are at risk for acute RV failure. In a patient with a shifted RV septum, further administration of intravenous fluid is not likely to improve cardiac output and could be harmful to the patient. RV dysfunction is almost always accompanied by a dilated IVC with diminished respirophasic variation. More advanced measures of RV systolic function include the tricuspid annular plane systolic excursion (TAPSE) using M-mode, the S′ velocity of the tricuspid annulus on tissue Doppler imaging, and the RV strain by speckle-tracking echocardiography. RV systolic pressure can be estimated from the velocity of the tricuspid regurgitant jet and is useful in evaluating patients with pulmonary hypertension or increased RV afterload, as well as assessing the response to pulmonary vasodilators such as nitric oxide and epoprostenol.

4. **Obstructive shock:** Low cardiac output (LVOT VTI <18 cm) despite adequate intravascular volume and normal underlying cardiac contractile function is characteristic of obstructive shock. Obstructive shock can be due to pulmonary embolism, pericardial effusion causing tamponade, tension pneumothorax, or outflow obstruction such as due to an intracardiac mass or thrombus. CCE can be used to confirm or exclude each of these diagnoses. A patient with a large pulmonary embolism will show signs of RV failure, including RV dilation and a large, noncollapsible IVC. The intraventricular septum will appear flattened ("D") during systole or diastole in the PSAX view, consistent with RV pressure or volume overload, respectively. **McConnell sign** is the presence of an akinetic or bulging mid-RV free wall and is a distinct finding in patients with acute pulmonary embolism. **Pericardial effusions** are typically diagnosed depending on hypoechoic fluid surrounding the heart and can be circumferential or localized. After cardiac surgery, tamponade may present with an isoechoic effusion secondary to clotting blood rather than the usual hypoechoic effusion. CCE showing pericardial effusion in a patient who is hypotensive should prompt a careful evaluation for echocardiographic signs of tamponade. The best views to assess tamponade are the A4C and SC4C views. Right atrial collapse during ventricular systole and RV diastolic collapse are fairly sensitive and specific for tamponade, respectively. Limited IVC collapsibility (<50% with inspiration or sniff) is also a sensitive marker of tamponade. There is normally a small degree of respirophasic variation of flow across both the tricuspid and mitral valves that becomes exaggerated in the presence of pericardial effusions due to impaired diastolic filling. These filling patterns can be assessed by measuring PWD across either the tricuspid or mitral valves and, in the presence of tamponade, should reveal increased right-sided filling velocities during inspiration and increased left-sided filling velocities during expiration. Initiation of positive pressure ventilation in a patient with suspected pericardial tamponade should be performed cautiously because decreased preload to the right ventricle from positive pressure ventilation may precipitate cardiovascular collapse. **Tension pneumothorax** should be assumed in patients with a large, noncollapsible IVC and the absence of lung sliding and a lung point sign on one side. Lastly, an intracardiac thrombus or mass can also cause obstructive shock and should be evident in multiple views before a diagnosis is made. Administration of contrast or

agitated saline may help distinguish thrombus or mass from the cardiac muscle itself. **Systolic anterior motion of the mitral** valve in patients with hypertrophic cardiomyopathy can cause significant LVOT obstruction that can be relieved by decreasing contractility, optimizing preload, increasing afterload, and decreasing heart rate.

B. Assessing Undifferentiated Respiratory Distress: Lung ultrasonography can be instrumental for investigating the cause of hypoxemia or dyspnea and to optimize mechanical ventilation in the patients who are critically ill. Given here are some specific applications for lung ultrasound encountered in the ICU setting.

1. **Pneumothorax:** When the space between the parietal pleura and the visceral pleura becomes air-filled, normal pleural sliding is absent on ultrasound exam. Loss of lung sliding can be a sign of pleural pathology and pneumothorax. Loss of lung sliding is also seen in lung collapse and in patients who have undergone pleurodesis. When visualized with M-mode, the "**stratosphere sign**" or "**barcode sign**" appears, wherein horizontal, laminar artifact appears throughout the image—much like the thin, linear clouds in the stratosphere or the thin lines on a barcode. Imaging of a **lung point** in pneumothorax can help define the physical limit of air in the space between the parietal and visceral pleura. Lung point refers to the physical point where the absence of lung sliding transitions into an area of regular, consistent lung sliding. The identification of a lung point using lung ultrasound confirms the diagnosis of a pneumothorax.
2. **Pleural effusion:** Pleural effusions are typically best seen with the phased-array probe and appear as hypoechoic spaces between the chest wall and the consolidated lung tissue beneath. Often, the lung tissue itself appears as a hyperechoic tail of tissue floating in the effusion (Figure 3.2C). It is important to delineate the boundaries of the effusion (the diaphragm below, visible lung tissue, and the chest wall) to avoid misidentification of ascitic fluid or pericardial fluid as a pleural effusion.
3. **Interstitial syndrome:** Alveolar-interstitial syndrome refers to the presence of alveolar or interstitial pathology in which there is an obliteration of the normal air-filled alveolar architecture due to fluid extravasation. It is defined by the presence of multiple B-lines on lung ultrasound and may be seen in a variety of lung pathologies including acute respiratory distress syndrome, pneumonia, cardiogenic pulmonary edema, and pneumonitis. Studies have shown that the number of B-lines within an ultrasound image correlates with the amount of extravascular fluid present in the lung. In severe lung pathology, B-lines can be so numerous that they create a confluent hyperechoic artifact that moves with respiration. The absence of B-lines in any lung field can essentially rule out alveolar-interstitial syndrome as a cause of acute hypoxemia, and instead suggests the presence of another entity such as pulmonary embolism, intracardiac shunting, or mainstem intubation.
4. **Ventilation optimization:** Lung and cardiac ultrasound can be utilized to optimize ventilation strategies in patients who are critically ill. A patient who is intubated with B-lines in multiple lung fields would likely benefit from increased positive end-expiratory pressure (PEEP) in addition to further diuresis. In a patient who fails to wean from mechanical ventilation, it may be useful to perform an echocardiographic assessment of diastology to evaluate for elevated left atrial pressures which may contribute to a patient's failure to wean from the ventilator. Patients with elevated left atrial pressure may require further diuresis and optimization of their volume status to facilitate successful liberation from the ventilator.

V. OTHER APPLICATIONS OF POINT-OF-CARE ULTRASOUND IN THE INTENSIVE CARE UNIT

A. Focused Assessment With Sonography for Trauma Exam: The FAST exam allows for rapid diagnosis of fluid (hemorrhage) in the intraperitoneal, retroperitoneal, and pericardial spaces. This exam can be completed using the curvilinear or phased-array probe. The goal of the FAST exam is to rapidly identify significant bleeding, which may suggest the need for emergent intervention (laparotomy or angioembolization). The FAST exam looks for free fluid in four areas: the perihepatic and hepatorenal space, the pelvis, the perisplenic space, and the pericardial space. The hepatorenal space is the most posterior portion of the upper abdominal cavity in a supine patient. The probe should be placed in the right posterior axillary line at the level of the 11th to 12th ribs. A perisplenic scan is accomplished by placing the probe in the left upper quadrant at the left posterior axillary line between the 10th and 11th ribs (Figure 3.3). The pelvis is scanned by placing the probe midline and superior to the pubic symphysis. Finally, the pericardial space is evaluated by placing the probe inferior to the xiphoid process and angling it upward and to the left toward the heart.

B. Detection of Deep Venous Thrombosis: Venous thrombosis and pulmonary embolism are common in ICUs and contribute substantially to patient morbidity. Studies have shown that intensivist-performed compression ultrasound is sensitive and specific in the diagnosis of proximal lower extremity deep venous thrombosis (DVT) compared with a formal vascular ultrasound (that included compression, color augmentation, and spectral Doppler ultrasound). In addition, CCUS results in significant time savings (diagnoses were made >12 hours earlier when using bedside ultrasound compared with formal ultrasound). Compression ultrasound involves scanning the lower extremity veins (common femoral, superficial femoral, and popliteal veins) and compressing them enough to cause venous collapse. Lack of compressibility in any of these major veins suggests the presence of a DVT.

C. Intracranial Pressure Measurement: Measurement of optic nerve sheath diameter by CCUS has been shown to correlate with radiologic signs and symptoms of increased intracranial pressure (ICP). An optic nerve sheath diameter of more than 5 mm correlates with an ICP greater than 20 mm Hg. Measurement of optic nerve sheath diameter should be performed with sterile ultrasound transmission gel and a sterile ultrasound probe sheath. Using the linear 5- to 10-MHz probe, the eye should be imaged through closed eyelids. Optic nerve sheath diameter measurements should be taken 3 mm behind the globe where ultrasound contrast is the greatest and measurements are therefore more reproducible. Note that this exam should not be performed in the presence of ocular injury.

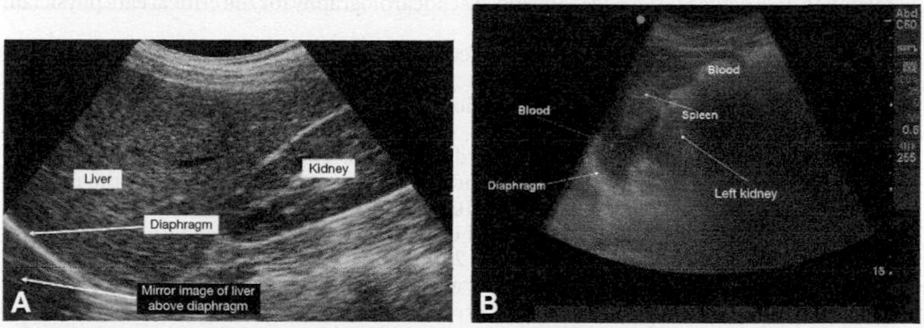

FIGURE 3.3 Selected images from a focused assessment with sonography for trauma (FAST) exam. **(A)** Normal ultrasound view of the Morrison pouch. A mirror-image artifact of the liver is present above the hyperechoic diaphragm. **(B)** FAST exam of perisplenic space showing hemoperitoneum.

D. Airway Ultrasound: Occasionally, auscultation and end-tidal carbon dioxide fail to provide adequate proof that an endotracheal tube is in correct position. This is especially true in situations of hemodynamic collapse when end-tidal carbon dioxide may be absent because of circulatory failure. CCUS can provide visualization of the endotracheal tube and/or cuff, providing confirmation of tube positioning. This exam is best performed using the linear probe and scanning from above the thyroid cartilage and down to the sternal notch. The frontal and lateral walls of the trachea should be visible as well as portions of the endotracheal tube provided it is in the correct location. Lung ultrasound showing the presence of bilateral lung sliding can provide further confirmation of correct endotracheal tube positioning, whereas unilateral lung sliding may raise concern for mainstem intubation.

E. Procedural Guidance: The use of ultrasound has become routine for the placement of central venous and arterial catheters, thoracentesis, paracentesis, and other bedside procedures in the ICU. There is now an abundance of data supporting the claim that many of these procedures can be performed faster and more safely under ultrasound guidance. Detailed description on the use of ultrasound for these various procedures is beyond the scope of this chapter.

Acknowledgments

We gratefully acknowledge previous edition authors Drs. Kenneth Shelton and Kate Riddell because portions of their chapter were retained in this revision.

Selected Readings

Austin DR, Chang MG, Bittner EA. Use of handheld point-of-care ultrasound in emergency airway management. *Chest.* 2021;159:1155-1165.

Brown SM, Sekiguchi H, Pinsky MR. A new era in critical care ultrasound: professionalization. *Ann Am Thorac Soc.* 2017;14:1747-1749.

Cheung AT, Savino JS, Weiss SJ, et al. Echocardiography and hemodynamic indexes of left ventricular preload in patients with normal and abnormal ventricular function. *Anesthesiology.* 1994;81:376-387.

Kimberly HH, Shah H, Marill K, et al. Correlation of optic nerve sheath diameter with direct measurement of intracranial pressure. *Acad Emerg Med.* 2008;15:201-204.

Koenig SJ, Narasimhan M, Mayo PH. Thoracic ultrasonography for the pulmonary specialist. *Chest.* 2011;140:1332-1341.

Kory PD, Pellecchia CM, Shiloh AL, et al. Accuracy of ultrasonography performed by critical care physicians for the diagnosis of DVT. *Chest.* 2011;139:538-542.

Lichtenstein DA. Ultrasound in the management of thoracic disease. *Crit Care Med.* 2007;35:S250-S261.

Narasimhan M, Koenig SJ, Mayo PH. Advanced echocardiography for the critical care physician: part 1. *Chest.* 2014;145:129-134.

Narasimhan M, Koenig SJ, Mayo PH. Advanced echocardiography for the critical care physician: part 2. *Chest.* 2014;145:135-142.

Raphael DT, Conrad FU. Ultrasound confirmation of endotracheal tube placement. *J Clin Ultrasound.* 1987;15:459-462.

Salen PN, Melanson SW, Heller MB. The focused abdominal sonography for trauma (FAST) examination: considerations and recommendations for training physicians in the use of a new clinical tool. *Acad Emerg Med.* 2000;7:162-168.

Via G, Hussein A, Wells M, et al. International evidence-based recommendations for focused cardiac ultrasound. *J Am Soc Echocardiogr.* 2014;27:683.e1-683.e33.

Vieillard-Baron A, Millington SJ, Sanfilippo F, et al. A decade of progress in critical care echocardiography: a narrative review. *Intensive Care Med.* 2019;45:770-788.

Volpicelli G, Elbarbary M, Blaivas M, et al. International evidence-based recommendations for point-of-care lung ultrasound. *Intensive Care Med.* 2012;38:577-591.

Werner SL, Smith CE, Goldstein JR, et al. Pilot study to evaluate the accuracy of ultrasonography in confirming endotracheal tube placement. *Ann Emerg Med.* 2007;49:75-80.

4 Airway Management

Takashi Sakano and Edward A. Bittner

See Video 4.1 on **Patient Positioning** and Video 4.2 on **Direct Laryngoscopy**

I. INTRODUCTION

Endotracheal intubation is indicated in the setting of acute respiratory failure (hypoxemic or hypercarbic) when noninvasive positive pressure ventilation (NIPPV) or high-flow nasal cannula (HFNC) has failed or is contraindicated or there is obtundation (Glasgow Coma Scale [GCS] score <8), airway obstruction, or anticipation of compromised airway patency due to trauma, edema, or other etiologies. This chapter reviews airway evaluation, advanced airway placement/maintenance, and evaluation for withdrawal of advanced airway support.

II. INDICATIONS FOR ADVANCED AIRWAY

Intact respiratory function requires a central drive to breathe, appropriate respiratory neuromuscular function, a patent upper airway, the ability to protect the airway from aspiration, and effective ventilation and perfusion matching. Placement of an endotracheal tube (ETT) allows ventilation of a patient who lacks a respiratory drive, can support the work of breathing in a patient who is weak, provides an opening through an upper airway that may be prone to collapse, mitigates large-volume aspiration, and, using positive pressure, reexpands atelectatic lung regions that contribute to ventilation/perfusion mismatch.

III. ASSESSMENT OF THE NEED FOR AN ADVANCED AIRWAY

A. Cardiopulmonary Resuscitation: Per advanced cardiac life support (ACLS) guidelines, bag-valve mask ventilation with 100% inspired oxygen is required. If bag-valve mask ventilation is inadequate, an advanced airway (ETT, supraglottic airway [SGA]) should be placed without interruption of chest compressions.

B. Decreased Level of Consciousness: Intubation may be required because of airway obstruction, decreased respiratory drive, and risk of aspiration. Although GCS less than 8 is classically taught as an indication for intubation, significant risk of aspiration exists with GCS scores greater than 8, and thus the presence of gastroesophageal reflux disease (GERD), esophageal sphincter dysfunction, and full stomach may justify intubation in a patient who is stuporous.

C. Pulse Oximetry: Continuous monitoring aids in the assessment of patients with hypoxia. Although more quantifiable and reliable than the appearance of cyanosis, there is no number that absolutely warrants intubation. Oxygen saturations below 88% usually require evaluation and may require intervention.

D. Respiratory Patterns

1. **Respiratory rate (RR)/Tidal volume (TV)**
   a. **↓RR/↑TV:** central cause (central nervous system [CNS] disorder, opiate effect)
   b. **↑RR/↑TV:** increased work of breathing to overcome changes in lung compliance (pulmonary edema, pneumothorax, alveolar consolidation, acute respiratory distress syndrome [ARDS]) or need for greater levels of ventilation (CO_2 production, sepsis, increased dead space)
   c. **↑RR/⇔TV:** other etiologies such as pain, bladder distension, and anxiety

2. **Symmetry:** The chest and abdomen should expand together with inspiration. Discordant movement may be seen during active exhalation, airway obstruction, and cervical spine paralysis with preserved diaphragm function. Pneumothorax, hemothorax, flail chest, splinting, and large bronchial obstructions can cause right/left asymmetry.
3. **Accessory muscle use:** Sternocleidomastoid and scalene muscle utilization suggests increased work of breathing and respiratory muscle fatigue/weakness. Firing of the external oblique muscles can signal active exhalation, a sensitive but not specific sign of respiratory distress.
4. **Inspiratory/expiratory timing**
   a. **Long inspiratory time:** upper airway or extrathoracic obstruction
   b. **Long expiratory time:** intrathoracic obstruction and/or bronchospasm
   c. **Inspiratory/expiratory pauses:** Sustained apnea necessitates intubation but periodic breathing does not usually require intubation, although the cause should be investigated.
5. **Auscultation/tactile exam**
   a. **Upper airway obstruction:** Stridor, absent breath sounds, and lack of air movement from mouth/nose suggest upper airway obstruction (jaw thrust, chin lift, nasal airway may alleviate).
   b. **Other:** Wheezing, rales, and absent breath sounds may indicate bronchospasm, pulmonary edema/consolidation, or pneumothorax, respectively.

E. Ventilation/Oxygenation Data

1. **Arterial blood gas (ABG):** Oxygen and carbon dioxide tensions and pH should be used to assess severity of disease and the success/failure of clinical interventions. It should not substitute for clinical judgment or delay critical interventions but remains the most reliable test for oxygenation and ventilation.
2. **Co-oximetry:** Evaluation of arterial blood, or via noninvasive multiwavelength oximeters, can assay methemoglobinemia, carboxyhemoglobinemia, and desaturated blood.
3. **Failed NIPPV:** Bilevel positive airway pressure (BiPAP) ventilation and continuous positive airway pressure (CPAP) ventilation can help avoid endotracheal intubation in patients with respiratory failure secondary to chronic obstructive pulmonary disease (COPD) and acute cardiogenic pulmonary edema. Lack of improvement justifies endotracheal intubation.

IV. PREPARATION FOR PLACEMENT OF AN ADVANCED AIRWAY

A. Physical Exam/Patient History: A brief airway exam and history are necessary to minimize the chance of failing to ventilate/intubate, to predict the need for advanced intubation techniques, and to be aware of potential complications.

1. **Airway anatomy:** Less than three fingerbreadths thyromental distance, small mouth opening, large incisors, limited ability to protrude the mandible, a large tongue, elevated Mallampati score, short neck, and limited cervical mobility may all contribute to difficult visualization of the glottis with laryngoscopy and should be checked.
2. **Potential difficulty with mask ventilation:** Facial hair, edentulousness, obesity, male gender, history of sleep apnea, and neck irradiation portend difficult mask ventilation.
3. **Data on prior intubation attempts:** If time permits, review old records for difficulty with prior intubation attempts and successful rescue techniques.
4. **Allergies:** Review for contraindications to the use of standard induction and maintenance drugs.
5. **Coagulation status:** Time permitting, a review of platelet count, prothrombin time/partial thromboplastin time (PT/PTT), and current anticoagulation therapy is worthwhile because profound anticoagulation may prohibit

nasal airway manipulation given the risk of bleeding. The provider should be aware of the potential for bleeding with multiple intubation attempts.

6. **Neuromuscular status**
   a. Patients with burns, crush injuries, prolonged immobility (>5 days), extensive upper motor neuron injury (such as debilitating stroke), denervation injuries, and myopathies are at risk for hyperkalemic arrest with the use of succinylcholine. Rocuronium is a viable alternative for intubation.
   b. Cervical spine instability may require flexible fiberoptic or video laryngoscopic (eg, GlideScope [Verathon]) intubation to minimize cervical manipulation.
   c. Increased intracranial pressure (ICP), presence of intracranial aneurysms, intracranial hemorrhage, and symptoms of cerebral ischemia/infarct should be noted and may affect choice of induction medications.
7. **Cardiovascular history:** Angina/ischemia, arrhythmias, valvular disease, left or right ventricular dysfunction, pulmonary or systemic hypertension, and aneurysms should be noted given the risk of cardiovascular collapse with common induction agents.
8. **Aspiration risk:** Recent gastric feeding, GERD, hemoptysis, emesis, bowel obstruction, obesity, pregnancy, and depressed mental status increase aspiration risk and may require rapid sequence intubation (RSI).
9. **Hemodynamic stability:** Note vasopressor requirements, work of breathing, blood pressure, heart rate, and oxygen saturation. Instability may require judicious use of induction agents.

B. **Choice of Advanced Airway Placement Technique:** Options include direct laryngoscopy, video-assisted laryngoscopy, nasotracheal intubation, flexible fiberoptic intubation (FOI; nasal/oral), and/or SGA placement.

1. **Direct laryngoscopy:** performed with a laryngoscope and direct visualization of the glottis
   a. **Advantages:** can be performed quickly with minimal equipment
   b. **Disadvantages:** uncomfortable for patients who are awake and difficult with unfavorable airway anatomy or cervical spine instability requiring cervical spine fixation
2. **Video-assisted laryngoscopy:** Modified laryngoscopy blades with an anteriorly angled camera at the blade tip are commonly used in the setting of predicted or encountered difficult direct laryngoscopy because of anterior/superior larynx, small mouth opening, obesity/redundant laryngeal soft tissue, or limited cervical mobility. Available devices include the C-Mac (Karl Storz) and the GlideScope.
   a. **Advantages:** similar intubation mechanics to direct laryngoscopy with the advantage of an improved view of an anterior/superior glottis because of an angled blade-tip camera
   b. **Disadvantages:** not always available in critical care units, cost, fragility, need for power source, limited portability, and impaired visualization in the presence of blood or secretions
3. **Nasotracheal intubation:** performed when the oral opening is insufficient for direct glottis visualization, in neck instability, and when access to a non-instrumented oral cavity is desired while maintaining an advanced airway
   a. **Advantages:** more easily tolerated by patients who are minimally sedated when compared with orotracheal intubation. It can be performed on patients with an unfavorable airway anatomy, in the sitting position to improve spontaneous respiratory mechanics/minimize aspiration, and without general anesthesia or paralytic agents.
   b. **Disadvantages:** Technically challenging and spontaneous respiration must be present to guide blind placement via breath sounds for blind intubation. Placement under direct visualization with Magill forceps

negates many advantages over orotracheal intubation. Contraindications include coagulopathy or planned anticoagulation/thrombolysis, nasal polyps, basilar skull fracture, and immunocompromise given the increased risk of sinusitis. ETT diameter may be limited given the nasal passage size.

4. **Flexible FOI:** Insertion of an ETT over a flexible fiberscope with glottis visualization can be performed via the oral or nasal cavity.
   a. **Advantages:** can intubate patients with unfavorable airway anatomy with minimal cervical manipulation. Fiberoptic visualization of the ETT tip upon airway exit can confirm accurate placement depth.
   b. **Disadvantages:** Technically difficult, equipment intensive, and visualization may be difficult with bleeding/excess secretions/distorted anatomy given the decreased ability to suction or manipulate the airway.
5. **Supraglottic airway:** SGAs are the category of airway rescue devices that are inserted into the pharynx for unobstructed ventilation. The laryngeal mask airway (LMA) is a commonly used SGA. As part of the American Society of Anesthesiologists' (ASA) difficult airway algorithm, an SGA may be used as an emergency airway, especially as a bridge to endotracheal intubation. Some SGAs allow intubation through their lumens.
   a. **Advantages:** rapid/easy placement in a majority of patients
   b. **Disadvantages:** not a long-term airway management strategy, decreased protection against aspiration, not tolerated by patients who are minimally sedated, and risk of gastric insufflation with positive pressure ventilation if not placed appropriately. SGA devices are ineffective for patients with upper airway edema.

C. **Monitors/Equipment:** Essential monitors during acute airway management include pulse oximetry, blood pressure, electrocardiography (ECG), and capnography (colorimetric or continuous). All equipment must be ready for immediate use (a handy mnemonic is iSOAP).

1. ***I*ntravenous (IV) access:** Adequate IV access should be available before intubation except in emergent cases such as cardiac arrest, which may necessitate intubation before IV access is obtained.
2. ***S*uction:** A functioning Yankauer or tonsil-tip suction device must be available.
3. ***O*xygen:** An in-wall or tank oxygen (full) source and functioning bag-valve mask must be available for proper oxygenation.
4. ***A*irway:** A laryngoscope (eg, Miller 2 or Macintosh 3 for adults, Miller 1 or Macintosh 2 for pediatrics), correctly sized ETT(s) (eg, 8.0 for men and 7.5 for women, see subsequent text for pediatrics) with stylet inserted and intact cuff must be available.
   a. **Pediatric ETT:** Recent literature supports the use of cuffed ETTs when ETT diameter is greater than 3.5 mm and the practice of inflating the cuff until a leak is present at 20 cm H_2O. If no cuff leak exists at 20 cm H_2O, downsize the ETT diameter by 0.5 mm and repeat leak test (Table 4.1).
5. ***P*harmacology:** An induction agent, a muscle relaxant, maintenance agent, vasopressor, vagolytic, and an antihypertensive agent should be immediately available.
6. See Table 4.2.

V. INTUBATION TECHNIQUES

Successful intubation requires optimal patient positioning, adequate preoxygenation (if possible), and proper intubation technique.

A. **Patient Positioning:** Time to optimize position for intubation is well spent and should not be overlooked (▶ Video 4.1: **Patient Positioning**).

TABLE 4.1 Endotracheal Tube Sizes

Age	Size (ID, mm)—Uncuffed	Size (ID, mm)—Cuffed
Preterm	2.5	
1000 g		
1000-2500 g		
Neonate to 6 mo	3.0	
6 mo to 1 yr	3.0-3.5 3	0-3.5
1-2 yr	3.5-4.0	3.0-4.0
>2 yr	4.0-5.0	3.5-4.5
	(Age in yr + 16)/4	(Age in yr/4) + 3

TABLE 4.2 Contents of Emergency Airway Kit

Airway Equipment	Pharmacologic Agents
ETT with stylet (6.0, 7.0, 7.5 mm ID)	Propofol
Laryngoscope handles (2—long, short)	Etomidate
Laryngoscope blades (C-Mac 3, Miller 2)	Ketamine
NPA	Midazolam
OPA (No. 3, No. 5)	Fentanyl
Bougie	Hydromorphone
LMA (No. 4)	Rocuronium
Syringes (3, 5, 10, 30 mL)	Succinylcholine
Tape	Phenylephrine
End-tidal CO_2 detector	Ephedrine
IV catheters (14-20 gauge)	Glycopyrrolate
Surgical lubricant	Esmolol
Portable videolaryngoscope	
Scalpel	

ETT, endotracheal tube; ID, internal diameter; IV, intravenous; LMA, laryngeal mask airway; NPA, nasopharyngeal airway; OPA, oropharyngeal airway.

1. **Bed position in room:** Move the head of the bed away from any walls, remove headboard, and bring the patient's head to the edge of the bed. If the headboard cannot be removed, place the patient diagonally on the bed for improved airway access.
2. **Bed height:** Elevate the bed so that the patient's pharynx is between the operator's umbilicus and xiphoid process. The semi-Fowler position (the head and trunk raised to between 15 and 45 degrees) or slight reverse Trendelenburg position may be beneficial to maximize oxygenation and minimize aspiration risk.
3. **Align pharyngeal, laryngeal, and oral axes:** In the supine position, the laryngeal, pharyngeal, and oral axes are not parallel (Figure 4.1A), inhibiting glottis visualization. Creating the "sniffing position" with neck flexion via blankets under the occiput (Figure 4.1B) and head extension on the atlantoaxial joint (Figure 4.1C) will align the three axes. Figure 4.1C illustrates the ideal position where the laryngeal, pharyngeal, and oral axes are nearly parallel.
4. **Patients undergoing trauma:** All such patients who have not received definitive cervical spine clearance via National Emergency X-Radiography Utilization Study (NEXUS) criteria or Canadian C-spine rules, computed tomography

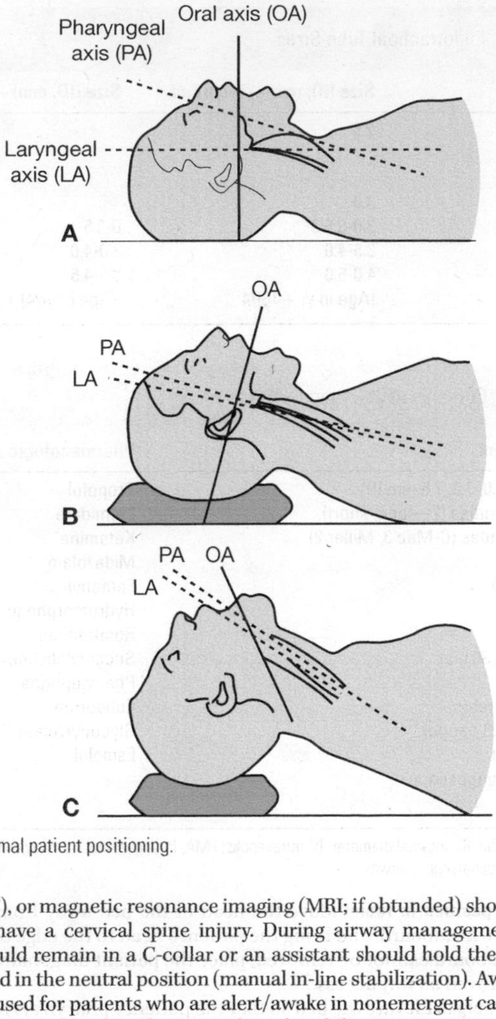

FIGURE 4.1 Optimal patient positioning.

(CT), or magnetic resonance imaging (MRI; if obtunded) should be assumed to have a cervical spine injury. During airway management, the patient should remain in a C-collar or an assistant should hold the patient's neck/head in the neutral position (manual in-line stabilization). Awake FOI should be used for patients who are alert/awake in nonemergent cases, whereas direct orotracheal intubation with neck stabilization is appropriate in all other cases. Note that bag-mask ventilation may result in cervical manipulation.

B. Preoxygenation: Replacement of functional residual capacity (FRC) nitrogen with oxygen is critical before intubation to maximize the reservoir of oxygen and delay the time until critical desaturation. This is especially relevant with patients who are obese and they should be preoxygenated to an end-tidal oxygen level greater than 85%.

1. **Patient who is awake/alert:** Tightly seal the bag-valve mask over the nose and mouth, provide 100% oxygen at high flows greater than 10 L/min, encourage TV breathing for 3 minutes, or vital capacity breathing if time limited, and use gentle chin-lift/jaw thrust maneuvers as needed to ensure airway patency. Postinduction, maintain airway seal and patency during the time between induction and intubation because apneic oxygenation can maintain oxygenation.

2. **Patient who is obtunded:** Without adequate respiratory effort, 8 to 10 breaths/min of positive pressure ventilation/support with a bag-valve mask at 100% oxygen is required for preoxygenation. Airway adjuncts to ensure airway patency such as an oropharyngeal airway (OPA) or a nasopharyngeal airway (NPA) may be required if bag-valve mask ventilation with head positioning and chin-lift/jaw thrust maneuvers is ineffective.
   a. **Oropharyngeal airway (OPA):** provided in three adult sizes (sizes 3, 4, 5—80, 90, 100 mm, respectively), which is the distance from the tip to flange. Proper size can be estimated by measuring the distance from earlobe to the ipsilateral corner of the lip. The distal tip is inserted facing upward against the hard palate and then rotated 180 degrees to advance into the posterior pharynx. An OPA that is too short may cause obstruction by pressing the tongue into the posterior pharynx, whereas an OPA that is too long may push the epiglottis against the glottis opening. An OPA may cause laryngospasm or emesis in a patient who is conscious or semiconscious.
   b. **Nasopharyngeal airway (NPA):** optimal for use in patients with obstructions who have intact oropharyngeal reflexes or minimal mouth opening when bag-valve mask ventilation is inadequate. NPAs are sized for adults by internal diameter (6-9 mm), should be inserted into the naris parallel to the hard palate after lubrication, and advanced until the flange rests on the outer naris. Use the largest diameter that will fit into the naris with minimal resistance. Bleeding tendency is a relative contraindication to NPA placement, whereas basilar skull fractures are a more absolute contraindication to NPA placement. NPAs are less likely to induce vomiting and are better tolerated than are OPAs in those who are awake/minimally obtunded.
   c. Preoxygenation is less effective in patients that are critically ill because of the presence of intrapulmonary shunts, decreased FRC, and increased oxygen consumption. Use of noninvasive ventilation or HFNCs may be beneficial for reducing the prevalence and magnitude of desaturation.

C. **Orotracheal Intubation:** Direct laryngoscopy, video-assisted laryngoscopy, and flexible FOI are common methods for oral ETT placement.

1. **The laryngoscope:** Direct visualization of the glottis can be achieved using a laryngoscope with either a Macintosh or Miller blade. Some laryngoscopes have the light emitted from a bulb on the blade; some fiberoptic systems have the light source in the handle, with the light carried to the blade tip. Nonfiberoptic handles and blades are not compatible with fiberoptic handles and blades. It is critical to ensure the system works before use (Figure 4.2).
   a. **Laryngoscope handle:** provides a place to apply a firm grip with the left hand
   b. **Macintosh blade:** a curved blade that is inserted into the vallecula (the space between the base of the tongue and the pharyngeal surface of the epiglottis). Upward pressure against the hyoepiglottic ligament elevates the epiglottis, exposing the glottis. Sizes range from No. 0 to No. 4, with No. 3 as the most commonly used blade in adults. Its deep flange provides more room for ETT passage when compared with a Miller blade (▶ Video 4.2: **Direct Laryngoscopy**).
   c. **Miller blade:** A straight blade whose tip is inserted underneath the laryngeal surface of the epiglottis and lifted to expose the glottis. The smaller flange provides less space for ETT placement. Sizes range from No. 0 to No. 3, with No. 2 being the most common size for adults.
2. **Endotracheal tube:** Choose an appropriate-size ETT (eg, 7.5 for women, 8.0 for men) and insert a malleable stylet, making sure that the tip of the stylet does not extend past the tip of the ETT. Bending the tube/stylet 40 to 80 degrees anteriorly 2 to 3 inches from the tip of the ETT ("hockey stick") may

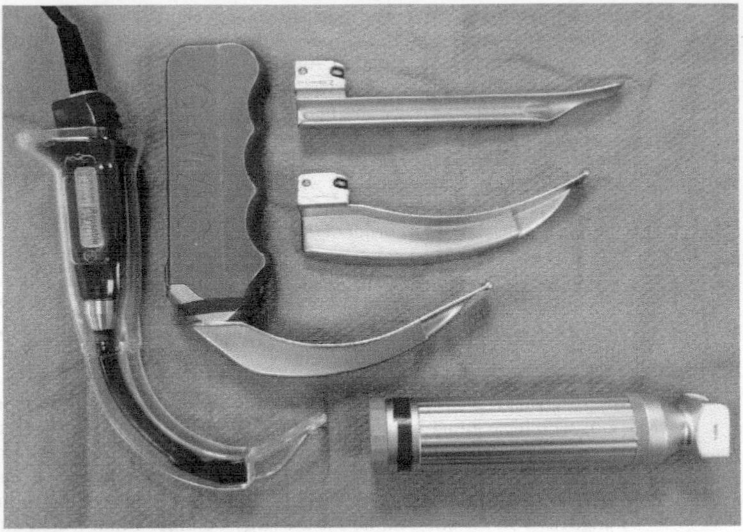

FIGURE 4.2 *Laryngoscopes (clockwise from bottom left: GlideScope, C-Mac, Miller 2, Macintosh 3, laryngoscope handle.)*

aid in the passage of the ETT along the posterior surface of the epiglottis if glottis visualization is suboptimal. Deflate the cuff before insertion.

3. **Direct laryngoscopy:** With the patient in optimal "sniffing" position and anesthetized, take the laryngoscope in your left hand near the meeting of the handle and blade and use your right hand to open the mouth via a scissoring maneuver during which you place your right thumb on the patient's right lower premolars and your right index finger on the right upper premolars, and press your thumb and index finger in opposing directions. With the mouth open, insert the laryngoscope blade in the right side of the mouth, and if using a Macintosh blade, use the curve of the blade to follow the tongue to its base while simultaneously using the flange to sweep the tongue to the left. Once the epiglottis is visualized, place the tip of the blade anteriorly into the vallecula. If using a Miller blade, advance the tip of the blade to the base of the epiglottis along its laryngeal surface; note that the tongue sweep will be much more difficult. Using either blade, following correct tip placement, lift the handle along its long axis to elevate the epiglottis for direct glottis visualization. Take care not to lever the laryngoscope handle with the maxilla as a fulcrum because damage to the maxillary incisors may result.
   a. If the glottis cannot be visualized, attempt the following:
      1. Suction or manually extract any obstructing material.
      2. Utilize external laryngeal manipulation to move the larynx posteriorly or laterally into the field of view.
      3. Improve positioning with neck flexion and head extension.
      4. Change to a straight blade if the epiglottis is obstructing the view.
   b. If the glottis remains obscured, remove the laryngoscope, resume bag-valve mask ventilation, and consider other approaches to securing the airway.
4. **ETT insertion:** While maintaining direct visualization of the glottis, hold the ETT in your right hand like a pencil and insert it into the right side of the

mouth through the vocal cords. Following visualization of the cuff passing fully through the glottis, stop advancement, remove the stylet, and inflate the cuff with a volume of air that allows for no air leak with 20 cm H_2O of positive pressure ventilation. Tube depth should be measured at the upper incisors, with an approximate proper depth of 21 cm for women and 23 cm for men.

5. **Video-assisted laryngoscopy:** The use of video laryngoscopy systems may be helpful with difficult airways because they facilitate glottis visualization unobtainable with direct laryngoscopy. Video laryngoscopy blades are available in designs similar to Macintosh blades, as well as with more anteriorly angled curvatures.
   a. **Video laryngoscope:** Load the handle/camera into a size 3 or 4 disposable video laryngoscope blade. Load a standard ETT with a stylet. A video laryngoscope with a more anteriorly angled blade requires a specialized stylet. Without this specialized stylet, passage of the ETT along the sharp curve of the anteriorly angled blade is nearly impossible. Following mouth opening as mentioned earlier, insert the video laryngoscope blade at the midline and advance the blade following the curvature of the tongue via rotation of the handle toward the nose until the base of the tongue is reached and the epiglottis can be seen. Continue advancement toward the epiglottis via rotation of the handle until visualization of the vocal cords. Keeping the vocal cords in the top one-third of the screen, insert the styleted tube into the right side of the mouth and advance along the curvature of the blade until the tip of the ETT is visualized on the screen. Advance the tube between the vocal cords using small rotations as needed and gradually begin to retract the stylet once the ETT tip is through the cords. Common errors are an inability to visualize the ETT tip by placing the camera too close to the glottis, excessively large rotations of the styleted ETT, and insertion of the video laryngoscope blade similar to direct laryngoscopy by not rotating the handle to follow the curvature of the blade and tongue.
   b. Many rigid fiberoptic (Bullard, Upsher) or video laryngoscopy systems are available (C-Mac, C-Mac D, GlideScope, King Vision, McGrath). Each system has unique operating requirements.
6. **ETT placement confirmation:** A major complication that can occur during endotracheal intubation is esophageal intubation, which must be recognized quickly via the following confirmatory techniques. None alone will guarantee proper ETT placement and if any doubt exists regarding proper ETT placement, remove the ETT, initiate bag-valve mask ventilation, and attempt intubation a second time.
   a. **Direct visualization:** Watch the ETT pass through the glottis.
   b. **Chest rise:** Observe symmetric bilateral chest rise with positive pressure ventilation.
   c. **Water vapor:** Observe condensation in the ETT on expiration and its disappearance on inspiration.
   d. **Auscultation:** Listen for clear bilateral inspiratory breath sounds in the upper thorax and their absence in the stomach. Lack of breath sounds in the left thorax may suggest right mainstem intubation and the ETT should be retracted until bilateral breath sounds are confirmed.
   e. **CO_2 measurement:** A capnometer on the mechanical ventilator or a disposable colorimetric CO_2 detector should be used to confirm persistent end-tidal CO_2 on expiration. End-tidal CO_2 may be absent despite endotracheal placement without adequate cardiopulmonary circulation. Conversely, end-tidal CO_2 may transiently be present following esophageal intubation because of residual CO_2 in the stomach from mask ventilation and will gradually disappear.

f. **Ventilation and oxygenation:** Leave the patient under the care of others only after several minutes of adequate oxygenation and ventilation have been observed.

7. **Secure the ETT:** Tape the ETT to bony structures of the maxilla. Take care to avoid pinching the lip against the ETT with tape and note the depth of the ETT at the upper incisors in the chart while also summarizing the procedure and noting any complications.
8. **Chest radiograph:** Obtain a chest plain radiograph to confirm ETT placement. The tip of the ETT should be approximately 2 to 4 cm above the carina.

D. **Nasotracheal Intubation:** Endotracheal intubation via the nares is a technique to be used when an orotracheal tube is not feasible, such as the inability to open the mouth or predicted oral surgery. The technique is as follows:

1. **Nasal vasoconstriction:** To avoid excessive bleeding, nasal application of 0.25% to 1% phenylephrine solution or 0.05% oxymetazoline spray several minutes before nasal instrumentation is recommended.
2. **Antisialagogue:** 0.2 mg glycopyrrolate IV
3. **Anesthesia:** Apply cotton-tipped nasal swabs dipped in 4% lidocaine solution to both nares. Nebulized 2% lidocaine via facemask and gargling of 2% lidocaine for more distal airway anesthesia may be considered.
4. **Endotracheal tube (ETT):** A standard ETT or nasal RAE (Ring-Adair-Elwyn) tube can be used. Sizes to be considered are 7.0 to 7.5 mm for men and 6.0 to 6.5 mm for women. Standard depth measured at the nares is 26 cm for women and 28 cm for men. A flexible-tipped ETT may minimize airway trauma. Generously lubricate the ETT cuff but avoid lubrication in the lumen of the ETT (Figure 4.3).
5. **Naris dilation:** To dilate the nares and ensure patency, insert a well-lubricated NPA of the largest diameter that does not meet resistance. The inner diameter of the NPA should be no smaller than that of the ETT. Remove the NPA before intubating.

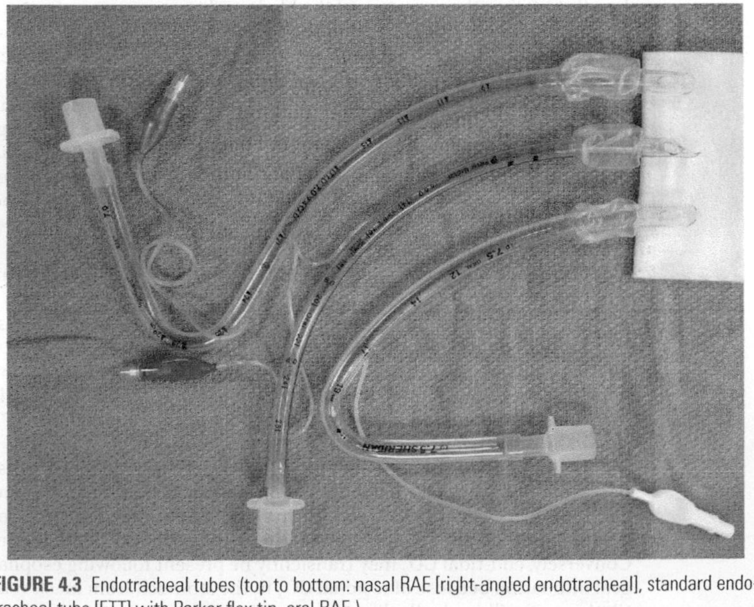

FIGURE 4.3 Endotracheal tubes (top to bottom: nasal RAE [right-angled endotracheal], standard endotracheal tube [ETT] with Parker flex tip, oral RAE.)

6. **Nasal ETT insertion basics:** Insert the ETT perpendicular to the plane of the face and parallel to the hard palate. If resistance is met in the pharynx, the ETT may be impacting the posterior pharyngeal wall and the ETT should be retracted, the neck extended, and the ETT readvanced. Do not advance against resistance.
7. **Blind nasal ETT placement:** When intubating a patient who is spontaneously breathing, the operator can advance the ETT while listening for breath sounds at the proximal end of the ETT, which should become louder as the glottis nears. Sudden loss of breath sounds suggests placement in the esophagus, piriform recess, or vallecula, whereas a cough, condensation on the interior of the ETT, and loss of voice suggests endotracheal intubation. Common maneuvers to correct placement errors are the following:
   a. Neck extension and/or cricoid pressure can move the larynx posteriorly and direct the ETT away from the esophagus.
   b. Neck flexion can direct the ETT away from the vallecula.
   c. Tilting (not rotating) the head toward the naris chosen for intubation and rotating the ETT toward the midline directs the tube away from the piriform recess.
   d. Inflate the cuff to move the tip of the ETT off the posterior pharyngeal wall in a patient with an anterior larynx, making sure to deflate the cuff before passage through the cords.
8. **Direct visualization:** In a patient who is anesthetized, following insertion of the ETT into the oropharynx via the naris, direct laryngoscopy is performed and Magill forceps are used to guide the ETT through the vocal cords under direct visualization. The ETT should be grasped proximally to the cuff to prevent cuff damage.
9. **Fiberoptic intubation:** A flexible fiberoptic bronchoscope can be inserted into the lumen of the ETT and used to guide the ETT through the glottis (technique described later).

E. **Fiberoptic Intubation:** Intubation with a flexible fiberoptic bronchoscope is recommended in cases of predicted difficult airways (abnormal airway anatomy, neck/head flexibility limitations) and can be performed awake or asleep via the nasal or oral routes with similar technique.

1. **Preparation**
   a. Consider preprocedure administration of 0.2 mg glycopyrrolate IV to minimize oral secretions.
   b. Connect the bronchoscope to a video screen or an eye piece and ensure proper white balance/focus. (Adult size will have greater resolution than does the pediatric size.)
   c. Lubricate the fiberoptic bronchoscope.
   d. Remove the stylet from an ETT with an inner diameter larger than the bronchoscope diameter, advance the bronchoscope through the ETT, and secure (lightly tape) the proximal end of the ETT to the proximal end of the bronchoscope.
   e. Connect suction tubing to the suction port of the bronchoscope.
   f. Minimize bronchoscope tip condensation by touching the tip of the bronchoscope to the patient's tongue or using a defogging solution.
2. **Anesthesia:** Proper local anesthesia is critical for an FOI performed with a patient who is awake. Nasal anesthesia is described earlier; and for oral anesthesia, the operator may consider nebulized lidocaine via facemask, lidocaine liquid gargling, gradual advancement of an OPA coated with 4% lidocaine paste (as the patient tolerates), or sequential administration of lidocaine delivered via an atomizer. Glossopharyngeal, superior laryngeal, and transtracheal blocks are more advanced techniques (out of the scope of this book). Care must always be taken to avoid local anesthetic toxicity.

3. **Oral insertion:** While holding the proximal end of the bronchoscope with the dominant hand and the distal end with the nondominant hand, an assistant should insert an Ovassapian airway or pull the tongue out of the mouth to maximize space in the oropharynx. Keeping the bronchoscope straight at all times, insert the tip into the mouth and feed it slowly forward with the nondominant hand. On reaching the base of the tongue, the tip should be flexed anteriorly and advanced toward the epiglottis. Slide the tip underneath the epiglottis, advance through the glottis after visualization, and advance distally in the trachea until 3 to 4 cm above the carina. If visualization becomes unclear at any point, retract the bronchoscope until landmarks are recognized and reattempt placement. Once the bronchoscope is intratracheal, an assistant should advance the ETT over the bronchoscope to the standard depth. If resistance is met, rotate the ETT 90 degrees to place the bevel of the tube in a more favorable position. After ETT advancement, firmly hold the ETT and retract the bronchoscope making sure to visualize that the tip of the ETT is intratracheal at the appropriate depth.
4. **Nasal insertion:** The technique/preparation is identical to that for oral insertion, except entry is via the naris. Insert the bronchoscope perpendicular to the face and advance only when the lumen of the naris is clearly visualized. Lubricating the ETT cuff before insertion is advised.

F. **Supraglottic Airway:** There are a variety of different SGAs, each with its own system of utilization. Because the LMA is most commonly used, it is described here. The LMA does not protect against aspiration and should not be placed in a patient with intact airway reflexes.

1. **Sizes:** LMAs come in sizes 1 to 5 depending on patient size, with the most common adult sizes being No. 3 through No. 5.
2. **Insertion:** Generously lubricate the LMA cuff, place your index finger in the angle between the cuff and connecting tube, and using pressure with the index finger, advance along the hard palate until the cuff lodges into the pharynx. Inflate or deflate the cuff such that a leak begins to appear with positive pressure of 20 cm H_2O.
3. **Common errors**
   a. Forcing the tip of the LMA superiorly into the nasopharynx
   b. Folding the epiglottis over the trachea
   c. Folding the tip of the cuff upon itself
   d. Lateral rotation of the cuff within the oropharynx
4. **Specialized supraglottic airways**
   a. **Intubating SGA (Air Q, Mercury Medical):** lumen large enough for passing ETT blindly or with fiberoptic visualization after SGA placement (Figure 4.4).
   b. **Blind insertion airway device (BIAD; Combitube):** a single-lumen tube with esophageal and pharyngeal balloons that, when inflated, allow ventilation from a port between the balloon sites. Used in emergency settings

G. **Cricothyrotomy:** When endotracheal intubation, LMA placement, and mask ventilation fail to provide adequate ventilation, cricothyrotomy should be performed emergently.

1. **Needle cricothyrotomy:** Puncture the cricothyroid membrane with a 14-G IV catheter attached to a syringe and advance until air is aspirated from the trachea. Remove the needle, secure the catheter with your hand, and attach the catheter via tubing to either a jet ventilator or wall oxygen supply. Cyclically deliver oxygen, anticipating that it may not be possible for exhalation to occur but oxygenation may be possible. Avoid elevated intrathoracic pressures. Backup personnel should be summoned immediately, including those with surgical airway expertise.

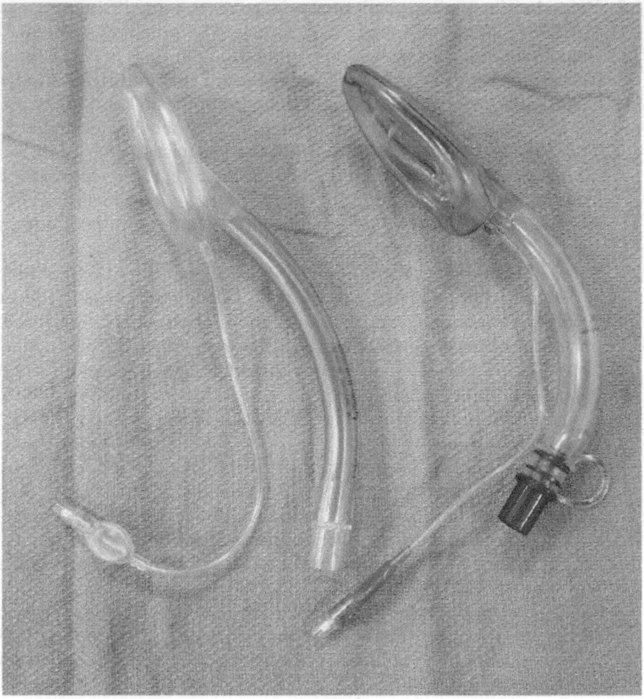

FIGURE 4.4 Supraglottic airways (left to right: LMA Unique, Air-Q intubating LMA.)

2. **Surgical cricothyrotomy:** Using a scalpel, incise the skin and subcutaneous tissue at the cricothyroid notch until piercing the cricothyroid membrane. Expand the membrane bluntly or with the scalpel and insert either a small tracheostomy tube (No. 4-6) or a No. 6 to 6.5 ETT cut near its distal end into the trachea.
3. **Complications:** Bleeding, subcutaneous/mediastinal emphysema, tracheal mucosal trauma, and barotrauma from inadequate expiration can all occur from cricothyrotomy and jet ventilation. These techniques should only be used temporarily while a more definitive surgical airway is achieved.

H. Emergent Tracheostomy: requires time and surgical equipment and may take longer for placement. Its use as an emergent procedure depends on the operator and the equipment available.

VI. INTUBATION PHARMACOLOGY

Hypnotics, neuromuscular blockers, analgesics, and local anesthetics are the primary agents used during endotracheal intubation.

A. Hypnotics/Amnestics: used to prevent consciousness and recall

1. **Propofol (γ-aminobutyric acid [GABA-A] agonist):** 1 to 2 mg/kg IV for induction, although care must be taken in patients who are hemodynamically unstable given its ability to decrease systemic vascular resistance (SVR) and inotropy.

2. **Midazolam (benzodiazepine):** titrated via 0.5- to 1-mg IV incremental doses to achieve sedation/anterograde amnesia without major hemodynamic effects. Onset is within 60 to 90 seconds and duration **is 20 to 60 minutes.**
3. **Dexmedetomidine (α-2 agonist):** 1 µg/kg IV over 10 minutes, followed by an infusion of 0.4 µg/kg/h. Side effects include hypotension and bradycardia, and induction is much more prolonged than with the abovementioned agents.
4. **Ketamine (*N*-methyl-D-aspartate [NMDA] antagonist):** 2 mg/kg IV for induction, and common side effects include nystagmus, tonic-clonic movements, hypertension, and vivid nightmares. It produces a dissociative anesthesia, often with eyes open, and benzodiazepines are commonly administered concomitantly to avoid nightmares.
5. **Etomidate (GABA-A agonist):** 0.5 mg/kg IV for induction and primarily only used in patients who are hemodynamically unstable given the side effects, which include adrenal suppression, myotonic movements, and pain on injection.

B. Neuromuscular Blockers (Neuromuscular Blocking Drugs [NMBDs]): All drugs in this class induce paralysis, respiratory arrest, abolishment of airway reflexes, and vocal cord relaxation. Concomitant sedation is required and intubation or mask ventilation must be achieved in a timely manner because the patient will remain in respiratory arrest.

1. **Depolarizing NMBDs (succinylcholine):** Following a 1-mg/kg IV intubating dose, fasciculations appear within 30 seconds, at which point the patient is ready for intubation. Succinylcholine has been the drug of choice for RSI but the operator must be aware of the contraindications (history of malignant hyperthermia, neuromuscular disease, upper motor neuron injury, burns, or immobility), given the risk of hyperkalemia.
2. **Nondepolarizing NMBDs:** For emergent intubation without succinylcholine, 1.2 mg/kg IV of rocuronium is recommended. Rocuronium use for RSI has increased with the availability of sugammadex, which can reverse deep neuromuscular blockade.

C. Analgesics: Intubation is a noxious stimulus that can induce a significant stress response. Opioids and local anesthetics can blunt the sympathetic response to intubation.

1. **Opioids:** Fentanyl 50 to 500 µg IV provides rapid analgesia (peak within 3-5 minutes) and cough suppression during intubation with a brief duration of action (30-60 minutes). Morphine 2 to 10 mg IV has a much slower onset (peak >30 minutes) and longer duration of action (3-4 hours). Hydromorphone 0.5 to 2 mg IV has an intermediate onset (peak 10-20 minutes) and duration (2-3 hours).
2. **Local anesthetics:** Topical local anesthetics (gargled lidocaine, nebulized lidocaine, and benzocaine spray may all provide analgesia for endotracheal intubation, although care must be taken to avoid accidental local anesthetic overdose/toxicity with unmetered use.
3. **Nerve blocks:** Glossopharyngeal, superior laryngeal, and transtracheal nerve blocks can be used for analgesia but should be avoided in patients with coagulopathies.

D. Cardiovascular Drugs

1. **β-Blockers:** Esmolol 10 to 100 mg IV may be titrated to minimize tachycardia from sympathetic surge following endotracheal intubation.

E. Vasopressors: Phenylephrine (80-160 µg IV), ephedrine (5-10 mg IV), and epinephrine (10-20 µg) can be titrated to minimize blood pressure and heart rate lability during induction.

VII. SPECIAL INTUBATING CIRCUMSTANCES

A. Rapid Sequence Intubation (RSI): In patients with a full stomach or high risk of gastric aspiration, an RSI is indicated to minimize the time between airway reflex inhibition and endotracheal intubation. In quick succession, an analgesic (fentanyl), hypnotic (propofol, ketamine, etomidate), and NMBD (succinylcholine, rocuronium) are provided in sequence and intubation is achieved as rapidly as possible. Cricoid pressure has been considered a standard of care, but given a lack of evidence of its value, and potential to complicate laryngoscopy, many clinicians are abandoning the use of cricoid pressure. Bag-valve mask ventilation is generally avoided to minimize gastric insufflation and the risk of regurgitation, although it should be used if intubation is not immediately successful or if rapid/severe oxygen desaturation occurs. Nasogastric tube insertion and decompression should be used for preventing pulmonary aspiration when time and circumstances allow in patients with a high risk of aspiration or gastric distension undergoing RSI.

B. Difficult Intubation: defined as the inability to place an ETT after three attempts by an experienced laryngoscopist. The ASA's difficult airway algorithm provides a framework for predicted and unpredicted difficult airways (Figure 4.5). In cases of difficult intubation, backup personnel should be summoned immediately, including those with surgical airway expertise.

1. **Predicted:** On the basis of airway exam, body habitus, lack of neck mobility, and many other clinical factors, a difficult airway may be predicted before any attempt at laryngoscopy. The safest approach is to maintain

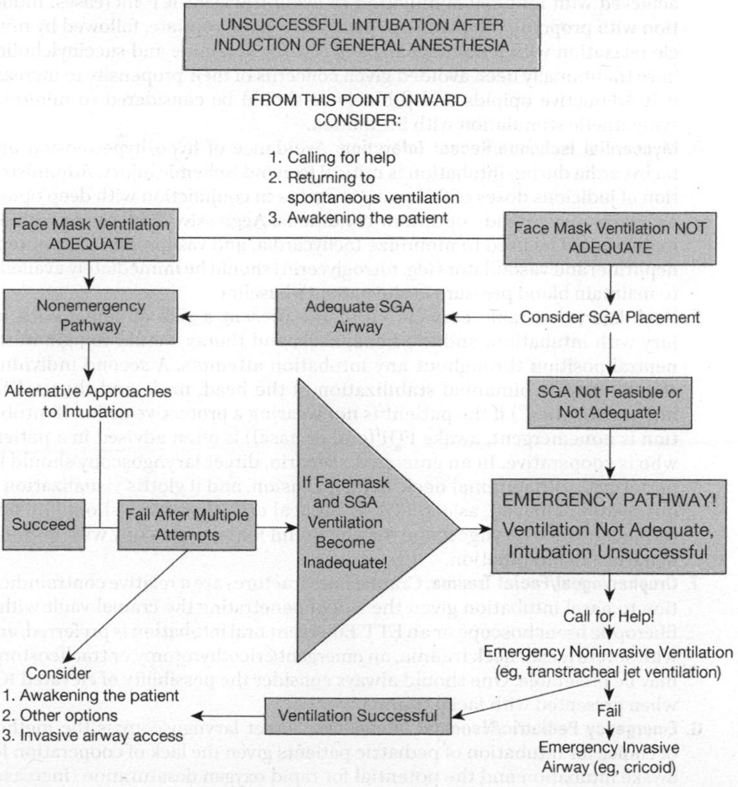

FIGURE 4.5 Difficult airway algorithm. SGA, supraglottic airway. (Redrawn and simplified from Apfelbaum JL, Hagberg CA. 2022 American Society of Anesthesiologists practice guidelines for management of the difficult airway. *Anesthesiology.* 2022;136:31-81.)

spontaneous respiration and to perform an awake FOI (described earlier), blind nasal intubation, or elective surgical airway under sedation. If induction of general anesthesia is needed, personnel capable of performing an emergent surgical airway should be present in the event that endotracheal intubation is not achieved rapidly.

2. **Unpredicted:** When intubation attempts have failed and spontaneous/assisted respirations are absent, an airway emergency is in progress and the next step is the placement of an SGA. If ventilation is successful, the SGA can be used as a bridge to endotracheal intubation. If ventilation via SGA is unsuccessful, a surgical cricothyrotomy should be performed by trained personnel. If no persons with surgical expertise are available, needle cricothyrotomy should be performed, followed by jet ventilation. Subcutaneous emphysema and bleeding after needle cricothyrotomy may make subsequent surgical cricothyrotomy impossible.
3. The **MACOCHA score** may be helpful in predicting difficult intubation in the critically ill. It consists of patient, pathology, and operator-related factors: 6 patient (**M**allampati score III or IV, obstructive sleep **A**pnea syndrome, reduced mobility of **C**ervical spine, limited mouth **O**pening), 2 pathology (**C**oma, severe **H**ypoxia), and 1 operator (non**A**nesthesiologist) factors.

C. Increased ICP: Airway management in patients with elevated ICP should be achieved with minimal stimulation to avoid transient ICP increases. Induction with propofol, thiopental, or etomidate is appropriate, followed by muscle relaxation with a nondepolarizing NMBD. Ketamine and succinylcholine have traditionally been avoided given concerns of their propensity to increase ICP. Adjunctive opioids and β-blockade should be considered to minimize sympathetic stimulation with intubation.

D. Myocardial Ischemia/Recent Infarction: Avoidance of hypo/hypertension and tachycardia during intubation is critical to avoid ischemic injury. Administration of judicious doses of IV hypnotic agents in conjunction with deep opioid analgesia may provide optimum conditions. Aggressive β-blockade with esmolol should be used to minimize tachycardia, and vasopressors (eg, norepinephrine) and vasodilators (eg, nitroglycerin) should be immediately available to maintain blood pressure at the patient's baseline.

E. Neck Injury: Unstable cervical vertebrae present a risk of spinal cord injury with intubation, and the head, neck, and thorax should remain in the neutral position throughout any intubation attempts. A second individual should provide bimanual stabilization of the head, neck, and thorax ("in-line stabilization") if the patient is not wearing a protective collar. If intubation is nonemergent, awake FOI (oral or nasal) is often advised in a patient who is cooperative. In an emergent scenario, direct laryngoscopy should be performed with minimal neck/head extension, and if glottis visualization is not readily achieved, asleep FOI or surgical cricothyrotomy should be performed. A video laryngoscope may be useful for laryngoscopy with minimal head/neck manipulation.

F. Oropharyngeal/Facial Trauma: Cranial base fractures are a relative contraindication to nasal intubation given the risk of penetrating the cranial vault with a fiberoptic bronchoscope or an ETT. Emergent oral intubation is preferred; and with severe facial/neck trauma, an emergent cricothyrotomy or tracheostomy may be preferable. One should always consider the possibility of elevated ICP when presented with facial trauma.

G. Emergency Pediatric/Neonatal Intubations: Direct laryngoscopy is the method of choice for intubation of pediatric patients given the lack of cooperation for awake intubation and the potential for rapid oxygen desaturation (increased oxygen consumption). A low-pressure high-volume (Hi-Lo) cuffed tube (size as previously discussed) is preferable and the cuff should be inflated such that a leak occurs at approximately 20 cm H_2O to prevent mucosal ischemia and to reduce the risk of tracheomalacia and tracheal stenosis because the tracheal cartilage in prepubertal children is not fully developed.

H. Common Complications of Intubation

1. **Hypertension/tachycardia:** Stimulation from laryngoscopy and ETT insertion can produce profound tachycardia and hypertension.
2. **Hypotension:** Severe hypotension can occur following induction of a patient in respiratory distress. In addition to the SVR lowering and negative inotropic effects of many induction agents, the removal of the drive to breathe and its sympathetic stimulation, combined with hyperinflation from mask ventilation and the resultant preload reduction, can cause profound hypotension.
3. **Bradycardia:** Vagal responses to laryngoscopy can be seen.

I. Gastric Aspiration: At highest risk are patients with a full stomach or who are not completely paralyzed before laryngoscopy.

VIII. ENDOTRACHEAL AND TRACHEOSTOMY TUBES

A. ETT Materials: Most ETTs are made from polyvinyl chloride (PVC). Specialized tubes designed to resist infection, resist airway fires, or resist mechanical obstruction due to kinking are available.

B. Cuff Designs

1. **Low pressure/high volume (Hi-Lo):** Found on standard disposable ETTs, these cuffs are highly compliant, conform to the irregular tracheal wall, and are less likely to cause tracheal mucosal ischemia at cuff pressures less than 30 cm H_2O.
2. **High pressure/low volume:** Found on specialty ETTs, the small area of contact with the tracheal wall, the high pressure required to achieve appropriate cuff inflation, and the required deformation of the tracheal wall to achieve an effective seal all place the trachea at risk for mucosal ischemia.
3. **Low profile (Lo-Pro):** Often used in pediatrics, these Hi-Lo tubes have cuffs that lie closer to the ETT for ease of visualization during intubation.

C. Preformed ETT: designed to move the ETT away from the surgical field

1. **Oral RAE:** ETT with an acute curvature at the proximal end for placement inferiorly along the chin
2. **Nasal RAE:** ETT with less acute curvature closer to the proximal end and exits the naris superiorly

D. Supraglottic Suction Tubes: designed to reduce ventilator-associated pneumonia by facilitating the removal of secretions that pool above the ETT cuff

E. Tracheostomy Tubes: available in many sizes, designs, and brands. Key design differences include cuffed/noncuffed, inner cannula/single lumen, fenestrated/nonfenestrated, and metal/PVC/silicone.

1. **Sizes:** vary depending on manufacturer and style of tube
2. **Obturator:** a relatively rigid stylet used to aid the insertion of a tracheostomy tube. It fits in the lumen of the tracheostomy tube and is removed following insertion.
3. **Inner cannula:** a disposable or reusable cannula that reduces the inner diameter of the tracheostomy tube but allows for cleaning by removal/replacement of the cannula, thus minimizing the risk of obstruction
4. **Key features**
    a. **Cuffed:** used for patients requiring mechanical ventilation. Phonation can be achieved with fenestration.
    b. **Uncuffed:** mostly used in patients who are nonventilated at low aspiration risk and allows coughing/phonation around the tube. Often worn over a long period of time. Should not be used if mechanical ventilation is needed

IX. ENDOTRACHEAL AND TRACHEOSTOMY TUBE MAINTENANCE

A. General Care

1. **Suctioning:** The pharynx and trachea of patients who are intubated may need periodic suctioning to clear secretions.
2. **Cuff pressure:** Pressure should be less than 25 to 30 cm H_2O to avoid mucosal damage and should be monitored routinely. A dedicated ETT cuff monitor (Posey Cufflator Endotracheal Tube Manometer) or a central venous pressure (CVP) transducer can be used.
3. **Securing the ETT:** Tape or a dedicated holder can be used to secure the ETT and should be reapplied/adjusted as needed. With oral tubes, lip impingement should be avoided. With nasal tubes, the patient should routinely be assessed for sinusitis, otitis media, and naris ischemia/necrosis.

B. Common Endotracheal and Tracheostomy Tube Problems

1. **Cuff leak:** noted via audible flow of air around the anterior portion of the ETT cuff during positive pressure ventilation while the patient is supine, often with delivered TVs less than expected. Leaks can often be repaired via reinflation with a small volume of air but large leaks generally require urgent reintubation. Common causes of persistent large-volume cuff leak are supraglottic cuff position, cuff damage, and tracheal dilatation.
   a. **Supraglottic cuff position:** A cuff that is above the vocal cords can be seen on chest radiograph or laryngoscopy and is fixed via cuff deflation and ETT advancement.
   b. **Damaged cuff system:** The cuff or its inflation system may slowly or quickly leak air. In either case, ETT replacement is needed and the level of urgency depends on the speed of the leak.
   c. **Tracheal dilatation:** An ETT with a cuff that is unable to seal a widened tracheal lumen will need to be replaced with an ETT with a larger volume air-filled cuff or a foam cuff tube (Bivona Fome-Cuff). This scenario is seen as a leak with a widened trachea on chest radiograph.
2. **Mainstem intubation:** Following initial intubation or subsequent position changes, the ETT may migrate such that the tip is in the left or right mainstem bronchus. High airway pressures and desaturation may occur. Confirmation is via unilateral breath sounds and chest radiograph and the problem can be fixed via cuff deflation and retracting the ETT to the appropriate depth.
3. **Airway obstruction:** Triggering of the high airway pressure or low-volume alarm in the absence of obvious changes in pulmonary compliance/bronchial obstruction suggests ETT obstruction. Common causes are ETT kinking and secretions. Head/neck manipulation may relieve positional ETT kinks, whereas suctioning via soft suction catheter may relieve obstructing secretions. A kinked ETT will not let a soft suction catheter pass. In either case, if manual ventilation is not possible, immediate ETT replacement is required.
4. **Malpositioned tracheostomy tube:** Pressure from the tracheostomy tube on the anterior or posterior tracheal walls can damage the tracheal mucosa, cause obstruction, and predispose to decannulation.
5. **Dislodged tracheostomy tube:** A fresh tracheostomy tract typically takes 7 to 10 days to mature and attempted reinsertion of a dislodged tube via the surgical stoma can create a false lumen, with disastrous consequences when positive pressure ventilation is resumed. Patients whose tracheostomy tubes are dislodged before maturation of the surgical stoma should receive bag-valve mask ventilation and/or prompt orotracheal intubation, rather than an attempt at reinsertion of the dislodged tube at the bedside
6. **Airway bleeding:** Return of blood during airway suctioning requires prompt evaluation. The primary etiologies are repeated trauma from suctioning

and mucosal erosion, both of which must be evaluated. Fiberoptic bronchoscopy can be used to examine the airway for trauma. If bleeding is persistent or without a clear source, evaluation by an otolaryngologist is advised. If bleeding is minimal, the airway will require time to heal, and the irritant should be removed, either from less frequent suctioning or replacement of the tracheostomy tube or ETT distal to the lesion. Bleeding from a tracheostomy tube can be particularly dangerous, with the risk of erosion into mediastinal vessels causing exsanguination and/or clotting with ETT obstruction, or a trachea-esophageal fistula causing aspiration and/or airway obstruction. In cases of persistent obstruction/bleeding from a tracheostomy, urgent laryngotracheal intubation followed by surgical evaluation/exploration is indicated.

C. ETT Replacement: often required in the setting of mechanical ETT failure, size inadequacy, and location (oral vs nasal) changes. Techniques for tube exchange include direct laryngoscopy, bronchoscopy, and use of a tube exchanger.

1. **Direct laryngoscopy:** reintubation as previously described. Useful in patients without a prior difficult airway and minimal airway trauma/edema
2. **Bronchoscopy:** After loading a fresh ETT on a flexible bronchoscope, the bronchoscope is advanced via the nasal or oral route until the glottis is visualized, all the while maintaining ventilation by the intact old ETT. With glottis visualization, the old ETT cuff is deflated and the bronchoscope tip is passed around the deflated cuff into the trachea. Maintaining tracheal visualization, an assistant removes the old ETT followed by advancement of the fresh ETT into the trachea over the bronchoscope.

D. Tube Exchanger: A long, malleable stylet can be inserted blindly into the existing ETT and advanced to the appropriate tracheal depth using the depth markers. Once advanced to the appropriate depth, the old ETT can be removed over the stylet and the new ETT, blindly or under direct laryngoscopy, can be advanced into the trachea over the exchange stylet. Some specialized tube exchangers have a small lumen through which the patient can be oxygenated or jet ventilated. Tube exchangers that have larger lumens may be advanced over a bronchoscope.

X. TRACHEOSTOMY

Tracheostomy can be performed safely at the bedside as a percutaneous procedure or in the operating room as an open surgical procedure. Most bedside tracheostomies are performed using a modified Ciaglia technique, which utilizes sequential wire-guided plastic or balloon tracheal dilators before tracheostomy tube placement.

A. Advantages Over Oral Endotracheal Tubes

1. Decreased sedation requirement
2. Decreased risk of laryngeal damage/dysfunction
3. Reduced work of breathing
4. Improved oral/pharyngeal hygiene
5. Potential for phonation when the cuff is deflated

B. Disadvantages

1. Potential for tracheal stenosis at stoma site
2. Stoma infection
3. Erosion of neighboring vascular tissue leading to hemorrhage
4. Scarring and/or granulation tissue formation at stoma site
5. Operative complications

C. Timing of Placement: Given the risk of laryngeal damage with prolonged translaryngeal intubation, a tracheostomy should be considered after 7 to 10 days of oral intubation.

D. Tracheostomy Tube Change: Replacing a tracheostomy tube may be required because of improper size, malposition, or failure. Given the difficulty with decannulation of a fresh tracheostomy tract and the risk of a false tract creation, it is advisable to wait until the tract is 7 to 10 days old before attempting a tracheostomy tube exchange. If it is necessary to change within 7 to 10 days of initial cannulation, exchange should be made over a malleable stylet, equipment for laryngotracheal intubation should be readily available, and, preferably, the surgeon who initially placed the tracheostomy tube should be present in case surgical reexploration is necessary.

1. Technique

a. Be fully prepared for emergent laryngotracheal intubation.
b. Preoxygenate with 100% oxygen.
c. Clean the tracheostomy site with chlorhexidine and suction the trachea with a soft suction catheter.
d. Check that the new tracheostomy tube is mechanically intact and that the cuff inflates appropriately. Insert the obturator within the lumen to ensure a smooth distal surface for cannulation.
e. Deflate the cuff on the existing tube and remove the tube using the natural angulation of the tube. Slight resistance may be felt as the deflated cuff passes through the anterior tracheal wall.
f. Insert the new tracheostomy tube/obturator smoothly into the existing stoma along the curvature of the tube, being careful to avoid excessive resistance, which is suggestive of a new tract.
g. Inflate the cuff, if present, on the replacement tracheostomy and remove the obturator.

E. Manually ventilate with 100% oxygen and ensure proper placement as described previously.

XI. EXTUBATION

Removal of a laryngotracheal ETT or tracheostomy tube in the intensive care unit (ICU) is indicated once the patient is able to ventilate, oxygenate, clear secretions, and protect the airway without support.

A. Criteria

1. Subjective criteria

a. Underlying disease process improving
b. Appropriate cough/gag with airway suctioning

2. Objective criteria

a. GCS greater than 13, minimal sedation
b. Hemodynamically stable
c. SaO_2 greater than 90%, PaO_2 greater than 60 mm Hg, PaO_2/FIO_2 greater than 150
d. Positive end-expiratory pressure (PEEP) less than 5 to 8 cm H_2O
e. FIO_2 less than 0.4 to 0.5
f. $PaCO_2$ less than 60 mm Hg
g. pH greater than 7.25

3. Ventilator criteria (during spontaneous breathing trial [SBT])

a. Rapid shallow breathing index (RSBI: RR/VT) less than 105
b. Negative inspiratory force (NIF) greater than 20 cm H_2O
c. TVs greater than 5 mL/kg
d. Vital capacity greater than 10 mL/kg
e. RR less than 30

B. Devices that may aid in transition to decannulation of a tracheostomy tube:

1. Fenestrated cuffed tracheostomy tube: With the balloon down, inner cannula removed, and speaking valve in place, the airway is not protected but the patient can be tested for tolerance to decannulation.

2. **Small/cuffless tracheostomy tube:** A small diameter cuffless tracheostomy tube has insignificant airway resistance and performs as a guard against ventilatory failure and as a conduit for tracheal suctioning while the patient is evaluated for decannulation tolerance.

Speech and Swallow Evaluation: A modified barium swallow exam can elucidate potential causes of aspiration and a speech therapist can provide recommendations for aspiration risk minimization following extubation.

Selected Readings

American Heart Association. *Advanced Cardiovascular Life Support Provider Manual.* American Heart Association; 2020.

Apfelbaum JL, Hagberg CA, Connis RT, et al. 2022 American Society of Anesthesiologists practice guidelines for management of the difficult airway. *Anesthesiology.* 2022;136:31-81.

Cote CJ, Lerman J, Anderson B, eds. *A Practice of Anesthesia for Infants and Children.* 6th ed. Elsevier/Saunders; 2019:257.

Higgs A, McGrath BA, Goddard C, et al. Guidelines for the management of tracheal intubation in critically ill adults. *Br J Anaesth.* 2018;120:323-352.

Kornas RL, Owyang CG, Sakles JC, et al. Evaluation and management of the physiologically difficult airway: consensus recommendations from Society for Airway Management. *Anesth Analg.* 2021;132 395-405.

Longnecker DE, Mackey SC, Newman MF, et al. *Anesthesiology.* 3rd ed. McGraw-Hill; 2018:498.

MacIntyre NR, Cook DJ, Ely EW Jr, et al. Evidence-based guidelines for weaning and discontinuing ventilatory support: a collective task force facilitated by the ACCP, AARC, and the ACCCM. *Chest.* 2001;120(6 suppl):375S-395S.

5 Mechanical Ventilation

Carolyn J. La Vita

I. MECHANICAL VENTILATION

Mechanical ventilation provides artificial support of breathing and gas exchange.

A. Indications

1. Hypoventilation

- **a. Evaluation: Arterial pH** should be evaluated for evidence of hypoventilation. Chronic compensated hypercapnia is a stable condition that usually does not require mechanical ventilatory support and therefore arterial partial pressure of carbon dioxide ($PaCO_2$) is not useful in isolation.
- **b. Hypoventilation resulting in an arterial pH of less than 7.30** is often considered an indication for mechanical ventilation, but patient fatigue and associated morbidity must be considered and may prompt initiation of mechanical ventilation at a higher or lower pH.
- **c. Noninvasive ventilation (NIV)** may be considered for hypoventilation due to chronic obstructive pulmonary disease (COPD) or obesity hypoventilation syndrome (OHS).

2. Hypoxemia

- **a. Supplemental oxygen** should be administered to all patients with hypoxemia to attain arterial oxygen saturation by pulse oximetry (Spo_2) greater than 90% regardless of diagnosis (eg, appropriate oxygen therapy should not be withheld from patients with hypercapnia and COPD).
- **b.** Patients with **hypoxemic respiratory failure** due to atelectasis and/or pulmonary edema may benefit from **continuous positive airway pressure (CPAP)** administered noninvasively by face mask.
- **c. Endotracheal intubation and mechanical ventilation** should be considered for severe hypoxemia (Spo_2 <90% at a fraction of inspired oxygen [FIO_2] = 1.0) unresponsive to more conservative measures and can be considered earlier for lung protection if acute respiratory distress syndrome (ARDS) is suspected.

3. Respiratory fatigue

- **a.** Tachypnea, dyspnea, use of accessory muscles, nasal flaring, diaphoresis, and tachycardia may be an indication for mechanical ventilation before abnormalities of gas exchange occur.

4. Airway protection

- **a.** Mechanical ventilation may be initiated in patients who require endotracheal **intubation for airway protection**, even in the absence of respiratory abnormalities (eg, increased aspiration risk due to decreased mental status or massive upper gastrointestinal [GI] bleed).
- **b. The presence of an artificial airway** is not an absolute indication for mechanical ventilation (eg, many patients with a long-term tracheostomy do not require mechanical ventilation).

B. Goals of Mechanical Ventilation

1. Provide adequate alveolar oxygenation and ventilation.
2. Avoid alveolar overdistension.
3. Maintain alveolar recruitment.
4. Promote patient-ventilator synchrony.

5. Avoid incomplete exhalation, and thus generation of auto–positive end-expiratory pressure (PEEP; as a function of mechanical ventilator settings).
6. Use the lowest possible FIO_2.

II. THE VENTILATOR SYSTEM

A. The Ventilator is powered by gas pressure and electricity. Gas pressure provides the energy required to inflate the lungs (Figure 5.1).

1. Gas flow is controlled by **inspiratory and expiratory valves.** The electronics (microprocessor) of the ventilator controls these valves so that gas flow is determined by ventilator settings.
   a. **Inspiratory phase:** The inspiratory valve opens and controls gas flow and/or pressure, and the expiratory valve is closed.
   b. **Expiratory phase:** The expiratory valve opens and controls PEEP, and the inspiratory valve is closed.

B. The Ventilator Circuit delivers flow between the ventilator and the patient.

1. Owing to gas compression and the elasticity of the circuit, part of the gas volume delivered from the ventilator is not received by the patient. This **compression volume** is typically about 3 to 4 mL for every cm H_2O inspiratory pressure—most modern generation ventilators compensate for the compression volume.
2. The volume of the circuit containing gas that the patient rebreathes during the respiratory cycle is **mechanical dead space.** Mechanical dead space should be as low as possible. This is particularly an issue when low tidal volumes are used.

C. Gas Conditioning

1. **Filters** are placed in the inspiratory and expiratory limbs of the circuit.
2. **The inspired gas** is actively or passively humidified.
   a. **Active humidifiers** pass the inspired gas over a heated water chamber for humidification. Some also use a **heated circuit** to regulate airway temperature to a set point and to decrease condensate within the circuit. Active humidifiers can adjust well to temperature changes in the patient environment.
   b. **Passive humidifiers** (artificial noses or heat and moisture exchangers) are inserted between the ventilator circuit and the patient. They trap heat and humidity in the exhaled gas and return that on the subsequent inspiration. Passive humidification is satisfactory for many patients, but it is less effective than is active humidification, increases the resistance to inspiration and expiration, and increases mechanical dead space.

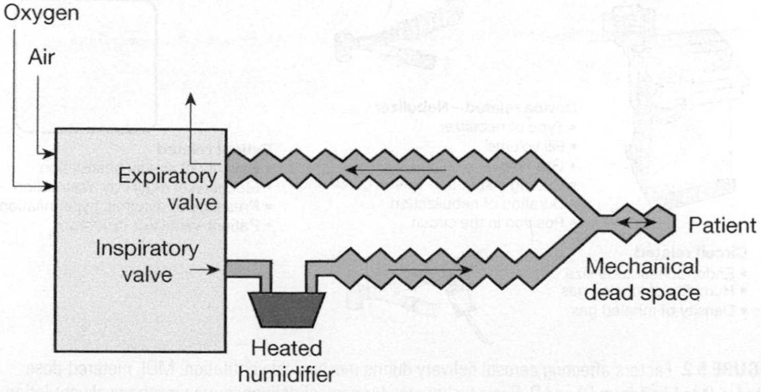

FIGURE 5.1 Simplified block diagram of a mechanical ventilator system.

c. The presence of **water droplets** in the inspiratory circuit near the patient (or in the proximal endotracheal tube if a passive humidifier is used) suggests that the inspired gas is adequately humidified.

D. Delivery of Inhaled Medications and Gases During Mechanical Ventilation

1. Inhaled medications can be delivered by **metered-dose inhaler** or **nebulizer** during mechanical ventilation. Dry powder inhalers cannot be adapted to the ventilator circuit. Inhaled gases (eg, inhaled nitric oxide [NO]) can be added directly to the inhaled gas mixture.
2. A variety of factors influence aerosol delivery during mechanical ventilation (Figure 5.2).
3. With careful attention to technique, either inhalers or nebulizers can be used effectively during mechanical ventilation.
4. The mesh nebulizer is commonly used because it overcomes issues with the use of jet nebulizers (mostly related to additional gas flow into the circuit) and is cost-effective compared with hydrofluoroalkane (HFA) metered-dose inhalers.
5. Mixtures of helium and oxygen (heliox) can also be delivered into the ventilator circuit. However, gases with physical characteristics different from oxygen and air have the potential to interfere with ventilator function.

III. CLASSIFICATION OF MECHANICAL VENTILATION

A. Negative Versus Positive Pressure Ventilation

1. The **iron lung** and **chest cuirass** create negative pressure around the thorax during the inspiratory phase. Although useful for some patients with a neuromuscular disease requiring long-term ventilation, these devices are almost never used in the intensive care unit (ICU).
2. **Positive pressure ventilation** applies pressure to the airway during the inspiratory phase, via invasive or noninvasive interface.
3. **Exhalation** occurs passively with both positive pressure ventilation and negative pressure ventilation.

B. Invasive Ventilation Versus NIV

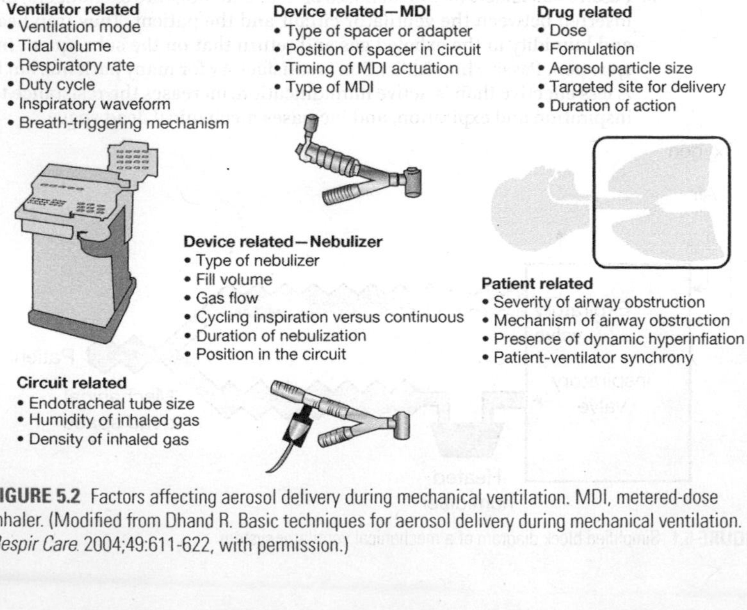

FIGURE 5.2 Factors affecting aerosol delivery during mechanical ventilation. MDI, metered-dose inhaler. (Modified from Dhand R. Basic techniques for aerosol delivery during mechanical ventilation. *Respir Care.* 2004;49:611-622, with permission.)

1. **Invasive ventilation** is delivered through an endotracheal tube (orotracheal or nasotracheal) or a tracheostomy tube.
2. Although mechanical ventilation through an artificial airway remains the standard in the patients who are most acutely ill, **NIV** is preferred in some patients such as those with an exacerbation of COPD, those with acute cardiogenic pulmonary edema, or those who are immunocompromised with acute respiratory failure. NIV is also useful to prevent postextubation respiratory failure, particularly in those patients with underlying lung disease and those who are obese. There are many patients, however, in whom NIV is not appropriate.
   a. NIV can be applied with a nasal mask, oronasal mask, nasal pillows, total face mask, or a helmet. Oronasal masks and total face masks are preferred in patients who are acutely ill and dyspneic, in whom mouth leak is often problematic.
   b. Although bilevel ventilators are most commonly used for NIV, any ventilator can be used to provide this therapy. Current generation ventilators designed for critical care have both invasive and noninvasive modes, and some have good leak-compensation algorithms.
   c. **Pressure support (PS)** is most commonly used for NIV. For bilevel ventilators, this is achieved by setting inspiratory positive airway pressure **(IPAP)** and expiratory positive airway pressure **(EPAP)**. The difference between IPAP and EPAP is the level of PS.
   d. An algorithm for the use of NIV (including evaluation of contraindications) in the critical care setting is provided in Figure 5.3.

C. Full Versus Partial Ventilatory Support

1. **Full ventilatory support** provides the entire minute ventilation, with little interaction between the patient and the ventilator. This usually requires sedation and sometimes neuromuscular blockade. Full ventilatory support is indicated for patients with severe respiratory failure, patients who are hemodynamically unstable, patients with complex acute injuries while they are being stabilized, and all patients receiving treatment for paralysis from high cervical spinal injury.
2. **Partial ventilatory support** provides a variable portion of the minute ventilation, with the remainder provided by the patient's inspiratory effort. The patient-ventilator interaction is important during partial ventilatory support.
   a. Partial ventilatory support is indicated for patients with moderately acute respiratory failure or patients who are recovering from respiratory failure.
      1. **Advantages** of partial ventilatory support include avoidance of muscle weakness during long periods of mechanical ventilation, preservation of the ventilatory drive and breathing pattern, decreased requirement for sedation and neuromuscular blockade, a better hemodynamic response to positive pressure ventilation, and better ventilation of dependent lung regions.
      2. **Disadvantages** of partial ventilatory support include a higher work of breathing (WoB) for the patient and difficulty achieving lung-protective ventilation if the patient has a strong respiratory drive.

IV. THE EQUATION OF MOTION

A. Delivery of gas into the lungs is determined by the interaction between the ventilator, respiratory mechanics, and respiratory muscle activity, which is described by the **equation of motion** of the respiratory system:

$$P_{vent} + P_{mus} = V_T/C + \dot{V} \times R$$

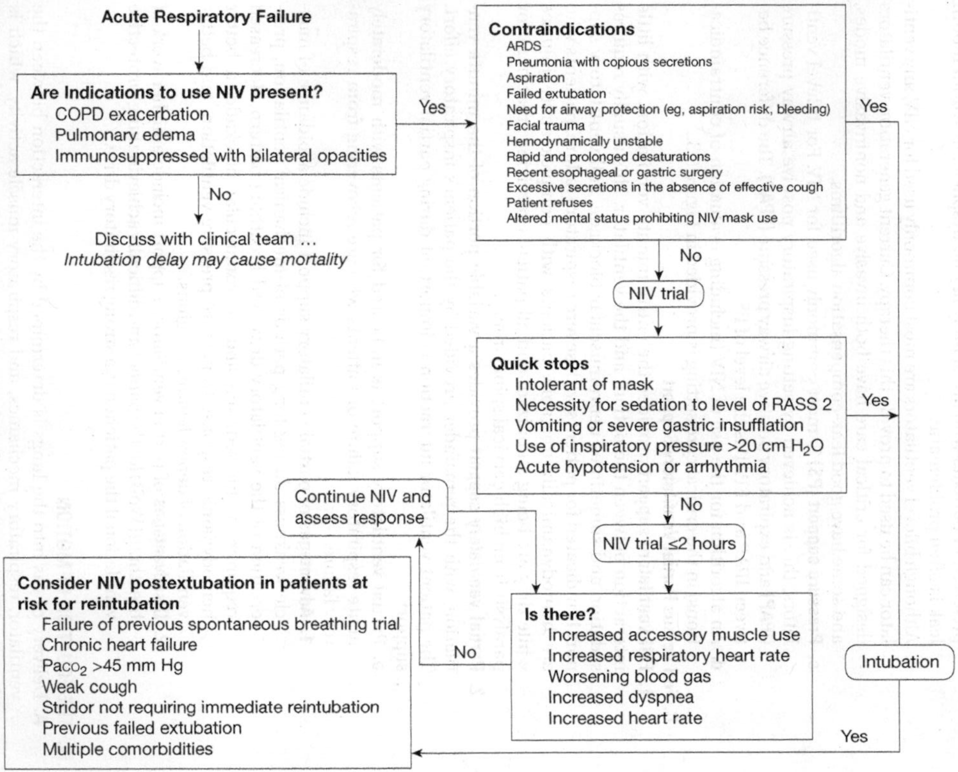

FIGURE 5.3 An algorithm for application of noninvasive ventilation. ARDS, acute respiratory distress syndrome; COPD, chronic obstructive pulmonary disease; NIV, noninvasive ventilation; RASS, Richmond Agitation Sedation Scale.

where P_{vent} is the pressure applied by the ventilator, P_{mus} is the pressure generated by the respiratory muscles, V_T is tidal volume, C is compliance, $\dot{V}$ is gas flow, and R is airways resistance.

1. Pressure generated from either the respiratory muscles (spontaneous breathing) or ventilator (full ventilatory support), or both (partial ventilatory support), applied to the respiratory system results in gas flow into the lungs.
2. For a given pressure, gas flow is opposed by airways resistance and the elastance (inverse of compliance) of the lungs and chest wall.
3. Larger tidal volumes, lower compliance, higher flow, and higher resistance all require a higher pressure.

V. PHASE AND CONTROL VARIABLES

A. The **trigger variable** starts the inspiratory phase.
   1. The trigger variable determines when the ventilator initiates a breath.
   2. The ventilator detects patient inspiratory effort by either a pressure change (**pressure trigger**) or a flow change (**flow trigger**).
   3. The **trigger sensitivity** is set to both prevent excessive patient effort and avoid autotriggering. Pressure trigger sensitivity is commonly set at 0.5 to 2 cm H_2O, and flow trigger sensitivity is set at 2 to 3 L/min.
      a. Autotrigger can be caused by artifacts such as cardiac oscillations and leaks. This is corrected by making the trigger less sensitive.
      b. Ineffective trigger can be due to neuromuscular disease or auto-PEEP. Switching the trigger variable is rarely effective to deal with failed triggers.
   4. Pressure triggering and flow triggering are equally effective if sensitivity is optimized and closely monitored.

B. The **control variable** remains constant throughout inspiration. The most common of these are volume control (VC), pressure control (PC), and adaptive control (Table 5.1).
   1. **Volume control:** Despite the name, the ventilator actually controls flow (the time derivative of volume) to maintain a **constant delivered tidal volume** regardless of airways resistance or respiratory system compliance.
      a. A decrease in respiratory system compliance or an increase in airways resistance results in an increased peak inspiratory pressure during VC. Decreased compliance also results in an increased plateau pressure (Pplat; the pressure during an inspiratory pause when the flow is zero).
      b. With VC, the **inspiratory flow is fixed** regardless of patient effort. This unvarying flow may induce patient-ventilator dyssynchrony.
         1. Inspiratory flow patterns during VC include **constant flow** (rectangular wave; Figure 5.4) or **descending-ramp flow** (Figure 5.5).
         2. Use of the constant-flow waveform results in a higher peak pressure, which is largely borne by the airways and not the alveoli.
         3. Use of a descending-ramp waveform results in maximal flow early in the breath when lung volume is minimal. This reduces peak pressures but decreases expiratory time, which may increase the risk of auto-PEEP and dynamic hyperinflation.
      c. The **inspiratory time** during VC is determined by inspiratory flow, the inspiratory flow pattern, and tidal volume.
      d. VC is preferred when an assured minute ventilation or tidal volume is desirable (eg, avoiding hypercarbia in patients with intracranial hypertension or preventing overdistension in ARDS).

TABLE 5.1 Comparison of Several Breath Types During Mechanical Ventilation

	Pressure control ventilation	Volume control ventilation	Adaptive control ventilation	Pressure support ventilation	Proportional assist ventilation
Tidal volume	Variable	Set	Minimum set	Variable	Variable
Peak inspiratory pressure	Limited by pressure control setting	Variable	Variable	Limited by pressure support setting	Variable
Plateau pressure	Limited by pressure control setting	Variable	Variable	Limited by pressure support setting	Variable
Inspiratory flow	Descending; variable	Set; constant or descending ramp	Descending; variable	Variable	Variable
Inspiratory time	Set	Set (flow and volume settings)	Set for adaptive pressure control; variable for adaptive pressure support	Variable	Variable
Respiratory rate	Minimum set (patient can trigger)	Minimum set (patient can trigger)	Minimum set for adaptive pressure control; not set for adaptive pressure support	Variable; rate not set	Variable; rate not set

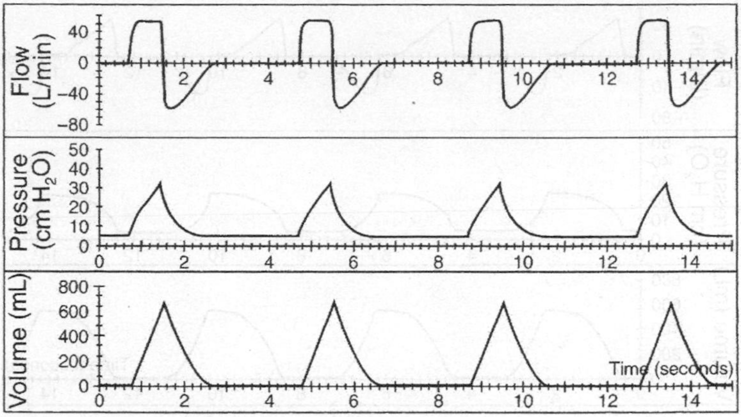

FIGURE 5.4 Constant-flow volume ventilation.

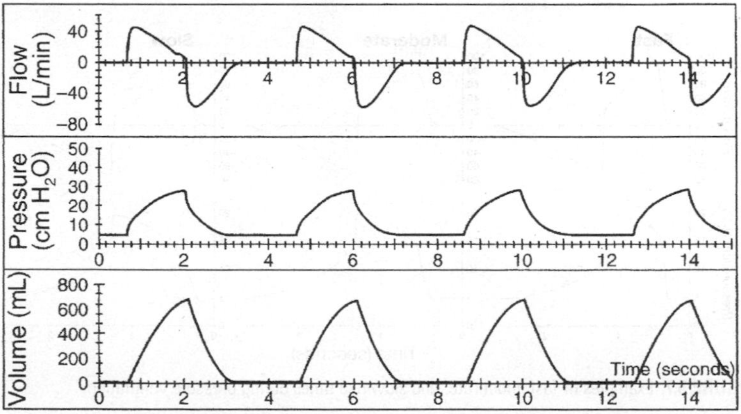

FIGURE 5.5 Descending-ramp volume ventilation.

2. Pressure control

a. With PC (Figure 5.6), **the pressure applied to the airway is constant** regardless of the airways resistance or respiratory system compliance.

b. The inspiratory flow during PC is exponentially descending and determined by the PC setting, airways resistance, and respiratory system compliance. With low respiratory system compliance (eg, ARDS), flow decreases rapidly. With high airways resistance (eg, COPD), flow decreases slowly.

c. Some ventilators allow the adjustment of the **rise time**, which is the pressurization rate of the ventilator at the beginning of the inspiratory phase (Figure 5.7). The rise time is the amount of time required for the PC level to be reached after the ventilator is triggered.

A rapid rise time delivers more flow at the initiation of inhalation, which may be useful for patients with a high respiratory drive.

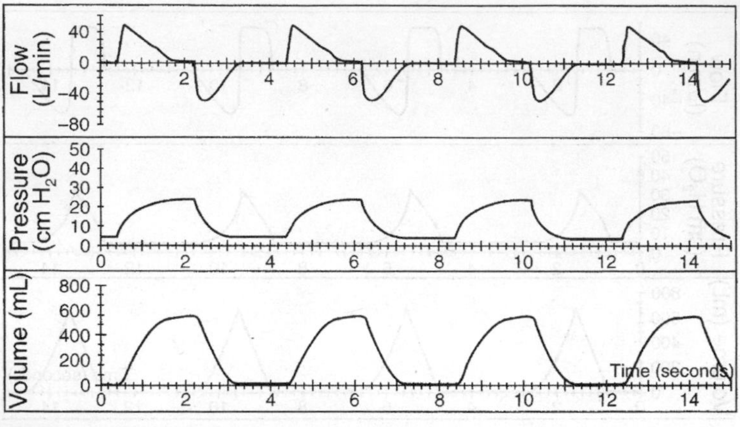

FIGURE 5.6 Pressure-controlled ventilation.

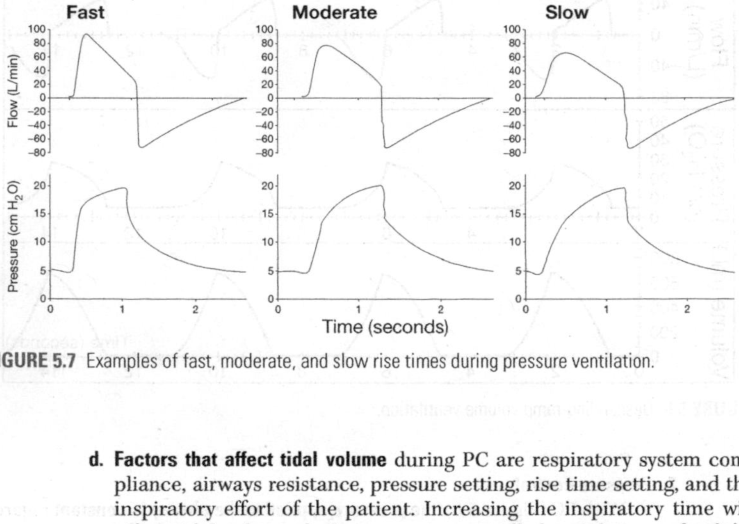

FIGURE 5.7 Examples of fast, moderate, and slow rise times during pressure ventilation.

d. **Factors that affect tidal volume** during PC are respiratory system compliance, airways resistance, pressure setting, rise time setting, and the inspiratory effort of the patient. Increasing the inspiratory time will affect tidal volume during pressure-controlled ventilation only if the end-inspiratory flow is not zero. Once the flow decreases to zero, no additional volume is delivered.

e. Unlike VC, **inspiratory flow is affected by patient effort**—increased patient effort will increase the flow from the ventilator and thereby the delivered tidal volume. This may improve patient-ventilator synchrony, but results in unpredictable tidal volumes and the potential for overdistension.

f. With PC, **the inspiratory time is set** on the ventilator.

1. If the inspiratory time is set to be longer than the expiratory time, pressure-controlled inverse ratio ventilation (PCIRV) results. This strategy has been used to improve oxygenation in patients with ARDS but has generally fallen out of favor in recent years because it has not been shown to improve patient outcomes and can adversely affect hemodynamics.

2. PC can be desirable for improving patient-ventilator synchrony but this is controversial. It is also used as an alternative to PS when a fixed inspiratory time or rate is desired.

3. **Adaptive control**

a. With adaptive control, the breath is ventilator- or patient triggered, pressure limited, and ventilator- or patient cycled. With adaptive PC, the pressure limit is not constant, but varies breath to breath on the basis of a comparison of the set and delivered tidal volume.

b. Although the ventilator is capable of controlling only pressure or volume at any time, adaptive control combines features of PC (variable flow) and VC (constant tidal volume) (Table 5.1).

c. **Pressure-regulated volume control (PRVC on Servo, Viasys, NKV-550), AutoFlow (Draeger), and VC+ (Puritan-Bennett)** are trade names that function in a similar manner. With this form of adaptive PC, the PC level increases or decreases in an attempt to deliver the desired tidal volume.

d. With **volume support (VS)**, the PS level varies on a breath-to-breath basis to maintain a desired tidal volume. Each breath is patient triggered. If the patient's effort increases (increased tidal volume for the set level of pressure support ventilation [PSV]), the ventilator decreases the support of the next breath. If the compliance or patient effort decreases, the ventilator increases the support to maintain the set volume. This combines the attributes of PSV with the guaranteed minimum tidal volume.

e. The clinical utility of adaptive control is yet to be determined and has potential drawbacks:

1. Tidal volumes may exceed the desired tidal volume if the patient makes vigorous inspiratory efforts, which could result in overdistension lung injury.
2. If the tidal volume exceeds the target volume, the ventilator will decrease the level of PS. This may increase the patient's WoB in the setting of increased respiratory demand.
3. If the lungs become stiffer (ie, compliance decreases) and the tidal volume does not meet the target, the ventilator will increase the pressure, which could result in overdistension lung injury.

4. The choice of VC, PC, or adaptive control usually is the result of clinician familiarity, institutional preferences, and personal bias.

C. **Cycle** is the variable that terminates inspiration, which is commonly time (VC or PC) or flow (PSV).

VI. BREATH TYPES DURING MECHANICAL VENTILATION

A. **Spontaneous Breaths** are triggered and cycled by the patient.

B. **Mandatory Breaths** are either triggered by the ventilator or the patient and cycled by the ventilator.

VII. MODES OF VENTILATION

The combination of the various possible breath types and phase variables determines the mode of ventilation (Table 5.1). There are many modes of ventilation, and their nomenclature can be confusing because manufacturers often use different names for similar ventilation modes. Only a few of the more commonly used modes are discussed in the following section.

A. Continuous Mandatory Ventilation (CMV) or Assist-Control (A/C) Ventilation

1. Every breath is a mandatory breath type (Figure 5.8). Although CMV is more descriptive, the terms CMV and A/C are used interchangeably.
2. **The patient can trigger** additional breaths but always receives at least the set respiratory rate.

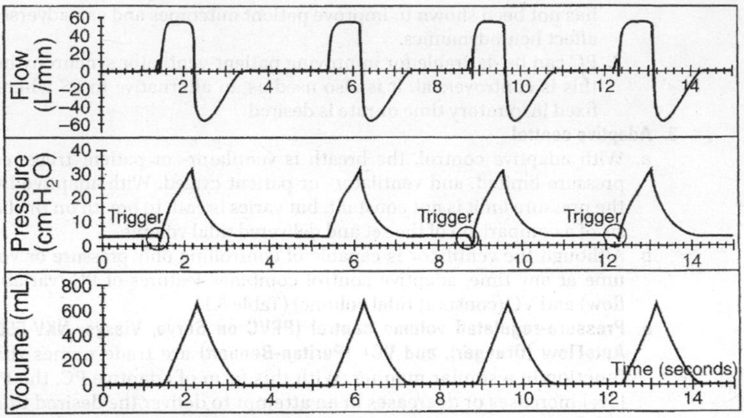

FIGURE 5.8 Continuous mandatory ventilation (assist-control ventilation).

3. All breaths, whether ventilator triggered or patient triggered, are VC, PC, or adaptive control (ie, all breaths are the same).
4. Triggering at a rapid rate may result in hyperventilation, hypotension, and dynamic hyperinflation (auto-PEEP).

B. Continuous Spontaneous Ventilation: With continuous spontaneous ventilation modes, all breaths are triggered and cycled by the patient. There is no set rate, inspiratory time, or expiratory time. If the patient effort ceases (ie, due to sedation, clinical deterioration) for a predetermined time interval (apnea delay), the ventilator will deliver support in an A/C mode.

1. **Continuous positive airway pressure:** During CPAP, the ventilator provides no inspiratory assist.
   a. Strictly speaking, CPAP applies a positive pressure to the airway. However, current ventilators allow the patient to breathe spontaneously without applying positive pressure to the airway (CPAP = 0).
   b. CPAP can be applied to an endotracheal tube/tracheostomy tube (invasive) or to a face mask (noninvasive).
2. **Pressure support (PS)**
   a. **The patient's inspiratory effort is assisted** by the ventilator at a preset pressure with PS. All breaths are spontaneous breath types (Figure 5.9) and supported by equal inspiratory pressure level.
   b. A pressure **rise time** can be set during PS, similar to PC ventilation.
   c. Because the ventilator delivers only patient-triggered breaths, appropriate apnea alarms must be set on the ventilator. The lack of a backup rate may result in apnea and sleep-disordered breathing in some patients.
   d. The ventilator cycles to the expiratory phase when the flow decreases to a predetermined value (eg, 5 L/min or 25% of the peak inspiratory flow). **If the patient actively exhales**, the ventilator may pressure cycle to the expiratory phase. The ventilator may not cycle correctly **in the presence of a leak** (eg, bronchopleural fistula or mask leak with NIV). A secondary time cycle will terminate inspiration at 3 to 5 seconds (depending on the ventilator, sometimes adjustable).
   e. Some ventilators allow the clinician to **adjust the flow cycle** criteria during PS (Figure 5.10). This allows adjustment of the inspiratory time to better coincide with the patient's neural inspiration (thus avoiding active exhalation or double triggering). If the ventilator is set to cycle at a greater percentage of peak flow, the inspiratory time is decreased.

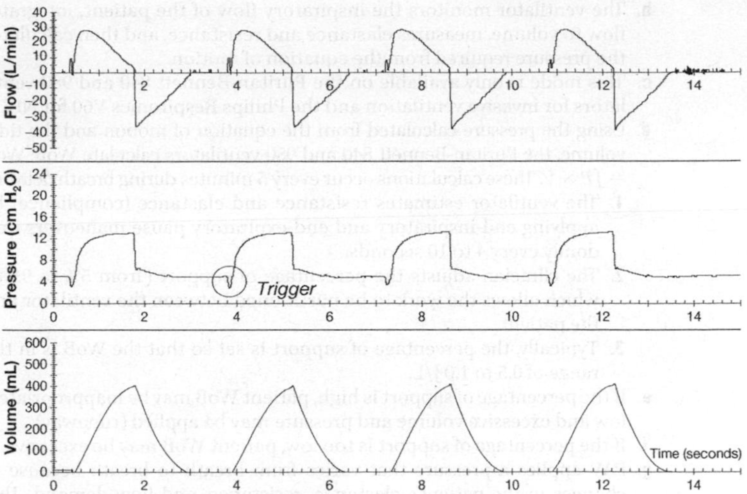

FIGURE 5.9 Pressure support ventilation.

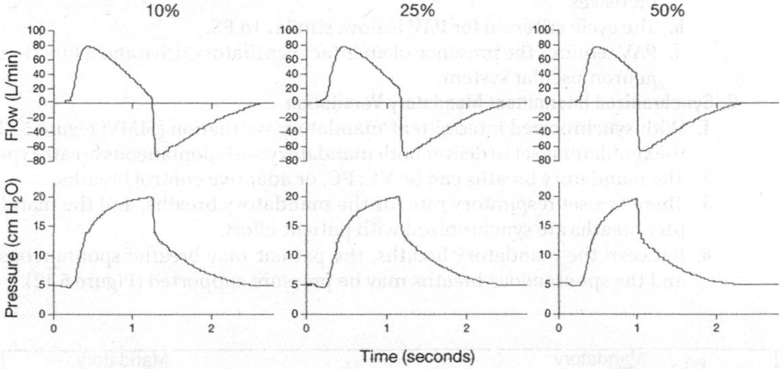

FIGURE 5.10 Examples of pressure support ventilation with termination flows of 10%, 25%, and 50% of peak flow.

Conversely, if the ventilator is set to cycle at a lower percentage of the peak flow, the inspiratory time is increased. As a general rule, a higher flow cycle is necessary for obstructive lung disease and a lower flow cycle is necessary for restrictive lung disease (eg, patients recovering from acute lung injury [ALI]).

f. The tidal volume, inspiratory flow, inspiratory time, and respiratory rate may vary from breath to breath with PS.

g. **Tidal volume** is determined by the level of PS, rise time, lung mechanics, and the inspiratory effort of the patient.

h. With a strong respiratory drive, the resultant tidal volume and transpulmonary pressure may not be lung protective.

3. Proportional assist ventilation

a. Proportional assist ventilation (PAV) provides ventilatory support as a proportion of the patient's calculated WoB.

b. The ventilator monitors the inspiratory flow of the patient, integrates flow to volume, measures elastance and resistance, and then calculates the pressure required from the equation of motion.
c. This mode is only available on the Puritan-Bennett 840 and 980 ventilators for invasive ventilation and the Philips Respironics V60 for NIV.
d. Using the pressure calculated from the equation of motion and the tidal volume, the Puritan-Bennett 840 and 980 ventilators calculate WoB: WoB $= \int P \times V$. These calculations occur every 5 minutes during breath delivery.
   1. The ventilator estimates resistance and elastance (compliance) by applying end-inspiratory and end-expiratory pause maneuvers randomly every 4 to 10 seconds.
   2. The clinician adjusts the percentage of support (from 5% to 95%), which allows the work to be partitioned between the ventilator and the patient.
   3. Typically, the percentage of support is set so that the WoB is in the range of 0.5 to 1.0 J/L.
e. If the percentage of support is high, patient WoB may be inappropriately low and excessive volume and pressure may be applied (runaway).
f. If the percentage of support is too low, patient WoB may be excessive.
g. PAV applies a pressure that varies from breath to breath because of changes in the patient's elastance, resistance, and flow demand. This differs from PS, in which the level of support is constant regardless of demand, and VC, in which the level of support decreases when demand increases.
h. The cycle criterion for PAV is flow, similar to PS.
i. PAV requires the presence of an intact ventilatory drive and a functional neuromuscular system.

C. Synchronized Intermittent Mandatory Ventilation

1. With synchronized intermittent mandatory ventilation (SIMV; Figure 5.11), the ventilator is set to deliver both mandatory and spontaneous breath types.
2. The mandatory breaths can be VC, PC, or adaptive control breaths.
3. There is a set respiratory rate for the mandatory breaths, and the mandatory breaths are synchronized with patient effort.
4. Between the mandatory breaths, the patient may breathe spontaneously and the spontaneous breaths may be pressure supported (Figure 5.12).

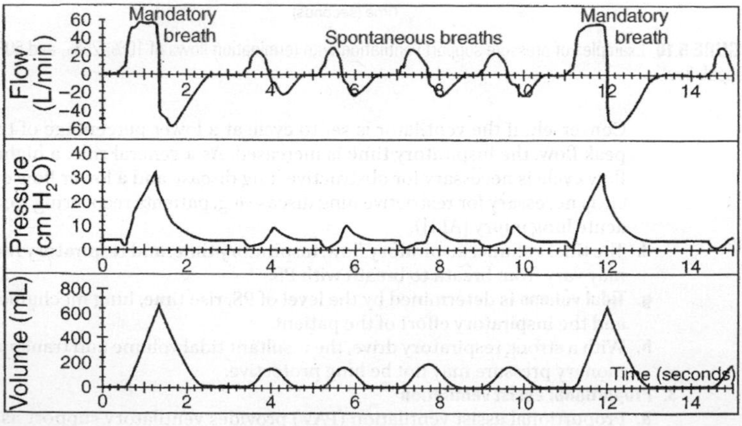

FIGURE 5.11 Synchronized intermittent mandatory ventilation.

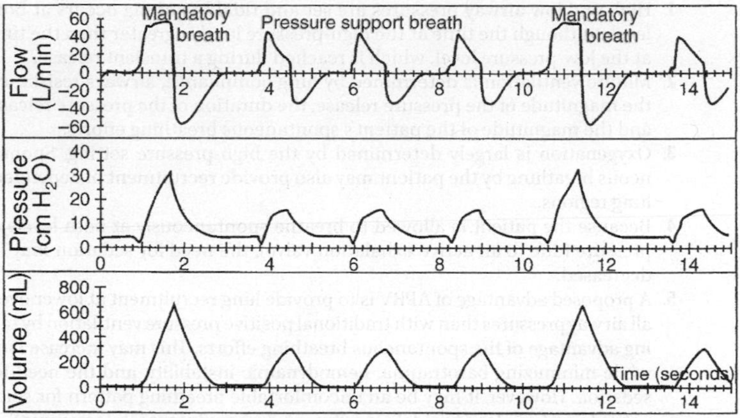

FIGURE 5.12 Synchronized intermittent mandatory ventilation with pressure support.

5. The patient's inspiratory efforts may be as great during the mandatory breaths as the spontaneous breaths. It is therefore a myth that SIMV rests the patient during the mandatory breaths and allows active contraction of the muscles of the respiratory system only during spontaneous breaths.
6. The different breath types during SIMV may induce patient-ventilator asynchrony.
7. Note that CMV and SIMV become synonymous if the patient is not triggering the ventilator (eg, with neuromuscular blockade).

D. Airway Pressure Release Ventilation (APRV) allows spontaneous breathing at alternating high and low CPAP levels (Figure 5.13). On some ventilators, APRV is achieved using modes called BiLevel (Puritan-Bennett) or BiVent (Maquet).

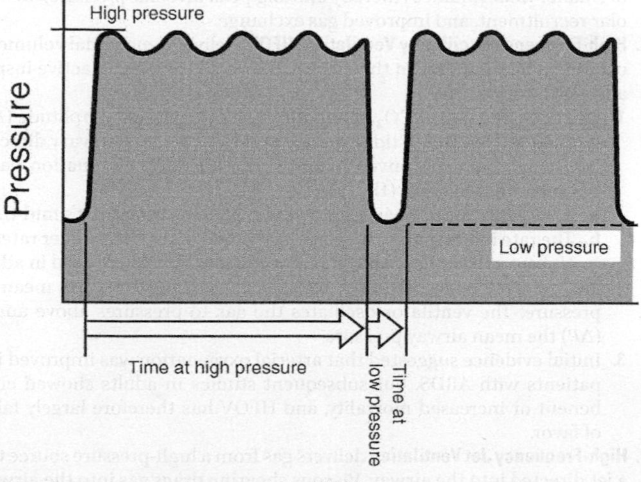

FIGURE 5.13 Airway pressure release ventilation (APRV).

1. High and low airway pressures are set and tidal breathing occurs at both levels, although the time at the high-pressure level is greater than the time at the low-pressure level, which is reached during a transient release.
2. Minute ventilation is determined by lung compliance, airways resistance, the magnitude of the pressure release, the duration of the pressure release, and the magnitude of the patient's spontaneous breathing efforts.
3. Oxygenation is largely determined by the high-pressure setting. Spontaneous breathing by the patient may also provide recruitment of dependent lung regions.
4. Because the patient is allowed to breathe spontaneously at both levels of pressure (due to an active exhalation valve), the need for sedation may be decreased.
5. A proposed advantage of APRV is to provide lung recruitment at lower overall airway pressures than with traditional positive pressure ventilation by taking advantage of the spontaneous breathing efforts. This may increase $Pa{O_2}$ while minimizing barotrauma, hemodynamic instability, and the need for sedation. However, it may be an uncomfortable breathing pattern for some patients and can lead to tidal recruitment-derecruitment (atelectrauma).
6. Of concern is the potential for overdistension during tidal breathing at the high-pressure level.
7. Depending on the ventilator brand, APRV may be applied using BiLevel, BIPAP, BiVent, BiPhasic, PCV+, or DuoPAP.
8. Evidence is lacking for improved outcomes with the use of APRV.

E. The choice of the mode of ventilation depends on the capability of the ventilator, the experience and preference of the clinician, and, most important, the needs of the patient. Rather than relying on a single best mode of ventilation, one should determine the mode that is most appropriate for each individual situation. However, the more complex and adaptive modes of ventilation have not consistently been shown to improve outcomes.

VIII. HIGH-FREQUENCY VENTILATION

A. With high-frequency ventilation (HFV), the patient is ventilated with higher than normal rates (ie, >60/min) and smaller tidal volumes (<5 mL/kg).

B. Theoretic advantages include a lower risk of alveolar overdistension because of smaller tidal volumes (thereby limiting peak alveolar pressure), better alveolar recruitment, and improved gas exchange.

C. **High-Frequency Oscillatory Ventilation (HFOV)** delivers small tidal volumes by oscillating a bias gas flow in the airway. The oscillator has an active inspiratory and expiratory phase.

1. The determinants of CO_2 elimination are the pressure amplitude (ΔP) and frequency (Hz). HFOV tidal volume and CO_2 elimination vary directly with ΔP. In contrast to conventional ventilation, CO_2 elimination varies inversely with frequency (Hz).
    a. ΔP is set to induce wiggling that is visible to the patient's mid-thigh.
    b. The rate is adjustable from 3 to 15 Hz (180-900/min). Higher rates (12-15 Hz) are used in neonates and lower rates (3-6 Hz) are used in adults.
2. The primary determinant of oxygenation during HFOV is mean airway pressure. The ventilator oscillates the gas to pressures above and below (ΔP) the mean airway pressure.
3. Initial evidence suggested that arterial oxygenation was improved in some patients with ARDS, but subsequent studies in adults showed either no benefit or increased mortality, and HFOV has therefore largely fallen out of favor.

D. **High-Frequency Jet Ventilation** delivers gas from a high-pressure source through a jet directed into the airway. Viscous shearing drags gas into the airway.

1. Tidal volume is determined by the driving pressure, inspiratory time, catheter size, and respiratory system mechanics.
2. Mean airway pressure is controlled by driving pressure, inspiratory:expiratory (I:E) ratio, and PEEP.
3. High-frequency jet ventilation uses rates of 240 to 660 breaths/min.
4. In the United States, jet ventilators are occasionally used in operating rooms and neonatal ICUs, but rarely used in adult ICUs.

E. High-Frequency Percussive Ventilation, also called volumetric diffusive respiration, uses a sliding nongated venturi to separate inspired and expired gases and provide PEEP. It is commercially available only on the Percussionaire volumetric diffusive respirator (VDR) ventilator.

1. Minute ventilation is controlled by respiratory rate and peak inspiratory pressure.
2. Respiratory rates of 180 to 600 breaths/min are used.
3. Oxygenation is determined by peak inspiratory pressure, I:E ratio, and PEEP.
4. High-frequency percussive ventilation has popularity in the care of patients with burn injury despite lack of high-level evidence reporting better outcomes.

IX. SPECIFIC VENTILATOR SETTINGS

A. A Tidal Volume target of 4 to 8 mL/kg predicted body weight (PBW) is used. Ideal body weight (IBW) is determined by the height and sex of the patient. The terms predicted body weight (PBW) and ideal body weight (IBW) can be used synonymously.

$$\text{Male patients: PBW} = 50 + 2.3 \times [\text{height (inches)} - 60]$$

$$\text{Female patients: PBW} = 45.5 + 2.3 \times [\text{height (inches)} - 60]$$

1. Lower tidal volumes decrease the risk and extent of alveolar overdistension and **ventilator-induced lung injury (VILI)**.
2. Use a tidal volume of 6 mL/kg (4-8 mL/kg) for patients with **ARDS**.
3. Accumulating *evidence supports the use of tidal volumes* of less than 8 mL/kg for all patients who are mechanically ventilated.
4. Monitor the **Pplat** and consider tidal volume reduction if the Pplat is greater than 30 cm H_2O.
   a. Because lung injury is a function of transalveolar pressure, a higher Pplat may be acceptable if pleural pressure is increased (eg, obesity or abdominal hypertension).
   b. Lower Pplat is desirable and may be associated with improved outcomes.
   c. With a strong inspiratory effort, transalveolar pressure may be injurious despite that airway pressure is acceptable (eg, during PC or PS).
5. Tidal volume may also be adjusted to minimize **driving pressure** (Pplat − PEEP). An individual subject meta-analysis suggests that tidal volume and PEEP should be selected such that the driving pressure is less than 15 cm H_2O; a higher driving pressure increases the mortality risk.

B. Respiratory Rate

1. The respiratory rate and tidal volume determine **minute ventilation.**
2. Set the rate at 15 to 25/min to achieve a minute ventilation of 8 to 12 L/min.
   a. With low tidal volumes and a low pH, a higher respiratory rate may be necessary.
   b. A lower respiratory rate (and longer expiratory phase) may be necessary to avoid air trapping and dynamic hyperinflation.
   c. In the recovery phase, spontaneous modes (eg, PS, PAV) can be used to allow the patients to choose their own respiratory rate.

3. Adjust the rate to achieve the desired pH and $PaCO_2$.
4. **A high minute ventilation** (>10 L/min) requirement may be required for increased carbon dioxide production or high dead space.

C. **I:E Ratio**

1. **Inspiratory time** can be directly set or determined by flow, tidal volume, and flow pattern; it is not directly set with all modes of ventilation.
2. **Expiratory time** is determined by the inspiratory time and respiratory rate and is not directly set in any mode of ventilation.
3. The expiratory time generally should be longer than the inspiratory time (eg, I:E of 1:2).
4. **The expiratory time should be lengthened** (eg, higher inspiratory flow, lower tidal volume, lower respiratory rate) if positive pressure ventilation causes a blood pressure drop or if auto-PEEP is present. If air trapping is significant and accompanied by an acute drop in blood pressure, the patient may be temporarily disconnected from the ventilator (about 30 seconds) to allow exhalation and then reconnected. If such maneuver is therapeutic, ventilator settings should be adjusted to reduce auto-PEEP and resultant hemodynamic compromise.
5. **Inspiratory time can be lengthened** to increase mean airway pressure and may thus improve oxygenation in some patients by limiting derecruitment.
   a. With other options to increase mean airway pressure (eg, increased PEEP), there is little role for an inverse I:E (ie, inspiratory time longer than expiratory time).
   b. When long inspiratory times are used, auto-PEEP can develop and hemodynamics must be closely monitored.

D. **Oxygen Concentration (FIO_2)**

1. Initiate mechanical ventilation with an FIO_2 of 1.0.
2. Titrate the FIO_2 using pulse oximetry. A target SpO_2 of 88% to 95% is usually acceptable.
3. Severe, persistent hypoxemia (requiring FIO_2 >0.60) usually indicates the presence of shunt (intrapulmonary or intracardiac).

E. **Positive End-Expiratory Pressure**

1. **Appropriate levels of PEEP** increase the functional respiratory capacity, decrease intrapulmonary shunt, and improve lung compliance (by preventing derecruitment).
   a. Because lung volumes are typically decreased with acute respiratory failure, it is reasonable to use a PEEP of at least 5 cm H_2O with the initiation of mechanical ventilation for most patients.
   b. **Maintaining alveolar recruitment** in disease processes such as ARDS may decrease the likelihood of ventilator-associated lung injury.
   c. Although higher levels of PEEP often increase PaO_2, evidence has not shown that higher levels of PEEP (compared with modest levels of PEEP) decrease mortality.
2. A number of methods have been used to titrate the best level of PEEP in patients with ALI.
   a. PEEP can be titrated with a goal to allow a decrease in FIO_2 to 0.6 or less.
   b. PEEP can be set according to a table of FIO_2/PEEP combinations to achieve an SpO_2 of 88% to 95%, as was done in the ARDSNet trials.
   c. PEEP can be set 2 to 3 cm H_2O above the lower inflexion point of the pressure-volume curve to prevent end-tidal derecruitment. However, this is difficult to measure reliably in patients who are critically ill.
   d. PEEP can be set to achieve the best respiratory system compliance. The best compliance can be determined from either an incremental or a decremental PEEP trial. A decremental PEEP trial may theoretically achieve a greater lung volume for a given level of PEEP but may result in progressive derecruitment over time if adequate time for equilibration is not spent at each PEEP level.

e. PEEP can be adjusted to the best stress index, as assessed from the slope of the pressure-time curve during constant-flow volume ventilation. This may require special software and can be difficult to estimate at the bedside.

f. PEEP can be titrated with an esophageal balloon in place to measure esophageal pressure (Pes) as a proxy for pleural pressure. The goal with this method is to set PEEP equal to or greater than Pes to prevent end-tidal derecruitment.

g. PEEP can be titrated by monitoring percentage of inflation and ventilation distribution via electrical impedance tomography (EIT).

h. There is little evidence that any approach to setting PEEP is superior to another in terms of patient outcomes.

i. Modest levels of PEEP (8-12 cm H_2O) should be used for mild ARDS and higher levels of PEEP (12-20 cm H_2O) should be used for moderate and severe ARDS.

3. In patients with COPD, PEEP may be used to counterbalance auto-PEEP, thereby decreasing the WoB and improving the patient's ability to trigger the ventilator.

4. In patients with left ventricular failure, PEEP may improve cardiac performance by decreasing venous return and left ventricular afterload.

5. Adverse effects of PEEP

a. PEEP may **decrease cardiac output** by decreasing venous return. Hemodynamics should be monitored during PEEP titration.

b. High levels of PEEP may result in **alveolar overdistension** during the inspiratory phase. It may be necessary to decrease the tidal volume with high PEEP.

c. PEEP may **worsen oxygenation with focal lung disease** because it results in a redistribution of pulmonary blood flow from overdistended lung units to the unventilated lung units. PEEP may also worsen oxygenation with cardiac shunt (eg, patent foramen ovale).

X. COMPLICATIONS OF MECHANICAL VENTILATION

A. Ventilator-Induced Lung Injury

1. Overdistension injury (volutrauma) occurs if the lung parenchyma is subjected to an abnormally high transpulmonary pressure.

a. Overdistension injury produces inflammation and increased alveolar-capillary membrane permeability.

b. Tidal volume should be limited to 4 to 8 mL/kg of IBW (yet lower 4-6 mL/kg of IBW in patients with ALI/ARDS) and Pplat limited to 30 cm H_2O (or lower) to prevent overdistension injury.

c. Because the risk of overdistension lung injury is related to transpulmonary pressure, higher Pplats may be acceptable if pleural pressure is increased (eg, abdominal distension, chest wall burns, chest wall edema, obesity).

2. Pressure-related injury (barotrauma) occurs when the airways and alveoli are subjected to high transmural pressures, resulting in extravasation of gas through the bronchovascular sheath into the pulmonary interstitium, mediastinum, pericardium, peritoneum, pleural space, and subcutaneous tissue.

a. Manifestations of barotrauma include **tension pneumothorax**, which should be suspected if there is a sudden increase in peak inspiratory pressure or sudden desaturation or hemodynamic instability in a patient who is mechanically ventilated.

b. Barotrauma can occur with spontaneous breathing (eg, spontaneous pneumothorax in status asthmaticus) but is classically associated with high airway pressures in a patient who is mechanically ventilated.

c. High transpulmonary pressures may promote alveolar injury **in the absence of high airway pressures** (eg, strong inspiratory effort on PC or PS).

3. Derecruitment injury (atelectrauma) occurs if there is cyclic alveolar opening and closing with tidal breathing.

- **a.** This injury may be avoided using appropriate levels of PEEP to maintain alveolar recruitment. In ARDS, this may require 8 to 20 cm H_2O, and sometimes more depending on pleural pressure.

4. Oxygen toxicity

- **a.** High concentrations of oxygen for long periods may cause lung damage, worsen $\dot{V}/\dot{Q}$ matching, and promote atelectasis.
- **b.** Although the precise role of oxygen toxicity in patients with respiratory failure is unclear, it is prudent to reduce the FIO_2 to the minimum necessary to maintain adequate arterial oxygenation (usually SpO_2 88%-95%), although some patients tolerate lower SpO_2.
- **c.** Appropriate levels of inspired oxygen should never be withheld for fear of oxygen toxicity.

B. Patient-Ventilator Asynchrony

1. Trigger asynchrony refers to the inability of the patient to trigger the ventilator.

- **a.** Trigger asynchrony may be due to an **insensitive trigger setting** on the ventilator, which is corrected by adjusting the trigger sensitivity. This is commonly seen in patients with neuromuscular diseases or critical illness myopathy.
- **b.** Flow trigger instead of pressure trigger can be tried, although this rarely solves the problem.
- **c.** A common cause of trigger asynchrony is the presence of **auto-PEEP**. If auto-PEEP is present, the patient must generate enough inspiratory effort to overcome the auto-PEEP before triggering can occur. This can be addressed by reducing the auto-PEEP (eg, administer bronchodilators, increase expiratory time). Setting the extrinsic PEEP to equal auto-PEEP can improve trigger synchrony.
- **d.** Autotrigger is another form of asynchrony. In this case, the ventilator is triggered by an artifact other than the patient's inspiratory effort. Examples include oscillations in the flow or pressure at the proximal airway due to the heart beating against the lungs or a leak causing the airway flow or pressure to change.

2. Flow asynchrony

- **a.** During VC, flow is fixed and may not meet the patient's inspiratory flow demands. The inspiratory pressure waveform will demonstrate a characteristic scalloped pattern if the patient makes excessive inspiratory effort.
- **b.** Flow asynchrony may be improved during VC ventilation by increasing the inspiratory flow or changing the inspiratory flow pattern.
- **c.** Changing VC to PC or PS, in which flows are variable, may also be helpful. However, this runs the risk of overdistension due to high tidal volumes if the patient generates a strong inspiratory effort.

3. Cycle asynchrony occurs when the patient's expiratory effort begins before or after the end of the inspiratory phase set on the ventilator. Cycle asynchrony can occur if the inspiratory time is inappropriately short or long. This is corrected by adjusting the inspiratory time.

- **a.** If the inspiratory flow is too high or the inspiratory time setting is too short, the patient may double trigger the ventilator.
  - **1.** This can be addressed during VC by reducing the flow setting or adding an inspiratory pause.
  - **2.** During PC, this can be addressed by setting a longer inspiratory time.
- **b.** If the inspiratory flow is too low or the inspiratory time setting is too long, the patient may actively exhale.
  - **1.** This can be addressed during VC using a higher inspiratory flow.
  - **2.** On PC, this is addressed by setting a shorter inspiratory time.
- **c.** When PSV is used in patients with high airways resistance and high lung compliance (eg, COPD), it may take a long time for inspiratory flow

to decrease to the flow cycle criteria set in the ventilator. The patient may therefore actively exhale to terminate the inspiratory phase.

1. This can be corrected using a PC rather than a PS setting. The inspiratory time is then set so that inspiratory flow does not reach zero.

2. Most ventilators allow the clinician to adjust the termination flow during PS to improve synchrony.

3. This problem may improve with the use of a lower PS setting.

4. Reducing airways resistance (eg, with bronchodilators, secretion clearance) can resolve this problem.

4. Asynchrony can be the result of acidosis, pain, and anxiety. These nonventilator factors should also be considered when asynchrony is present. Sedation and paralysis may be required in some patients.

C. Auto-PEEP

1. Auto-PEEP is the result of gas trapping (dynamic hyperinflation) due to insufficient expiratory time and/or increased expiratory airflow resistance. The pressure exerted by this trapped gas is called auto-PEEP or intrinsic PEEP.

2. The increase in alveolar pressure due to auto-PEEP may adversely affect hemodynamics by reducing venous return.

3. The presence of auto-PEEP can produce trigger dyssynchrony, as discussed earlier.

4. Detection of auto-PEEP

a. Some ventilators allow auto-PEEP to be measured directly.

b. In patients who are spontaneously breathing, auto-PEEP can be measured using an **esophageal balloon.**

c. The **patient's breathing pattern** can be observed. If exhalation is still occurring when the next breath is delivered, auto-PEEP is present.

d. If flow graphics is available on the ventilator, it can be observed that **expiratory flow** does not return to zero before the subsequent breath is delivered.

e. Inspiratory efforts **that do not trigger the ventilator** suggest the presence of auto-PEEP.

5. Factors affecting auto-PEEP

a. Physiologic factors: A high airways resistance increases the likelihood of auto-PEEP.

b. Ventilator factors: A high tidal volume, high respiratory rate, or prolonged inspiratory time increases the likelihood of auto-PEEP. Reducing minute ventilation and increasing expiratory time decreases the likelihood of auto-PEEP.

D. Hemodynamic Perturbations

1. Positive pressure ventilation increases intrathoracic pressure and **decreases venous return.** Right ventricular filling is limited by the reduced venous return and cardiac output therefore decreases.

2. When alveolar pressure exceeds pulmonary venous pressure, pulmonary blood flow is affected by alveolar pressure rather than left atrial pressure, producing an **increase in pulmonary vascular resistance.** Consequently, right ventricular afterload increases and right ventricular ejection fraction falls.

3. Left ventricular filling is limited by reduced right ventricular output and decreased left ventricular diastolic compliance.

4. Increased right ventricular size affects left ventricular performance by shifting the interventricular septum to the left.

5. Intravascular volume resuscitation counteracts the negative hemodynamic effects of PEEP.

6. Increased intrathoracic pressure may **improve left ventricular ejection fraction and stroke volume, reducing afterload.** This beneficial effect may be significant in patients with poor ventricular function.

E. Infection-Related, Ventilator-Associated Complications: See **Chapter 12.**

Selected Readings

Amato MBP, Meade MO, Slutsky AS, et al. Driving pressure and survival in the acute respiratory distress syndrome. *N Engl J Med.* 2015;372:747-755.

Branson RD, Johannigman JA. What is the evidence base for the newer ventilation modes? *Respir Care.* 2004;49:742-760.

Brower RG, Lanken PN, MacIntyre N, et al. Higher versus lower positive end-expiratory pressures in patients with the acute respiratory distress syndrome. *N Engl J Med.* 2004;351:327-336.

Chatburn RL. Classification of ventilator modes: update and proposal for implementation. *Respir Care.* 2007;52:301-323.

Dhand R. Inhalation therapy in invasive and noninvasive mechanical ventilation. *Curr Opin Crit Care.* 2007;13:27-38.

Fan E, Needham DM, Stewart TE. Ventilatory management of acute lung injury and acute respiratory distress syndrome. *JAMA.* 2005;294:2889-2896.

Ferguson ND, Cook DJ, Guyatt GH, et al. High-frequency oscillation in early acute respiratory distress syndrome. *N Engl J Med.* 2013;368:795-805.

Habashi NM. Other approaches to open-lung ventilation: airway pressure release ventilation. *Crit Care Med.* 2005;33(3 suppl):S228-S240.

Hess DR. Ventilator waveforms and the physiology of pressure support ventilation. *Respir Care.* 2005;50:166-186.

Hess DR, Thompson BT. Patient-ventilator dyssynchrony during lung protective ventilation: what's a clinician to do? *Crit Care Med.* 2006;34:231-233.

Lellouche F, Mancebo J, Jolliet P, et al. A multicenter randomized trial of computer-driven protocolized weaning from mechanical ventilation. *Am J Respir Crit Care Med.* 2006;174:894-900.

MacIntyre NR. Is there a best way to set positive expiratory-end pressure for mechanical ventilatory support in acute lung injury? *Clin Chest Med.* 2008;29:233-239.

Meade MO, Cook DJ, Guyatt GH, et al. Ventilation strategy using low tidal volumes, recruitment maneuvers, and high positive end-expiratory pressure for acute lung injury and acute respiratory distress syndrome: a randomized controlled trial. *JAMA.* 2008;299:637-645.

Mercat A, Richard JC, Vielle B, et al. Positive end-expiratory pressure setting in adults with acute lung injury and acute respiratory distress syndrome: a randomized controlled trial. *JAMA.* 2008;299:646-655.

Myers TR, MacIntyre NR. Respiratory controversies in the critical care setting. Does airway pressure release ventilation offer important new advantages in mechanical ventilator support? *Respir Care.* 2007;52:452-460.

NIH/NHLBI ARDS Network. Ventilation with lower tidal volumes as compared with traditional tidal volumes for acute lung injury and the acute respiratory distress syndrome. *N Engl J Med.* 2000;342:1301-1308.

Nilsestuen JO, Hargett KD. Using ventilator graphics to identify patient-ventilator asynchrony. *Respir Care.* 2005;50:202-234.

Ramnath VR, Hess DR, Thompson BT. Conventional mechanical ventilation in acute lung injury and acute respiratory distress syndrome. *Clin Chest Med.* 2006;27:601-613.

6

Hemodynamic Management

Diana Barragan Bradford and Aranya Bagchi

I. HEMODYNAMIC PERTURBATIONS

Hemodynamic perturbations are common during intensive care unit (ICU) admission. Both hypotensive and hypertensive emergencies threaten cardiovascular system's ability to provide sufficient oxygen and metabolic substrates to meet the demands of the body's tissues. In the event that supply is insufficient to meet demand, pathophysiologic alterations lead to the clinical manifestations of progressive end-organ damage, be it neurologic, cardiovascular, pulmonary, renal, gastrointestinal, hematologic, or musculocutaneous. The goal of the hemodynamic management of such patients is to maintain end-organ oxygenation and perfusion in order to preserve function.

II. SHOCK

It is a state of inadequate tissue perfusion, leading to tissue hypoxia and organ dysfunction. In its early stages, shock may be *compensated*: potent neurohumoral reflexes, including activation of the sympathetic nervous system and the renin-angiotensin-aldosterone system, act to maintain a supply of oxygen sufficient to meet cellular demands. With the failure of these reflexes, however, shock becomes *progressive* and, ultimately, *irreversible*: as demand for intracellular energy outstrips supply, anaerobic metabolism predominates and lactic acid production rises, membrane-associated ion transport pumps fail, the integrity of cell membranes is compromised, and cell death ensues. Shock is classified according to one of four mechanisms: hypovolemic, cardiogenic, obstructive, or distributive. The first three mechanisms may be categorized as states of *hypodynamic* shock, whereas the last may be categorized as a state of *hyperdynamic* shock. It is important to emphasize that multiple mechanisms of shock may coexist in one patient—for example, a patient with poor cardiac function may also be vasoplegic. Therefore, in addition to the traditional classification of shock, it may be useful to identify the primary physiologic derangements causing shock in that patient. The basic determinants of hemodynamics are heart rate, rhythm, preload (right heart vs left heart), systemic vascular resistance, pulmonary vascular resistance, and myocardial contractility. For example, two patients with a similarly low cardiac output and cardiogenic shock, but one with predominantly right ventricular dysfunction and the other with left ventricular dysfunction, will need to be managed differently—the identification of primary physiologic derangements in each case may help personalize the management of shock. Table 6.1 shows typical physiologic derangements in the different types of shock.

A. Types of Shock

1. **Hypovolemic shock** occurs with the depletion of effective intravascular volume, due to insufficient intake, excessive loss, or both. Common causes include dehydration, acute hemorrhage, gastrointestinal and renal losses, and interstitial fluid redistribution occurring in the context of severe tissue trauma, burn injuries, or pancreatitis. Hemorrhage is the most common cause of shock in trauma patients. In the authors' experience, systems classification of hemorrhage, such as by the American College of Surgeons, provide little practical value. Following principles of damage control resuscitation are more useful in the management of hemorrhagic shock.

TABLE 6.1 Hemodynamic Parameters in Shock

Type of shock	Preload		Afterload		Contractility	
	Right ventricle (CVP)	Left ventricle (PAOP)	PVR	SVR	RV	Left ventricle
Hypovolemic	↓	↓	↔/↑	↑	↑	↑
Cardiogenic						
Predominantly RV failure	↑	↓	↔/↑	↑	↓	↔/↑
Predominantly LV failure	↑	↑	↑	↑	↔/↓	↓
Severe diastolic dysfunction	↑	↑	↔/↑	↔/↑	↔/↑	↔/↑
Obstructive						
Pulmonary embolism	↑	↓	↑	↑	↓	↔/↑
Cardiac tamponade	↑	↔/↑	↔/↑	↑	↔	↔
Distributive	↓	↓	↔/↑	↔/↓	↓	↓

CVP, central venous pressure; LV, left ventricle; PAOP, pulmonary artery occlusion pressure; PVR, pulmonary vascular resistance; RV, right ventricle; SVR, systemic vascular resistance.
The key hemodynamic findings in each category are highlighted in red. Note that although the **cardiac output** may increase in distributive shock (such as septic shock), **myocardial contractility** almost always decreases.

2. **Cardiogenic shock** is defined as persistent hypotension and inadequate tissue perfusion due to primary cardiac dysfunction occurring in the context of adequate intravascular volume and adequate or elevated left or right ventricular filling pressures. It may be caused by abnormalities of heart rate, rhythm, or contractility, although it occurs most commonly after extensive acute myocardial infarction (AMI) or ischemia leading to left or right ventricular failure. Other etiologies of cardiogenic shock include acute (eg, takotsubo) and chronic cardiomyopathies, myocarditis, and **myocardial contusion.**
3. **Obstructive shock** occurs as a result of an impediment to the normal flow of blood either to or from the heart, producing impairment of venous return or arterial outflow. Common causes include **tension pneumothorax, abdominal compartment syndrome, pulmonary embolism, and pericardial tamponade.** Uncontrolled and high levels of auto-PEEP may cause acute hypotension in certain circumstances.
4. **Distributive shock** is characterized by low afterload to the left ventricle (low systemic vascular resistance). Cardiac output may be impaired, normal or high. In the critical care setting, it is most commonly caused by sepsis. Other etiologies include neurogenic shock, anaphylaxis, adrenal insufficiency, hepatic failure, and high-output arteriovenous fistulae.

B. Monitoring in shock should be directed toward detecting, if not preventing, the progression of tissue hypoperfusion as well as toward assessing the adequacy of resuscitation. It is critical, although challenging, to accurately identify patients who are in subclinical shock (ie, those who have normal blood pressure but impaired tissue perfusion). Studies suggest that these patients are at a higher risk of dying than patients who are hypotensive but have preserved perfusion. The classification of shock proposed by the Society for

Cardiovascular Angiography and Intervention (SCAI) is one useful framework that can be applied to a broad range of patients, although it is designed specifically with cardiogenic shock in mind. It classifies shock into five categories—A (**At risk** for shock), B (**Beginning** shock), C (**Classical** shock), D (**Deteriorating** shock), and E (in **Extremis**). Figure 6.1 shows the stages of shock together with physiologic and laboratory correlates. Although some of the parameters described are more specific to cardiogenic shock, the scheme is useful in defining impaired tissue perfusion, which is applicable across all forms of shock.

It should be emphasized that most metrics used to monitor patients in shock are relatively insensitive and/or nonspecific. Clinicians should use as many data points as possible (history, physical examination, invasive monitoring, and laboratory data) in the management of their patients.

1. **Physical examination** of patients can be challenging and often unreliable. The authors' practice includes using point of care ultrasound (POCUS) to complement standard physical examination. Some clinical pearls: (a) a patient may have cool hands and feet, but if their calves and thighs are cool the clinician should be concerned; (b) A capillary refill time of greater than 3 seconds, and in particular, mottling of the skin are signs of concern.

SCAI Shock Classification (Modified)

SCAI SHOCK STAGE	DESCRIPTION	PHYSICAL EXAMINATION	BIOCHEMICAL MARKERS	HEMODYNAMICS
A At risk	Not currently experiencing signs or symptoms of CS, but at risk for its development	☐ Normal JVP ☐ Warm and well-perfused ☐ Strong distal pulses ☐ Normal mentation ☐ Clear lung sounds	☐ Normal lactate ☐ Normal (or at baseline) renal function	☐ SBP >100 mm Hg (or at baseline) ☐ CI ≥2.5 (if acute) ☐ CVP ≤10 ☐ PCWP ≤15 ☐ PA Sat ≥65%
B Beginning Shock	Clinical evidence of hemodynamic instability without hypoperfusion	☐ Elevated JVP (excluding hypovolemic shock) ☐ Warm and well-perfused ☐ Strong distal pulses ☐ Normal mentation ☐ Rales in lung fields	☐ Normal lactate ☐ Minimal acute renal function impairment ☐ Elevated BNP	☐ SBP <90 mm Hg, or MAP <60 mm Hg, or > 30 mm drop from baseline ☐ HR ≥100 bpm
C Classic Shock	Hypoperfusion requiring intervention (pharmacologic or mechanical) beyond volume resuscitation	☐ Volume overload (excluding hypovolemic shock) ☐ Altered mental status ☐ Cold and clammy ☐ Extensive rales ☐ Urine output <30 mL/h	☐ Lactate ≥2 ☐ CR 1.5 x baseline or >50% drop in GFR ☐ Increased LFTs ☐ Elevated BNP	☐ CI <2.2 (if invasive hemodynamics performed [strongly recommended]) ☐ PCWP >15
D Deteriorating	Failure of initial support strategy to restore perfusion	☐ Any of stage C and worsening (or not improving) signs/sx of hypoperfusion despite initial therapy	☐ Any of stage C and lactate rising and persistently ≥2 ☐ Deteriorating renal function ☐ Worsening LFTs ☐ Rising BNP	☐ Any of stage C and requiring escalating doses or increasing numbers of pressors or addition of MCS device to maintain perfusion
E Extremis	Acute or impending circulatory collapse	☐ Typically unconscious ☐ Near pulselessness ☐ Cardiac collapse ☐ Multiple defibrillations	☐ Lactate ≥8 ☐ CPR ☐ Severe acidosis (pH <7.2)	☐ Profound hypotension despite maximal hemodynamic support ☐ Need for bolus doses of vasopressors

FIGURE 6.1 Modified SCAI shock checklist. (Modified from Naidu SS, Baran DA, Jentzer JC, et al. SCAI SHOCK stage classification expert consensus update: a review and incorporation of validation studies. *J Am Coll Cardiol.* 2022;79(9):933-946, with permission from Elsevier.)

POCUS can be used to assess pulmonary edema (B lines), cardiac function, and central venous pressure (CVP) (based on inferior vena caval dynamics) more effectively than by physical examination. It is important to emphasize that patients who are hypoperfused (cool extremities, prolonged capillary refill time, and mottling) need expedited care. Available data strongly suggest that hypoperfused patients who are normotensive have worse outcomes than hypotensive patients who are adequately perfused. Standard monitors (continuous electrocardiogram [ECG], pulse oximetry, urinary output, noninvasive blood pressure, and temperature monitoring) should be used in every patient when possible. Some metrics (pulse oximeter-based oxygen saturation, capillary refill, and mottling) may be more prone to error in patients with dark skin—a higher index of suspicion and escalation to more invasive monitoring may be appropriate.

2. **Advanced monitoring of cardiac function and tissue perfusion** often requires the placement of invasive monitors (arterial line, central venous, or pulmonary arterial catheters) and includes both hemodynamic and metabolic indices, the utility of which are likely greater when followed over time rather than when examined at discrete time points. Echocardiography may be used both as a basic monitor (and a technique to extend the physical examination) and as an advanced monitor to assess quantitative metrics (see **Chapter 3**)
   a. **Echocardiography.** Basic echocardiography limited to five views—parasternal long axis, parasternal short axis, apical four-chamber, subcostal long axis, and inferior vena cava, and focusing on qualitative evaluation can help identify or exclude common causes of shock (severe hypovolemia, left or right ventricular dysfunction, acute valvular regurgitation, pericardiac tamponade, and severe pulmonary embolism). Advanced echocardiography can be used by qualified intensivists to measure the stroke volume and stroke volume index (SVI) and the medial E/e′ ratio among other quantitative measurements. Both SVI and the E/e′ ratio have been shown to be associated with worse outcomes in cardiogenic shock in a large study. These metrics are particularly useful in shock stages B-C, where they may be used to identify patients who might benefit from pulmonary artery catheter placement and management guided by advanced hemodynamic monitoring.
   b. **Hemodynamic indices.** Measurement of systemic blood pressure allows for a global rather than a regional assessment of the adequacy of tissue perfusion. Most patients in shock will have an **indwelling arterial cannula** placed for systemic blood pressure measurement (see **Chapter 1**). The need to infuse potent vasoactive medications, measure central venous oxygen saturation, and establish large-volume access frequently requires the placement of a **central venous catheter.** Placement of a **pulmonary artery (PA) catheter (PAC)** may further assist in the differential diagnosis of shock when the hemodynamic profile is not clear from peripheral assessment and may aid in monitoring cardiac responses (eg, PA occlusion pressure, cardiac output) to therapeutic interventions. Earlier clinical trials have demonstrated limited benefit for PAC placement, but it can be instrumental in guiding therapy among patients with undifferentiated or cardiogenic shock. A key benefit of using the pulmonary artery catheter is its ability to identify patients with right ventricular dysfunction greater than (or in addition to) severe left ventricular dysfunction. The CVP:PCWP ratio (normally <50%) and the Pulmonary Artery Pulsatility index (PAPi: PA pulse pressure ÷ CVP) have both been shown to identify right ventricular dysfunction.

Although invasive monitoring has fallen out of favor in many ICUs over the last decade, more recent evidence points to the value of invasive monitors. A high CVP (>12 mm Hg) is among the most reliable indicators of risk for acute kidney injury in both cardiogenic and septic shock. In addition, recent population-based retrospective studies have suggested that PAC-derived indices have led to increased utilization of mechanical circulatory support and improved survival in patients with severe cardiogenic shock, particularly in specialized centers. Although more data are required, PAC monitoring for severe cardiogenic shock is routine at our institution. Additional monitors (eg, esophageal Doppler monitors, arterial pulse waveform analysis) are now available to allow less-invasive assessment of cardiac output, stroke volume, and systemic vascular resistance (SVR) (see **Chapter 1**). The utility of these monitors in the management of severe shock is still unproven.

c. **Metabolic indices**

1. **Acidemia/Acidosis:** Metabolic acidemia (pH < 7.34) and metabolic acidosis (caused by anion gap-acidosis or nongap acidosis, conditions that can cause acidemia in the absence of respiratory compensation) may reflect a state of increased anaerobic metabolism and endogenous acid production occurring with progressive tissue hypoperfusion. It may also signal worsening renal and hepatic function and an inability to metabolize and clear the increasing endogenous acid load. Patients in shock often compensate for metabolic acidosis by increasing their minute ventilation and maintaining a normal pH. This should be kept in mind when intubation and mechanical ventilation are required because a "normal" minute ventilation postintubation may unmask significant acidemia.
2. **Serum lactate.** The physiology of lactic acidosis is complex. Although traditionally considered to be a marker of anaerobic metabolism, data in humans with severe septic shock (and in preclinical animal models) strongly suggest that aerobically generated lactate (through sympathetic stimulation of Na-K-ATPase) contributes to total lactate in most patients. Conversely, it is not unusual to encounter normal lactate values in patients with severe mesenteric ischemia and intestinal necrosis. Nonetheless, lactate values are strongly correlated with poor outcomes in patients who are critically ill, regardless of whether hyperlactatemia is associated with hypotension. Thus, early measurement and tracking of serial lactate levels are important in most patients with shock. The value of lactate clearance as a useful end point in resuscitation is, however, less well established.
3. **Mixed venous (SVO_2) and central venous ($ScVO_2$) oxygen saturations** reflect the balance between systemic oxygen delivery (DO_2) and systemic oxygen consumption (VO_2). When supply is insufficient to meet demand or demand exceeds supply, SVO_2 falls below the normal range of 65% to 75%. Given that SVO_2 reflects the balance between DO_2 and VO_2, it is affected by the variables that determine them, including body temperature, metabolic rate, hemoglobin concentration, arterial oxygen saturation (SaO_2, to a much greater degree than arterial oxygen partial pressure, which contributes only minimally to arterial oxygen content in most situations), and cardiac output. Therefore, when using the SVO_2 to estimate cardiac output, it is important to ensure that temperature, SaO_2 and Hb measurements are taken into account. Using the Fick equation to estimate CO allows the clinician to automatically factor in changes in Hb and SaO_2, and is encouraged (when using a PAC) over SVO_2 measurements. The Fick

equation does not factor in changes in oxygen consumption (from fever, hypothermia, or dysoxia), therefore should be used with caution when changes in Vo_2 are suspected. SVo_2 can be falsely elevated in septic shock secondary to mitochondrial dysfunction (cytopathic dysoxia).

4. Venous-arterial CO_2 difference (Pv-aco_2). Recent studies have provided data that suggest utility in monitoring the mixed venous to arterial Pco_2 difference, particularly in patients with pulmonary arterial catheters. In general, the lower the cardiac output, the higher this difference, although the relationship is not linear. An elevated or widening Pv-aco_2 in a patient with septic shock may suggest inadequate resuscitation. More data are required before target values of Pv-aco_2 can be recommended, and it is unclear if central venous CO_2 values can be substituted for mixed venous CO_2, precluding the widespread adoption of this metric.

C. Management of Shock

1. General principles. If shock is defined as a state of inadequate tissue perfusion and oxygenation, it makes sense that treatment should be aimed at increasing Do_2 while maintaining Vo_2.

a. Supplemental oxygen. Supplemental oxygen should be supplied and the institution of endotracheal intubation with controlled mechanical ventilation should be considered early. However, hyperoxia (defined in some studies as $Pao_2 > 300$ mm Hg) should be avoided, given the association of hyperoxia with worse outcomes in many conditions including acute myocardial infarction and cardiac arrest. In practice, targeting Sao_2 not higher than 92% to 94% and Pao_2 not greater than 120 mm Hg seem to be safe.

b. Circulation. Delivery of well-oxygenated blood to the tissues depends on an adequate cardiac output and driving pressure. Thus, fluid resuscitation plays an integral role in the treatment of shock. In the event that infusion of crystalloid, colloid, or blood products is insufficient to establish and maintain adequate systemic oxygen delivery, pharmacologic therapy with inotropes, and/or vasopressors may be required.

2. Fluid resuscitation is the cornerstone of the treatment of hypotension and shock. Its aim is both to increase effective circulating intravascular volume and, through the Frank-Starling mechanism, to increase cardiac ventricular preload and therefore cardiac output. Unfortunately, it is often difficult to predict whether, and by how much, the **cardiac output will increase in response to volume loading.** Although inadequate fluid replacement may result in continued tissue hypoperfusion and the progression of shock, **overly aggressive resuscitation may result in heart failure** and pulmonary and tissue edema, which in turn will further compromise tissue perfusion and possibly increase mortality. The fluids available for resuscitation include crystalloids, colloids, and blood products; however, the optimal choice of fluid remains controversial. **In most ICU patients, fluid resuscitation should be limited to those who have been identified to be likely to be "responders" to the volume challenge.** Recommendations for indiscriminate fluid administration, such as 30 mL/kg of crystalloids to all patients with septic shock, although part of some guidelines, should be discouraged in favor of a more thoughtful approach to resuscitation.

a. Crystalloids. The most commonly used crystalloid solutions are **lactated Ringer** and 0.9% **"normal" saline solutions,** which are inexpensive, easily stored, and readily available. There are data to suggest that in most cases, lactated Ringer is a preferable crystalloid over 0.9% saline, as too much chloride may lead to hyperchloremic acidosis and risk increasing renal dysfunction. Of note, hyperkalemia or acute kidney injury are

not contraindications to the administration of lactated Ringer or other balanced electrolyte solutions. Patients with traumatic brain injuries or those that need hyperosmolar therapies are an exception and should be resuscitated with 0.9% saline.

b. Colloids include both natural and synthetic solutions. Because of their high molecular weight and increased osmotic activity, colloids remain in the intravascular space longer than crystalloids and thus require less volume to achieve the same hemodynamic goals.

1. **Human albumin** is derived from pooled human plasma and is available as 5% and 25% solutions in normal saline. Heat treatment eliminates the risk of transmission of viral infections. Although there is no evidence of harm from the use of albumin as a resuscitation fluid (except perhaps in head injury victims), no clear benefit has been shown either and its relatively high cost limits its widespread use. Relatively weak data support the use of albumin in patients with septic shock and patients with severe hypoalbuminemia.
2. **Synthetic colloids** include **dextran** and **hydroxyethyl starch (HES).** Because of their antigenicity and high incidence of anaphylactic and anaphylactoid reactions, the dextrans have largely been replaced by starch-based compounds. **Hydroxyethyl starches** are high-polymeric glucose compounds available with a variety of mean molecular weights and molar substitution patterns and dissolved in normal saline or sodium lactate. Fluid resuscitation with HES has been associated with an increased need for renal replacement therapy. Based on these results, the use of HES in patients with severe sepsis and septic shock is strongly discouraged.

c. Blood products. Although not recommended for pure volume expansion due to their potential for disease transmission, immunosuppression, transfusion reaction, and transfusion-related acute lung injury, as well as their limited availability and high cost, administration of packed red blood cells may be indicated to improve systemic oxygen delivery. **Current practice has trended toward steadily more restrictive transfusion, and transfusion triggers between 7 and 8 g/dL are recommended in most patients that are not actively bleeding.** This includes patients with sepsis, GI bleeding, postcardiac surgery, and even those with acute myocardial ischemia. In the latter population, a recent randomized controlled trial (RCT) in more than 600 patients showed that a transfusion trigger of 8 g/dL was noninferior to a transfusion trigger of 10 g/dL in patients with acute myocardial infarction. A larger RCT is currently underway. In our institution, the use of a transfusion trigger >8 g/dL has become exceedingly uncommon in the absence of active bleeding.

3. Specific considerations

a. Hypovolemic shock. Because hypovolemic shock entails a reduction in effective intravascular volume, it would seem logical that its treatment would involve rapid and early-volume resuscitation. However, in the case of hemorrhagic shock with ongoing blood loss, aggressive fluid administration prior to definitive hemostasis may increase bleeding from disrupted vessels and promote the progression of tissue hypoperfusion. As such, delayed and initially limited, rather than immediate and vigorous, fluid resuscitation may be beneficial. It must also be kept in mind that massive hemorrhage also involves loss of platelets and coagulation factors, such that balanced infusions of packed red blood cells and fresh frozen plasma may be required. As is the case with any massive transfusion, care must be taken to guard against the development of the lethal triad of cold, coagulopathy, and acidemia.

b. Cardiogenic shock. Unlike the highly robust evidence base for most cardiologic disorders, data-driven therapies for patients with cardiogenic shock are relatively scarce. Optimal pharmacologic therapy (most effective pressors, inotropes, etc.) remains undefined, leading to significant heterogeneity in clinical practice. Abnormalities in rate, rhythm, contractility, and valvular mechanics associated with cardiogenic shock may require a host of specialized interventions, ranging from pacemaker and defibrillator placements to antithrombotic therapy, percutaneous coronary intervention with angioplasty, stenting, open coronary revascularization, mechanical support with intra-aortic balloon counterpulsation devices, and even left ventricular assist devices (see **Chapter 18**). The choice of mechanical circulatory support devices also largely depends on local institutional experience rather than outcomes-based data. As an example, the use of the intra-aortic balloon pump remains popular in the United States despite the presence of high-quality data, suggesting a minimal impact on outcomes in postmyocardial infarction cardiogenic shock.

c. Obstructive shock requires specific interventions targeted to the cause of blood flow impairment. Tension pneumothorax is treated with needle decompression followed by tube thoracostomy, abdominal compartment syndrome is treated with surgical decompression, pulmonary embolism is treated with supportive care and may involve the use of thrombolysis or surgical embolectomy, cardiac tamponade is treated with pericardiocentesis, auto-PEEP requires temporary suspension of mechanical ventilation and adjustment of ventilator settings.

d. Distributive shock. In the critical care setting, distributive shock is most commonly caused by *systemic inflammatory response syndrome* (inflammation) or *sepsis*. Guidelines for the management of **severe sepsis** and **septic shock** are reviewed in **Chapter 12.** In brief, appropriate initial management rests upon the triad of early broad-spectrum antimicrobial therapy, hemodynamic resuscitation, and source control. **Anaphylactic shock** is another form of distributive shock resulting from an acute, immunoglobulin E (IgE)–mediated reaction involving the release of multiple inflammatory mediators from mast cells and basophils. Initial management requires immediate identification and discontinuation of the suspected antigen, prompt provision of ventilatory and cardiovascular support, and pharmacologic therapy directed at the immune mediators of the symptomatology, including epinephrine, the histamine H_1- and H_2-receptor blockers diphenhydramine and ranitidine, respectively, and corticosteroids.

III. PHARMACOLOGIC THERAPIES OF HYPOTENSION AND SHOCK

When appropriate fluid replacement fails to restore adequate blood pressure and tissue perfusion, pharmacologic therapy with vasopressors and/or inotropes is required. What counts as "appropriate fluid replacement" is difficult to quantify. If arterial pressures and perfusion parameters are normal, then there is no need to target an arbitrary CVP (eg, there is no basis for a target CVP of 8-12 mm Hg recommended by some guidelines). Persistent metabolic acidemia, elevated serum lactate levels, and depressed SVO_2/Fick Cardiac Output suggest the need for further pharmacologic intervention, although the choice of a specific agent will depend on the clinical context. Tables 6.2 and 6.3 summarize the common vasopressor and inotropic agents, including their receptor-binding affinity and major hemodynamic effects and side effects.

TABLE 6.2 Commonly Used Vasopressor and Inotropic Agents: Receptor Selectivity

Drug	α_1	α_2	β_1	β_2	DA	Other
Phenylephrine	+++++	0	0	0	0	
Ephedrine	+++	0	+++	++	0	
Vasopressin	0	0	0	0	0	V_1/V_2
Dopamine[a]	+++	0	++++	++	+++++	
Norepinephrine	++++	0	+++	+	0	
Epinephrine	+++++	+++	++++	+++	0	
Isoproterenol	0	0	+++++	+++++	0	
Dobutamine	+	0	+++++	+++	0	
Milrinone						

α_1, α_1 receptor; α_2, α_2 receptor; β_1, β_1 receptor; β_2, β_2 receptor; DA, dopamine receptors; V_1/V_2, vasopressin receptors; 0, zero receptor affinity; + through +++++, minimal to marked receptor affinity.
[a]Effects of dopamine vary with dose, from predominantly DA agonism at low doses to predominantly α agonism at high doses.

TABLE 6.3 Commonly Used Vasopressor and Inotropic Agents: Hemodynamic Effects and Major Clinical Side Effects

Drug	HR	MAP	CO	SVR	Renal blood flow	Side effects
Phenylephrine	↓	↑↑↑	↓	↑↑↑	↓↓↓	Reflex bradycardia, HTN, peripheral and visceral vasoconstriction
Ephedrine	↑↑	↑↑	↑↑	↑	↓↓	Tachycardia
Vasopressin	0	0	0	↑	↑	Peripheral and visceral vasoconstriction
Dopamine[a]	↑↑	↑	↑↑↑	↑	↑↑↑	Arrhythmias
Norepinephrine	↓	↑↑↑	↑/↓	↑↑↑	↓↓↓	Arrhythmias
Epinephrine	↑↑	↑	↑↑	↓/↑	↓↓	HTN, arrhythmias, cardiac ischemia
Isoproterenol	↑↑↑	↓	↑↑↑	↓↓	↓/↑	Arrhythmias
Dobutamine	↑	↑	↑↑↑	↓	↑	Tachycardia, arrhythmias
Milrinone	0	↓	↑↑	↓↓↓	↓	Arrhythmias, hypotension
Levosimendan	0	↓	↑↑	↓↓↓	↓	Tachycardia, hypotension

0, zero receptor affinity; ↓↓↓ through ↑↑↑, decrease through increase in effect; CO, cardiac output; HR, heart rate; HTN, hypertension; MAP, mean arterial pressure; SVR, systemic vascular resistance.
[a]Effects of dopamine vary with dose, from predominantly DA agonism at low doses to predominantly α agonism at high doses.

An important point to emphasize is that the initiation of vasoactive agents should never be delayed purely because of the lack of central venous access. Multiple studies support the safety of peripherally administered vasoactive agents (sometimes at lower concentrations than their centrally administered counterparts).

A. **Non–Catecholamine Sympathomimetic Agents** are synthetic drugs used primarily as vasopressors. They are classified according to their affinity for activation of **α- and/or β-adrenergic receptors.**
   1. **Phenylephrine** is a selective α_1 adrenergic agonist that causes arterial vasoconstriction. By increasing SVR, it rapidly raises mean arterial pressure, although reflex bradycardia may cause a reduction in cardiac output.

Because of its rapid onset and its ease of titration, phenylephrine is often used as a first-line, temporizing agent to treat hypotension. Its indications include hypotension secondary to peripheral vasodilatation, such as following the administration of potent hypnotic medications or epidural local anesthetics. Because of its pure vasoconstrictive effect, phenylephrine may be poorly tolerated in patients with compromised left ventricular function.

2. **Ephedrine** is a direct and indirect α- and β-adrenergic agonist that causes an increase in heart rate and cardiac output with modest vasoconstriction. As such, its hemodynamic profile is similar to that of epinephrine, although much less potent.
3. **Arginine vasopressin (AVP)** (antidiuretic hormone [ADH]) is a nonapeptide hormone endogenously synthesized in the hypothalamus and stored in the posterior pituitary. In addition to its roles in osmoregulation and volume regulation, which are mediated through the **V_2 receptors**, AVP acts through **V_1 receptors** to increase arteriolar smooth muscle tone and thus SVR. Although vasopressin levels in hypovolemic (hemorrhagic) and cardiogenic shock are appropriately elevated, serum levels in patients with septic shock have been found to be inappropriately low. Vasopressin may be used in vasodilatory shock other than sepsis states, such as after cardiac surgery. The optimal dosing of vasopressin is unclear. Some practitioners use a fixed dose (either 0.03 or 0.04 U/min as a "replacement strategy"). The authors prefer to use vasopressin as a titrated vasoactive medication with a dose-response range, and doses of 0.01 to 0.06 U/min are common in our institution. Some studies, including the recent vasopressin versus noradrenaline as initial therapy in septic shock (VANISH) and vasopressin versus norepinephrine in vasoplegic shock after cardiac surgery (VANCS) trials provide support for this strategy. Careful monitoring for digital and organ ischemia should be maintained when using vasopressin (as indeed with high doses of any vasopressor agent). Because vasopressin is reported to have a greater effect on the systemic circulation compared to the pulmonary circulation, it may be a preferred vasopressor in patients with right ventricular dysfunction, in whom increases in pulmonary vascular resistance (PVR) may be detrimental.

B. Catecholamines include endogenous compounds **dopamine, norepinephrine,** and **epinephrine** and synthetic compounds such as **isoproterenol** and **dobutamine.**

1. Endogenous

a. Dopamine is the immediate precursor to norepinephrine and epinephrine. Its actions vary with its dosing. At low doses, it affects primarily dopaminergic receptors in splanchnic, renal, coronary, and cerebral vascular beds, leading to vasodilatation and increased blood flow. At intermediate doses, dopamine increasingly stimulates β_1-adrenergic receptors producing positive inotropic and chronotropic effects. At high doses, α_1-adrenergic effects predominate, causing an increase in SVR. However, its use in patients in shock is limited by its arrhythmogenicity. Norepinephrine has been found to be superior to dopamine in a large head-to-head comparison. The same study found dopamine to be associated with higher mortality in an a priori defined group of patients with cardiogenic shock. However, the definition of cardiogenic shock in the study was imprecise. Dopamine may be useful when chronotropy would be beneficial, as in symptomatic bradycardia.

b. Norepinephrine is an endogenous catecholamine with both α- and β-adrenergic activity. Its potent vasoconstrictive and inotropic effects frequently make it the drug of choice to treat hemodynamically unstable patients who require the support of both vascular tone and myocardial contractility. Compared with epinephrine, it lacks β_2 activity. Norepinephrine was found to be superior to dopamine in an RCT, as mentioned earlier. A systematic review of 11 RCTs comparing norepinephrine and dopamine in septic shock found that norepinephrine was associated with lower mortality and a lower risk of arrhythmias compared to dopamine. Thus, norepinephrine is the recommended first-line vasopressor in septic shock.

c. **Epinephrine** is the primary endogenous catecholamine produced by the adrenal medulla. As mentioned earlier, epinephrine has potent α_1, β_1, and β_2 activities, which together act to increase heart rate and contractility. It is the mainstay of cardiopulmonary resuscitation and second-line vasopressor in the treatment of septic shock when an additional agent is needed to achieve hemodynamic goals. Its effect on BP is caused by positive inotropic and chronotropic effects and to vasoconstriction in vascular beds, especially the skin, mucosae, and kidney. Its strong β_2 effect promotes bronchodilation and blocks mast cell degranulation, making it the drug of choice for **anaphylaxis.**

2. **Synthetic**

a. **Isoproterenol** is a pure β-adrenergic agonist whose β_1 effects increase heart rate, contractility, and cardiac output. Because of its β_2 activation, both diastolic and mean arterial pressures may slightly decrease. The combination of increased cardiac work and decreased diastolic pressures may compromise coronary perfusion and lead to myocardial ischemia, particularly in patients with preexisting coronary artery disease. Despite these limitations, isoproterenol may be useful in cases of cardiogenic shock in heart transplant recipients, where the donor organ is denervated and will only respond to direct-acting sympathomimetic agents.

b. **Dobutamine** is another synthetic catecholamine with predominantly β activity. With its high affinity for β_1 receptors, dobutamine is a potent inotrope with moderate chronotropic effects. The β_2 effects of dobutamine produce a modest decrease in SVR. Taken together, dobutamine's potent inotropic and slight vasodilatory effects make it a suitable agent for patients with cardiogenic shock with depressed left ventricular function, elevated filling pressures, and increased SVR.

C. **Phosphodiesterase-III (PDE-III) Inhibitors**, such as amrinone, **milrinone,** and enoximone exert their effects by inhibiting PDE-III, an enzyme especially abundant in vascular smooth muscle and cardiac tissues, where it increases cAMP levels, which in turn leads to increased chronotropy and inotropy. Amrinone has been largely replaced by milrinone due to its shorter duration of action, easier titratability, and decreased risk of thrombocytopenia. Milrinone is indicated for IV administration in patients with acute heart failure and may be of some benefit to patients with right heart failure secondary to elevated PA pressures. Milrinone is administered with a loading dose of 50 μg/kg followed by a continuous infusion of 0.25 to 0.7 μg/kg/min. In practice, particularly in ICUs, a loading dose is rarely, if ever used. The elimination half-life of milrinone is about 2.3 hours and is significantly prolonged in patients with impaired renal function and those on renal replacement therapy (RRT), making dobutamine a preferable initial inotrope in this population. The arrhythmogenicity of dobutamine and milrinone were similar in a well-conducted trial (The dobutamine compared with milrinone (DOREMI) trial), but milrinone appears more likely to cause vasodilatation and hypotension than dobutamine. Enoximone is not available in the United States.

D. **Calcium Sensitizers.** The calcium sensitizer **levosimendan** stabilizes the conformational change in troponin C as it binds to calcium, thus facilitating myocardial cross-bridging and augmenting contractility. Its unique promise was the ability to increase inotropy without significantly increasing myocardial energy consumption, which was unfortunately not borne out in clinical trials. The levosimendan for the prevention of acute organ dysfunction in sepsis (LEOPARDS) trial suggested worse outcomes with levosimendan in patients with septic shock (longer duration of mechanical ventilation and ICU stay) and is not recommended for this use. Levosimendan is approved in Europe for the treatment of acute decompensated heart failure but is not available in the United States.

E. Adjunct Treatments for Refractory Shock:

1. Steroids. Use of steroids in shock varies widely across the intensive care committee. The value of laboratory testing (the cosyntropin stimulation test) is unclear. Consensus guidelines recommend the use of relatively low dose (200 mg/day of hydrocortisone in divided doses or continuous infusions) steroids started early (within 6 hours) in patients on high doses of norepinephrine (>0.25 μg/kg/min). A meta-analysis aggregating more than 7000 patients has found no mortality benefit, but a more rapid resolution of shock and less time on mechanical ventilation with steroids. The most common adverse effects are hyperglycemia and hypernatremia. There is a risk of increased muscle weakness with steroids, but there does not appear to be an increase in the risk of infections.
2. Sodium bicarbonate. Empiric treatment of metabolic acidemia has been controversial. Based on the results of the BICAR-ICU study, treatment of significant acidemia (pH < 7.20) may be beneficial, particularly in patients with acute kidney injury (AKI). It is important to ensure that the patient has the ventilatory capacity to eliminate the CO_2 generated by bicarbonate treatment to prevent worsening of acidemia.
3. Methylene blue. Methylene blue (MB) inhibits nitric oxide–mediated vasodilatation primarily by inhibiting soluble guanylate cyclase. Data supporting the use of methylene blue in vasoplegic shock are modest. It is used as a rescue therapy in vasoplegic shock from sepsis or following cardiopulmonary bypass (bolus dose 1.5 mg/kg, with or without subsequent infusion). It is renally cleared, and although data are scarce, it's uncertain whether continuous venovenous hemofiltration (CVVH) can clear MB. Therefore, although a bolus dose of MB can be used in most patients, the use of a continuous infusion is probably not advisable in patients with AKI or renal replacement. If possible, following pulmonary arterial pressures is advisable, given a risk of worsening PVR. MB should not be used in patients at risk for serotonin syndrome (ie, patients on selective serotonin reuptake inhibitors [SSRIs] or antibiotics such as linezolid) and in patients with G6PD deficiency.
4. Hydroxocobalamin is approved for the treatment of cyanide toxicity. It can also be used as a rescue medication in severe vasoplegic shock (5 g IV over 15 minutes). Its mechanism of action is not well defined but may include reducing nitric oxide–induced vasodilatation by inhibiting nitric oxide synthase enzymes. Hydroxocobalamin turns the urine a dark purple and interferes with a number of laboratory assays for 12 to 48 hours after administration.
5. Angiotensin II is a naturally occurring hormone with potent vasopressor effects. A synthetic human preparation is now available. Given very little collective experience with angiotensin II in patients with shock and its expense, it is considered a rescue agent for refractory shock when it is available.
6. Vitamin C. Interest in vitamin C for shock (particularly septic shock) surged after a 2017 report that claimed dramatic mortality benefits in septic shock with a regimen that included vitamin C, thiamine, and hydrocortisone. Since then, however, multiple well-designed RCTs have tested the efficacy of vitamin C alone as well and in combination with thiamine and hydrocortisone in septic shock with no evidence of benefit. At this time, vitamin C is not recommended as an adjunct in patients with shock.

IV. HYPERTENSION

As was the case with shock, hypertensive crises may also compromise blood flow and the delivery of oxygen to tissues, complicating the care of patients and necessitating treatment in a higher-acuity critical care setting. According to the 2020 International Society of Hypertension Global Hypertension Practice Guidelines, patients with **substantially elevated** and with evidence of acute or progressive end-organ damage are classified as having a **"hypertensive emergency"** and require immediate blood pressure reduction, albeit not necessarily to normal ranges, to limit end-organ damage. Patients with substantially elevated BP who lack acute hypertension-mediated organ damage (structural and functional changes in arteries or end-organs) are not considered a hypertensive emergency and can typically be treated with oral antihypertensive therapy.

A. The **clinical presentation** of hypertensive emergencies largely reflects the macro- and microvascular consequences of compromised tissue perfusion and oxygenation.

1. **Neurologic**: encephalopathy with the symptoms and signs of increased intracranial pressure secondary to cerebral hyperperfusion, including headache, nausea, vomiting, visual disturbances, papilledema, altered mental status, confusion, obtundation, localized or generalized seizure activity, intracranial hemorrhage, and stroke
2. **Cardiovascular**: angina, acute coronary syndrome with electrocardiographic and enzymatic evidence of ischemia and/or AMI, acute heart failure, and acute aortic dissection
3. **Respiratory**: dyspnea, acute pulmonary edema, respiratory failure
4. **Renal**: oliguria, acute renal failure
5. **Obstetric:** severe preeclampsia, HELLP (**h**emolysis, **e**levated **l**iver enzymes, and **l**ow **p**latelets) syndrome, eclampsia
6. **Hematologic**: hemolytic anemia, coagulopathy

B. Management: The goal of therapy is to limit end-organ damage and restore the balance between tissue oxygen supply and demand. Rapid and excessive reduction in blood pressure may compromise organ blood flow and precipitate cerebral, coronary, or renal ischemia. Therefore, it is best to manage patients with hypertensive emergencies with continuous intravenous infusions of easily titratable, short-acting agents, such as esmolol, clevidipine, nitroglycerine (NTG), and sodium nitroprusside (SNP). There is a lack of RCT data to provide clear-cut guidance on BP targets and times within which these should be achieved. In the case of hypertensive emergencies not complicated by recent ischemic stroke or acute aortic dissection, a general goal is to reduce blood pressure by 15% to 20% within 30 to 60 minutes, provided the patient remains clinically stable. If these changes are well tolerated, further reduction toward a normal blood pressure can be made over the course of the next 24 to 48 hours.

1. **Acute ischemic stroke.** In patients who have suffered an acute ischemic stroke, higher pressures may be tolerated in an attempt to improve perfusion to metabolically compromised tissues. For patients not eligible for thrombolytic therapy (see **Chapter 30**) and lacking evidence of other end-organ involvement, the American Stroke Association recommends pharmacologic intervention for systolic blood pressure (SBP) >220 mm Hg and/or diastolic blood pressure (DBP) >140 mm Hg, aiming for a 10% to 15% reduction in blood pressure. Patients eligible for thrombolytic therapy require intervention for SBP >185 mm Hg and DBP >110 mm Hg.
2. **Acute aortic dissection.** For patients with acute aortic dissections, various consensus guidelines recommend achieving an SBP between 100 and 120 mm Hg, provided that symptoms and signs of neurologic and/or renal compromise do not develop. In general, the goals of pharmacologic

intervention are to reduce the force of left ventricular contraction and to decrease the rate of rise of the aortic pulse pressure wave (ie, the "dP/dT") while maintaining the blood pressure as low as possible without compromising organ function. If the strength of left ventricular contraction can be reduced and the rate of rise of arterial pressure as a function of time mitigated, the risk of dissection extension and rupture may be minimized.

C. **Pharmacologic Therapies**

1. **Vasodilators**

a. **Sodium nitroprusside** is a potent arterial and (to a lesser extent) venous vasodilator. Its rapid onset and short duration of action make it ideal for continuous infusion. **Central administration** is preferred. The normal dose range is 20 to 200 µg/min. Because SNP is photodegradable, protection with foil wrapping is necessary. **Adverse effects** include **cyanide toxicity**—free cyanide ions (CN^-) bind to cytochrome oxidase and uncouple oxidative metabolism, causing tissue hypoxia. At low infusion rates, cyanide can be converted to thiocyanate (by thiosulfate and rhodanase), which is less toxic than CN^-. The risk of cyanide and thiocyanate toxicity is dose dependent and increases with renal impairment. **Signs of cyanide toxicity** include tachyphylaxis, increased mixed venous PaO_2, and metabolic acidosis. Cyanide neutralization can be achieved by two different strategies: facilitating cyanide metabolism through two nontoxic pathways (sodium nitrite and sodium thiosulfate) or by directly binding to the cyanide molecule (hydroxocobalamin). **Sodium nitrite** increases the production of methemoglobin, and **sodium thiosulfate** provides additional sulfur donors that transform cyanide to thiocyanate which is then renally excreted. **Hydroxocobalamin** combines with cyanide to form cyanocobalamin (vitamin B_{12}), which is excreted by the kidneys. The current consensus recommends the use of hydroxocobalamin as a first choice whenever it is available. Other potential adverse effects of nitroprusside infusion include increased intracranial pressure with cerebral vasodilatation, intracoronary steal with coronary vasodilatation, and impairment of hypoxic pulmonary vasoconstriction, worsening ventilation-perfusion matching, and worsening hypoxemia. **Rebound hypertension** may occur when SNP is abruptly discontinued.

b. **Nitroglycerine** is a venous and (to a lesser extent) arterial vasodilator. By dilating venous capacitance vessels, NTG reduces preload and offloads the heart, decreasing ventricular end-diastolic pressure, myocardial work, and myocardial oxygen demand. At the same time, NTG dilates large coronary vessels and relieves coronary artery vasospasm, promotes the redistribution of coronary blood flow to ischemic regions, and decreases platelet aggregation, all of which serve to improve myocardial oxygen supply. NTG's salutary effects on the balance between supply and demand of myocardial oxygen render it of particular use in hypertensive emergencies associated with acute coronary syndromes or acute cardiogenic pulmonary edema. **IV administration** of NTG is easy to titrate to effect and is the preferred route for critically ill patients. Common rates of infusion range from 25 to 1000 µg/min. Because NTG is absorbed by polyvinyl chloride IV tubing, its dose may decrease after 30 to 60 minutes, once the IV tubing is fully saturated. **Hypotension, reflex tachycardia**, and **headache** are common side effects. **Tachyphylaxis** is common with continuous exposure to the drug.

c. **Nicardipine** is a second-generation dihydropyridine calcium-channel blocker that causes vascular and coronary vasodilation through the relaxation of vascular smooth muscle. The reduction in afterload and cardiac work accompanied by coronary vasodilatation and increased coronary blood flow make nicardipine useful in hypertensive crises associated with angina and coronary artery disease. The normal dose range is 5 to 15 mg/h. The development of reflex tachycardia may limit its benefit in some patients. A newer, third-generation dihydropyridine, **clevidipine**, has recently received Food and Drug Administration (FDA) approval for the treatment of perioperative hypertension. An ultra-short-acting and selective arteriolar vasodilator, clevidipine, reduces afterload and increases cardiac output without causing reflex tachycardia. It is metabolized by erythrocyte esterases so that its clearance is not prolonged in cases of renal or hepatic dysfunction. Both drugs can impair hypoxic pulmonary vasoconstriction and worsen hypoxemia.

d. Fenoldopam is an arteriolar vasodilator acting primarily as a δ_1 dopamine receptor agonist. At low doses (up to 0.04 μg/min), it results in renal vasodilation and natriuresis without systemic hemodynamic effects. At higher doses, it is a potent antihypertensive. Its onset is within 5 minutes and its duration of action is 30 to 60 minutes. In addition to its antihypertensive effects, fenoldopam has been shown to improve creatinine clearance in severely hypertensive patients with and without impaired renal function. Its administration may lead to increased intraocular pressure and so should proceed with caution in patients with glaucoma.

e. Hydralazine is an arteriolar vasodilator with a not well-understood mechanism of action. Its delayed onset of action (5-15 minutes) makes it difficult to titrate in most hypertensive emergencies. It is often used on an as-needed basis (10-20 mg IV) as an additional means of controlling BP high points. High doses may be accompanied by immunologic reactions, including a lupus-like syndrome with arthralgias, myalgias, rashes, and fever.

2. Adrenergic inhibitors

a. Labetalol is a selective β_1- and nonselective α-antagonist with an **α- to β-blocking ratio of 1:7** following IV administration. With this receptor profile, labetalol reduces arterial pressure and SVR while largely maintaining heart rate, cardiac output, and coronary and cerebral blood flow. Initial IV doses of 5 to 10 mg can be increased to 15 to 20 mg in 5-minute intervals and followed by a continuous infusion of 1 to 5 mg/min.

b. Esmolol is a short-acting β_1-selective antagonist with a rapid onset of action lending to its ease of titratability. As is the case with clevidipine, it contains an ester linkage that is rapidly hydrolyzed by erythrocyte esterases. In cases of hypertensive emergencies complicating and complicated by acute aortic dissection, esmolol is frequently the α-blocker of choice to combine with a vasodilator such as nitroprusside to achieve hemodynamic control.

Selected Readings

De Backer D, Cecconi M, Chew MS, et al. A plea for personalization of the hemodynamic management of septic shock. *Crit Care.* 2022;26(1):372. Published December 1, 2022. doi:10.1186/s13054-022-04255-y

Ducrocq G, Gonzalez-Juanatey JR, Puymirat E, et al. Effect of a restrictive vs liberal blood transfusion strategy on major cardiovascular events among patients with acute myocardial infarction and anemia: the REALITY Randomized Clinical Trial. *JAMA.* 2021;325(6):552-560. doi:10.1001/jama.2021.0135

Garan AR, Kanwar M, Thayer KL, et al. Complete hemodynamic profiling with pulmonary artery catheters in cardiogenic shock is associated with lower in-hospital mortality. *JACC Heart Fail.* 2020;8(11):903-913. doi:10.1016/j.jchf.2020.08.012

Gordon AC, Mason AJ, Thirunavukkarasu N, et al. Effect of early vasopressin vs norepinephrine on kidney failure in patients with septic shock: the VANISH Randomized Clinical Trial. *JAMA*. 2016;316(5):509-518. doi:10.1001/jama.2016.10485

Hajjar LA, Vincent JL, Barbosa Gomes Galas FR, et al. Vasopressin versus norepinephrine in patients with vasoplegic shock after cardiac surgery: the VANCS Randomized Controlled Trial. *Anesthesiology*. 2017;126(1):85-93. doi:10.1097/ALN.0000000000001434

Jaber S, Paugam C, Futier E, et al. Sodium bicarbonate therapy for patients with severe metabolic acidaemia in the intensive care unit (BICAR-ICU): a multicentre, open-label, randomised controlled, phase 3 trial. *Lancet*. 2018;392(10141):31-40. doi:10.1016/S0140-6736(18)31080-8

Jentzer JC, Wiley BM, Anavekar NS, et al. Noninvasive hemodynamic assessment of shock severity and mortality risk prediction in the cardiac intensive care unit. *JACC Cardiovasc Imaging*. 2021;14(2):321-332. doi:10.1016/j.jcmg.2020.05.038

Kraut JA, Madias NE. Lactic acidosis. *N Engl J Med*. 2014;371(24):2309-2319. doi:10.1056/NEJMra1309483

Levy B, Gibot S, Franck P, Cravoisy A, Bollaert PE. Relation between muscle Na+K+ ATPase activity and raised lactate concentrations in septic shock: a prospective study. *Lancet*. 2005;365(9462):871-875. doi:10.1016/S0140-6736(05)71045-X

Mathew R, Di Santo P, Jung RG, et al. Milrinone as compared with dobutamine in the treatment of cardiogenic shock. *N Engl J Med*. 2021;385(6):516-525. doi:10.1056/NEJMoa2026845

Nagendran M, Russell JA, Walley KR, et al. Vasopressin in septic shock: an individual patient data meta-analysis of randomised controlled trials. *Intensive Care Med*. 2019;45(6):844-855. doi:10.1007/s00134-019-05620-2

Naidu SS, Baran DA, Jentzer JC, et al. SCAI SHOCK stage classification expert consensus update: a review and incorporation of validation studies: this statement was endorsed by the American College of Cardiology (ACC), American College of Emergency Physicians (ACEP), American Heart Association (AHA), European Society of Cardiology (ESC) Association for Acute Cardiovascular Care (ACVC), International Society for Heart and Lung Transplantation (ISHLT), Society of Critical Care Medicine (SCCM), and Society of Thoracic Surgeons (STS) in December 2021. *J Am Coll Cardiol*. 2022;79(9):933-946. doi:10.1016/j.jacc.2022.01.018

Ospina-Tascón GA, Umaña M, Bermúdez WF, et al. Can venous-to-arterial carbon dioxide differences reflect microcirculatory alterations in patients with septic shock? *Intensive Care Med*. 2016;42(2):211-221. doi:10.1007/s00134-015-4133-2

Rossello X, Bueno H, Gil V, et al. Synergistic impact of systolic blood pressure and perfusion status on mortality in acute heart failure. *Circ Heart Fail*. 2021;14(3):e007347. doi:10.1161/CIRCHEARTFAILURE.120.007347

Rygård SL, Butler E, Granholm A, et al. Low-dose corticosteroids for adult patients with septic shock: a systematic review with meta-analysis and trial sequential analysis. *Intensive Care Med*. 2018;44(7):1003-1016. doi:10.1007/s00134-018-5197-6

Unger T, Borghi C, Charchar F, et al. 2020 International society of hypertension global hypertension practice guidelines. *Hypertension*. 2020;75(6):1334-1357. doi:10.1161/HYPERTENSIONAHA.120.15026

7 Sedation and Analgesia

Lukas H. Matern and Ryan J. Horvath

I. PRINCIPLES OF SEDATION AND ANALGESIA

Effective sedation and analgesia can substantially impact the clinical and functional outcomes of the critically ill. It is therefore essential that intensivists develop a thorough knowledge of sedative pharmacology and the principles regarding its use. This chapter begins with a brief overview of the objectives of analgosedation regimens, provides up-to-date evidence on drug monitoring and dosing, and outlines common medications and techniques aimed at optimizing analgesia and sedation in critical care settings.

A. Many patients are admitted to the intensive care unit (ICU) with respiratory failure requiring endotracheal intubation and mechanical ventilation, resulting in the need for management of anxiety and pain. In addition, there are a myriad of other potential sources of discomfort that the patients who are critically ill may experience. Goals of sedation for these patients may include reducing pain and distress, easing adaptation to invasive and noninvasive mechanical ventilatory support, lowering oxygen consumption and carbon dioxide production, stabilizing hemodynamics, and protecting patients with brain injury from the development of edema or ischemia. The high prevalence of chronic psychiatric sequelae in ICU survivors further underscores the importance of providing adequate sedation. For example, one study found that 85% of the critically ill reported significant anxiety during their ICU stay, which persisted a year after discharge in 62% of survivors. The growing number of research has also suggested that sedation is often overused and may cause a wide array of complications.

B. The complex interrelationship of pain, agitation, and delirium—sometimes termed the **ICU triad**—demands an individualized approach to assessment and management. Numerous variables linked to a patient's unique set of chronic comorbidities and acute illnesses may impact each component of the triad. Thus, the optimal management plan for a patient who is critically ill often includes both analgesic and sedative agents in a combinatorial **analgosedation** regimen to mitigate contributors to the ICU triad. For example, in the case of trauma with numerous rib fractures, a patient who is mechanically ventilated may benefit from analgesia provided by a thoracic epidural infusion of dilute bupivacaine with hydromorphone while a propofol infusion may then be added to improve tolerance of positive pressure ventilation.

C. Analgosedation should be targeted to the goal of optimizing patient stability and comfort while minimizing the risk of adverse cardiopulmonary, neuromuscular, and psychiatric drug effects. Although general analgosedation algorithms such as that used at our institution (Figure 7.1) provide a broad framework and facilitate decision-making, one-size-fits-all sedation protocols do not clearly reduce the duration of mechanical ventilation or improve outcomes. The goals of sedation should be revisited often within a multidisciplinary ICU team and should evolve in tandem with the patient's clinical status.

D. Some patients with severe respiratory failure may require deep sedation with or without neuromuscular blockade to facilitate lung-protective ventilation. In these

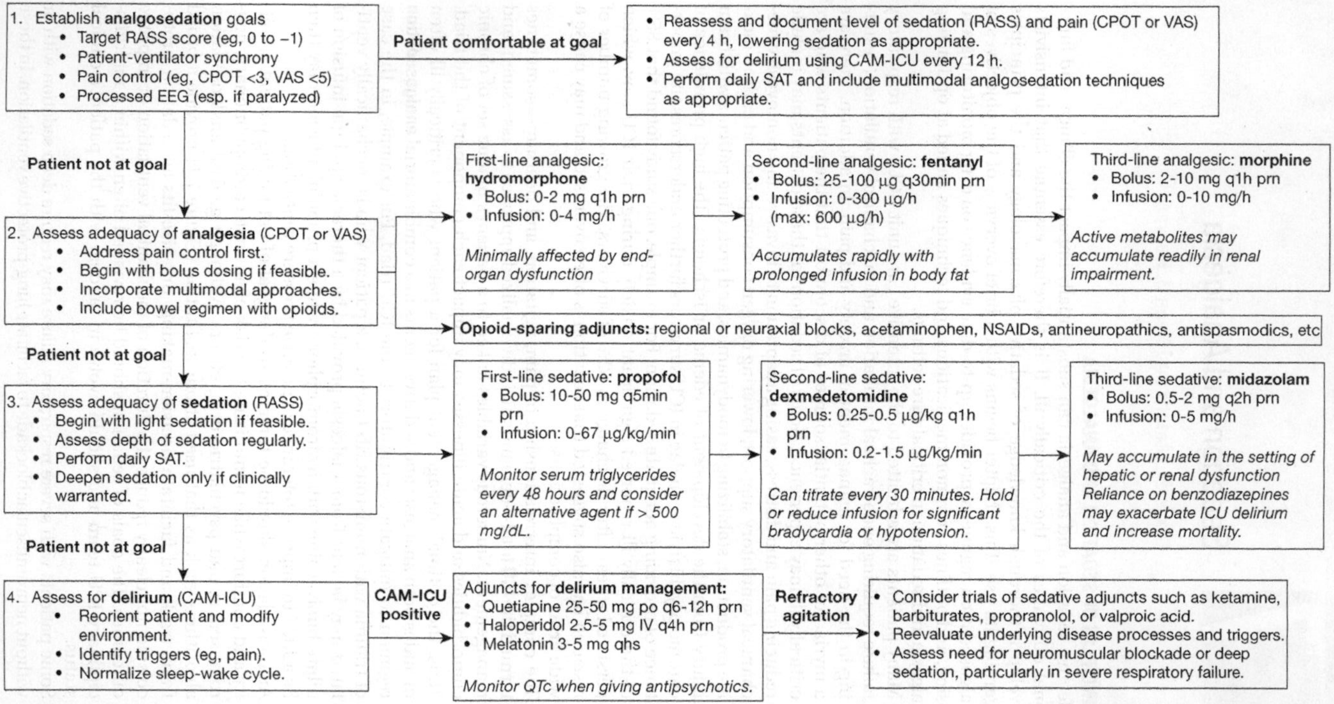

FIGURE 7.1 General stepwise approach to analgosedation. CAM-ICU, confusion assessment method-intensive care unit; CPOT, Critical Care Pain Observation Tool; EEG, electroencephalogram; NSAIDs, nonsteroidal anti-inflammatory drugs; po, orally; prn, as needed; q, every; RASS, Richmond Agitation Sedation Scale; SAT, spontaneous awakening trial; VAS, visual analog scale.

patients, the respiratory depressant effects of agents such as propofol and opioid infusions may be beneficial for reducing the respiratory drive to achieve ventilator-patient synchrony until gas exchange improves. In addition, deeper planes of sedation may be required to lower intracranial pressure in patients with brain injury, to abort seizure activity, or to prevent awareness during neuromuscular blockade. It should be emphasized that neuromuscular blocking agents do not confer amnesia, so adequate sedation is required to prevent awareness in patients who are pharmacologically paralyzed. Many patients who are not paralyzed but are receiving mechanical ventilation require sedation for comfort and anxiolysis while remaining conscious enough to communicate their needs.

E. In contrast, patients accustomed to mechanical ventilation may require little to no sedation. In certain extreme cases, such as for patients in a persistent vegetative state or coma, sedation may not be required. Over the past decade, numerous studies have reported on the benefits of lighter sedation or nonsedation of patients undergoing mechanical ventilation. In one high-profile trial, patients randomized to a "no sedation" group were liberated from mechanical ventilation and discharged from the ICU significantly earlier compared to patients receiving protocolized sedation, although the "no sedation" group exhibited a higher incidence of delirium. This finding of increased delirium has subsequently been examined in a larger trial conducted by the same group, which found no meaningful differences in primary end points between patients who are sedated and nonsedated. The nonsedated are better able to interact with ICU staff and are thus more likely to participate in physical therapy and mobilization, which has similarly been associated with shorter duration of mechanical ventilation, reduced delirium, and accelerated recovery from critical illness.

F. Reduced levels of sedation may also help mitigate delirium in the ICU. **Delirium** is a cognitive disturbance with an acute onset and fluctuating clinical course. The reported incidence of delirium in the ICU ranges from 11% to 87%. Common risk factors include age older than 65 years, male sex, dementia, prior history of delirium, immobility, dehydration, coexisting medical conditions, treatment with psychoactive and anticholinergic drugs, and malnutrition. Other modifiable risk factors include the use of physical restraints, higher doses of sedative-hypnotics and opioids, active infection, recent surgery, uncontrolled pain, and disruption of a normal sleep cycle. Limiting the administration of medications known to potentiate disorientation—such as benzodiazepines and anticholinergics—may reduce ICU delirium.

II. MONITORING AND TITRATION OF SEDATIVES

Unmonitored or improperly calibrated sedation strategies may predispose patients to delirium, posttraumatic stress disorder (PTSD), prolonged mechanical ventilation, or increased mortality. Unfortunately, our observation has been that many clinicians aggressively sedate patients early in their ICU course and may maintain an unnecessarily deep plane of sedation. An ideal strategy instead incorporates scale-directed titration and regular interruption of sedation. The **Richmond Agitation Sedation Scale (RASS)** (Table 7.1) remains one of the most widely used instruments to determine a patient's level of sedation. By establishing a RASS goal, nurses and bedside clinicians can titrate a patient's sedation to a measurable target.

A. Continuous Versus Intermittent Dosing of Sedatives and Analgesics

1. Continuous sedative or opioid infusions may provide a stable level of analgosedation. However, the clinical duration of the action of certain common agents (eg, fentanyl and midazolam) markedly increase with prolonged infusion compared with bolus dose or intermittent administration. The **context-sensitive half-time (CSHT)** describes the period required for the plasma drug concentration to decline by 50% after a continuous infusion is stopped. For many sedatives, the CSHT increases with the duration of infusion until drug redistribution mechanisms are saturated, and it may be markedly greater than the simple elimination half-life of a given drug.

TABLE 7.1 The Richmond Agitation Sedation Scale (RASS)

Descriptor	Definition	Points
Combative	Overtly combative, violent, or immediately dangerous to staff	+4
Very agitated	Aggressive, pulls or removes tube(s) or catheter(s)	+3
Agitated	Frequent nonpurposeful movements, fighting ventilator	+2
Restless	Anxious, but movements are not aggressive or vigorous	+1
Alert and calm		0
Drowsy	Not fully alert, but exhibits sustained awakening (eye opening/eye contact) to voice (>10 s)	−1
Light sedation	Briefly awakens with eye contact to voice (<10 s)	−2
Moderate sedation	Movement or eye-opening to voice (but no eye contact)	−3
Deep sedation	No response to voice, but movement or eye-opening to physical stimulation	−4
Unarousable	No response to voice or physical stimulation	−5

Adapted from Sessler CN, Gosnell MS, Grap MJ, et al. The Richmond agitation-sedation scale: validity and reliability in adult intensive care unit patients. *Am J Respir Crit Care Med.* 2002;166:1338-1344.

2. Despite the ongoing popularity of continuous sedative infusions, bolus administration of analgesics and sedative agents often provides increased flexibility in achieving a patient's sedation and analgesia goals. For instance, intermittent intravenous (IV) doses of short-acting opioids or sedatives may allow a patient to remain stably sedated through periods of increased stimulation. A common example is as-needed dosing of fentanyl—a drug that would otherwise exhibit a prolonged CSHT if infused continuously—to permit a patient to tolerate repositioning or other care intervention. Another ancillary benefit of intermittent sedative dosing is an overall decrease in the quantity of medication administered, a consideration that may become particularly salient when drug shortages arise.

B. Scheduled Interruption of Sedation

1. Regular interruption of continuous sedation, also termed a **spontaneous awakening trial (SAT)**, may decrease the duration of mechanical ventilation, lower the quantity of medication administered, mitigate delirium, and improve clinical outcomes. The development of encephalopathy, drug-induced respiratory depression, muscle wasting, and constipation can also be minimized with daily SATs. Daily interruption of sedative medications may also facilitate recognition of the point at which analgosedation should be weaned.
2. If long-term sedation is required for a patient who is mechanically ventilated, the coordination of a daily SAT with a **spontaneous breathing trial (SBT)** has also been shown to reduce mortality in patients in the ICU. Coupling SAT and SBT may also be helpful in allowing assessment of a patient's progress toward liberation from invasive ventilatory support.

C. Weaning From Sedation

1. Weaning refers to the gradual discontinuation of analgesics and sedatives when these are no longer clinically indicated. A plan for weaning from analgosedation is best established early in the patient's ICU stay and readdressed in step with an evolving clinical trajectory. Although there is no single weaning strategy that is clearly superior for all patients, the intensivist must guard against withdrawal syndromes and abrupt weaning of prolonged sedation, which can result in significant harm. Several strategies for safe weaning from opioids and common sedatives are outlined in Figure 7.2.

Opioid weaning

- Options: Reduce infusion directly or replace with enteral opioids.
    - Once oral replacement is initiated, reduce opioid infusion by 25% per dose until off.
- Monitor for withdrawal symptoms.

If severe withdrawal symptoms (eg, psychomotor agitation, tachycardia, hypertension, abdominal cramps) emerge: (1) treat with clonidine or as-needed opioid bolus doses and (2) maintain infusion rate or taper dose until symptoms are controlled before weaning further.

Methadone taper method (preferred for opioid-tolerant patients)
Caution with prolonged QTc and hepatic impairment, particularly given variable pharmacokinetics.

Sample oral methadone taper: 10 mg q8h × 48 h, 7.5 mg q8h × 48 h, 5 mg q8h × 48 h, 5 mg q12h × 24 h, 2.5 mg q12h × 24 h, then off.

Oral equivalent taper method (preferred for opioid-naive patients)
Consider if hydromorphone infusion <1.5 mg/h or fentanyl <150 mcg/min.

Sample oral hydromorphone taper: 8 mg q4h × 48 h, 6 mg q4h × 48 h, 4 mg q4h × 24 h, 4 mg q6h × 24 h, then transition to prn dosing.

Infusion taper method
Wean infusion by 25% per day. Once at low rate, transition to standing or as-needed IV equianalgesic boluses.

Dexmedetomidine weaning

- Options: Reduce infusion directly or transition to clonidine.
- Monitor for signs and symptoms of withdrawal, especially rebound hypertension and tachycardia.

Oral clonidine taper method
Initiate oral clonidine and increase with each dose to a maximum of 0.6 mg q8h.

- If dexmedetomidine < 0.7 μg/kg/h: start clonidine 0.1 mg q8h.
- If dexmedetomidine > 0.7 μg/kg/h: start clonidine 0.2 mg q8h.

Sample oral clonidine taper (after dexmedetomidine infusion is off for 24 h): 0.3 mg q8h × 24 h, 0.2 mg q8h × 24 h, 0.1 mg q8h × 24 h, 0.1 mg q12h × 24 h, then off.

Infusion taper method
Wean infusion by 25% every 6 h. Once at low rate, discontinue or transition to as-needed clonidine dosing.

Midazolam weaning

- Options: Reduce infusion directly or replace with enteral benzodiazepines.
    - Once oral replacement is initiated, reduce midazolam infusion by 25% per dose until off.
- Monitor for withdrawal symptoms*.

*If severe withdrawal symptoms (eg, seizures or psychosis) emerge, treat with bolus doses of lorazepam (0.5-2 mg IV or po prn). Maintain infusion at same rate or taper dose until symptoms are controlled for 12-24 h before weaning further.

Infusion taper method
Divide total daily dose of midazolam by 6 for daily lorazepam dose. Divide total lorazepam dose to allow for a q4-6h dosing regimen.

Sample lorazepam taper (from midazolam at 3 mg/h): 3 mg q6h × 24 h, 2 mg q6h × 24 h, 1 mg q6h × 24 h, 1 mg q8h × 24 h, 1 mg q12h × 12 h, then off

Phenobarbital taper method
Give loading dose of 5-10 mg/kg IBW, then 1-3 mg/kg IBW doses q8-12h. Wean midazolam by 25% after loading and by 25% with each subsequent dose.

Infusion taper method
Wean infusion by 25% per day, then transition to standing or as-needed midazolam boluses.

FIGURE 7.2 Sample weaning strategies for opioids, dexmedetomidine, and midazolam. IBW, ideal body weight; IV, intravenous; po, orally; prn, as needed; q, every.

III. SEDATIVE MEDICATIONS

Sedative agents may be defined as drugs that are capable of depressing consciousness via their interactions with the central nervous system. Sedatives thus directly benefit the patient by reducing awareness, alleviating anxiety and agitation, and producing variable degrees of amnesia. However, it should be noted that most sedatives increase the risk of respiratory complications resulting from a depressed ventilatory drive, respiratory muscle weakness and atrophy, dampened protective airway reflexes, and upper airway obstruction. Therefore, patients who are critically ill and not receiving mechanical ventilation should be closely monitored by trained personnel while receiving sedation and appropriate respiratory support should be readily available when deeper levels of sedation are necessary. Further agent-specific considerations are outlined subsequently.

A. Propofol

1. Propofol remains one of the most widely used sedatives in critical care medicine. It is a GABAergic (γ-aminobutyric acid) agent that rapidly crosses the blood-brain barrier because of its lipophilicity. After bolus administration, propofol exhibits an onset of action within seconds and a duration of action between 10 and 15 minutes. These pharmacokinetic characteristics are particularly favorable for patients who require frequent neurologic assessments. Multiple studies have shown that propofol-based sedation is associated with a shorter time to mental status recovery, more rapid liberation from mechanical ventilation, and greater cost-effectiveness when compared to benzodiazepine-based sedation in the ICU. However, long-term infusions may cause propofol to accumulate within lipid stores and greatly increase its duration of effect.
2. The most notable hemodynamic consequence of propofol use is dose-dependent hypotension, which may be the result of systemic vasodilation and, to a lesser extent, myocardial suppression. Because of its lipophilicity, propofol is also uniquely formulated within a lipid-rich emulsion. Serum triglycerides should therefore be monitored every 3 to 7 days while the patient receives a continuous propofol infusion because cases of propofol-induced pancreatitis from hypertriglyceridemia have been documented. Of note, propofol's lipid emulsion provides the patient with approximately 1.1 kcal/mL and should be counted as a caloric source when formulating nutritional plans.
3. Propofol infusion syndrome (PRIS) is a rare but potentially lethal complication of prolonged or high-dose propofol infusion. PRIS is characterized by bradyarrhythmias, myocardial depression, profound metabolic acidosis, rhabdomyolysis, and shock. PRIS is most frequently reported among children who are critically ill, particularly those with traumatic brain injury receiving high doses of propofol, although it has been reported in adults as well. The clinician should maintain an appropriate index of suspicion when monitoring for this complication, which may entail regular measurement of serum pH, lactate, and creatinine kinase when a prolonged propofol infusion is required.

B. Dexmedetomidine

1. Dexmedetomidine is a highly selective α_2-adrenergic receptor agonist. Stimulation of the 2A variant of the α_2 receptor produces sedation, anxiolysis, and modest analgesia, whereas stimulation of the 2B variant induces peripheral vasoconstriction, yields more robust analgesia, and suppresses shivering. Unlike many sedatives, dexmedetomidine does not powerfully depress ventilation at usual doses and some degree of autonomic arousal may occur during administration. These properties allow for a more awake, interactive, and easily mobilized patient, and studies have indicated that the use of this agent may be associated with a shorter time to ventilator

liberation and a decreased length of stay in the ICU. Dexmedetomidine is approved for short-term sedation (<24 hours). However, it has been studied over longer periods at dosages that exceed the proprietary upper limit of 0.7 μg/kg/h. In early trials involving higher infusion rates, dexmedetomidine was safe and at least as effective as lorazepam and midazolam in providing targeted sedation and was associated with fewer days on the ventilator and in the ICU. Compared to other sedative-hypnotics, it may also result in a lower incidence of delirium.

2. A recent randomized controlled trial found that the use of high-dose dexmedetomidine (1-1.5 μg/kg/h) as a primary sedative did not confer any clinically meaningful benefits over a "usual care" approach including propofol, midazolam, and other agents. In fact, more than 70% of patients in the dexmedetomidine arm required propofol supplementation to reach the targeted sedation goal, and the primary use of dexmedetomidine was associated with higher rates of adverse hemodynamic events such as significant hypotension and bradycardia. The use of high-dose dexmedetomidine infusions should therefore be considered carefully depending on the patient's clinical status and ICU needs.

3. Dexmedetomidine is most commonly used in short-term sedation for patients who are otherwise ready to be extubated but cannot safely be weaned from other sedative-hypnotics because of delirium or agitation. A loading dose of 0.25 1 μg/kg can reduce the time required to achieve target serum concentrations of dexmedetomidine, although bolus administration is best supervised by an experienced clinician because of its association with bradycardia. A reasonable alternative to a bolus dose of dexmedetomidine is to initiate an infusion at 0.6 to 0.7 μg/kg/h and adjust the infusion rate by 0.1 to 0.2 μg/kg/h at intervals no more frequent than every 30 minutes. This approach may minimize hemodynamic fluctuations. Owing to frequent dosage adjustments during this transition, a protocolized approach can help guide bedside staff in optimizing safety while achieving the intended sedation target.

4. Dexmedetomidine doses exceeding 1.5 μg/kg/h offer minimal benefit over lower infusion rates. Other sedatives, analgesic adjuncts, or antipsychotics should be incorporated into the patient's regimen to augment the effects of dexmedetomidine if this rate is reached. Withdrawal syndromes characterized by agitation and tachycardia may result from the discontinuation of a long-term infusion. If a component of symptomatic withdrawal is suspected, a taper including the administration of clonidine—a less potent and less selective α_2-adrenergic receptor agonist—may be initiated. Reliance on dexmedetomidine only as a primary sedative is often limited by its inability to produce deep sedation as well as by adverse effects such as hypotension and bradycardia. When significant bradycardia arises, the most effective intervention is to interrupt the infusion and administer atropine or glycopyrrolate to normalize the heart rate as needed. Although dexmedetomidine is considered neutral with respect to the patient's ventilatory drive at usual doses, higher infusion rates or large boluses may blunt the respiratory drive and precipitate upper airway obstruction when the airway is not secured. Finally, drug-induced hyperthermia related to dexmedetomidine has been documented and may prompt an unnecessary workup for fever in a patient who is critically ill.

C. Ketamine

1. Ketamine produces rapid-onset sedation as well as analgesia mainly via antagonism of glutamatergic *N*-methyl-D-aspartate (NMDA) receptors in the central nervous system. To a lesser extent, ketamine may also act on minor opioid receptors. Ketamine sedation is characterized as a unique dissociative state, one in which the patient's level of consciousness is depressed despite disinhibition of cortical activity. During the administration of ketamine-based sedation, patients may exhibit nystagmus and a trance-like cataleptic state. However, ketamine is notable for its ability to produce effective and relatively balanced analgosedation—including amnesia, decreased awareness, and pain relief in tandem. Ketamine can thus serve as an effective opioid-sparing primary analgesic or adjunct for painful procedures such as debridement and dressing changes.

2. Even at subanesthetic plasma concentrations, ketamine decreases opioid requirements, prevents the development of opioid-induced hyperalgesia, and may reduce opioid tolerance. This makes it useful in patients receiving chronic opioid therapy. Ketamine also maintains relative hemodynamic stability by decreasing catecholamine reuptake and indirectly increasing sympathetic tone. Unlike most other sedatives, ketamine preserves normal airway reflexes, maintains spontaneous ventilation, and promotes bronchodilation. A patient may receive a low-dose ketamine infusion (between 1 and 5 μg/kg/min) without significant respiratory depression. Of note, because the NMDA receptor is blocked in its resting conformation by a magnesium ion, magnesium repletion or supplementation may potentiate the effects of ketamine.
3. Several significant downsides to ketamine-based sedation may restrict its use. Although ketamine tends to produce relative hypertension and tachycardia via its indirect sympathomimetic effects, it may also act as a negative inotrope in patients who are catecholamine depleted, such as those with decompensated heart failure. Ketamine is further associated with hypersalivation and distressing emergence phenomena, which may result in confusion, nightmares, and audiovisual hallucinations. Fortunately, emergence phenomena are rarely reported with low-dose ketamine infusions (<5 μg/kg/min) and can be curtailed with judiciously dosed amnestic agents such as midazolam.

D. Benzodiazepines

1. Benzodiazepines are potent anxiolytic, amnestic, and sedative medications. They potentiate the activation of central $GABA_A$ receptors and produce highly dose-dependent effects. These drugs also possess anticonvulsant properties and are useful in the management of seizures and alcohol withdrawal. Although benzodiazepines—particularly midazolam—were used as first-line sedatives in the past, studies have shown that infusions of benzodiazepines for primary ICU sedation are associated with slow awakening, delayed tracheal extubation, and impaired assessment of neurologic function. Furthermore, benzodiazepines may produce paradoxical agitation and confusion in older patients, and they have been associated with the development of ICU delirium. Patients receiving prolonged benzodiazepine infusions are also at risk for withdrawal on discontinuation and slow weaning may be required.
2. The two most frequently administered benzodiazepines in the ICU are midazolam and lorazepam. **Midazolam** is a potent, short-acting benzodiazepine with an onset of action within 1 to 3 minutes of injection. Midazolam exhibits lipophilic properties in vivo and accumulates in adipose tissues. As a result, extensive reservoirs of midazolam may develop after prolonged infusion, particularly in the obese, producing extended sedation because of ongoing drug redistribution. In addition, midazolam is degraded to active metabolites that may accumulate in the setting of renal failure. Patients receiving midazolam may develop tachyphylaxis more rapidly than do those receiving other benzodiazepines, requiring escalating doses to sustain a desired clinical effect. Because of concerns surrounding unpredictable

awakening after prolonged infusion, midazolam is recommended only for short-term sedation (no more than 48 hours). **Lorazepam**, although rarely administered as an infusion, is less lipophilic than midazolam. Therefore, an IV bolus of lorazepam will demonstrate a slower onset of action but will not result in bioaccumulation to the same degree. Lorazepam undergoes hepatic glucuronidation to an inactive metabolite and is thus the preferred benzodiazepine for patients with renal failure.

E. Volatile Anesthetics

1. Modern volatile anesthetics—including **isoflurane**, **sevoflurane**, and **desflurane**—belong to a unique class of medications that are delivered via anesthesia machines or ventilators with specialized vaporizers and inhaled along with a carrier gas. Although these agents depress consciousness via mechanisms that remain incompletely characterized, the best available evidence suggests that volatile anesthetics bind with low affinity to a variety of targets, activating inhibitory receptors (eg, $GABA_A$ and glycine) while blocking certain excitatory pathways. Volatile anesthetic pharmacology is complex and beyond the scope of this chapter. For the purposes of this discussion, it is sufficient to recognize that, when appropriate equipment is used, volatile anesthetics are highly predictable in their pharmacokinetics, are eliminated independently of hepatorenal function, and may be easily monitored and titrated.
2. Clinical interest in the incorporation of volatile anesthetics into intensive care is not new. This interest has been spurred by characteristics of modern volatile anesthetics including rapid, predictable onset and offset times; a favorable combination of analgesia, amnesia, and muscle relaxation; and relative hemodynamic stability without the need for excess fluid administration. There is also evidence that volatile anesthetics reduce pulmonary inflammation, and their bronchodilatory effects—which may be particularly desirable in patients with obstructive lung pathology—are thoroughly established.
3. The ease of volatile anesthetic delivery in ICU settings has been enhanced by the development of adaptable **anesthetic-conserving devices (ACDs)**, which act as portable vaporizer modules and have been approved in several countries outside of the United States. However, notable limitations persist surrounding the use of volatile anesthetics in the ICU, including the need for specialized equipment, expanded training of bedside staff, requirements for waste gas scavenging, and the risk of rare but severe adverse reactions such as malignant hyperthermia.
4. Volatile anesthetic-based sedation in the ICU increased during the COVID-19 pandemic. The increase in volatile anesthetic use was motivated by shortages of mechanical ventilators for large numbers of patients admitted to critical care settings, which drove many hospitals to employ anesthesia machines as ICU ventilators, as well as shortages of more common sedative agents. One retrospective study found that the use of isoflurane was associated with decreased utilization of IV analgesic and sedative agents such as hydromorphone and propofol, whereas a separate small-scale analysis found that oxygenation was improved in a small cohort of patients with COVID-19-related acute respiratory distress syndrome (ARDS) who received isoflurane for sedation. Although such findings are encouraging, significant further study in this area remains to be performed.

F. Other Sedative Agents and Adjuncts

1. Older sedatives such as **barbiturates**, which potentiate GABA receptors at a separate site relative to benzodiazepines, are now infrequently used for primary ICU sedation. However, the properties of long-acting barbiturates

continue to be useful in alcohol withdrawal syndromes, and **phenobarbital** is routinely employed for this purpose at our institution (see **Chapter 31**). Barbiturates may also be useful in reducing cerebral metabolic demand under specific circumstances.

2. **Antipsychotics** comprise a class of agents that primarily antagonize central dopaminergic (D_2) receptors, thus interrupting subcortical pathways that may exacerbate agitation and delirium. Although not used to achieve sedation primarily, the first-generation antipsychotic **haloperidol** is a high-potency drug that can be given intermittently to alleviate symptoms of hyperactive delirium. Repeated or high doses of haloperidol may be associated with acute dystonic reactions and other extrapyramidal adverse effects. The second-generation antipsychotic agent **quetiapine** is a lower potency agent that is often tolerated well with fewer extrapyramidal symptoms. However, antipsychotics may prolong the QT interval and carry an association with increased mortality in older patients treated for psychotic symptoms in the setting of dementia.
3. A broad array of other medications can be used off-label to complement a light to moderate sedation regimen or promote sleep. For example, small-scale studies suggest that the administration of scheduled **melatonin** in the evening to stabilize the circadian rhythm may be modestly effective in reducing ICU delirium. Agents such as **trazodone** and **mirtazapine** are also employed to enhance nighttime sedation and alleviate anxiety. However, use of these medications is not supported by strong evidence of clinical benefit, and adverse effects such as hypotension and metabolic disturbances may be observed in association with their use.

IV. PAIN MANAGEMENT

Pain is a prominent cause of distress in patients in the ICU. Such pain may arise from an underlying condition—such as operative wounds, burns, bone fractures, bowel obstruction, pancreatitis, and so on—or from routine ICU-related care itself—including endotracheal intubation, physical therapy, repositioning, dressing changes, or prolonged immobility. It is estimated that up to 70% of patients will experience at least moderate pain during an ICU stay. Patients with inadequate pain control are at risk for the development of acute stress disorder and PTSD, and pain may trigger or exacerbate delirium. In addition, nociceptive stimulation may adversely affect a patient's hemodynamics and make tight control of blood pressure and heart rate difficult. Accordingly, pain should be addressed to ensure patient comfort and reduce adverse events. The ongoing management of any preexisting chronic pain must also be taken into consideration to prevent a patient from experiencing additional distress while receiving critical care.

Pain assessment and management in the ICU may be complicated by a patient's inability to communicate effectively because of sedation, neuromuscular blockade, or cognitive impairment arising from delirium or encephalopathy. To address this problem, several observational scales have been developed to facilitate pain assessment. For those who are unable to self-report or describe pain but who have intact motor function and observable behaviors, the validated **Critical Care Pain Observation Tool (CPOT)** is a reliable behavioral pain scale for patients in the ICU. The CPOT includes four behavioral categories: (i) facial expression, (ii) body movements, (iii) muscle tension, and (iv) ventilator compliance in patients who are ventilated. Each of these four indicators is scored from 0 to 2 with the assumption that a relationship exists between each score and the intensity of pain, yielding a useful composite score between 0 and 8.

Although opioids are the mainstay of pain control in the ICU, it is increasingly recognized that patients may benefit from a thoughtful approach to **multimodal analgesia**. Such a regimen may consist of a scheduled or an as-needed opioid in combination with nonopioid adjuncts or regional analgesics such as those described subsequently.

A. Opioids: Opioids comprise a large class of powerful analgesics and serve as the most commonly used pain medications in the ICU. Their primary mechanism of action involves stimulation of inhibitory opioid receptors, thus dampening and altering neurologic responses to pain. The available evidence suggests that opioids act on the substantia gelatinosa in the dorsal horn of the spinal cord to reduce nociceptive inputs to the central nervous system. Opioids also appear to produce descending inhibitory modulation of nociceptive transmission and alter central pain processing.

Activation of opioid receptors in the brain and spinal cord can result in significant respiratory depression and sedation. Patients with sleep apnea or other hypoventilation syndromes are particularly susceptible to respiratory depression and hypercapnia when receiving opioids. Because opioid receptors are distributed throughout the enteric nervous system, opioids also decrease intestinal motility, increase transit time, and may ultimately produce constipation and ileus. Opioid-induced bowel hypomotility may delay the tolerance of enteral nutrition, prolong a patient's hospital stay, and even predispose patients to the reflux of enteral tube feeds with consequent aspiration. Therefore, a bowel regimen incorporating at least two laxative agents should be prescribed preemptively in patients requiring high or prolonged doses of opioid analgesics. Neurotoxicity is increasingly reported as an additional complication of opioid use, particularly among older adults, those with hepatorenal impairments, those with baseline neurocognitive disorders, and those receiving larger doses of opioids. Reported symptoms of opioid-induced neurotoxicity may include rigidity, myoclonus, and hyperalgesia.

When possible, opioids given by mouth or through an enteral tube offer several theoretical advantages over parenteral opioids, including convenience, lower rates of infectious complications, and improved maintenance of mucosal structure and function, which may prevent gut atrophy and resulting bacterial translocation into the bloodstream. The primary disadvantage of enteral opioid therapy is variable gastrointestinal bioavailability and, consequently, an increased time to peak clinical effect.

Prolonged opioid therapy may lead to progressive tolerance, ultimately resulting in dose escalation to maintain analgesia. **Opioid rotation** (eg, transitioning from oral oxycodone to morphine) may partially offset the accumulation of tolerance in patients requiring prolonged opioid courses because incomplete cross-tolerance is observed between specific opioid agents. Because abrupt cessation of prolonged opioid therapy may also produce a highly distressing withdrawal syndrome, gradual discontinuation (eg, with an **opioid taper**) is recommended for patients who have developed significant tolerance. Because of the wide array of potential adverse effects associated with opioid administration, a thorough understanding of drug pharmacology should guide the selection of the specific agent used. Key considerations relating to common opioids are detailed here.

1. **Morphine** is a naturally occurring opioid often regarded as the standard to which other opioids are compared. It has a time to onset of 5 minutes and a peak effect observed between 15 and 40 minutes after IV administration, with a variable duration of action of 2 to 5 hours. Intermittent IV doses of 2 to 10 mg or continuous infusion rates of 1 to 3 mg/h are often adequate to relieve moderate to severe pain in the average opioid-naive adult. The dose required for a given patient depends on factors such as tolerance as well as metabolic and excretory capacity. Morphine undergoes hepatic conjugation to morphine-3-glucuronide, a major metabolite with potentially neurotoxic effects, and morphine-6-glucuronide, which possesses 20 to

40 times the analgesic potency of morphine itself. Both metabolites are eliminated via the kidney and may accumulate in patients with renal impairment. For this reason, alternative opioids are often preferred in patients who are critically ill with acute or chronic kidney injury.

2. **Hydromorphone** is a semisynthetic opioid with 5 to 7 times greater potency than morphine. It also produces its clinical effects more rapidly because it requires only 10 to 20 minutes to reach a peak and exhibits a duration of action between 3 and 6 hours. Although it is more lipid soluble than is morphine, hydromorphone does not accumulate significantly in adipose tissue compared to highly lipophilic agents such as fentanyl. Hydromorphone undergoes hepatic conversion to a major metabolite, hydromorphone-3-glucuronide, that can produce neuroexcitatory symptoms such as myoclonus, allodynia, or seizures when renal elimination is ineffective. Therefore, although it is generally safe for hydromorphone to be given as a continuous infusion even in patients with moderate renal impairment, caution should be taken in patients with severely reduced kidney function.
3. **Fentanyl** has a potency approximately 100 times greater than that of morphine. It is a highly lipid-soluble synthetic opioid with rapid onset (~2-3 minutes) and brief duration of action (20-30 minutes) when administered as an IV bolus. With repeated injections or continuous infusion, large stores of fentanyl may accumulate in adipose tissue. These reserves of opioids must later be redistributed and metabolized to terminate the clinical action of the drug, which may lead to markedly prolonged effects after discontinuation. However, fentanyl lacks renally excreted active metabolites, making it an ideal analgesic agent for patients with severe renal impairment.
4. **Remifentanil** is a synthetic opioid with an even more rapid onset of action and shorter duration than that of fentanyl. In contrast to other opioids, remifentanil is metabolized to inactive breakdown products by nonspecific esterases in the plasma, red blood cells, and interstitial tissues, so its effects are not significantly altered by hepatic or renal failure. The CSHT of remifentanil is also consistently brief (~4 minutes) even after an infusion of long duration. However, opioid-induced hyperalgesia—a paradoxically increased sensitivity to pain—may occur in patients receiving prolonged remifentanil infusions, limiting its utility in the ICU.
5. **Methadone**, although approximately equipotent with respect to morphine, varies widely in its effects between patients. Importantly, it is unique in its ability to act on multiple targets, functioning as an antagonist at the NMDA receptor and producing some serotonergic effects. It exhibits a variable but generally long duration of 15 to 40 hours, although its clinical effects may appear to wear off earlier in the critically ill. Methadone is used primarily in patients who have developed tolerance to long-term opioid therapy because it counteracts both opioid-induced hyperalgesia and withdrawal symptoms. It is also useful when incorporated into an opioid taper.
6. **Meperidine**, a low-potency synthetic opioid, is generally avoided as a primary analgesic in the critically ill because of its association with myocardial depression and off-target effects. Because of its structural resemblance to atropine, meperidine also possesses vagolytic properties and may cause tachycardia and hypotension. It is rarely used in the ICU other than in the treatment of shivering. Meperidine's major metabolite, normeperidine, may also accumulate in renal failure and has been associated with seizure activity due to neuroexcitation.

B. Nonopioid Analgesics: Exclusive reliance on opioids for pain control may predispose patients to the wide array of drug complications described earlier. This highlights the importance of including opioid-sparing medications in a comprehensive analgosedation plan. The following section provides a partial overview of commonly prescribed analgesic adjuncts, although it should be noted that sedatives with intrinsic analgesic effects (such as dexmedetomidine, which are discussed elsewhere in this chapter) may be included in this category as well.

1. **Acetaminophen:** Acetaminophen (also known as paracetamol) is a centrally active antipyretic and analgesic used to treat mild to moderate pain. It is an attractive adjunct in many patients because of its availability, reliable dosing, favorable safety profile in controlled settings, and multiple formulations (ie, oral, rectal, and IV). When combined with an opioid, acetaminophen also produces a greater analgesic effect than do higher doses of the opioid alone. The total daily dose of acetaminophen should not exceed 4 g, and the drug should be dosed carefully in patients with existing hepatic dysfunction.
2. **Nonsteroidal anti-inflammatory drugs:** Nonsteroidal anti-inflammatory drugs (NSAIDs) are a useful class of analgesic and anti-inflammatory agents that remain highly effective and widely available. These medications exert their effects through the inhibition of proinflammatory prostaglandin synthesis. Of the NSAIDs, **ketorolac** (often referred to by its common trade name, *Toradol*) is the most potent parenteral NSAID currently available. The usual dose of ketorolac is 15 to 30 mg IV every 6 to 8 hours, with higher doses generally conferring a longer duration of action. The analgesic efficacy of 30 mg of ketorolac is similar to that of 10 mg of morphine, although a ceiling effect may be reached at doses of 15 mg. However, ketorolac—as with other NSAIDs—is associated with risks of gastrointestinal bleeding, renal injury, and platelet dysfunction. Reduced baseline renal function, hypovolemia, and advanced age increase the risk of NSAID nephrotoxicity. To minimize such adverse effects, ketorolac should be administered for no more than 3 days at a time. By comparison, **ibuprofen** and **naproxen** are the most common enteral NSAIDs given in the United States. These agents are significantly less potent than is ketorolac but share a similar side effect profile. The typical analgesic dose of ibuprofen is 400 to 600 mg every 6 to 8 hours, whereas naproxen has a longer duration of action and may be dosed at 250 to 500 mg every 12 hours.
3. **Antineuropathic drugs:** A variety of medications are currently used primarily to target neuropathic pain such as that arising from postherpetic neuralgia, radiculopathy, or diabetic neuropathy. However, these agents may be useful adjuncts as part of an opioid-sparing or multimodal approach to analgesia in the critically ill. Many antineuropathic agents produce sedation particularly in combination with opioids. **Gabapentin**, which was originally developed as an anticonvulsant, has efficacy in the treatment of various neuropathic pain syndromes. A common initial dose of gabapentin is 300 mg every 8 to 12 hours, although dose escalation up to 1200 mg is possible.
4. **Antispasmodic drugs:** Antispasmodic agents act via several different pathways to reduce muscle tension and alleviate myofascial pain. Although evidence of its clinical efficacy in patients who are critically ill remains limited, the antispasmodic agent **tizanidine** has gained popularity as an adjunct within a multimodal pain regimen. Similar to dexmedetomidine, tizanidine acts via agonism of α_2-adrenergic receptors. A common starting dose is 2 to 4 mg in the evening, although twice-daily dosing is also possible. Sedation and hypotension are the most common adverse effects at increased doses.
5. IV **lidocaine** may be a useful adjunct in alleviating pain in patients tolerant to opioids. Topical agents (eg, menthol-based creams and lidocaine patches) may be helpful in reducing highly localized and superficial pain, while nonpharmacologic techniques such as cold application or the delivery of transcutaneous electrical nerve stimulation (TENS) may also be effective in certain situations.

C. Regional Analgesia: Regional anesthesia consists of infiltrating a peripheral nerve with an anesthetic agent and blocking transmission to avoid or relieve pain. Regional analgesia may be further subdivided into neuraxial modalities, such as epidural or spinal (intrathecal) anesthetics, and peripheral nerve blocks.

1. **Neuraxial analgesia** can powerfully and rapidly alleviate severe pain, particularly when adequate relief cannot be achieved by oral and IV analgesics alone. For example, it has been demonstrated that a **continuous epidural infusion**, when compared with IV opioid therapy, provides superior relief of thoracoabdominal pain resulting from surgery or trauma and has a number of other ancillary benefits including earlier mobility, relative cardiopulmonary stability, reduced incidence of ileus, and a lower risk of venous thromboembolism. These benefits are countered by the potential risks of sympathectomy, motor block, urinary retention, and rare but catastrophic neurologic injury. Notably, epidural analgesia has been associated with a reduction in mortality for patients with multiple rib fractures in some studies. Thoracic paravertebral catheters, although less effective than are epidural catheters, have been associated with improved pulmonary function in patients with rib fractures while producing a lower risk of hypotension and preserving respiratory strength.
2. **Peripheral nerve blocks** may also be used to relieve pain that is relatively localized to an extremity or specific anatomic distribution. For instance, upper extremity analgesia may be achieved through placement of an infraclavicular catheter, whereas a sciatic or femoral catheter provides durable lower extremity analgesia. The placement of peripheral nerve blocks may be safer relative to the use of neuraxial analgesia in patients who are anticoagulated or coagulopathic. Nonetheless, site-specific adverse effects must be considered when placing a peripheral nerve block. For example, a single-injection block or catheter near the proximal brachial plexus carries a high risk of phrenic nerve blockade, which produces hemidiaphragmatic paralysis that may be poorly tolerated in a patient with limited ventilatory capacity. Continuous blockade of an extremity also commonly limits patient mobility and may mask limb-threatening complications such as acute compartment syndrome. Therefore, the use of peripheral nerve blocks in the ICU remains limited to select circumstances.

V. NEUROMUSCULAR BLOCKADE

If patient-ventilator synchrony cannot be achieved through optimal analgosedation alone, neuromuscular blockade (ie, chemical paralysis) may be a reasonable intervention for the critically ill who require mechanical ventilation for refractory or severe respiratory failure (ie, P/F ratio <120-150) receiving >60% FIO_2 and a positive end-expiratory pressure (PEEP) >10 cm H_2O.

A. It is imperative to maintain a deep level of sedation to prevent awareness during the period of paralysis. Although current technology is not infallible, it is reasonable to titrate analgosedation according to a **processed electroencephalogram** (eg, bispectral index or SedLine monitor) to achieve a higher likelihood of adequate sedation during paralysis.

B. The neuromuscular blocking agent **cisatracurium**, a drug that undergoes predictable nonenzymatic degradation in the plasma, is commonly used for patients in the ICU who require neuromuscular blockade. The infusion rate of cisatracurium should be titrated depending on peripheral nerve monitoring. Typically, a moderately dense neuromuscular blockade—in which a cisatracurium infusion is targeted to one to three visible or palpable twitches in response to a **train-of-four (TOF)** stimulus—is sufficient. If patient-ventilator synchrony cannot be achieved via a moderate degree of neuromuscular blockade, it may be useful to titrate the infusion to achieve deeper paralysis. A deep blockade is characterized by the absence of visible or palpable twitches in response to plain TOF stimulation, whereas one to two twitches can still be elicited in response to a TOF stimulus after a 50-Hz tetanic stimulus is applied.

C. The need for chemical paralysis should be reevaluated every 12 hours, ideally during multidisciplinary rounds. If the patient's hypoxemia has improved, an attempt should be made to discontinue the cisatracurium infusion. If patient-ventilator asynchrony recurs, neuromuscular blockade may be reestablished. Once neuromuscular blockade is no longer indicated, it should be discontinued promptly and the level of sedation should be lightened or reduced accordingly.

Selected Readings

Baumgartner L, Lam K, Lai J, et al. Effectiveness of melatonin for the prevention of intensive care unit delirium. *Pharmacotherapy*. 2019;39(3):280-287.

Block BM, Liu SS, Rowlingson AJ, et al. Efficacy of postoperative epidural analgesia: a meta-analysis. *JAMA*. 2003;290:2455-2463.

Carson SS, Kress JP, Rodgers JE, et al. A randomized trial of intermittent lorazepam versus propofol with daily interruption in mechanically ventilated patients. *Crit Care Med*. 2006;34(5):1326-1332.

Girard TD, Kress JP, Fuchs BD, et al. Efficacy and safety of a paired sedation and ventilator weaning protocol for mechanically ventilated patients in intensive care (awakening and breathing controlled trial): a randomized controlled trial. *Lancet*. 2008;371:126-134.

Hanidziar D, Baldyga K, Ji CS, et al. Standard sedation and sedation with isoflurane in mechanically ventilated patients with coronavirus disease 2019. *Crit Care Explor*. 2021;3(3):e0370.

Hughes CG, Mailloux PT, Devlin JW, et al. Dexmedetomidine or propofol for sedation in mechanically ventilated adults with sepsis. *N Engl J Med*. 2021;384(15):1424-1436.

Hughes MA, Glass PS, Jacobs JR. Context-sensitive half-time in multicompartment pharmacokinetic models for intravenous anesthetic drugs. *Anesthesiology*. 1992;76:334–341.

Kress JP, Pohlman AS, O'Connor M, et al. Daily interruption of sedative infusions in critically ill patients undergoing mechanical ventilation. *N Engl J Med*. 2000;342:1471-1477.

Lonardo NW, Mone MC, Nirula R, et al. Propofol is associated with favorable outcomes compared with benzodiazepines in ventilated intensive care unit patients. *Am J Respir Crit Care Med*. 2014;189(11):1383-1394.

Martyn JAJ, Mao J, Bittner EA. Opioid tolerance in critical illness. *N Engl J Med*. 2019;380(4):365-378.

Mehta S, Cook D, Devlin JW, et al. Prevalence, risk factors, and outcomes of delirium in mechanically ventilated adults. *Crit Care Med*. 2015;43(3):557-566.

Mikkelsen ME, Christie JD, Lanken PN, et al. The adult respiratory distress syndrome cognitive outcomes study: long-term neuropsychological function in survivors of acute lung injury. *Am J Respir Crit Care Med*. 2012;185(12):1307-1315.

Olsen HT, Nedergaard HK, Strøm T, et al. Nonsedation or light sedation in critically ill, mechanically ventilated patients. *N Engl J Med*. 2020;382(12):1103-1111.

Pandharipande PP, Pun BT, Herr DL, et al. Effect of sedation with dexmedetomidine vs lorazepam on acute brain dysfunction in mechanically ventilated patients: the MENDS randomized controlled trial. *JAMA*. 2007;298:2644-2653.

Reade MC, Finfer S. Sedation and delirium in the intensive care unit. *N Engl J Med*. 2014;370(5):444-454.

Riker RR, Shehabi Y, Bokesh PM, et al. Dexmedetomidine vs. midazolam for sedation of critically ill patients. *JAMA*. 2009;301:489-499.

Schweickert WD, Pohlman MC, Pohlman AS, et al. Early physical and occupational therapy in mechanically ventilated, critically ill patients: a randomized controlled trial. *Lancet*. 2009;373(9678):1874-1882.

Sessler CN, Gosnell MS, Grap MJ, et al. The Richmond agitation-sedation scale: validity and reliability in adult intensive care unit patients. *Am J Respir Crit Care Med*. 2002;166:1338-1344.

Shehabi Y, Howe BD, Bellomo R, et al. Early sedation with dexmedetomidine in critically ill patients. *N Engl J Med*. 2019;380(26):2506-2517.

Sigakis MJ, Bittner EA. Ten myths and misconceptions regarding pain management in the ICU. *Crit Care Med*. 2015;43(11):2468-2478.

Strøm T, Martinussen T, Toft P. A protocol of no sedation for critically ill patients receiving mechanical ventilation: a randomised trial. *Lancet*. 2010;375(9713):475-480.

Wongtangman K, Grabitz SD, Hammer M, et al. Optimal sedation in patients who receive neuromuscular blocking agent infusions for treatment of acute respiratory distress syndrome-A retrospective cohort study from a New England Health Care Network. *Crit Care Med*. 2021;49(7):1137-1148.

8 Fluids, Electrolytes, and Acid-Base Management

Gina H. Sun and Yvonne Lai

Optimal management of fluids, electrolytes, and acid-base status in patients who are critically ill requires a general understanding of their normal composition and regulation. Disease processes, trauma, and surgery can all affect the manner by which the body controls its fluid balance and electrolytes.

I. FLUID COMPARTMENTS

A. The Total Body Water (TBW) ranges from 50% to 70% of the body mass and is determined by lean body mass, sex, and age (Table 8.1). There is an inverse relationship between TBW and percentage body fat because of the low water content of adipose tissues.

B. Compartments of TBW

1. The **intracellular** compartment is approximately 66% of TBW (~40% of body mass).
2. The **extracellular** compartment is approximately 34% of TBW (~20% of body mass) and can be further divided into the following:
   - **a.** The **intravascular** compartment, composed of plasma. It is approximately 5% of total body mass.
   - **b.** The **extravascular** compartment, composed of interstitial fluid, lymph, bone fluid, fluids of the various body cavities, and mucosal/secretory fluids. The extravascular compartment represents approximately 15% of total body mass.
   - **c.** The **third space**, an ill-defined space invoked to account for otherwise inexplicable fluid losses in the perioperative period or in patients who are critically ill. It may be considered "nonfunctional" interstitial fluid that cannot equilibrate with the circulating blood volume. However, many experts doubt the existence of a discrete third space.

C. Ionic Composition of the Fluid Compartments: Various physiologic terms describe the concentrations of ions in a solution.

1. **Molarity:** Moles of solute per liter of solution
2. **Molality:** Moles of solute per kilogram of solvent
3. **Osmolarity:** Osmoles per liter of solution. The number of osmoles is determined by multiplying the number of moles of solute by the number of freely

TABLE 8.1 Total Body Water as a Percentage of Body Weight (%)

	Male	Female
Thin	65	55
Average	60	50
Obese	55	45
Neonate	75-80	
First year	65-75	
Ages 1-10 yr	60-65	
Ages 10 yr to adult	50-60	

dissociated particles from one molecule of solute. For example, 1 mole of NaCl will yield 2 osm in solution.

4. **Osmolality:** Osmoles per kilogram of solvent
5. Electrolytes in physiology are generally described in terms of milliequivalents per liter (mEq/L). The fluids of each compartment are electrically neutral. Average concentrations of each electrolyte in various compartments are given in Table 8.2.

D. Movement of Water in the Body

1. Water is generally readily permeable through cell membranes and moves freely throughout the different fluid compartments. Movement of water is largely determined by **osmotic pressure** and **hydrostatic pressure.** The osmotic pressure depends on the number of osmotically active molecules in solution.
2. The movement of water between the interstitial and intravascular compartments within the extracellular space is described by **Starling's equation**:

$$Q_f = K_f\left[(P_c - P_i) - \sigma(\text{pi}_c - \text{pi}_i)\right]$$

where Q_f is the fluid flux across the capillary membrane; K_f is a constant reflecting the permeability of capillaries to water and their surface area; P_c and P_i are the hydrostatic pressures in the capillary and interstitium, respectively; σ is the reflection coefficient (see subsequent text); and pi_c and pi_i are the colloid osmotic pressures in the capillary and interstitium, respectively.

   a. Large, negatively charged intravascular proteins to which vascular membranes are impermeable are responsible for the osmotic pressure gradient between intravascular and interstitial compartments. This component of osmotic pressure, known as **oncotic pressure** or **colloid osmotic pressure**, contributes a small amount to the total osmotic pressure of the fluids. The positive ions that are associated with the negatively charged proteins also contribute to the osmotic pressure. **Albumin** is the predominant type of protein responsible for the oncotic pressure, accounting for approximately two-thirds of the total oncotic pressure. Cells do not contribute to the oncotic pressure.

   b. The **reflection coefficient** (σ) describes the permeability of plasma proteins across a specific capillary membrane. It ranges from 0 (completely

TABLE 8.2 Fluid Electrolyte Composition of Body Compartments

	Plasma (mEq/L)	Interstitial (mEq/L H_2O)	Intracellular[a] (mEq/L H_2O)
Cations			
Na	142	145	10
K	4	4	159
Ca	5	5	<1
Mg	2	2	40
Anions			
Cl	104	117	3
HCO_3	24	27	7
Proteins	16	<0.1	45
Others	9	9	154

[a]Intracellular electrolytes are difficult to measure, and most of the measurements are from myocytes, which may or may not be applicable to other cell types.

permeable) to 1 (impermeable) and varies in different disease states; it is approximately 0.7 in healthy tissues.

c. Edema occurs when the rate of interstitial fluid accumulation is greater than the rate of interstitial fluid removal by the lymphatic system.

II. FLUID DEFICITS AND REPLACEMENT THERAPY

A. Fluid Volume Deficits and appropriate fluid therapy are dependent on the source and type of fluid loss. Because all membranes are permeable to water, fluid deficits in one compartment will affect all other compartments. Fluid losses can be broadly classified on the basis of the initial source of loss. Fluid losses also lead to electrolyte abnormalities.

1. Intracellular fluid (ICF) compartment deficits arise from **free water loss.**

a. Sources of free water loss include the following:

1. Insensible losses through the skin and respiratory tract

2. Renal losses secondary to the inability to reabsorb water, such as in neurogenic or nephrogenic diabetes insipidus (DI; see **Section III.C**)

b. With free water loss, both intracellular and extracellular volumes decrease in proportion to their volumes in the body; therefore, two-thirds of the loss will be intracellular. Similarly, **free water replacement** will be distributed in proportion to their volumes in the body; only one-third of the administered free water will end up in the extracellular space and even less will enter the intravascular space.

c. Therapy includes replacement of water with either **hypotonic saline** (5% dextrose in water with 0.45% sodium chloride solution) or **free water** (5% dextrose in water). Electrolytes (especially sodium) must be monitored with therapy.

2. Extracellular fluid (ECF) compartment deficit

a. In general, ECF losses are isotonic. Losses may occur in each compartment, and fluid losses from one compartment are rapidly reflected in others.

b. Clinical manifestations of ECF losses are notoriously variable. Although textbooks routinely refer to clinical findings associated with quantified losses (3%-5% losses leading to dry mucous membranes and oliguria, to over 10%-20% losses leading to circulatory collapse), these signs are frequently unreliable. See the discussion on intravascular fluid deficit in **Section II.A.3.**

c. Causes of ECF losses include blood loss, vomiting, diarrhea, and "third spacing."

1. Replacement of ECF volume loss usually requires isotonic salt solutions. Volumes required to replace ECF deficits can vary considerably among patients on the basis of the inciting event and comorbid processes.

3. Intravascular fluid (plasma volume) deficit

a. Intravascular volume deficits will lead to interstitial fluid depletion as the two compartments equilibrate. It should be noted that with acute blood loss, laboratory values such as hemoglobin levels are not accurate indices of the severity of blood loss until equilibration with the ECF compartment has taken place.

b. The clinical utility of classifications based on percentage volume loss and clinical manifestations (such as the Advanced Trauma Life Support [ATLS] classification of hemorrhage) is questionable because signs of bleeding, including tachycardia, diaphoresis, and so forth, are extremely variable. Perhaps the most relevant clinical feature associated with intravascular volume loss is **orthostatic hypotension** (or **orthostatic tachycardia**) in a patient who is relatively stable. In a patient who is unstable, clinicians should use a combination of **noninvasive** and **invasive methods**

to assess blood volume and "**fluid responsiveness," the ability of volume administration to increase cardiac output significantly.** For a discussion of static and dynamic parameters predicting fluid responsiveness, see **Chapters 1** and **3.** Patients should be resuscitated early and aggressively—however, reliance on static numbers (eg, 30 mL/kg crystalloid) or goals (eg, give fluids until central venous pressure [CVP] is 8-12 mm Hg) should be avoided in favor of frequent reassessment of both parameters of fluid responsiveness and global/regional perfusion indices.

B. Fluid Replacement Therapy (see **Chapter 33**)

1. **Crystalloid solutions** (see Table 8.3 **for the composition of commonly used crystalloids**)
   a. **Maintenance fluids** are used to replace constitutive losses of fluids and electrolytes via urine, sweat, respiration, and the gastrointestinal (GI) tract.
      1. **Insensible water losses** include normal losses by skin and lungs, and total approximately 600 to 800 mL/d. **Sensible losses** of water include losses from the kidneys and GI tract. The obligate minimal urine output is 0.3 mL/kg/h and the average urine output is 1 mL/kg/h in an average 70-kg person (~1700 mL/d).
      2. **General guidelines for hourly maintenance fluid replacement** based on body weight (note that these guidelines should be tempered by frequent assessment of the patient's volume status):
         a. 0 to 10 kg: 4 mL/kg/h
         b. 11 to 20 kg: 40 mL/h + 2 mL/kg/h for each kilogram above 10 kg
         c. Greater than 20 kg: 60 mL/h + 1 mL/kg/h for each kilogram above 20 kg
      3. **Maintenance fluid composition:** In general, **hypotonic maintenance fluids** are used to replace insensible losses. Additional losses from other sources are often present in patients who are critically ill (eg, through drains, fistulas, etc) and require **isotonic fluid repletion.**
   b. For ECF repletion and intravascular fluid deficit (blood loss), isotonic solutions are used. The goal of **replacement fluid therapy** is to correct abnormalities in volume status or serum electrolytes. Because electrolytes are permeable through capillary membranes, crystalloids will rapidly redistribute from the intravascular compartment throughout the entire ECF, in the normal distribution of 75% extravascular to 25% intravascular.
2. **Colloid solutions** (see Table 8.4 **for the composition of commonly used colloids**). Colloid solutions are most commonly used for intravascular volume expansion. Unlike crystalloid solutions, the colloid elements do not freely

TABLE 8.3 Composition of Crystalloid Solutions

	Na	Cl	K	Ca	Buffer	Dextrose	pH	Osmolarity
D5W	0	0	0	0	0	5	4.5	252
D5 0.45% NaCl	77	77	0	0	0	5	4.0	406
0.9% NaCl	154	154	0	0	0	0	5.0	308
7.5% NaCl	1283	1283	0	0	0	0	5.0	2567
Lactated Ringer's	130	109	4	3	28[a]	0	6.5	273

Na, Cl, K, Ca, and buffer concentrations are in milliequivalents per liter; dextrose is in grams per 100 mL. D_5W, 5% dextrose in water; D_5 0.45% NaCl, 5% dextrose in water with 0.45% sodium chloride solution.
[a]Lactate.

TABLE 8.4 Physiologic and Chemical Characteristics of Colloid Solutions

Fluid	Average molecular weight (kDa)	Oncotic pressure (mm Hg)	Serum half-life (h)
5% albumin	69	20	16
25% albumin	69	70	16
6% hetastarch	450	30	2-17

cross intact capillary membranes and therefore do not redistribute as readily into the entire ECF compartment in the absence of a severe capillary leak state. Colloids have been thought to have a number of important potential advantages over crystalloids, although clinical evidence for these advantages is weak.

a. More effective volume expansion and less edema formation

b. Better at maintaining endothelial integrity

c. Improved microcirculation

d. Less immunomodulation

e. The chief disadvantage of colloids is their **significantly higher cost compared** with crystalloids (see subsequent text for the harmful effects specific to the hydroxyethyl starches [HESs]).

3. Transfusions of blood and blood components are important for maintaining the oxygen-carrying capacity of blood and for coagulation. A detailed discussion of transfusions as a part of fluid management can be found in **Chapter 33.**

a. Transfusion should be restricted in patients who are critically ill but are not actively bleeding and do not have evidence of ongoing myocardial ischemia.

b. Patients needing massive transfusion should be transfused early with a 1:1:1 ratio of packed red blood cells (PRBCs) to fresh frozen plasma (FFP) to platelets for the best outcomes (see **Chapter 33**).

4. Clinical use—crystalloids versus colloids: The controversy over the ideal resuscitation fluid is an old one and is unlikely to be definitively answered in the near future. Nonetheless, in the past decade, a number of large, well-designed trials have provided some guidelines for evidence-based fluid resuscitation—the recommendations given here are based on our interpretation of these trials.

a. Crystalloids

1. The initial choice of resuscitation fluid should almost always be a crystalloid. In spite of the expected advantages of colloids at volume expansion, the data show only a 30% to 40% decrease in total volumes infused with colloid-based resuscitation compared with crystalloids (rather than the expected 3-fold difference) over days to weeks.

2. Normal saline (NS) contains 154 mEq/L of sodium chloride, which is relatively hyperchloremic compared to plasma. Large-volume resuscitation with NS can be associated with greater hyperchloremic metabolic acidosis.

3. Because of these, lactated Ringer's (LR, or a balanced crystalloid) may be preferred in most instances to NS, even in the presence of renal dysfunction. LR contains 4 mEq/L of potassium but can still be safe in patients with hyperkalemia and renal dysfunction, with data showing that the crystalloid does not significantly increase potassium levels. NS-induced hyperchloremic metabolic acidosis can worsen hyperkalemia. In addition, accumulating evidence suggests that excessive chloride administration may be associated with worse renal outcomes and, perhaps, increased mortality.

4. The choice between NS and balanced crystalloid should be individualized. A patient with hypernatremia may benefit from LR. However, in patients with neurologic injury who would benefit from relative hypernatremia, resuscitation with NS is recommended.

b. Colloids: Colloids are rarely used as first-line intervention for volume resuscitation. Colloid solutions include albumin and hyperoncotic starches (pentastarch and HESs).

1. **HESs are contraindicated in patients with severe sepsis** and septic shock. There is high-quality evidence linking HES solutions and worse renal injury and mortality in patients with sepsis. It is probably prudent to altogether avoid HES solutions in patients who are critically ill.
2. Albumin is safe in most patients who are critically ill (**with the exception of those with head injury, in whom it has been associated with increased mortality**). The administration of albumin is not associated with improved outcomes in the broad population of patients who are critically ill. However, there are some groups of patients in whom albumin should be considered:
   a. Patients with liver disease and cirrhosis undergoing large-volume paracentesis
   b. Patients with septic shock and hypoalbuminemia. A recent study showed that keeping serum albumin levels greater than 3 g/dL was associated with a mortality benefit in patients with septic shock (subgroup analysis of the albumin Italian outcome sepsis [ALBIOS] trial).

III. ELECTROLYTES AND ELECTROLYTE ABNORMALITIES: SODIUM

A. The normal range of serum (plasma) sodium concentration is 135 to 145 mEq/L. Abnormalities in serum sodium suggest abnormalities in both water and sodium balance.

B. Hyponatremia is defined by a serum sodium of less than 135 mEq/L. Severe hyponatremia can cause central nervous system (CNS) and cardiac abnormalities, such as seizures and dysrhythmias. Hyponatremia can be classified on the basis of concomitant plasma tonicity.

1. **Isotonic hyponatremia** (~290 mOsm/kg H_2O) occurs when there are elevated levels of other ECF constituents such as protein and lipids. This form of hyponatremia is also known as **pseudohyponatremia** and is an artifact of measurement due to lipid and protein displacement of volume for a given volume of plasma. Therapy for this hyponatremia is not required.
2. **Hypertonic hyponatremia** is due to the movement of intracellular water into the extracellular compartment under the influence of **osmotically active substances** (eg, glucose, mannitol) with consequent dilution of ECF sodium. A common example of hypertonic hyponatremia is seen with **hyperglycemia**, which can decrease serum sodium concentration by approximately 1.6 mEq/L for each 100 mg/dL of blood glucose. Treatment includes removal of the osmotically active substance and restoration of volume.
3. **Hypotonic hyponatremia** is the most common form of hyponatremia. This type of hyponatremia is due to higher TBW relative to total body sodium. Hypotonic hyponatremia is further classified on the basis of the ECF volume status (hypovolemic, hypervolemic, and isovolemic). In all three scenarios, the extracellular compartment volume status does not always correlate with the intravascular or effective arterial volume status.

a. **Hypovolemic hypotonic hyponatremia** can result from renal or nonrenal causes. In either case, water and salt are lost, but the loss of sodium is greater than the loss of water.
   1. **Renal causes** include the use of diuretics (particularly thiazide diuretics), osmotic diuresis, mineralocorticoid deficiency/hypoaldosteronism, hypothyroidism, and, rarely, renal salt-wasting nephropathy, cerebral salt-wasting syndrome, and certain types of renal tubular acidosis (RTA).
   2. **Nonrenal causes** include fluid losses from the GI tract, skin (burns), cerebral salt-wasting syndrome, and intravascular volume depletion via third spacing.
   3. Renal and nonrenal causes can be distinguished by urine electrolytes. A urine sodium of greater than 20 mEq/L suggests a renal etiology, whereas a urine sodium of less than 10 mEq/L suggests a nonrenal etiology.
   4. **The goal of therapy is to replace extracellular volume with isotonic sodium solutions** and to allow for appropriate renal free water excretion.

b. **Hypervolemic hypotonic hyponatremia** is associated with congestive heart failure (CHF), renal failure with nephritic/nephrotic syndrome, and cirrhosis.
   1. **Mechanism:** In these disease processes, the effective arterial intravascular volume is low even if the total blood volume is normal or increased. The activation of the renin-angiotensin-aldosterone system and the sympathetic nervous system and the release of antidiuretic hormone (ADH) lead to oliguria and salt retention. The result is expansion of ECF volume.
   2. **Manifestations** include edema, elevated jugular venous pressure, pleural effusions, and ascites.
   3. The **goal of therapy** is to control the primary disease process. Fluid and salt restriction and the use of diuretics may also be appropriate.

c. **Euvolemic hypotonic hyponatremia**
   1. **Causes:** Syndrome of inappropriate ADH secretion (SIADH), psychogenic polydipsia, medications (eg, oxytocin), physiologic nonosmotic stimulus for ADH release (eg, nausea, anxiety, pain), hypothyroidism, and adrenal insufficiency
   2. Causes of SIADH include neurologic (head injury, subarachnoid hemorrhage, intracranial surgery), pulmonary (pneumonia, chronic obstructive pulmonary disease [COPD], tuberculosis), malignancies, major surgeries (postoperative pain and nausea stimulate ADH secretion), and medications (desmopressin, cyclophosphamides, tricyclic antidepressants [TCAs], selective serotonin reuptake inhibitors [SSRIs]). It is important to **distinguish SIADH** from **cerebral salt-wasting syndrome**, a form of hypovolemic hyponatremia associated with head injury. Volume status is the only way to distinguish between these two conditions in patients with traumatic brain injury who are hyponatremic.

4. **Therapy for hyponatremia**

a. **General guidelines:** Most patients with hyponatremia have a chronic electrolyte abnormality and will be mostly asymptomatic. Thus, if these patients require treatment, it entails a slow correction through fluid restriction (euvolemic or hypervolemic etiology) or isotonic saline/oral salt tablets (hypovolemic or diuretic-related etiology). More aggressive therapy should be instituted in patients with symptomatic or severe hyponatremia, which includes hypertonic saline and, potentially, vasopressin receptor antagonists.

b. Treatment of underlying disease: If the patient is hyponatremic from adrenal insufficiency, administer glucocorticoids that will directly suppress the release of ADH. If the patient is hyponatremic because of reversible causes of SIADH (eg, nausea, pain, anxiety), treat the underlying cause first. Iatrogenic/drug causes of hyponatremia should be approached by stopping the offending medication first.

c. Fluid restriction is an appropriate intervention for euvolemic and hypervolemic hyponatremia. The amount of fluid restriction is dependent on the level of urine output, but in general, restriction to 50% to 60% of daily fluid requirements is the initial goal.

d. Urgent intervention is required in patients with symptomatic hyponatremia (nausea, vomiting, lethargy, altered level of consciousness, and seizures). The sodium deficit can be calculated as follows:

$$\text{Sodium deficit} = \text{TBW} \times 140 - [\text{Na}]_{\text{serum}}$$

The rate of correction of the serum sodium is important and must be tailored to the individual patient. Both delayed and rapid correction can be associated with neurologic injury. Safe correction can be achieved with **hypertonic saline (3% NaCl)** in patients with euvolemia and with **infusion of NS** in patients with hypovolemia. The rate of infusion should result in a correction of serum sodium of 1 to 2 mEq/L/h for the first 24 hours or until the serum sodium reaches a level of 120 mEq/L, and then be reduced to a correction rate of 0.5 to 1 mEq/L/h.

e. The **vaptans** are active nonpeptide vasopressin receptor antagonists that are used in the treatment of euvolemic and hypervolemic hyponatremia, including for patients with chronic heart failure, cirrhosis, SIADH, or hyponatremia from other causes. Experience with these agents is limited, particularly in patients in the intensive care unit (ICU).

C. Hypernatremia is defined by a serum sodium of greater than 145 mEq/L. Hypernatremia is also a description of total body sodium content relative to TBW and can exist in hypovolemic, euvolemic, and hypervolemic states. Hypernatremia may be due to TBW loss (more common) or increased salt intake without water. In all cases, the serum is hypertonic. Clinical manifestations of hypernatremia include tremulousness, irritability, spasticity, confusion, seizures, and coma. Symptoms are more likely to occur when the rate of change is rapid. When the change is gradual and chronic, cells in the CNS will increase cellular osmolality, thereby preventing cellular water loss and dehydration. This process starts approximately 4 hours after the onset and stabilizes in 4 to 7 days. This change in CNS cellular osmolality is an important concept when considering therapy.

1. Hypovolemic hypernatremia

a. Caused by the loss of hypotonic fluids through renal (eg, osmotic diuresis and drug induced) or nonrenal (eg, skin or GI losses) sources. There is a loss of water and salt, with a greater proportion of water loss, which results in a decrease in the ECF volume and the effective arterial blood volume. Osmotic diuresis through the kidneys can be due to glucose, mannitol, or urea. GI losses include vomiting or osmotic diarrhea, whereas skin losses include burns or perspiration.

b. It is recommended that isotonic saline be used for initial volume repletion, followed by hypotonic crystalloid solutions, such as 0.45% NS.

2. Hypervolemic hypernatremia is caused by excess sodium and usually results from the infusion or intake of solutions with high sodium concentration. The acute salt load leads to intracellular dehydration with ECF expansion, which can cause edema or heart failure. The goal of therapy is to remove the excess sodium; this can be accomplished using nonmedullary gradient-disrupting diuretics (eg, thiazides).

3. **Euvolemic hypernatremia**
   a. Caused by the loss of free water through renal (eg, osmotic diuresis and drug induced) or nonrenal (eg, excessive insensible loss through skin or respiration) sources.
   b. Measuring urine osmolality (Uosm) is important. Nonrenal processes are associated with a high Uosm (>800 mOsm/kg H_2O) caused by a release of ADH in response to plasma tonicity, whereas renal processes are associated with a low Uosm (~100 mOsm/kg H_2O) because of the lack or inability of the kidneys to respond to ADH.
   c. In most cases of hypernatremia from free water loss, the intravascular and ECF volumes appear normal because there is no gain or loss of total body sodium. Therapy involves the replacement of free water.
   d. Central and nephrogenic DI (see **Chapter 26**) are among the renal causes of euvolemic hypernatremia. Evaluation of urinary osmolality (usually Uosm is less than the plasma osmolality) and the response to ADH may help determine the site of the lesion.
      1. **Central (neurogenic) DI** can be caused by pituitary damage from tumor, trauma, surgery, granulomatous disease, and idiopathic causes. Central DI is treated with desmopressin (intranasal, 5-10 µg daily or twice daily).
      2. **Nephrogenic DI** can be caused by severe hypokalemia with renal tubular injury, hypercalcemia, chronic renal failure, interstitial kidney disease, and drugs (eg, lithium, amphotericin, demeclocycline). Therapy includes correcting the primary cause if feasible and possibly free water repletion.
4. **Free water deficit** and correction of hypernatremia

$$\text{Free water deficit} = \text{TBW}^*\{1-(140/[\text{Na}])\}$$

The correction of hypernatremia should occur at approximately 1 mEq/L/h. Approximately one-half of the calculated water deficit is administered during the first 24 hours and the rest over the following 1 to 2 days. Aggressive correction is dangerous, especially in chronic hypernatremia because rapid correction can cause cerebral edema. Rapid correction is reasonable if the hypernatremia is acute (<12 hours). Neurologic status should be carefully monitored while correcting sodium derangements and the rate of correction decreased if there is any change in neurologic function.

IV. POTASSIUM

A. In an average adult, the total body potassium is approximately 40 to 50 mEq/kg. Most of the potassium is in the intracellular compartment. In general, intake and excretion of potassium are matched. The electrocardiogram (**ECG**) is useful in diagnosing true potassium imbalance because the level of polarization of an excitable cell and its ability for repolarization are determined by the extracellular and intracellular potassium concentrations.

B. **Hypokalemia:** serum potassium of less than 3.5 mEq/L. A general rule is that a 1 mEq/L decrease in serum potassium represents approximately a total body potassium deficit of 200 to 350 mEq.

1. **Causes of hypokalemia**
   a. Transcellular redistribution (increased entry into cells mostly through increased Na+/K+-ATPase pump activity)

1. **Alkalemia** (a 0.1-0.7 mEq/L change per 0.1 U change in pH)
2. Increased circulating **catecholamines** via β_2-adrenergic receptors
3. Increased **insulin**

b. Renal-associated causes

1. Without hypertension
   a. With **acidosis**
      i. DKA, RTA types 1 and 2
   b. With **alkalosis**
      i. Diuretics
      ii. Vomiting
      iii. Nasogastric suction (leading to hyperaldosteronism)
      iv. Transport defects—thick ascending limb (Bartter syndrome), cortical collecting duct (Gitelman syndrome)
2. With hypertension
   a. Renal artery stenosis
   b. Hyperaldosteronism due to tumor (Conn syndrome, adrenal adenoma)
   c. Glucocorticoid-mediated hyperadrenalism
   d. Pseudo-hyperadrenalism
      i. Licorice ingestion
      ii. Cushing syndrome
      iii. Liddle syndrome

c. Hypomagnesemia
d. Acute leukemia
e. Excessive GI losses
f. Dietary
g. Lithium toxicity
h. Hypothermia

2. **Manifestations** of hypokalemia include myalgias, cramps, weakness, paralysis, urinary retention, ileus, and orthostatic hypotension. **ECG manifestations**, in order of progression of worsening hypokalemia, are decreased T-wave amplitude, prolonged QT interval, U wave, dragging of ST segment, and increased QRS duration. **Arrhythmias** are common, including atrial fibrillation, premature ventricular beats, supraventricular and junctional tachycardia, and Mobitz I second-degree atrioventricular block (see **Chapter 17**).
3. **Therapy: IV potassium replacement** is appropriate in patients who have severe hypokalemia or who cannot take oral preparations. The rate of replacement should be governed by the clinical signs. The recommended maximal rate of infusion is 0.5 to 0.7 mEq/kg/h, with continuous ECG monitoring. **Hypomagnesemia** should be corrected before potassium repletion (see **Section IV.C**).

C. Hyperkalemia: serum potassium of greater than 5.5 mEq/L

1. **Causes** of hyperkalemia
   a. Hemolysis of sample
   b. Leukocytosis (white blood cell count >50 000/mm^3)
   c. Thrombocytosis (platelet count >1 000 000/mm^3)
   d. Transcellular redistribution
      1. Acidemia
      2. Insulin deficiency, hyperglycemia, hyperosmolality
      3. Drugs (digitalis, β-blockers, succinylcholine)
   e. Malignant hyperthermia
   f. Cell necrosis (rhabdomyolysis, hemolysis, burns)
   g. Increased intake via replacement therapy and transfusions
   h. Decreased renal potassium secretion
      1. Renal failure

2. Hypoaldosteronism
3. Drugs: heparin, angiotensin-converting enzyme inhibitors, and potassium-sparing diuretics

2. **Manifestations** of hyperkalemia include muscle weakness and cardiac conduction disturbances. **ECG changes** include atrial and ventricular ectopy (serum potassium of 6-7 mEq/L), shortened QT interval, and peaked T waves. Worsening hyperkalemia will lead to widening of the QRS and, eventually, **ventricular fibrillation.**
3. Therapy for hyperkalemia is emergent in the presence of ECG changes, particularly when serum potassium is greater than 6.5 mEq/L. Continuous ECG monitoring is recommended. Therapy should begin in an ICU if the potassium levels show an increasing trend, even in the absence of ECG changes (see **Chapter 23, Section VII.C**). Treatment modalities include cell membrane stabilizers (calcium gluconate), promoting transcellular shift (insulin with glucose, β_2 agonists), and decreasing total body potassium (loop diuretics, Kayexalate, dialysis).

V. ELECTROLYTE ABNORMALITIES: CALCIUM, PHOSPHORUS, AND MAGNESIUM

A. Calcium acts as a key signaling element for many cellular functions and is the most abundant electrolyte in the body. Normal values of total serum calcium range from 8.5 to 10.5 mg/dL (4.5-5.5 mEq/L). However, because calcium is bound to protein (~40%), the appropriate range of total serum calcium that can provide for adequate ionized calcium is dependent on the total serum calcium and the amount of serum protein (particularly albumin). The **ionized calcium** provides a better functional assessment, with **normal values ranging from 4 to 5 mg/dL (2.1-2.5 mEq/L or 1.05-1.25 mmol/L)**. Direct measurement of ionized calcium is commonly available and is superior to "corrected" calcium values based on albumin levels. Ionized calcium can be affected by the pH of the serum, with acidemia leading to higher ionized calcium and alkalemia to lower ionized calcium. Modulators of calcium homeostasis include parathyroid hormone (PTH) and 1,25-dihydroxyvitamin D, which increase calcium levels, and calcitonin, which decreases calcium levels.

1. **Hypercalcemia** (see **Chapter 26**): A total serum calcium of greater than 10.5 mg/dL (5.5 mEq/L or 2.6 mmol/L) or ionized calcium of greater than 5.0 mg/dL (2.5 mEq/L or 1.25 mmol/L)
   - **a. Causes** of hypercalcemia
     1. Primary hyperparathyroidism
     2. Immobilization
     3. Malignancy (bone destruction from metastases or hormone secretion)
     4. Granulomatous diseases (tuberculosis, sarcoidosis), secondary to increased 1,25-dihydroxyvitamin D production by the granulomatous tissue
     5. Thyrotoxicosis
     6. Primary bone reabsorption abnormalities (Paget disease)
     7. Adrenal insufficiency
     8. Pheochromocytoma
     9. Milk-alkali syndrome: high intake of calcium (>5 g/d)
     10. Drugs (thiazides, vitamin D, lithium, estrogens)
   - **b. Diagnosis**
     1. **PTH levels:** low in malignancy-associated hypercalcemia and high in primary, secondary, and tertiary hyperparathyroidism
     2. **1,25-dihydroxyvitamin D levels:** elevated in granulomatous disease
     3. **PTH-related protein:** elevated in malignancy-associated hypercalcemia (breast, lung, thyroid, renal cells)
     4. **Protein electrophoresis:** monoclonal band associated with myeloma

5. **Thyroid-stimulating hormone (TSH)**
6. **Chest radiographs:** Evaluate for malignancy and granulomatous disease.

c. **Manifestations:** Hypercalcemia will affect multiple organ systems, including neurologic, cardiovascular, renal, GI, and musculoskeletal. The patient may exhibit muscle weakness, lethargy, and, possibly, coma. ECG abnormalities include bradycardia, shortened QT interval, increased PR and QRS intervals, and atrioventricular block. Polyuria, nephrolithiasis, and nephrogenic DI are common. GI manifestations include nausea/vomiting, constipation, and pancreatitis.

d. **Treatment** is described in detail in **Chapter 26**. Here, we summarize the main considerations. Treatment should be initiated if neurologic symptoms are present, total serum calcium is greater than 12 to 13 mg/dL, or calcium/phosphate product is greater than 75.

1. First, begin immediate hydration with NS to restore volume status and decrease serum calcium concentration by dilution.
2. After establishing euvolemia, a loop diuretic can be added to NS with the goal of generating a urine output of 3 to 5 mL/kg/h.
3. Other electrolytes should be repleted.
4. Hemodialysis, if the abovementioned therapy is ineffective
5. The use of pamidronate, calcitonin, and glucocorticoids is described in detail in **Chapter 26**. Calcium channel blockers can also be used to treat the cardiotoxic effects of **hypercalcemia**.

2. **Hypocalcemia** (see **Chapter 26**): an ionized calcium of less than 4 mg/dL (2.1 mEq/L or 1.05 mmol/L)

a. **Causes of hypocalcemia**

1. **Sequestration of calcium** can be caused by hyperphosphatemia (from renal failure), pancreatitis, intravascular citrate (from PRBCs), and alkalemia.
2. **PTH deficiency** can be caused by surgical excision of the parathyroid gland, autoimmune parathyroid disease, amyloid infiltration of the parathyroid gland, severe hypermagnesemia, hypomagnesemia, HIV infection, and hemochromatosis.
3. **PTH resistance** is due to congenital abnormality or secondary to hypomagnesemia.
4. **Vitamin D deficiency** is caused by malabsorption, poor nutritional intake, liver disease, anticonvulsants (phenytoin), inadequate sunlight, and renal failure.
5. **Inappropriate calcium deposition** can be due to formation of complex with phosphorus in hyperphosphatemic states (rhabdomyolysis), acute pancreatitis, and post-parathyroidectomy.
6. **Sepsis** and **toxic shock syndrome**

b. **Manifestations** of hypocalcemia include generalized excitable membrane irritability leading to paresthesias and progressing to tetany and seizures. The classic physical examination findings include **Trousseau sign** (spasm of the upper extremity muscles that causes flexion of the wrist and thumb with extension of the fingers and can be elicited by occluding the circulation to the arm) and **Chvostek sign** (contraction of the ipsilateral facial muscles elicited by tapping over the facial nerve at the jaw). **ECG changes** include prolonged QT and heart block. Respiratory manifestations include apnea, bronchospasm, and laryngeal spasm (typically seen after thyroidectomy or parathyroidectomy surgery). Anxiety and depression may also be seen as neurologic manifestations of hypocalcemia.

c. **Diagnosis**

1. Confirm true hypocalcemia by checking ionized calcium and pH.
2. Rule out hypomagnesemia.
3. Check PTH level; if low or normal, hypoparathyroidism may be involved; if high, check for phosphorus level. A low phosphorus level

suggests pancreatitis or vitamin D deficiency, whereas a high phosphorus level suggests rhabdomyolysis or renal failure.

d. **Therapy for hypocalcemia:** Infusion of calcium at 4 mg/kg of elemental calcium with either **10% calcium gluconate** (93 mg of calcium/10 mL) or **10% calcium chloride** (272 mg of calcium/10 mL). A bolus should be followed by an infusion because the bolus will increase the ionized form of calcium for 1 to 2 hours. To avoid precipitation of calcium salts, **intravenous (IV) calcium solutions should not be mixed with IV bicarbonate solutions**. Calcium chloride is caustic to peripheral veins and should be given via central venous access if possible. Suspected vitamin D or PTH deficiency is treated with calcitriol (0.25 µg, up to 1.5 µg po once a day). Oral calcium repletion with at least 1 g of elemental calcium a day should be given along with vitamin D therapy.

B. Phosphorus exists mainly as a free ion in the body. Approximately 0.8 to 1 g of phosphorus is excreted in the urine per day. Phosphorus excretion is affected by PTH (which inhibits proximal and distal nephron phosphorus reabsorption), vitamin D, high dietary phosphorus intake, cortisol, and growth hormone.

1. **Hypophosphatemia** occurs in 10% to 15% of patients who have been hospitalized.
   a. **Causes**
      1. **Gastrointestinal:** malnutrition, malabsorption, vitamin D deficiency, diarrhea, and use of aluminum-containing antacids
      2. **Renal losses:** primary hyperparathyroidism, renal transplantation, ECF expansion, diuretics (acetazolamide), Fanconi syndrome, post–obstructive uropathy and post–acute tubular necrosis (ATN), glycosuria, DKA
      3. **Redistribution:** alkalosis, post–alcohol withdrawal, parenteral hyperalimentation, burns, and continuous venovenous hemofiltration
   b. **Manifestations** usually occur when phosphorus is less than 1.0 mg/dL.
      1. **Neurologic:** metabolic encephalopathy
      2. **Muscular:** myopathy, respiratory failure, cardiomyopathy
      3. **Hematologic:** hemolysis, white blood cell dysfunction
   c. **Diagnosis**
      1. Urinary phosphorus less than 100 mg/d suggests GI losses.
      2. Urinary phosphorus greater than 100 mg/d suggests renal wasting.
      3. Elevated serum calcium suggests hyperparathyroidism.
      4. Elevated PTH suggests primary or secondary hyperparathyroidism or calcipenic rickets.
   d. **Treatment**
      1. Increase oral intake to 1000 mg/d.
      2. Elemental phosphorus: 450 mg per 1000 kcal of hyperalimentation
      3. Dose of IV phosphorus should not exceed 2 mg/kg (0.15 mmol/kg) of elemental phosphorus.
2. **Hyperphosphatemia**
   a. **Causes**
      1. **Renal:** decreased glomerular filtration rate (GFR), increased tubular reabsorption, hypoparathyroidism, pseudohypoparathyroidism, acromegaly, thyrotoxicosis
      2. **Endogenous:** tumor lysis, rhabdomyolysis
      3. **Exogenous:** vitamin D administration, phosphate enemas
   b. **Manifestations** are related to hypocalcemia due to calcium phosphate deposition and decreased renal production of 1,25-dihydroxyvitamin D.
   c. **Treatment**
      1. Phosphate binders to reduce GI absorption
      2. Volume expansion and dextrose 10% in water with insulin may reduce acutely elevated phosphorus levels.
      3. Hemodialysis and peritoneal dialysis

C. Magnesium: Serum magnesium is maintained between 1.8 and 2.3 mg/dL (1.7-2.1 mEq/L); 15% is protein bound.

1. **Hypermagnesemia** is rare in patients with normal renal function. It is defined as greater than 2.5 mg/dL.
   a. **Causes**
      1. Acute and chronic renal failure
      2. Magnesium administration for toxemia of pregnancy, magnesium-containing antacids and laxatives
      3. Hypothyroidism
      4. Lithium toxicity
   b. **Manifestations**
      1. Cardiac dysrhythmias and hypotension
      2. Decreased neuromuscular transmission
      3. CNS dysfunction: confusion, lethargy
      4. Respiratory depression
   c. **Treatment**
      1. IV calcium
      2. Hemodialysis to remove magnesium in renal failure
2. **Hypomagnesemia** is defined as serum magnesium less than 1.8 mg/dL.
   a. **Causes**
      1. **Gastrointestinal**
         a. Decreased intake (chronic alcoholism)
         b. Starvation
         c. Magnesium-free enteral feedings
         d. Decreased GI intake because of nasogastric suction and malabsorption
      2. **Renal losses**
         a. Diuretic therapy
         b. Post–obstructive diuresis
         c. Recovery (polyuric phase) from ATN
         d. DKA versus hypercalcemia
         e. Primary hyperaldosteronism
         f. Bartter syndrome and Gitelman syndrome
         g. Aminoglycoside, cisplatin, and cyclosporine nephrotoxicity
   b. **Manifestations**
      1. Hypokalemia and hypocalcemia; hypokalemia is the result of excess urine losses, which can only be corrected with magnesium repletion.
      2. ECG changes mimic hypokalemia.
      3. Digoxin toxicity is magnified by hypomagnesemia.
      4. Neuromuscular fasciculations with Chvostek and Trousseau signs may be present.
   c. **Treatment** for hypomagnesemia should be initiated when ECG changes and/or signs of tetany are present.
      1. **Intravenous:** with $MgSO_4$, 6 g in 1 L of 5% dextrose in water over 6 hours
      2. **Oral:** with magnesium oxide, 250 to 500 mg 4 times a day

VI. ACID-BASE PHYSIOLOGY

Acid-base homeostasis is essential for maintaining life. Significant acid-base derangements have major physiologic consequences that can be life-threatening. However, it is the primary cause of the derangement that largely determines prognosis. There are three major methods for quantifying acid-base disorders: the **physiologic** approach, the **base excess** approach, and the **physicochemical** (or **Stewart**) approach. In this section, we present a systematic approach to acid-base disorders relying primarily on the physiologic approach.

A. Physiologic Approach to Acid-Base Disturbances: The physiologic approach uses the carbonic acid-bicarbonate system:

$$H^+ + HCO_3^- \leftrightarrow H_2CO_3 \leftrightarrow H_2O + CO_2$$

A primary change in $Paco_2$ causes a secondary (compensatory) response in the HCO_3^- concentration and vice versa. Because the concentration of hydrogen ions in plasma is very low (~40 nEq/L), the pH (the negative logarithm of the hydrogen ion concentration) is used clinically. H_2CO_3 is in equilibrium with the dissolved CO_2. The **Henderson-Hasselbalch equation** describes the relationship between the pH, $Paco_2$, and HCO_3^-:

$$pH = 6.1 + \log\left\{\left[HCO_3^-\right] / \left(0.03 \times Paco_2\right)\right\}$$

Because pH = $-\log[H^+]$, the equation can be rearranged (this form is also known as the **Henderson equation**):

$$\left[H^+\right] = 24 \times (Paco_2 / [HCO_3^-])$$

The equation can be used to verify the reliability of a blood gas value, using the $Paco_2$ from the blood gas result and an HCO_3^- from a simultaneously drawn metabolic panel (the HCO_3^- value reported in a blood gas is calculated, not measured). The $[H^+]$ is roughly estimated by adding or subtracting 10 nEq/L per change in 0.1 pH units from 40 nEq/L. The four primary acid-base disorders comprise two metabolic disorders (acidosis and alkalosis) and two respiratory disorders (acidosis and alkalosis). The terms **acidemia** and **alkalemia** describe the state of the pH, whereas the terms **acidosis** and **alkalosis** describe the processes leading to these pH states.

B. A Systematic Approach to the Diagnosis of Acid-Base Disorders: All steps listed here are often not necessary. However, this approach enables an efficient and thorough evaluation of patients with complex acid-base abnormalities.

1. **History and physical examination:** A thorough clinical evaluation often provides important diagnostic clues. The medical history, including medications being taken, may predispose a patient toward specific acid-base disturbances. Vital signs and neurologic, pulmonary, and GI signs and symptoms may indicate the severity of the disturbance as well as point to the type of acid-base disorder.
2. Determine the **primary acid-base disorder:** The pH defines whether the patient is **acidemic** (pH $<$7.35) or **alkalemic** (pH $>$7.45). The serum $[HCO_3^-]$ (measured separately on a metabolic panel) determines whether there is a **metabolic acidosis** ($[HCO_3^-]$ less than 22 mEq/L), or a **metabolic alkalosis** ($[HCO_3^-]$ greater than 28 mEq/L). The $Paco_2$ defines the presence of a **respiratory acidosis** ($Paco_2$ $>$45 mm Hg) or **respiratory alkalosis** ($Paco_2$ $<$35 mm Hg).
3. Define the **secondary** (or **compensatory**) **response:** The **predicted** $Paco_2$ for a given $[HCO_3^-]$ or vice versa can be calculated (Table 8.5). The presence of a **mixed acid-base disorder** (ie, two or more coexisting acid-base disturbances) is suggested if the measured value is greater or less than predicted. For example, a patient with a pH of 7.16 with a $[HCO_3^-]$ of 12 mEq/L has a primary metabolic acidosis. The predicted $Paco_2$ for this patient would be 26 mm Hg. If the actual $Paco_2$ is 40 mm Hg, the patient has a superimposed respiratory acidosis (even though the $Paco_2$ is "normal").

TABLE 8.5 Simple Acid-Base Disorders and Compensatory Changes

Disorder	Mechanism	Primary disturbance	Compensation	Compensatory change
Metabolic acidosis, pH <7.35	H^+ retention or production; HCO_3^- loss	↓ HCO_3^- from 24 mEq/L	↓ $Paco_2$	$\Delta Paco_2 = 1.2 \times \Delta HCO_3^-$ (or $1.5 \times HCO_3^- + 8 \pm 2$)
Metabolic alkalosis, pH >7.45	HCO_3^- retention or production; H^+ loss	↑ HCO_3^- from 24 mEq/L	↑ $Paco_2$	$\Delta Paco_2 = 0.7 \times HCO_3^- + 20 \pm 1.5$
Respiratory acidosis, pH <7.35	$Paco_2$ retention	↑ $Paco_2$ from 40 mm Hg	↑ HCO_3^-	Acute: $\Delta HCO_3^- = 0.1 \times \Delta Paco_2$; $\Delta pH = 0.08/10$ mm Hg $\Delta Paco_2$ Chronic: $\Delta HCO_3^- = 0.4 \times \Delta Paco_2$; $\Delta pH = 0.03/10$ mm Hg $\Delta Paco_2$
Respiratory alkalosis, pH >7.45	Excessive $Paco_2$ reduction	↓ $Paco_2$ from 40 mm Hg	↓ HCO_3^-	Acute: $\Delta HCO_3^- = 0.2 \times \Delta Paco_2$; $\Delta pH = 0.08/10$ mm Hg $\Delta Paco_2$ Chronic: $\Delta HCO_3^- = 0.5 \times \Delta Paco_2$; $\Delta pH = 0.03/10$ mm Hg $\Delta Paco_2$

4. Calculate the **corrected anion gap (AG_{corr})**: For a metabolic acidosis, the anion gap (AG) is calculated ($[Na^+] - [Cl^-] - [HCO_3^-]$). The normal value is typically between 5 and 12 mEq/L, depending on the laboratory. Because albumin accounts for up to 75% of the AG, the AG should **always** be corrected for hypoalbuminemia (common in critically ill patients) to give the **corrected anion gap (AG_{corr} = AG + 2.5 × (4.0 − serum albumin [in g/dL])**).
5. Calculate the **delta-delta (Δ-Δ) or delta gap:** In patients with a high AG metabolic acidosis, calculating the delta gap may help diagnose a concomitant metabolic alkalosis or a non–AG metabolic acidosis. The delta gap is the comparison between the increase in AG_{corr} above the upper reference value (above 12 mEq/L) and the decrease in $[HCO_3^-]$ below the lower reference value (24 mEq/L). In theory, high AG acidosis is characterized by an increase in the AG_{corr} that is closely matched by a decrease in $[HCO_3^-]$. Thus, the delta gap is close to zero (0 ± 5 mEq/L) in pure AG acidosis. If the gap is greater than **6 mEq/L**, a **concomitant metabolic alkalosis** is present; if the gap is equal to or less than **6 mEq/L**, a **superimposed non–AG metabolic acidosis** is present.
6. Calculate the **urinary anion gap (UAG):** The UAG ($[Na^+] + [K^+] - [Cl^-]$) is a convenient surrogate for the excretion of urinary ammonium. The UAG is negative in extrarenal causes of non–AG acidosis (eg, diarrhea or ureteral diversion), whereas it is positive in conditions where urinary excretion of ammonium (as ammonium chloride) is impaired, such as renal failure, distal RTA, or hypoaldosteronism. In certain cases (urine pH >6.5, urinary $[Na^+]$ <20 mEq/L, polyuria), the **urine osmolal gap** may be more reliable.
7. Calculate the **serum osmolal gap:** In any patient with an unexplained high AG acidosis, a serum osmolal gap should be calculated because laboratory confirmation of toxic alcohol (or propylene glycol) intoxication is often not rapidly available and may require immediate treatment. The serum

osmolal gap is the difference between the measured and calculated serum osmolality (calculated serum osmolality = 2 × Na^+ (in mEq/L) + glucose (in mg/dL)/18 + blood urea nitrogen (BUN; in mg/dL)/2.8. Normal values are less than 10 mOsm/kg.

8. Measurement of **urinary [Cl^-]**: History and clinical examination are often sufficient to determine the causes of metabolic alkalosis. In case of ambiguity, urinary [Cl^-] may be measured. Urinary [Cl^-] less than 25 mEq/L is typically associated with gastric fluid losses (**chloride-responsive alkalosis**), whereas values greater than 40 mEq/L suggest inappropriate renal excretion of NaCl (eg, hyperaldosteronism or severe hypokalemia; **chloride-resistant alkalosis**).

C. Metabolic Acidosis is caused by a primary decrease in [HCO_3^-] because of one of three mechanisms: (a) increased usage of HCO_3^- for buffering of a strong acid (endogenous or exogenous), (b) GI or renal bicarbonate losses, and (c) dilution of the ECF by large volumes of non-bicarbonate-containing fluids (such as NS). Note that LR solution typically does not cause hyperchloremic acidosis because the administered lactate is rapidly metabolized by the liver to bicarbonate. Metabolic acidosis is classified as high AG or normal AG (Table 8.6).

D. High AG Metabolic Acidosis

1. **Lactic acidosis** is common in patients who are critically ill. Conventionally, lactic acidosis has been classified as type A (ie, associated with evidence of tissue hypoxia) and type B, or nonhypoxic (ie, liver disease, total parenteral nutrition, thiamine deficiency, DKA, medications [eg, epinephrine, metformin, propofol, iron, etc], intoxications [methanol, ethylene glycol, etc], and trauma). However, it has become clear in recent years that in patients with septic shock, a significant fraction of the lactate is generated aerobically via catecholamine-driven accelerated glycolysis and increased

TABLE 8.6 Classification of Metabolic Acidoses

Anion gap metabolic acidosis
Endogenous
Diabetic ketoacidosis; severe ketoacidosis (alcohol, starvation); uremia; lactate
Exogenous
Toxins
Ethylene glycol, methanol, salicylate
Non–anion gap metabolic acidosis
Gastrointestinal losses
Diarrhea; pancreatic, biliary, and enterocutaneous fistulas; ostomies
Ureterosigmoidostomy
Infusion and ingestion of chloride-containing salts; total parenteral nutrition; cholestyramine
Renal losses
Type I (distal) RTA
Type II (proximal) RTA
Type IV (hyperkalemic) RTA
Metabolic acidosis of renal failure

RTA, renal tubular acidosis.

activity of the Na^+/K^+-ATPase pump. Some clinically relevant points regarding lactic acidosis in patients who are critically ill are mentioned here:

a. Although the pathophysiology of hyperlactatemia is complicated, the evidence strongly suggests an **association between elevated lactate and a poor outcome.** This is true even in the presence of "high-normal" lactate levels (2-4 mmol/L) and even in the **absence of associated hypotension.**

b. The **AG_{corr}** and **base deficit do not reliably predict** increased lactate levels—they are sensitive but not specific. The advantage of the AG and base deficit is that they are routinely reported and can alert the clinician to the possibility of metabolic acidosis, but if lactic acidosis is suspected, the lactate level should be measured.

c. Some studies support using lactate clearance as a marker of adequate resuscitation. Given the complexity of lactate generation, however, it would be wise to consider the lactate levels in the context of the whole patient and not continue to administer fluids only because the lactate has not normalized.

2. **Diabetic ketoacidosis** (see **Chapter 26**): Insulin deficiency leads to excess hepatic ketone production and is treated by insulin administration. DKA is treated with IV insulin infusion and crystalloids to replace fluid losses from glycosuria-driven osmotic diuresis. Bicarbonate therapy is not recommended in children with DKA unless pH falls below 6.9 because of the association between bicarbonate treatment and cerebral edema. However, in adults, it is reasonable to individualize therapy (see subsequent text) rather than treat using arbitrary cutoffs. **Patients with a substantial hyperchloremic non–AG metabolic acidosis** can benefit from bicarbonate at higher pH values.

3. **Starvation ketoacidosis:** Ketones are present in serum and urine. Treatment includes refeeding and correction of associated metabolic and electrolyte abnormalities such as hypophosphatemia and hypokalemia.

4. **Alcoholic ketoacidosis:** Seen in patients with chronic alcoholism and binge drinking. **A high AG and a normal lactate level** in such a patient may be a clue to alcoholic ketoacidosis because the test widely used to detect ketonuria (the nitroprusside test) **detects only acetoacetate and not β-hydroxybutyrate,** the primary ketoacid seen in alcoholic ketoacidosis. Treatment includes IV hydration along with IV thiamine, glucose, and phosphorus administration.

5. **Intoxications and ingestions:** See **Chapter 31.**

E. Non–AG Metabolic Acidosis

1. **Nonrenal causes**

a. **GI losses:** often seen with severe diarrhea, ileus, enterocutaneous fistulas, ostomies, laxative abuse, and villous adenoma of the rectum. Therapy includes bicarbonate replacement. Volume replacement is also essential because avid sodium retention by the kidney decreases its ability to excrete hydrogen ions.

b. **Ureterosigmoidostomy:** Urinary diversion through the intestine can cause non–AG acidosis, hypokalemia, and, sometimes, hypocalcemia and hypomagnesemia. These abnormalities are less severe when urinary diversion is done with ileal conduits.

2. **Renal causes**

a. **Renal Tubular Acidosis**

1. **Type 1 (distal) RTA**

a. **Mechanisms:** impairment of the apical membrane H^+-ATPase and decreased ability to acidify urine

b. **Diagnosis:** positive UAG, urine pH greater than 5.5, low serum potassium, possible nephrocalcinosis and nephrolithiasis, filtered bicarbonate excreted less than 10%

c. **Therapy:** bicarbonate replacement (1-2 mEq/kg/24 h) and potassium replacement

2. **Type 2 (proximal) RTA**
   a. **Mechanisms:** impaired proximal bicarbonate absorption with bicarbonate wasting
   b. **Diagnosis:** UAG unreliable because of the presence of an additional anion (bicarbonate) in the urine; urine pH less than 5.5, low serum potassium; filtered bicarbonate excreted greater than 15%
   c. **Therapy:** high doses of bicarbonate (10-25 mEq/kg/24 h), potassium, calcium, and vitamin D supplementation
3. **Type 4 (hyperkalemic) RTA**
   a. **Mechanisms:** selective aldosterone deficiency (common in types 1 and 2 diabetic nephropathy) and hyporeninemic hypoaldosteronism
   b. **Diagnosis:** positive UAG, urine pH less than 5.5, high serum potassium, filtered bicarbonate excreted less than 10%
   c. **Therapy:** Treat hyperkalemia with exchange resins (as long as there is no ileus) and loop diuretics.
4. **Renal failure:** Renal failure can cause both a high AG acidosis and a non–AG acidosis. As the GFR falls below 30 to 40 mL/min, ammonium production falls below the level required to secrete the daily acid load, which is buffered by bicarbonate in the ECF, causing bicarbonate levels to fall. Non–AG acidosis due to chronic renal insufficiency may be treated by oral bicarbonate supplementation to reduce the adverse effects of prolonged acidosis—muscle wasting and bone demineralization.

F. **Physiologic Effects of Severe Acidemia**: Irrespective of the cause, accumulation of H^+ ions can have important consequences, most prominently affecting the cardiovascular system. These include decreased cardiac contractility, arteriolar dilatation, sensitization to ventricular arrhythmias, and decreased responsiveness to catecholamines. The result is often severe hemodynamic instability. Other adverse effects include hyperventilation (Kussmaul breathing), respiratory muscle fatigue, increased pulmonary vascular resistance, hyperkalemia, insulin resistance, obtundation, and coma.

G. **Symptomatic Management of Severe Acidemia:** Although the primary treatment of severe acidemia is the amelioration of the underlying condition causing the acidemia, it may be necessary to provide symptomatic treatment and improve extracellular and intracellular pH to avoid hemodynamic collapse while waiting for treatment of the underlying condition to take effect. Symptomatic treatment is often required when the pH is less than 7.15, and rarely if it is greater than 7.20. However, decisions must be individualized because certain comorbidities (eg, severe pulmonary hypertension with right ventricular dysfunction) may require symptomatic treatment at higher pH values.

a. **Bicarbonate administration** is often the initial buffer used to treat severe acidemia. The dose of bicarbonate is titrated to effect. Some have recommended the following formula to calculate the bicarbonate dose: **0.3 × weight (in kilograms) × base deficit**, provided as an infusion. However, bicarbonate administration has a number **of potential drawbacks**:
   1. Some patients cannot eliminate the excess CO_2 generated by bicarbonate administration (either because of respiratory fatigue or because of the limits of lung-protective ventilation), and in these patients, bicarbonate may exacerbate intracellular acidosis.
   2. Bicarbonate can stimulate glycolysis (by inducing phosphofructokinase) and increase lactate production.
   3. Bicarbonate may cause hypernatremia, hypervolemia, and hyperosmolality.

b. **Nonbicarbonate buffers** have been under investigation for many years, but only one—**THAM** (tris-hydroxymethyl-amino-methane)—is in clinical use. THAM is a more effective buffer than is bicarbonate (its pKa is 7.8, compared with a pKa of 6.3 for bicarbonate). It avoids a sodium load and does not generate CO_2; instead, it buffers H^+ by generating NH_3^+ that is eliminated by the kidneys. Thus, **preserved renal function** (or renal replacement therapy) is required for its efficacy but it is independent of pulmonary function. The initial dose of THAM (in milliliters, of a 0.3 molar solution) is calculated by weight (in kilograms) × base deficit. The maximum dose is 15 mmol/kg, although the maximum dose is seldom required. Side effects of THAM include respiratory depression (not an issue in patients who are mechanically ventilated), hypoglycemia, and venous irritation. Hyperkalemia has been documented with THAM, and it should not be used in the setting of renal failure (unless on replacement therapy) and hyperkalemia.

c. It should be noted that the data for the symptomatic treatment of acidemia are poor and no high-quality trials exist. Management is governed largely by physiologic principles.

H. Metabolic Alkalosis

1. **Causes**
   a. **GI losses:** H^+ losses from the upper GI tract due to vomiting or nasogastric suctioning
   b. **Diuretics** cause a **contraction alkalosis** (reduction of the ECF volume around existing bicarbonate concentrations because of the excretion of bicarbonate-free urine) along with chloride and potassium wasting, which alter normal renal handling of H^+ and bicarbonate.
   c. **Hyperaldosteronism** causes metabolic alkalosis by increasing H^+ losses at the distal nephron.
   d. **Other causes**
      1. Posthypercapneic alkalosis
      2. Hypokalemia
      3. Bicarbonate or citrate infusion: **Massive transfusion** can cause metabolic alkalosis (provided that the patient has been adequately resuscitated and has normal hepatic function) because of the citrate transfused with blood products.
2. **Management:** Chloride-responsive metabolic alkalosis (see **Section VI.B.8**) responds to volume repletion with NaCl solutions. Potassium repletion often ameliorates chloride-resistant alkalosis. Although treatment of symptomatic alkalosis with 0.1 normal (dilute) hydrochloric acid has been reported, it is extremely unusual in clinical practice.

I. Respiratory Acidosis is due to decreased CO_2 excretion resulting in a rising $PaCO_2$ and a compensatory decrease in $[HCO_3^-]$. Hypoventilation results from decreased ventilating capacity, either in patients who **cannot breathe** (eg, neuromuscular disease, respiratory fatigue, severe obstructive lung disease, etc) or in patients who **will not breathe** (eg, altered responsiveness of the respiratory center to $PaCO_2$ in patients who are narcotized). Treatment centers around the underlying disorder. Occasionally, patients with severe respiratory acidosis may require symptomatic therapy (see earlier text). A fascinating recent approach to symptomatic hypercapnea is the **partial extracorporeal removal of CO_2**, allowing the use of very low tidal volumes (~4 mL/kg) in acute respiratory distress syndrome (ARDS).

J. Respiratory Alkalosis is due to alveolar hyperventilation. Hyperventilation may be due to a metabolic cause (eg, fever), pain, anxiety, or neurogenic (eg, head injuries or strokes) in patients with normal pulmonary function. Patients with intrinsic lung disease (pneumonia or pulmonary embolism) may also present with hyperventilation. Management is directed at the underlying cause.

K. The Physicochemical (Stewart) Approach to Acid-Base Physiology: Critics of the physiologic approach argue that the bicarbonate buffer system is only one of numerous buffers in the body, and that changes in the bicarbonate buffers are reflective of the cumulative effect of multiple metabolic and respiratory processes. The Stewart physicochemical approach defines mathematically the determinants of the acid-base balance in aqueous solutions on the basis of the laws of mass action, conservation of mass, and conservation of charge. The Stewart approach defines **three independent variables**—namely, **Pa_{CO_2}, SID (strong ion difference)**, and A_{tot} **(total weak acids)**—that completely describe the acid-base status of a closed system. Other changes, including changes in $[H^+]$ and $[HCO_3^-]$, are secondary to changes in the independent variables. The details of the Stewart system are beyond the scope of this chapter. Its proponents believe that complex acid-base disorders are easier to understand and explain by the Stewart method and that it is mathematically sound. However, critics of the more complex Stewart method contend that there is no evidence that patient management using the Stewart approach produces superior results compared to the physiologic approach. For this reason, the physiologic approach continues to be the preferred method of diagnosing acid-base disturbances at the authors' institution.

Acknowledgments

The authors of this chapter gratefully acknowledge the contributions of Drs. Gauran and Steele, the authors of this chapter in the earlier (6th) edition.

Selected Readings

Berend K, de Vries APJ, Gans ROB. Physiological approach to the assessment of acid–base disturbances. *N Engl J Med.* 2014;371:432-445.

Caironi P, Tognoni G, Masson S, et al. Albumin replacement in patients with severe sepsis or septic shock. *N Engl J Med.* 2014;370:1412-1421.

Cerda J, Tolwani AJ, Warnock DG. Critical care nephrology: management of acid–base disorders with CRRT. *Kidney Int.* 2012;82:9-18.

Finfer S, Bellomo R, Boyce N, et al. A comparison of albumin and saline for fluid resuscitation in the intensive care unit. *N Engl J Med.* 2004;350:2247-2256.

Holmdahl MH, Wiklund L, Wetterberg T, et al. The place of THAM in the management of acidemia in clinical practice. *Acta Anesth Scand.* 2000;44:524-527.

Kraut JA, Madias NE. Differential diagnosis of nongap metabolic acidosis: value of a systematic approach. *Clin J Am Soc Nephrol.* 2012;7:671-679.

Kraut JA, Madias NE. Lactic acidosis. *N Engl J Med.* 2014;371:2309-2319.

Kurtz I, Kraut J, Ornekian V, et al. Acid–base analysis: a critique of the Stewart and bicarbonate-centered approaches. *Am J Physiol Renal Physiol.* 2008;294:F1009-F1031.

Perner A, Haase N, Guttormsen AB, et al. Hydroxyethyl starch 130/0.42 versus Ringer's acetate in severe sepsis. *N Engl J Med.* 2012;367:124-134.

Rastegar A. Use of the $\Delta AG/\Delta HCO_3$ ratio in the diagnosis of mixed acid–base disorders. *J Am Soc Nephrol.* 2007;18:2429-2431.

Yunos NM, Bellomo R, Hegarty C, et al. Association between a chloride-liberal vs chloride-restrictive intravenous fluid administration strategy and kidney injury in critically ill adults. *JAMA.* 2012;308:1566-1572.

9 Trauma

Katherine H. Albutt and Jonathan J. Parks

I. INTRODUCTION

Trauma is a leading cause of morbidity and mortality globally. According to the World Health Organization (WHO), road traffic injuries accounted for 1.25 million deaths in 2014, and trauma is expected to rise to the third leading cause of disability worldwide by 2030. The most common causes of mortality from trauma are hemorrhage, multiple organ dysfunction syndrome, and cardiopulmonary arrest. In the United States alone, more than 50 million patients receive some form of trauma-related medical care annually, and trauma accounts for approximately 30% of all intensive care unit (ICU) admissions. This chapter explains the initial evaluation of trauma patients, highlights some aspects of critical care unique to trauma patients, and addresses the care of specific commonly encountered injuries.

II. INITIAL EVALUATION AND PRIMARY SURVEY (THE ABCDEs)

It is essential that the ICU providers have some familiarity with the workup and management of the trauma patient before transfer to the ICU. The initial evaluation of the trauma patient begins in field. Whenever possible, emergency medical services (EMS) should notify the receiving hospital that a trauma patient is en route. This provides the receiving hospital with information and time that can be crucial to the management of the severely injured patient. A clear, simple, and organized approach is needed when managing a severely injured patient. The American College of Surgeons' Advanced Trauma Life Support (ATLS) course provides a standard algorithmic approach to the management of the trauma patient. Hemorrhage and respiratory compromise are the most common causes of preventable trauma deaths, and the initial evaluation is aimed at rapid identification of these entities. The primary survey consists of the following steps: (a) **A**irway assessment and protection; (b) **B**reathing and ventilation; (c) **C**irculation; (d) **D**isability; and (e) **E**xposure. It is worth noting that although these steps can be performed in sequence, in many settings with large teams they may be performed simultaneously.

A. Airway: Within minutes, severely injured patients can develop airway obstruction or inadequate ventilation leading to hypoxia and death within minutes. Airway obstruction is a major cause of preventable death among trauma patients. Definitive guidelines for tracheal intubation in trauma do not exist. When in doubt, it is generally best to intubate early, particularly in patients with hemodynamic instability or severely altered level of consciousness. Although an awake, talking patient has a stable airway, trauma to the neck (eg, injuries with bleeding, expanding hematoma, subcutaneous emphysema, etc) can quickly lead to airway compromise and respiratory collapse. In the unconscious patient, the airway must be protected immediately in an expedient yet controlled manner. See **Chapter 4** for an excellent review and the details of airway management, including rapid sequence intubation. Specific indications for securing the airway and considerations for managing the airway in trauma patients are described here.

1. **Indications for endotracheal intubation**
   a. Respiratory distress with signs of potential impending airway collapse such as stridor or crepitus, bleeding or expanding neck hematoma, or severe facial injury.
   b. **Glasgow Coma Scale (GCS)** $\leq$ 8.
2. **Special situations**
   a. **Head injury:** In these cases, it is important to minimize the intracranial hypertension associated with laryngeal stimulation, the hypotension sometimes associated with induction regimens, and hypoxemia because all of these can worsen outcome in head injury. No specific pharmacologic adjuncts have been proved effective.
   b. **Cervical spine injury:** In-line cervical spine stabilization should be maintained in almost all trauma patients. The presence of a cervical spine injury should be assumed in all blunt trauma patients until proved otherwise.
   c. **Basilar skull fracture:** Nasotracheal intubation should be avoided to prevent inadvertent passage of foreign bodies into the cranial vault.
   d. **Suspected laryngotracheal injury:** Consider awake fiberoptic intubation in the operating room for awake patients who are controlling their airway. Paralysis and direct laryngoscopy can precipitate an emergency. Whenever possible, surgical assistance should be available in case tracheostomy is required.
   e. **Maxillofacial injury:** In cases of severe maxillofacial injury, consider early placement of a surgical airway if orotracheal intubation fails.

B. Breathing: Once airway patency is ensured, the next step is to assess the adequacy of oxygenation and ventilation. Victims of trauma can present with varied pathology that will affect their breathing, including pneumothorax, hemothorax, aspiration, flail chest, and diaphragmatic rupture. Initial evaluation begins with a physical exam including auscultation of breath sounds bilaterally, observation of the chest to look for asymmetry or paradoxical motion, and palpation of the thorax to feel for crepitus or deformity. Monitoring instruments are placed (pulse oximeter, blood pressure cuff) and oxygen supplementation is provided. Additional adjuncts include portable chest x-ray and chest ultrasonography. Tension pneumothorax, massive hemothorax, and cardiac tamponade are immediate threats to life that should be identified at this stage of the primary survey. The most common initial interventions affecting breathing are tube thoracostomy and endotracheal intubation. In unstable patients with absent breath sounds, radiographic confirmation of pneumothorax or hemothorax is not necessary and only delays treatment; tube thoracostomy should be performed emergently. In cases of suspected pneumothorax or hemothorax without obvious signs on physical exam, either ultrasound or chest x-ray performed in the trauma bay can be used for immediate further evaluation. See the following sections on pneumothorax, hemothorax, and pulmonary contusion regarding further management of these injuries.

C. Circulation: Hemorrhage is the most common cause of circulatory compromise in trauma, as well as the most common preventable cause of mortality. Be alert for subtle signs of hemorrhagic shock, particularly in the older patients, who may be on cardiovascular medications that blunt such signs, and in young, healthy adults who may not present with obvious manifestations. Hypotension generally does not manifest until at least 30% of the patient's blood volume has been lost. Large-bore peripheral intravenous access should be obtained and transfusion begun if there is concern about hemorrhage. Hemodynamically significant bleeding can occur in five locations, which are evaluated as noted:

1. **External:** physical exam
2. **Thoracic cavity:** physical exam, chest x-ray, ultrasound, empiric chest tube placement
3. **Abdominal cavity:** physical exam, ultrasound (focused abdominal sonography for trauma [FAST] exam), diagnostic peritoneal aspiration
4. **Extraperitoneal pelvis:** physical exam, pelvic x-ray
5. **Thighs:** physical exam, x-ray

Other less common but important causes of circulatory compromise in trauma include tension pneumothorax, pericardial tamponade, and neurogenic shock. Pericardial tamponade, once suspected from vital signs and physical exam findings, is most frequently confirmed by ultrasound. Neurogenic shock from spinal cord injury is identified by the combination of hypotension with bradycardia, along with changes to the motor or sensory exam.

D. Disability: Once problems related to the airway, breathing, and circulation are addressed, perform a focused neurologic examination. This should include a description of the patient's level of consciousness using the GCS score, and assessments of pupillary size and reactivity, gross motor function, sensation, and presence or absence of any lateralizing symptoms.

E. Exposure: Be certain that the trauma patient is completely undressed and that the entire body is examined for signs of injury during the primary survey. Missed injuries pose a grave threat. Neglected regions often include the scalp, axillary folds, perineum, and the abdominal folds in obese patients. Penetrating wounds may be present anywhere. While maintaining cervical spine precautions, examine the patient's back; do not neglect examination of the gluteal fold and posterior scalp. Hypothermia should be prevented if possible and treated immediately once identified.

III. DIAGNOSTIC STUDIES AND THE SECONDARY SURVEY

A number of diagnostic studies should be obtained during or subsequent to the primary survey, including (a) plain films; (b) ultrasound (FAST exam); (c) laboratory studies (particularly a type and screen); and (d) electrocardiogram (ECG). A careful, head-to-toe secondary assessment (the secondary survey) is performed in all trauma patients determined to be stable on completion of the primary survey. The secondary survey includes a detailed history, a thorough and efficient physical examination, and targeted diagnostic studies. Once the secondary survey is complete, hemodynamically stable patients may be taken for additional imaging such as computed tomography (CT) scanning. Unstable patients should be transported to the operating room or angiography suite for further intervention.

IV. TRAUMA RESUSCITATION

A. Goals of Resuscitation: These are determined by the patient and the suspected injuries. Young healthy patients with suspected bleeding can undergo "permissive hypotension" while en route to definitive control of the bleeding source. If they are awake and alert, they have an acceptable blood pressure. If they are sedated, we select an arbitrary but relatively low systolic pressure goal of 90 mm Hg. Patients with suspected head injury or older patients who are more likely to have a higher baseline systolic pressure may not be candidates for this type of resuscitation strategy and have more standard resuscitation goals.

B. Choice of Resuscitation Fluid: Hypovolemia secondary to bleeding should be treated with blood products. "Balanced resuscitation" guides transfusion strategy, with delivery of blood components that in combination approaches the composition of whole blood as a target. Many centers employ a massive transfusion protocol to facilitate balanced resuscitation for severe hemorrhage needing more than 10 units. We never consider colloid (albumin) in patients with head injuries or burns and rarely use it in the initial resuscitation of any patient.

V. SPECIFIC INJURIES

A. Traumatic Brain Injury (TBI): For the critically ill TBI patient, a checklist approach to physiologic management goals may improve outcomes. Care is oriented at managing intracranial hypertension to prevent herniation. Current recommendations include the early placement of cerebrospinal fluid (CSF) drainage systems to lower intracranial pressure (ICP) in patients with an initial GCS less than 6 and utilizing ICP monitoring to reduce in-hospital and 2-week postinjury mortality in patients with severe TBI. ICP greater than 22 mm Hg should be treated because values above this level are associated with increased mortality, and recommended target cerebral perfusion pressure (CPP) is between 60 and 70 mm Hg. See **Chapter 10** for a thorough review of critical care of the neurologic patient. The latest Brain Trauma Foundation guidelines can be found at www.braintrauma.org.

B. Blunt Cerebrovascular Injury (BCVI): Severe acceleration/deceleration or flexion/extension forces can injure the intima of the carotid or vertebral vessels, resulting in thrombus formation and risk of emboli/stroke. Finding this injury requires a high index of suspicion because there are usually no clinical signs or symptoms until an often catastrophic stroke has occurred. The Eastern Association for the Surgery of Trauma (EAST) guidelines recommend using a screening protocol, such as the Denver or Memphis criteria, to detect BCVI in blunt polytrauma patients. Among patients with cervical spine injuries, screening CT angiography is recommended to detect BCVI. Antithrombotic therapy should be utilized in patients diagnosed with BCVI.

C. Pneumothorax

1. As previously stated, a patient with absent breath sounds and hypotension or respiratory distress should have a chest tube placed without waiting for imaging.
2. **Occult pneumothorax:** An "occult" pneumothorax is one that is found on CT but not seen on plain radiography. Previously, it was thought that any patient requiring positive pressure ventilation with a pneumothorax required tube thoracostomy. Randomized controlled trials have shown that positive pressure ventilation does not influence the progression of occult pneumothoraces. We no longer routinely place chest tubes for stable patients with occult pneumothoraces who will undergo positive pressure ventilation, but caregivers must be alert for progression, and we typically monitor these patients with serial chest x-rays.

D. Hemothorax: Posttraumatic hemothorax comes from the chest wall, lung, or intrathoracic vessels. Drainage allows for lung reexpansion and assessment of bleeding severity. Surgical intervention should be considered when the initial output is greater than 1500 mL, is greater than 200 mL/h over the first 4 hours, or there is hemodynamic instability because this degree of bleeding is less likely to stop spontaneously. If bleeding stops and chest x-ray shows persistent effusion, chest CT is useful to evaluate for retained hemothorax, which may be treated with intrapleural thrombolytics or thoracoscopic evacuation.

E. Rib Fracture: The presence of rib fractures should alert the intensivist to the potential for associated injuries including pneumothorax, hemothorax, pulmonary contusion, liver or spleen laceration, and diaphragmatic injury. Adequate pain control and pulmonary toilet are the cornerstones of rib fracture management. This can be accomplished with epidural, paravertebral, or intercostal nerve blocks, opioids, nonsteroidal anti-inflammatory medication, or combinations of these and other adjuncts. The goals should be normal tidal volumes, normal mobility, an effective cough, and secretion clearance. Patients with flail chest (two or more consecutive ribs fractured in two or more places) and respiratory failure or severe chest wall deformity may benefit from open reduction and internal fixation of rib fractures.

F. Pulmonary Contusion: This is more commonly seen associated with blunt traumatic injury to the chest wall. Unlike most sequelae of trauma, pulmonary contusions usually take 24 to 48 hours to "bloom" and fully manifest. Management includes minimizing fluid resuscitation, but even with careful fluid management, many patients will require intubation. Colloid resuscitation does not improve outcomes compared with crystalloid. Pulmonary contusion rarely presents as an isolated injury and is often associated with rib, diaphragm, and extrathoracic injuries.

G. Aortic Injury: This is usually related to a significant deceleration injury (fall from height or motor vehicle collision) resulting in a contained rupture of the aorta, most commonly immediately distal to the origin of the left subclavian artery. It is most often diagnosed by chest CT with intravenous contrast. Surgical control of a contained rupture is nonemergent if there are other pressing injuries, but tight "impulse control" of heart rate and blood pressure should be maintained until repair, which can usually be accomplished with an endovascular stent.

H. Blunt Cardiac Injury: This injury is associated with significant chest wall trauma and manifests as hypotension and/or new arrhythmias. More significant, time-sensitive injuries such as cardiac tamponade or tension pneumothorax must be ruled out before hypotension is attributed to blunt cardiac injury. Suspected blunt cardiac injury should be evaluated with an ECG and a serum troponin measurement. If both are normal, no blunt cardiac injury exists. If either an elevated troponin or a new arrhythmia is found, the patient should be admitted to a monitored bed for 24 hours. If either exists with hypotension or significant arrhythmias, the patient should be admitted to the ICU and undergo a transthoracic echocardiogram to look for a traumatic valvular lesion, tamponade, or segmental wall motion abnormality. Occasionally, inotropic support is required until the myocardium recovers.

I. Abdominal Solid Organ Injury: The spleen, liver, and kidneys are susceptible to injury (laceration, contusion, hematoma), particularly in blunt trauma. In the absence of hemodynamic instability or peritonitis, these injuries can be managed with serial abdominal exams and serial measurement of hematocrit. Large-bore intravenous lines and reversal of coagulopathy are important in managing these injuries. If there are signs of continued bleeding, these injuries can be managed by angioembolization or by surgery. There are no absolute values for minimum hematocrit, or number of units of transfused blood, or hemodynamic parameters to guide the decision to intervene on these injuries. Rather, the clinician must evaluate the entire patient and how the solid organ injury affects management.

J. Pelvic Fracture: These can cause significant bleeding and rapid decompensation, and management should focus on large-bore intravenous access and reversal of any coagulopathy. There are three modalities for managing severe bleeding from pelvic fractures: pelvic fixation, extraperitoneal pelvic packing, and bilateral internal iliac artery angioembolization. In unstable patients, they are often employed simultaneously. Patients with extraperitoneal packing will require reoperation for pack removal. Because angioembolization is typically done with absorbable gelatin foam, a small percentage of patients with recurrent bleeding will require repeat angioembolization.

K. Extremity Compartment Syndrome: This secondary injury is related to swelling, crush injury, or periods of ischemia with reperfusion (tourniquet application, vascular injury, long bone fracture with or without vascular injury). Clinically, compartment syndrome will present as a tense compartment The 6 Ps—pain, pallor, paresthesia, pulselessness, poikilothermia, and/or paralysis—in an awake, sober, and cooperative patient should raise your suspicion for a possible compartment syndrome. In patients with a decreased level of consciousness, the index of suspicion should remain high.

1. If there is any doubt about the diagnosis, compartment pressures can be measured directly with commercially available devices or with a transducer and large-bore needle. Although different thresholds have been proposed, urgent surgical decompression is usually required when compartment pressures reach 25 to 30 mm Hg and should be performed urgently.

L. **Cervical Spine Injury:** Most blunt trauma patients requiring ICU admission will have had a high-energy mechanism of injury, such that the possibility of cervical spine injury must be considered. Many patients will arrive to the ICU with a hard cervical collar in place to provide in-line stabilization. For patients who are clinically evaluable (not intoxicated, no distracting injury), the cervical spine can be cleared by physical exam alone. If there is no posterior midline tenderness or no pain or paresthesia with axial loading, flexion, extension, or rotation, there is no need for further evaluation. Patients who cannot be clinically cleared by exam should undergo CT of the cervical spine. When injuries are found, they can be treated appropriately (either with immobilization or surgery). When no injuries are found on CT, in-line stabilization is typically maintained until a clinical evaluation can be performed to assess for possible ligamentous injury. If patients are likely to be clinically evaluable shortly after CT is performed, it is appropriate to wait for the opportunity to examine them. If not, or if the physical exam is abnormal despite a normal CT scan finding, cervical spine magnetic resonance imaging (MRI) should be performed to evaluate for ligamentous injury. It should be performed as soon as feasible because prolonged cervical collar application is associated with a number of complications from pressure ulceration to ventilator-associated pneumonia.

VI. OTHER CONSIDERATIONS

A. **Thromboprophylaxis:** Trauma patients are at high risk for deep venous thrombosis (DVT) and pulmonary embolism. Because trauma can be associated with bleeding and significant tissue damage, there is occasionally confusion or reluctance about how or when to initiate thromboprophylaxis and what agents to use.

1. Mechanical prophylaxis is safe for virtually all patients and reduces the risk of DVT compared with no prophylaxis.
2. Pharmacologic prophylaxis is more effective than is mechanical prophylaxis.
3. Low-molecular-weight heparin (LMWH) is more effective than is unfractionated heparin.
4. Combined mechanical and pharmacologic prophylaxis is more effective than either alone.
5. Prophylactic inferior vena cava (IVC) filter placement has not been proved to be effective in trauma patients.
6. Immediate pharmacologic prophylaxis is safe in patients without a major hemorrhagic injury or intracranial hemorrhage.
7. Pharmacologic prophylaxis should generally be considered safe 48 hours after bleeding control in patients with hemorrhagic injuries or 48 hours after stable intracranial imaging in patients with intracranial hemorrhage.

B. **Damage Control:** Damage control surgery refers to the tactic of controlling bleeding and limiting contamination without necessarily performing definitive reconstruction at the time of initial operation in unstable trauma patients. This may involve using temporary packs to control bleeding, performing intestinal resection without anastomosis, or placing temporary intravascular shunts rather than performing bypass grafts. The ICU physician needs to understand the state of the incomplete anatomy (eg, cannot provide enteral feeding to a patient whose gastrointestinal [GI] tract is out of continuity) and the physiologic derangements (eg, hypothermia, coagulopathy) that need to be corrected to allow for definitive treatment of the patient's injuries.

C. Open Abdomen: After laparotomy for trauma, the abdominal cavity may be left open for one of two reasons: (a) closure may result in intra-abdominal hypertension or abdominal compartment syndrome or (b) a damage control operation was performed and early reoperation is anticipated to remove packs or definitively address injuries. The open abdomen is usually managed with a closed suction dressing. An open abdomen per se does not require neuromuscular blockade or cessation of enteral feeding. If the abdomen was left open because of concerns about compartment syndrome, multiple procedures may be required to achieve primary fascial closure. The key is to begin the closure process early before abdominal domain is lost. If physiologically tolerated, a negative fluid balance may also increase the rate of fascial closure.

D. Tertiary Survey: Patients undergo primary and secondary surveys as mentioned. Because these occur in the heat of the moment in the trauma bay, it is possible to miss non-life-threatening, but nonetheless significant, injuries. A repeated head-to-toe physical exam and review of systems (the "tertiary survey") have been shown to reduce the rate of missed injuries. Patients undergoing urgent interventions shortly after presentation who may have never had a complete secondary survey are at particularly high risk for missed injuries.

E. Antibiotic Prophylaxis: Trauma patients do not require antibiotic prophylaxis exceeding that of other critically ill or surgical patients. Penetrating injuries should undergo appropriate wound care and/or closure, but do not require prophylaxis. Periprocedural prophylaxis is appropriate for patients undergoing laparotomy or emergency tube thoracostomy, but even in the presence of hollow viscus injury, antibiotic administration should not be routinely extended beyond 24 hours.

VII. SUMMARY

The greatest immediate risks to trauma patients are hemorrhage and cardiopulmonary compromise, and the initial evaluation focuses on identifying and addressing these without the luxury of axial imaging. Once patients have been stabilized, further imaging and a tertiary survey are performed to identify all injuries. The bulk of critical care for trauma is identical to the care for any critically ill patient, but there are key differences in certain aspects of care. Commonly, different injuries present competing management priorities, requiring the intensivist to actively evaluate and manage the entire patient and entire injury burden.

10 Critical Care of the Neurologic Patient

Benjamin R. M. Brush and Sahar F. Zafar

I. INTRODUCTION

A. Common Problems and Diagnoses Requiring Neurocritical Care

1. Increased intracranial pressure (ICP) → requiring close monitoring, hyperosmolar therapy, and/or surgical intervention: related to edema (traumatic brain injury, strokes), lesions with mass effect (intracranial tumor, hematoma, or abscess), hydrocephalus (mass or blood obstructing ventricles, disturbances in cerebrospinal fluid (CSF) homeostasis), central nervous system (CNS) infections
2. Traumatic brain injury (TBI) → requiring ICP/multimodal monitoring, normothermia, surgical interventions, and often neuroprognostication. Indications for ICP monitoring in TBI:
   a. Severe TBI (GCS 3-8) and an abnormal computed tomography (CT) scan
   b. Severe TBI with a normal CT scan but presence of two of the following: age >40 years, unilateral or bilateral motor posturing, or systolic blood pressure (SBP) <90 mm Hg
3. Stroke → large-volume strokes usually involving the middle cerebral artery or posterior fossa and requiring monitoring for the development of malignant cerebral edema and subsequent hyperosmolar therapy and/or surgery. Additionally, patients with stroke may demonstrate dynamic changes in symptoms with blood pressure decreases and require temporary augmentation to allow collateral vessels to form.
4. Subarachnoid hemorrhage (SAH) → requiring close neurologic and hemodynamic monitoring including for vasospasm and delayed cerebral ischemia
5. Refractory seizures and status epilepticus → requiring intubation due to poor mental status, in the setting of sedating medications, or burst suppression, hemodynamic and metabolic monitoring
6. Infections of the CNS (meningitis, encephalitis) → requiring intubation due to poor mental status, ICP monitoring, seizure control, CSF diversion
7. Neuromuscular disease presenting with respiratory failure (Guillain-Barré syndrome/acute inflammatory demyelinating polyneuropathy [AIDP], myasthenia gravis, amyotrophic lateral sclerosis) → requiring mechanical ventilation, autonomic instability (in AIDP)
8. Toxidromes: serotonin syndrome, neuroleptic malignant syndrome, severe benzodiazepine or alcohol withdrawal → requiring seizure control, close hemodynamic and cardiac monitoring, thermoregulation, and intubation
9. Spinal cord injury → requiring close hemodynamic monitoring and management of autonomic dysregulation
10. Postoperative care of complex neurosurgical patients → requiring close monitoring of neurologic exam and hemodynamics
11. Cardiac or pulmonary failure in the context of neurologic injury
12. Impaired arousal with the inability to maintain patent airways or need for mechanical ventilation

B. General Principles of Neurocritical Care: multimodal neuromonitoring (see **Section II**), neuroprotection, intracerebral hemodynamics

II. MONITORING

The utility of an integrated multimodal approach to the decompensating neurologic patient has gained traction in recent years, although studies on any one metric have yet to show strong evidence in its support. Still, the consensus is that the use of multiple modalities and interpretation of trends is likely to be beneficial to patients, and trials are ongoing to evaluate this.

A. Neurologic Examination: In general, minimize sedation and follow serial bedside exams, monitoring relevant parameters such as cortical, brainstem, and spinal cord function. In patients with status epilepticus or patients requiring sedation for elevated ICPs or pharmacologic paralysis, the exam may be limited to checking brainstem reflexes or simply pupillary response. The exam should be documented and reported as mental status (level of alertness, orientation, attention, language: ability to express and comprehend), cranial nerves, strength, sensation, deep tendon reflexes, and coordination.

1. **Red Flags: Pupillary asymmetries** (make sure patient has not been exposed to pharmacologic stimuli such as atropine drops or nebulizers)—concerning for increasing ICP, ruptured posterior cerebral artery or posterior communicating artery aneurysm; **Cushing triad** (combination of elevated blood pressure, bradycardia, and irregular respiration)—concerning for increasing ICP; **impaired upgaze**—concerning for hydrocephalus; **decreasing NIFs/vital capacity or decreasing strength affecting the neck and bulbar muscles**—concerning for worsening neuromuscular failure; **meningismus**—concerning for SAH or CNS infection; **acute loss of reflexes and ascending paralysis**—concerning for progressive AIDP
2. **Start with a minimal stimulus** and then escalate as needed (whisper before yelling, give verbal commands before pinching). Note: If the patient has a gaze preference or neglect, stand on the side that the patient's gaze is turned toward.
3. **Cortical function:** In essentially all right-handed individuals and over 70% of left-handed individuals, **language is processed in the left hemisphere** and **attention in the right hemisphere**. The **motor cortex** (precentral gyrus) controls the **contralateral limbs. Sensation** is processed in the postcentral gyrus of the **contralateral hemisphere**. The frontal eye fields direct gaze to the contralateral side; therefore, a stroke (lack of stimulation on the affected side) drives gaze **toward** the side of the injury (eg, L-gaze deviation in an L-sided stroke) while a seizure (excessive stimulation on the affected side) drives gaze **away** from the point of onset (R-gaze deviation with L-sided seizure).
4. **Brainstem function:** The brainstem controls involuntary eye movements, pupillary function, facial sensation, and vital functions. Knowledge of its functions is critical in the evaluation of the comatose patient and the posterior circulation acute stroke syndromes (see Table 10.1).
5. **Spinal cord function:** In contrast to brainstem and cortical injuries, spinal cord injury often produces bilateral, symmetric impairment of the limbs but never facial weakness. Always distinguish anterior column function (strength, sensation of pin/temperature) from posterior column function (sensation of vibration, proprioception), document reflexes and sacral functions (anal sphincter tone, bulbocavernosus reflex). The aim of localization is to identify the highest level of injury.
   a. **Brown-Séquard syndrome** of hemicord dysfunction is characterized by ipsilateral loss of motor and proprioceptive functions and contralateral loss of pain and temperature (fibers carried in the spinothalamic tract decussate at the spinal cord level).
   b. **Anterior spinal artery syndrome** is characterized by bilateral symmetric motor weakness and dissociated sensory loss, with impairments in pain and temperature sensation and preservation of proprioception

TABLE 10.1 Common Findings in Brainstem Lesions

Lesion level	Common findings	Anatomic pathway
Midbrain	Midposition fixed pupils	Light reflex pathways
	Ophthalmoplegia	Oculomotor nuclei
	Hemiparesis, Babinski sign	Cerebral peduncles
High pons	Pinpoint, reactive pupils	Sympathetic fibers
	Internuclear ophthalmoplegia	Medial longitudinal fasciculus
	Facial weakness	Facial nerve
	Reduced corneal sensation	Trigeminal nerve
Low pons	Horizontal reflex gaze paralysis	Abducens nerve, horizontal gaze center
	Hemiparesis, Babinski sign	Corticospinal, corticobulbar tracts
Medulla	Disordered breathing	Respiratory center
	Hypotension, hypertension, dysrhythmias	Vasomotor center

and vibration (fibers for the latter are carried in the posterior column, which is supplied by the posterior spinal arteries). Thoracic and thoracoabdominal aortic aneurysm repair surgery is a risk factor for anterior spinal artery syndrome.

c. **Central cord syndrome** is common in syrinx or cervical injuries and characterized by motor and sensory impairment predominantly affecting the upper extremities.

d. **Cauda equina syndrome** is characterized by variable degrees of bilateral lower motor neuron weakness in the legs (sparing the arms), sensory loss of the lower extremities and sacrum, and dysfunction of the bowel and bladder.

B. ICP Monitoring

1. **Intracranial compliance:** The skull is a rigid box filled with incompressible brain parenchyma, blood, and cerebrospinal fluid (CSF). When the volume of one component increases, the others must adjust or there is a rapid rise in **ICP** (Figure 10.1) (eg, expanding edema pushes CSF from ventricles into subarachnoid space). **ICP** is normally less than 10 mm Hg (5-15 mm Hg); transient elevations up to 30 mm Hg are usually tolerated. Blood flow into the head is dependent on a pressure gradient where **cerebral perfusion pressure (CPP)** = Mean arterial pressure (MAP) − ICP. When ICP rises above 20 mm Hg (or CPP falls below 60 mm Hg), **cerebral blood flow (CBF)** may be inadequate. Additional pressure differentials may exist between compartments of the brain and can lead to clinical herniation even though measured or global ICP may not be significantly elevated.

2. **ICP-monitoring devices and potential complications**

a. **External ventricular drain (EVD):** usually placed in the right lateral ventricle. The ventricular catheter is connected to a pressure transducer. Risks include intracranial hemorrhage upon insertion and infection (increasing with the duration of catheter presence). Advantages: allows for drainage of CSF and can be recalibrated (leading to improved reliability over time).

b. **Fiberoptic intraparenchymal catheters:** (commonly called "bolts") inserted a few mm into the parenchyma through a burr hole usually ipsilateral to the lesion. Advantages: less invasive, lower bleeding, and infection risk. Disadvantages: cannot be recalibrated once placed, requires special

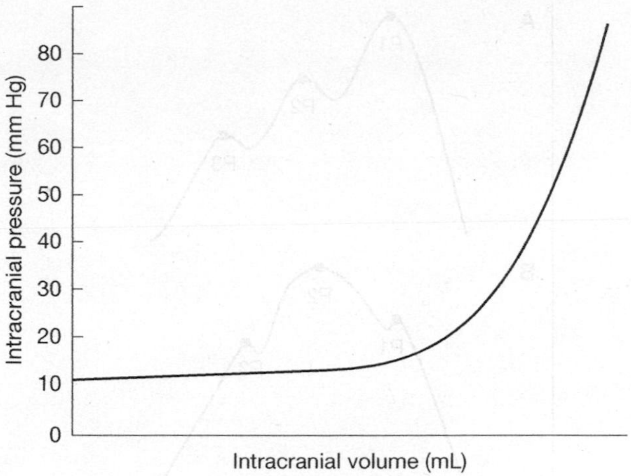

FIGURE 10.1 Intracranial compliance curve. In the normal ICP range, increases in intracranial volume produce minimal changes in ICP initially. Further small increases in intracranial volume at the "elbow" of the curve, however, can produce an abrupt increase in ICP. ICP, intracranial pressure.

signal transducing monitors, and may not be compatible with the available monitoring systems if patients are transferred between institutions. External transducers require periodic recalibration to remain accurate, sometimes called "zeroing" because of the task of zero calibrating to the level of the foramen of Monro.

c. In patients with temporal or posterior fossa lesions, high ICPs in the region of injury might not be accurately measured by the monitoring device as not all pressure is transmitted uniformly throughout compartments within the skull. Clinical judgment should be used when assessing the risk of herniation.

3. ICP waveforms

a. There are three components to an ICP wave: P1 (percussion wave) represents arterial pulsation, P2 (tidal wave) represents intracranial compliance, and P3 (dicrotic wave) represents aortic valve closure. Normally, P1 has the highest peak; if P2 >P1, there should be a concern for impaired intracranial compliance and increased ICP in the appropriate clinical context (Figure 10.2).

b. Lundberg A waves ("plateaus") are characterized by increased ICP lasting >5 minutes, at times up to hours. They are pathologic and strongly concerning for intracranial hypertension with the risk of herniation. Lundberg B waves are oscillations of ICP at a frequency of 0.5 to 2 waves/min. They have been noted in cerebral vasospasm and in the right clinical context can be associated with high ICP; at times they can progress to Lundberg A waves. Lundberg C waves are oscillations with a frequency of 4 to 8 waves/min. They have been noted in healthy individuals and are of unclear clinical significance.

C. Electroencephalogram (EEG): Continuous EEG is frequently used in the intensive care unit (ICU) to capture paroxysmal events, monitor patients with fluctuating or poor mental status (to evaluate the background and rhythm and assess for nonconvulsive status epilepticus), adjust therapy for ongoing seizures (including status epilepticus requiring burst suppression), patients requiring

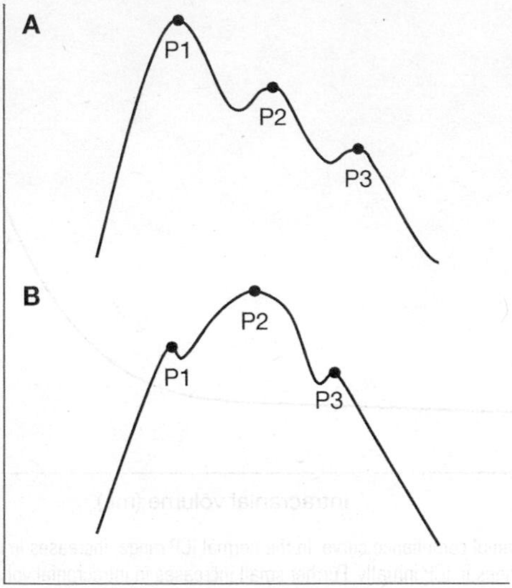

FIGURE 10.2 Intracranial pressure wave. **A:** Normal wave appearance. **B:** Decreased compliance. P1, percussion wave; P2, tidal wave; P3, dicrotic wave.

titration of automated external defibrillators (AEDs) under EEG surveillance, and sedation for refractory ICP. Quantitative EEG may also aid in detecting small changes in the EEG that can correlate with changes in ICP or impending ischemia. New modalities are emerging, such as the compressed spectral array, which transforms the EEG into a succinct graphic display of changes in frequency and amplitude, allowing a simplified yet efficient screening of continuous EEG data. Additional indications of continuous EEG include prognostication, particularly in cardiac arrest and anoxic brain injury patients, and ischemia detection, particularly in patients with aneurysmal SAH.

D. CSF Microdialysis: Microdialysis probes can be inserted into brain tissue and allow for serial sampling of physiologic markers such as glucose, lactate, pyruvate, amino acids as well as drug concentrations. These measurements depend on cerebral metabolism and may indicate impending cerebral ischemia and allow for more precise adjustments in medications such as antibiotics or insulin therapy. Still largely investigational studies are underway to explore their use.

E. Brain Tissue Oxygenation: Oxygen partial pressure measurements can be made using fiberoptic catheters placed within the brain tissue, usually as part of ICP-monitoring catheters. This monitor reports local brain tissue oxygen levels (goal >20) as well as temperature and in some cases pH. Adjustments in cerebral perfusion, systemic oxygenation, temperature management, and transfusion strategies can be made to optimize tissue oxygenation and showed promise in the phase II BOOST-II trial with BOOST-III now underway to evaluate clinical efficacy.

F. Jugular Bulb Oxygen Tension: Continuous monitoring of the jugular bulb oxygen saturation may provide information regarding hemispheric brain tissue oxygen extraction. Patients with jugular saturations below 50% (indicating a supply-demand mismatch) tend to have poor outcomes.

G. Pupillometry: Bedside handheld meters can quantify pupil size and speed of response to light. The Neurologic Pupil index™ (NPi) is a proprietary measure of pupil response but ranges from 0 to 4.9 and is abnormal when NPi <3. Constriction velocity (CV) can also be measured and is abnormal when CV <0.8 mm/s.

H. Optic Nerve Sheath Diameter: By placing an ultrasound probe over a patient's eye, the optic nerve sheath can be sonated and measured 3 mm behind the globe. As this is contiguous with the subarachnoid space, pressure fluctuations are transmitted down the sheath causing distension. A diameter of greater than 5 to 6 mm is associated with ICP >20.

III. NEUROIMAGING

A. Computed Tomography (CT): used routinely, in many ICUs as a portable scanner, to evaluate for gross pathology (such as intracranial hypertension [ICH], evolving strokes, mass lesions, edema, and hydrocephalus) or perform an interval screening (to assess the evolution of an ICH, large stroke, or midline shift). CT angiogram is used to assess for occlusion, stenoses, or aneurysm in the intracranial and neck vasculature. CT perfusion studies can differentiate stroke core from penumbra. Given the relatively large contrast load, it is prudent to assess renal function before ordering CT angiogram or perfusion. CT spine can help rule out fractures and misalignments.

Hypodense: Edema and ischemia

Hyperdense: blood and calcifications (the latter being brighter based on Hounsfield units)

B. Magnetic Resonance Imaging: allows for evaluation of the brain in greater detail compared to CT but takes longer time to complete (challenging in agitated patients as well as patients with high ICPs who cannot tolerate being in a flat position for the duration of the study) and requires careful screening for contraindications before the study. Indications include (1) evaluation of the extent of ischemia (stroke is apparent on diffusion-weighted sequences within minutes vs up to 6 hours on CT), (2) characterization of masses (extent of spread, extra vs intracranial location, pattern and degree of contrast enhancement, distinguishing tumor vs abscess, degree of surrounding edema), (3) underlying causes of an ICH, (4) degree of injury in traumatic and anoxic brain injury, (5) degree of ligamentous injury in spinal cord trauma as well as lesions in the spinal cord. MR angiogram can also further characterize vessels. In patients with renal failure, gadolinium use is contraindicated. However, vessel imaging can be obtained without giving IV contrast (time of flight sequence).

C. Transcranial Doppler (TCD): A bedside ultrasound-based study measuring the velocity of blood flow through the intracranial vasculature which is directly related to vessel diameter. It is most often used to monitor patients with SAH to assess for vasospasm (manifesting as increased velocities) but can also identify pathology within the circle of Willis (such as vascular stenoses, occlusions, turbulences, and retrograde flow) and has been correlated with ICP elevation.

D. Cerebral Angiography: Catheter-based angiography remains the gold standard to evaluate the intracranial and neck vessels in detail. It is performed to better characterize aneurysms and other vascular malformations (such as arteriovenous malformations [AVMs] and dural arteriovenous fistulas [AVFs]. Note: cavernomas are low-flow lesions that are not seen on angiography), to assess for suspected vasculitis and vasospasm. In many cases, vascular malformations or vasospasm can be treated during the procedure (eg, through coiling of the aneurysms or embolization of AVMs or intra-arterial administration of calcium channel blockers, respectively). **Mechanical thrombectomy** is now performed via catheter-based retrieval of clot in large intracranial vessels to abort strokes and has been shown beneficial up to 24 hours after last seen well when patients are selected appropriately.

E. Nuclear Medicine Blood Flow Imaging: useful for assessing cerebral perfusion in cases of suspected brain death, especially when factors that confound the clinical evaluation are present.

F. Positron Emission Tomography (PET) and Single Photon Emission Computed Tomography (SPECT): radioactive studies, used as adjunct tests to detect epileptic foci, assess cerebral vasculature and perfusion, and screen for dementia.

IV. BLOOD PRESSURE MANAGEMENT

A. Ischemic Stroke: In patients who suffer an acute ischemic stroke, in particular those with a large vessel occlusion, consider allowing blood pressure (BP) to autoregulate (stop antihypertensive agents on admission) at least for the first 24 to 48 hours. Assess carefully whether patients with a proximal vessel occlusion (PVO) or critical neck vessel stenosis have exam changes with varying BPs and treat with vasopressors as needed to maintain perfusion of the penumbra. After administration of IV tPA, SBP should be maintained at <180 and diastolic BP at <110 mm Hg. Following mechanical thrombectomy BP should be lowered to <140 mm Hg for complete recanalization and <160 mm Hg for partial recanalization, to avoid reperfusion injury and risk for hemorrhagic transformation.

B. Intracranial Hemorrhage

1. **Subdural and epidural hemorrhage, traumatic SAH:** SBP goal <140 mm Hg
2. **Aneurysmal SAH:** Maintain SBP <140 to 160 mm Hg until the aneurysm is secured (coiled or clipped) and then liberalize. If the patient develops vasospasm, vasopressors and volume resuscitation are used to maintain euvolemia and further increase the BP in an effort to maintain perfusion.
3. **Intraparenchymal hemorrhage:** Per American Heart Association guidelines, for SBP between 150 and 220 mm Hg and absence of contraindications to rapid BP treatment, targeting SBP <140 mm Hg is safe. The optimal blood pressure goal is not clear with recent INTERACT-2 suggesting that an SBP <140 mm Hg is probably safe and may be effective in improving functional outcome, while ATACH2 showed a higher risk for renal injury and no difference in outcomes with aggressive BP lowering. In some patients with chronically elevated BPs, SBPs should be controlled more cautiously to avoid end-organ damage due to decreased perfusion.

C. Hypertensive Encephalopathy and Posterior Reversible Encephalopathy Syndrome: Maintain SBP <140 mm Hg (with slower BP reduction in patients with chronically elevated BPs) and stop offending medications.

V. MANAGEMENT OF ELEVATED ICP

Treatment of increased ICPs should be initiated for sustained ICPs >20 mm Hg or in patients with relevant clinical pathology at risk for herniation. In general, the head of the bed should be elevated at 30° in patients at risk for high ICPs. Before central line placement, patients should be kept in that position until the last possible moment prior to puncture.

A. Osmotherapy: To date, mannitol is used more commonly than hypertonic saline (HTS); few studies have been performed to compare the two agents, with one recent article suggesting that HTS is more effective in lowering the ICP burden, leading to fewer days in the ICU. Avoid mannitol in patients with renal failure. HTS should be used with caution in patients with congestive heart failure as it can result in worsening volume overload: refer to **Section VII.C** for formula to calculate plasma osmolality.

1. **Hypertonic saline (HTS)** may also be used to reach the desired osmolality by directly affecting plasma sodium levels. When administering HTS solutions, frequent serum Na assessments are required to avoid a rapid change in plasma Na concentration (which can result in central pontine

myelinolysis). **NaCl at 3% concentration** can be given as either a bolus of 150 mL every 4 to 6 hours or as a continuous infusion of 0.5 to 1.0 mL/kg/h; **23.4% NaCl** is administered as a 30- to 60-mL IV bolus every 6 hours.

2. **Mannitol** (0.5-1.0 g/kg IV bolus every 4-6 hours) should be given to attain the minimum serum osmolality sufficient to produce the desired effects on the ICP, which often results in a stepwise increase in osmol gap (osmol gap = measured osm − calculated osm; normal <10). The goal of therapy can be continued until the osmol gap is equal to or greater than 15. Also, osmolality in excess of 320 mOsm/kg with mannitol does not produce incremental benefits and is often associated with an increased osmol gap and acute renal failure.

B. CSF Drainage: Draining even a small amount of CSF via the EVD catheter can significantly reduce ICP, especially with impaired intracranial compliance, although there is limited utility when the ventricles are collapsed.

C. Heavy Sedation and Paralysis: While sedation and paralysis are initially avoided in order to preserve the neurologic examination, they can be used in patients with increased ICP refractory to hyperosmolar therapy. Agitation, posturing, and coughing are subsequently diminished. Barbiturate coma should only be considered as a last resort because of the serious potential side effects and because the neurologic examination cannot be performed for several days or even longer. Continuous EEG should be considered to guide and monitor the depth of sedation.

D. Hypothermia: There are no clear data to suggest improvement of neurologic outcomes when cooling patients with high ICP, but some studies demonstrate a reduction of ICP. Although not a first-line therapy (given the need for increased sedation and hemodynamic changes, and potential effects on the clotting cascade), it can be used as an adjunctive treatment for increased ICP refractory to other medical management.

E. Hyperventilation: Hyperventilation decreases $PaCO_2$, which can induce constriction of cerebral arteries by alkalinizing the CSF. The resulting reduction in cerebral blood volume decreases ICP. However, with prolonged hyperventilation CBF returns to normal as the pH in the CSF is restored. Therefore, hyperventilation should only be used as a bridge to more definitive therapies.

F. Surgical Intervention:

1. If an underlying mass lesion (bleed, tumor, abscess, tension pneumocephalus) is contributing to the increase in ICP, urgent evacuation should be considered.
2. Decompressive hemicraniectomy, allowing for herniation of the swollen brain through the bone window to relieve pressure, can be considered with rapidly increasing ICP despite aggressive medical therapy. Yet, while this procedure may improve mortality, it has not been shown to improve functional outcome in edema related to TBI (RESCUEicp, DECRA) likely due to the already existing injury prompting the decompression. In patients with malignant middle cerebral artery (MCA) strokes, early decompressive hemicraniectomy within 48 hours can reduce mortality and may improve functional outcomes in younger patients (DESTINY, DECIMAL, HAMLET).
3. Suboccipital craniectomy is the removal of the skull overlying the cerebellum and is performed for cerebellar strokes or bleeds. Generally, patients with even large cerebellar strokes have a better prognosis from their stroke alone but a high risk of brainstem compression and hydrocephalus which would argue in favor of surgery.

G. Steroids: While corticosteroids are useful in the management of vasogenic edema associated with brain tumors or other conditions that disrupt the blood-brain barrier, their utility in treating other causes of increased ICP is quite limited. Studies of steroids in stroke, intracerebral hemorrhage, and head injury have not demonstrated benefit and may cause harm.

H. Medications That Influence ICP:

1. **Vasodilators** such as **hydralazine, sodium nitroprusside (SNP), nitroglycerin,** and, to a lesser degree, **nicardipine** can induce cerebral vasodilation. In patients with poor intracranial compliance, this can increase ICP.
2. **Barbiturates** such as **thiopental** and **pentobarbital**, although typically administered to lower ICP, are also potent antihypertensive agents, decreasing venous tone and cardiac contractility. This usually undesirable side effect may require the use of adrenergic agonists such as **phenylephrine** and **norepinephrine** to maintain adequate CPP.
3. **Hypo-osmolar and iso-osmolar solutions** such as lactated Ringer's solution and half normal saline in 5% dextrose (D_5 ½ NS) may exacerbate brain edema in the setting of osmotic diuretic therapy. **Glucose-containing solutions** may produce hyperglycemia and may lead to neurologic worsening after brain ischemia.

VI. MANAGEMENT OF STATUS EPILEPTICUS

Defined as tonic-clonic seizures lasting >5 minutes, or recurrent seizures without improvement in consciousness. Assess airway, breathing, and circulation. Antiseizure medication selection is based on ease of administration, patient comorbidities, and medication adverse effect profile. Continuous EEG monitoring should be considered for guiding the management of refractory and nonconvulsive status epilepticus.

1. Initial therapy (5-20 minutes)—First-line treatment typically benzodiazepines: Lorazepam 0.1 mg/kg IV (maximum 4 mg/dose); diazepam 0.15 to 0.2 mg/kg IV (maximum 10 mg/dose); midazolam 10 mg IM if >40 kg or 5 mg IM for 13 to 40 kg. If these drugs are not available: phenobarbital 15 mg/kg/dose IV single dose; rectal diazepam; nasal midazolam.
2. Second therapy phase (20-40 minutes)—fosphenytoin 20 mg PE/kg IV; valproic acid 40 mg/kg IV; levetiracetam 60 mg/kg IV (max dose 4500 mg); phenobarbital 15 mg/kg IV.
3. Third therapy phase/refractory status epilepticus (40-60 minutes)—If no response to first and second-line therapy, initiate anesthetics: propofol; midazolam; pentobarbital. Use continuous EEG to guide management.

VII. SODIUM AND WATER HOMEOSTASIS

A. Hyponatremia: In patients with elevated ICP, hyponatremia can significantly contribute to additional swelling and potentially increase the risk of herniation. It is therefore important to maintain an appropriate Na goal, determined by the patient's baseline Na level, degree of intracranial injury, and evolution in exam. Check urine Na and Osm (**before** initiating hyperosmolar therapy), volume status, fluid intake, and urine output to determine the underlying cause (volume depletion vs syndrome of inappropriate antidiuretic hormone [SIADH] vs salt wasting vs other etiologies).

1. **Intravascular volume depletion** remains a common cause of hyponatremia in the neurocritical care unit. Bladder catheterization and monitoring of central venous pressure (CVP) and plasma sodium are essential.
2. Cerebral injury may cause the release of **natriuretic factors**, leading to profound **salt wasting** that may require up to 200 mL/h of normal saline replacement or the use of 3% solution in continuous infusion in addition to fludrocortisone (0.1-0.3 mg by mouth once or twice a day). This is seen most often in vasospasm after SAH.
3. **SIADH** should be treated with fluid restriction when able but often hypovolemia must be avoided in neurologic patients due to risk of cerebral hypoperfusion (common in SAH, TBI, or postoperatively). Instead, treat with hypertonic saline (3%) or normal saline and loop diuretics.

B. Hypernatremia owing to Diabetes Insipidus (DI) may be seen after pituitary tumor resection, TBI, central herniation syndromes, and, occasionally, vasospasm following SAH. **Hypotonic fluids** and **vasopressin** therapy may be indicated, and hourly monitoring of urine output and specific gravity is required.

C. Osmotic Balance

$$\text{Plasma osmolality} = \left(2 \times \left[\text{Na}^+\right]\right) + [\text{BUN}]/2.8 + [\text{Glucose}]/18$$

where BUN is blood urea nitrogen and is normally 280 to 290 mOsm/kg.

VIII. TEMPERATURE REGULATION

A. Hyperthermia after brain injury is very common and has been shown to increase the release of excitatory neurotransmitters, further the breakdown of the blood-brain barrier, raise ICP, and worsen clinical outcomes. The source of fever should be properly investigated and appropriate therapy initiated promptly. Antipyretic measures, such as the administration of acetaminophen 650 mg every 4 to 6 hours, surface cooling (cooling blankets, ice packs), and/or intravascular cooling catheters, should be instituted. **Normothermia** (temperature 37 °C) should be maintained in all patients in the neuro ICU.

B. Shivering is a frequent problem with the above and should be addressed with magnesium infusion, meperidine 12.5 to 50 mg as needed to max 100 mg in 6 hours, buspirone 5 mg PO BID-TID, Propofol and/or Dexmedetomidine infusion, even paralysis if needed.

Induced hypothermia has been shown to be neuroprotective in global ischemic brain injury after cardiac arrest but not in focal brain injury as seen in TBI, ischemic stroke, and intracerebral hemorrhage. A large recent multicenter trial demonstrated that targeted hypothermia did not result in decreased mortality or improved functional outcomes compared with targeted normothermia (TTM2). Relative contraindications to cooling include intracranial hemorrhage, coagulopathies, active bleeding systemically, sepsis, and hemodynamic instability.

IX. GLUCOSE MANAGEMENT

Elevated blood glucose levels after acute brain and spinal cord injuries can increase tissue acidosis and edema in and around injured tissue and impair endogenous anti-inflammatory mechanisms of repair. **Hyperglycemia** has been shown to be a predictor of poor outcome in the ICU population and in many forms of acute brain injury. Hypoglycemia (<60 mg/dL) can also lead to focal neurologic deficits, seizures, as well as anoxic brain injury, and glucose levels should be acutely restored with a bolus of **50% dextrose solution (D_{50})** along with 100 mg IV **thiamine** to the severely malnourished patient to avoid the complication of Wernicke encephalopathy. Overall, the goal for care is to achieve normoglycemia (80-180 mg/dL) with the administration of insulin.

X. MECHANICAL VENTILATION IN THE NEURO ICU

A. Indications for Endotracheal Intubation: Impairment of airway reflexes occurs frequently in patients with neurologic compromise and predisposes the patient to aspiration as well as poor clearance of secretions.

1. **Neuromuscular respiratory failure** may be seen in amyotrophic lateral sclerosis, myasthenia gravis, AIDP, and critical care myopathy or polyneuropathy. Bedside pulmonary function testing (PFT) with a vital capacity of less than 20 cc/kg, negative inspiratory force of less negative than −30 cm H_2O (ie, −15 or closer to 0), or maximal expiratory force of less than 40 cm H_2O, suggests risk of imminent decline though vital capacity is the most reproducible. Appropriate patients may benefit from noninvasive ventilation such as BiPAP or high-flow nasal cannula, however, do not wait for arterial blood gas values to become abnormal before intubation.
2. **Transient apnea** in the setting of a self-limited generalized convulsion is not an indication for intubation or assisted ventilation.

B. Complications of Endotracheal Intubation include hypotension from anesthetic induction agents, reduced CBF, and increased ICP due to agitation or discomfort, or as a result of increased transthoracic pressure. To avoid worsening cerebral ischemia, particularly in the setting of acute stroke and a proximal vessel occlusion, the BP goals for the patient should be clarified and ideally maintained even during induction.

C. Considerations in Extubation: The ability to prevent aspiration and protect the airway is of utmost concern when extubating a patient who is neurologically ill. After confirming adequate cuff leak, oxygenation, and spontaneous ventilation to support independent respiratory function, the clinician should evaluate the capacity for adequate airway protection. Ideally, cough and gag reflexes should be present, and pharyngeal suctioning to keep the airway clear should not be needed more frequent than hourly and should not be increasing. In addition, careful evaluation of the swallowing and oral function should occur, especially in patients with facial weakness. Ask the patient to protrude the tongue, lick the lips, pucker the lips, and cough volitionally. Although the patient does not need to be neurologically intact for successful extubation, poor oral control may lead to rapid failure of extubation. Factors associated with successful extubation of neurologic patients in a prior study include intact gag, normal eye movements, ability to close eyes, and cough to command. In addition, because hypercapnia may be poorly tolerated in patients with significant brain edema or disturbed autoregulation, the patient should be able to maintain normocapnia without ventilatory assistance, and the period of peak anticipated brain swelling should have passed.

D. Permissive Hypercapnia is generally contraindicated in patients with intracranial hypertension or blood-brain barrier injuries because hypercapnia may result in unacceptable elevations of the ICP.

E. Spontaneous or Induced Hyperventilation causes acute cerebral vasoconstriction if the CO_2 reactivity is preserved, decreasing **cerebral blood volume (CBV)** and thereby ICP. If autoregulation is preserved, an increased CPP may restore the CBF. **The brain quickly equilibrates** to changes in P_{CO_2}. A new steady state is established within hours in most patients, and rebound may occur on return to normal respiration rate. **With excessive hypocapnia**, excessive vasoconstriction may produce regional or generalized cerebral ischemia. Lack of response to hyperventilation is a poor prognostic sign.

F. Neurogenic Pulmonary Edema: Within minutes to hours of CNS injury, there can be increased pulmonary interstitial and alveolar fluid (frequently seen in patients with SAH). This entity can be clinically difficult to distinguish from aspiration; however, fever and focal infiltrates are often absent. Although its precise pathophysiology is not completely understood, it is suggested that a massive sympathetic surge at the time of acute CNS injury may cause dramatically elevated pulmonary artery pressures and lead to capillary fracture with subsequent pulmonary edema, even though the pressures at the later time of measurement are no longer elevated. Supportive care and careful fluid management are required.

XI. BRAIN DEATH DETERMINATION

Driven by advances in critical care medicine such as mechanical ventilation as well as the evolution of organ donation, the concept of brain death was first established in the 1950-1960 and further defined over the following decades. Recommendations for minimum standards were reviewed most recently in *JAMA* in 2020, providing an algorithmic, unified, step-by-step approach to brain death determination. Before conducting the brain death assessment, reversible causes such as hypothermia, sedatives/paralytics/intoxication must be excluded. The key portions of brain death determination include the neurologic exam, confirming coma and absent brainstem reflexes, as well as the apnea test, demonstrating absence of spontaneous respirations despite an elevated P_{CO_2} after inducing apnea (Figure 10.3). In some cases, when the exam and/or apnea test are equivocal or cannot be performed properly, ancillary tests are used including digital subtraction angiography, nuclear medicine scan, and transcranial Doppler. Note that most institutions will have their own policy for confirming brain death.

Checklist for determination of brain death

Date and time____

Prerequisites (all must be checked)

- o Coma, irreversible and cause known
- o Neuroimaging explains coma
- o CNS depressant drug effect absent (toxicology screen/serum levels if indicated)
- o No evidence of residual paralytics (electrical stimulation if paralytics used)
- o Absence of severe acid-base, electrolyte, or endocrine abnormality
- o Normothermia or mild hypothermia (core temperature ≥ 36° C/96.8° F)
- o Systolic blood pressure > 100 mmHg
- o No spontaneous respirations

Examination (all must be checked)

- o Pupils nonreactive to bright light
- o Corneal reflex absent
- o Oculocephalic reflex absent (tested only if C-spine integrity ensured)
- o Oculovestibular reflex absent (30-50 mL ice water each ear, observe 1 min, 5 min between ears)
- o No facial movement to noxious stimuli at supraorbital nerve, temporo-mandibular joint
- o Gag reflex absent
- o Cough reflex absent to tracheal suctioning
- o Absence of motor response to noxious stimuli in all 4 limbs (spinally-mediated reflexes are permissible, posturing is not)

Apnea testing (all must be checked)

- o Patient is hemo-dynamically stable and euvolemic
- o Ventilator adjusted to provide normocarbia ($PaCO_2$ 35–45 mmHg)
- o Patient preoxygenated with 100% FiO_2 for > 10 min to PaO_2 > 200 mm Hg
- o Patient well-oxygenated with a PEEP of 5 cm H_2O
- o Provide oxygen via a suction catheter to the level of the carina at 10 L/min or attach T-piece with CPAP at 10 cm H_2O
- o Disconnect ventilator
- o Spontaneous respirations absent
- o ABG drawn at 5 minutes
- o ABG drawn at 10 minutes (reconnect ventilator)
- o $PaCO_2 \geq 60$ mmHg **or** ≥ 20 mmHg rise from baseline

Pre-test ABG: pH___ pCO_2____ pO_2____ **Post-test ABG:** pH___ pCO_2____ pO_2____@____min

OR:

- ¤ Apnea test aborted (cardiac ectopy, O_2 sat < 90%, SBP < 100 mmHg)

Ancillary testing (only 1 needs to be performed; to be ordered only if clinical examination cannot be fully performed due to patient factors, or if apnea testing inconclusive or aborted)

- ¤ Cerebral angiogram
- ¤ SPECT
- ¤ EEG
- ¤ TCD

Time of death (MM/DD/YY & 00:00) __________________ **due to**__________________ (etiology of coma)

Name of physician and signature

____

- ¤ attending neurologist/neurosurgeon
- ¤ neurocritical care fellow

FIGURE 10.3 Checklist for brain death determination criteria, excerpt from the MGH Brain Death Protocol, most recently revised 03/2011.

Selected Readings

Adams RD, Victor M. *Principles of Neurology*. McGraw-Hill; 1993.

Anderson CD, Bartscher JF, Scripko PD, et al. Neurologic examination and extubation outcome in the neurocritical care unit. *Neurocrit Care*. 2011;15(3):490-497.

Carney N, Totten AM, O'Reilly C, et al. Guidelines for the management of severe traumatic brain injury. *Neurosurgery*. 2017;80(1):6-15.

Cooper DJ, Rosenfeld JV, Murray L, et al. Decompressive craniectomy in diffuse traumatic brain injury. *N Engl J Med*. 2011;364(16):1493-1502. doi:10.1056/NEJMoa1102077

Dubourg J, Javouhey E, Geeraerts T, Messerer M, Kassai B. Ultrasonography of optic nerve sheath diameter for detection of raised intracranial pressure: a systematic review and meta-analysis. *Intensive Care Med*. 2011;37(7):1059-1068.

Fisher CM. The neurological examination of the comatose patient. *Acta Neurol Scand.* 1969;45(S36):5-56.

Glauser T, Shinnar S, Gloss D, et al. Evidence-based guideline: treatment of convulsive status epilepticus in children and adults: report of the Guideline Committee of the American Epilepsy Society. *Epilepsy Curr.* 2016;16(1):48-61.

Guarantors of Brain. *Aids to the Examination of the Peripheral Nervous System.* Bailliere Tindall; 1986.

Hutchinson PJ, Kolias AG, Timofeev IS, et al. Trial of decompressive craniectomy for traumatic intracranial hypertension. *N Engl J Med.* 2016;375(12):1119-1130.

Mangat HS, Chiu YL, Gerber LM, et al. Hypertonic saline reduces cumulative and daily intracranial pressure burdens after severe traumatic brain injury. *J Neurosurg.* 2015;122(1):202-210.

Nielsen N, Wetterslev J, Cronberg T, et al; TTM Trial Investigators. Targeted temperature management at 33°C versus 36°C after cardiac arrest. *N Engl J Med.* 2013;369(23):2197-2206.

Okonkwo DO, Shutter LA, Moore C, et al. Brain tissue oxygen monitoring and management in severe traumatic brain injury (BOOST-II): a phase II randomized trial. *Crit Care Med.* 2017;45(11):1907-1914.

Plum F, Posner JB. *Diagnosis of Stupor and Coma.* 3rd ed. FA Davis; 1982.

Ropper AH. *Neurological and Neurosurgical Intensive Care.* 4th ed. Raven; 2003.

Schwamm LH, Koroshetz WJ, Sorensen AG, et al. Time course of lesion development in patients with acute stroke: serial diffusion- and hemodynamic-weighted magnetic resonance imaging. *Stroke.* 1998;29(11):2268-2276.

Suarez JI, ed. *Critical Care Neurology and Neurosurgery.* Humana Press; 2004.

Wijdicks EF. *The Clinical Practice of Critical Care Neurology.* Lippincott-Raven; 1997.

Wijdicks EF. Determining brain death in adults. *Neurology.* 1995;45(5):1003-1011.

Wijdicks EF, Varelas PN, Gronseth GS, et al; American Academy of Neurology. Evidence-based guideline update: determining brain death in adults: report of the Quality Standards Subcommittee of the American Academy of Neurology. *Neurology.* 2010;74(23):1911-1918.

11 Nutrition in Critical Illness

Ander Dorken-Gallastegi and April E. Mendoza

I. INTRODUCTION

The delivery of calories and protein to a patient who is critically ill should be considered a high priority and integral to care. The goals of nutrition therapy include prevention of infectious morbidity, preservation of muscle mass, and prevention of metabolic complications. Choosing the appropriate route, timing, and dose of nutrition is crucial to achieving these goals.

II. PATHOPHYSIOLOGY OF NUTRITION IN CRITICAL ILLNESS

Postsurgical patients and patients who are critically ill are at risk for calorie-protein malnutrition. The response to illness includes increased energy expenditure, increased secretion of certain hormones (glucagon, glucocorticoids, catecholamines, vasopressin), and increase in inflammatory mediators (cytokines, acute-phase proteins).

A. Fluid shifts occur due to water retention and increased vascular permeability.

B. Increased glycogenolysis, gluconeogenesis, and insulin resistance result in hyperglycemia.

C. Skeletal muscle protein is catabolized for gluconeogenesis, resulting in protein depletion.

D. Resting energy expenditure remains elevated, and catabolism can continue for up to 3 weeks, even after resolution of the initial insult and despite adequate nutrition support.

III. ASSESSMENT OF NUTRITIONAL STATUS

The patients' medical history, nutritional intake history, physical exam, and laboratory data must be taken into account. The assessment of baseline nutritional status and malnutrition is difficult patients who are critically ill. The American Society for Parenteral and Enteral Nutrition (ASPEN) and the Society of Critical Care Medicine (SCCM) recommend the use of a nutritional risk assessment that incorporates the baseline nutritional status and disease severity such as the nutrition risk in critically Ill (NUTRIC) score or NRS-2002 score to identify patients who are at high risk of poor nutritional outcome and would benefit most from early and aggressive nutritional therapy (Tables 11.1 and 11.2). Neither body mass index nor serum protein levels (eg, prealbumin, albumin, CRP) are considered reliable markers of baseline nutritional status in patients who are critically ill.

A. Clinical History: Preexisting conditions such as unintentional weight loss, chronic disease, risk of aspiration, and alcohol abuse increase a patient's risk for protein-calorie malnutrition. The severity of the current illness, including the presence of fevers, burns, sepsis, or trauma, is associated with varying degrees of hypermetabolism and increased nutritional requirements.

B. Body Weight Measurements

1. Body mass index (BMI) = weight (kg)/(height [m])^2
2. Ideal body weight (IBW)
   - **a.** Men (kg) = 50 + 2.3 (height [inches] − 60)
   - **b.** Women (kg) = 45.5 + 2.3 (height [inches] − 60)

TABLE 11.1 Modified[a] NUTRIC Score

Variable	Points
Age (yr)	
<50	0
50-75	1
>75	2
APACHE-II score	
<15	0
15-19	1
20-27	2
≥28	3
SOFA score	
<6	0
6-9	1
≥10	2
Number of comorbidities	
0-1	0
≥2	1
Days in hospital to ICU admit	
0	0
≥1	1

A NUTRIC score of ≥5 represents high nutritional risk.

[a]The original NUTRIC score included IL-6 as a predictor variable. IL-6 was omitted from the "modified" NUTRIC score because it was noted that it made minimal contribution to the predictive power and it is not always readily available in clinical practice.

From Heyland DK, Dhaliwal R, Jiang X, Day AG. Identifying critically ill patients who benefit the most from nutrition therapy: the development and initial validation of a novel risk assessment tool. *Crit Care.* 2011;15:(6):1-11. doi:10.1186/CC10546; Rahman A, Hasan RM, Agarwala R, Martin C, Day AG, Heyland DK. Identifying critically-ill patients who will benefit most from nutritional therapy: further validation of the "modified NUTRIC" nutritional risk assessment tool. *Clin Nutr.* 2016;35(1):158-162. doi:10.1016/J.CLNU.2015.01.015

TABLE 11.2 NRS-2002 Score

Variable	Points
Nutritional Impairment	
None	0
Weight loss >5% in 3 mo *or* Food intake <50%-75% of normal requirement in the preceding week	1
Weight loss >5% in 2 mo *or* BMI 18.5-20.5 plus impaired general condition *or* Food intake 25%-60% of normal requirement in preceding week	2
Weight loss >5% in 1 mo (>15% in 3 mo) *or* BMI <18.5 plus impaired general condition *or* Food intake 0%-25% of normal requirement in preceding week	3
Severity of Disease	
Normal nutritional requirements	0
Hip fracture Chronic patients, in particular with acute complications: cirrhosis, COPD Chronic hemodialysis, diabetes, oncology	1

TABLE 11.2 NRS-2002 Score (*continued*)

Variable	Points
Major abdominal surgery, stroke	2
Head injury	
Bone marrow transplantation	3
Intensive care patients	
Age	
<70	0
≥70	1

COPD, chronic obstructive pulmonary disease.
An NRS score of ≥3 represents high nutritional risk.
Reprinted from Kondrup J, Ramussen HH, Hamberg O, et al. Nutritional risk screening (NRS 2002): a new method based on an analysis of controlled clinical trials. *Clin Nutr.* 2003;22(3):321-336. doi:10.1016/S0261-5614(02)00214-5, with permission from Elsevier.

3. The use of adjusted body weight is no longer recommended. The ASPEN & SCCM guidelines recommend the use of actual body weight in patients with a BMI up to 50. In patients with BMI >50, IBW should be used when a weight-based equation is used to determine daily caloric requirements (also see **Section XIII**).

C. Nutritional Laboratory Indices

1. Baseline electrolytes, glucose, and liver function tests should be obtained before initiation of nutrition therapy.
2. Albumin is a long-term marker of nutritional status with a half-life of approximately 21 days.
3. Prealbumin and transferrin are serum proteins with short half-lives (2-3 days and 8 days, respectively).
4. It is increasingly recognized that low albumin and prealbumin are more reflective of acute inflammation in the patient who is critically ill. For this reason, low or high levels should be interpreted with caution.
5. Trends over time are much more informative than single data points.

D. Resting Energy Expenditure: Energy requirements are difficult to estimate in the critically ill population. Predictive equations are commonly used but may over- or underestimate caloric requirements. Difficulties inherent to the surgical critically ill population include inaccurate weight assessments secondary to fluid resuscitation-related weight gain, inability to obtain an accurate nutrition history, and fluctuating metabolic needs throughout the course of illness.

1. Indirect calorimetry (IC), also referred to as metabolic cart, measures the ratio of carbon dioxide eliminated (vCO_2) to the oxygen consumed (vO_2) by the body. This is measured over a 10- to 30-minute period to calculate a respiratory quotient (RQ). Patients must be intubated, breathing low FIO_2 (<50%), and without chest tube leaks for this to be accurate. They also should be hemodynamically stable and on a stable nutrient regimen. Extracorporeal membrane oxygenation (ECMO) and extracorporeal carbon dioxide removal (ECCCO2R) interfere with IC measurements.
   a. IC is recognized as more accurate than predictive equations and is recommended by the SCCM, ASPEN, and European Society for Parenteral and Enteral Nutrition (ESPEN) to determine caloric need.
   b. A randomized controlled study (The Tight Calorie Control Study [TICACOS]) demonstrated superior outcomes when caloric prescription was guided by IC measurements.
   c. In the absence of IC, oxygen consumption (vO_2) measurements from pulmonary artery catheter or carbon dioxide production (vCO_2) measured from the ventilator can be used to predict resting energy expenditure and are proposed to be more accurate than predictive equations.

TABLE 11.3 Two Examples of Predictive Equations for the Estimation of Resting Energy Expenditure

Harris-Benedict equation	
Men	66.5 + (13.76 × weight in kg) + (5.003 × height in cm) − (6.755 × age in years)
Women	655 + (9.563 × weight in kg) + (1.850 × height in cm) − (4.676 × age in years)
Penn State equation	
(Harris-Benedict × 0.85) + (V_E × 33) + (T_{max} × 175) − 6433	

V_E: Minute ventilation (L/min).
T_{max}: Maximum body temperature in the previous 24 h (Celsius).

2. Several predictive equations have been published to predict resting energy expenditure (REE) such as the Harris-Benedict equation and the Penn State equation (Table 11.3).
3. Either predictive equations or weight-based equations such as 25 to 30 kcal/kg/d are considered sufficient per the 2019 ASPEN guidelines to determine energy needs in the intensive care unit (ICU) for patients with normal BMI. Weight-based equations should be modified in patients with obesity (also see **Section XIII**).

E. Protein Requirements: Protein is the most significant macronutrient in critical illness and may improve outcomes and reduce mortality. As a result of the catabolic state associated with critical illness, protein requirements in patients in ICU are unproportionally high compared to energy requirements. Protein supplementation is often needed in addition to standard formulas to meet daily goals.

1. The ASPEN guidelines recommend daily protein requirement calculation using a weight-based formula: 1.2 to 2 g/kg/d.

IV. COMPONENTS OF NUTRITION

Caloric requirements should be fulfilled with protein, carbohydrates, and fat.

A. Protein provides 4 kcal/g. Protein intake is critical for muscle anabolism and maintenance of a positive nitrogen balance. It should consist of both essential and nonessential amino acids.

B. Carbohydrates should fulfill between 40% and 60% of total caloric needs. They provide 3.4 kcal/g. Carbohydrate administration rate should be kept under 5 mg/kg/min.

C. Fat should provide 20% to 30% of total calories. Fat provides 9 kcal/g. Polyunsaturated fats are essential fatty acids and must be obtained from a dietary source. Propofol can be a considerable source of nonnutritional lipid intake in patients who are critically ill and should be accounted for in calculations.

V. INDICATIONS AND TIMING OF NUTRITIONAL SUPPORT

A. In patients who are critically ill at high nutritional risk (nutrition risk screening [NRS] 2002 ≥3 or NUTRIC ≥5), nutritional support therapy should be initiated in the form of enteral feeding, within 24 to 48 hours of ICU admission if there are no contraindications. Recent meta-analyses suggest that early initiation of enteral nutrition (EN) in patients who are critically ill is associated with lower mortality and infectious complications compared to later delivery of EN.

1. Early EN has been shown to be beneficial in ICU populations in whom it was previously thought to be harmful such as severe acute pancreatitis, open abdomen, and post-gastrointestinal (GI) surgery.
2. Current evidence suggests that EN is safe and beneficial in these settings as luminal nutrients have been demonstrated to enhance splanchnic perfusion.

3. Enteral feeding in patients who are hemodynamically unstable, particularly in the setting of escalating or high vasopressor requirements, remains controversial. Main concerns for EN in patients with uncontrolled shock are splanchnic steal phenomenon (increase in intestinal blood flow in the setting of impaired systemic circulation) and the rare but catastrophic complication of mesenteric ischemia. Major nutritional societies (ASPEN, SCCM, and ESPEN) recommend that EN should be withheld until the patient is fully resuscitated and/or hemodynamically stable. EN may be safe in patients who are stabilized on low-medium dose of vasopressors (norepinephrine <0.3 μg/kg/min). In case of any sign of intolerance in patients receiving concomitant EN and vasopressor support, EN should be withheld, and symptoms should be cautiously evaluated for potential signs of mesenteric ischemia.

B. Specialized nutrition therapy may not be required for the first week of hospitalization in patients without high nutritional risk (NRS 2002 <3 or NUTRIC <5) at baseline, considering the risk associated with placement of enteral delivery devices and the lack of evidence suggesting that aggressive nutritional supplementation is associated with improved outcomes in this population. In such cases, voluntary intake should be encouraged, nutritional risk should be reassessed daily, and nutrition therapy should be initiated if indications arise.

VI. ENTERAL NUTRITION

A. EN is preferred over parenteral nutrition (PN) in patients with a functional GI tract. EN reduces infectious complications, improves wound healing, decreases GI mucosal permeability (and bacterial translocation), supports intestinal villous integrity, enhances the intestinal mucosa–associated immune system, preserves microbiome balance, and is more cost effective than PN.

B. Even in patients unable to tolerate EN at sufficient rates to fulfill their caloric needs, "trophic" tube feeds (10-20 mL/h) can provide nonnutritional benefits such as maintaining mucosal integrity, immune function, and preventing ileus.

C. The European Society for Intensive Care Medicine (ESICM) and ESPEN recommend withholding EN in the following conditions:

- Uncontrolled shock with escalating pressor requirements
- Uncontrolled, severe hypoxemia, hypercapnia, or acidosis
- Active upper GI bleeding
- Overt bowel ischemia
- Abdominal compartment syndrome
- Gastric residual volumes (GRV) greater than 500 mL for longer than 6 hours. Although this is controversial, ASPEN does not recommend the routine assessment of GRV.

D. For patients who have contraindications for or who cannot tolerate EN, PN may be required. For previously well-nourished patients at low nutritional risk who cannot meet nutritional needs with EN, late initiation of PN (after day 8) has been shown to be associated with fewer infections, enhanced recovery, and decreased cost compared to early initiation (within 48 hours).

VII. DELIVERY ROUTE OF ENTERAL NUTRITION

A. In the majority of patients who are critically ill, EN can be initiated into the stomach for practical reasons and to avoid delays in the initiation of EN.

B. Postpyloric feeding (formula delivered directly into the duodenum or jejunum) should be considered in patients at high risk for aspiration and patients with poor tolerance for gastric EN. Major risk factors for aspiration in patients who are critically ill are discussed later (under **Section XV**). In most patients, the delivery of EN should not be delayed solely to obtain postpyloric access.

1. Placement of postpyloric tubes may be done blindly, endoscopically, or with fluoroscopic guidance.

2. Blind **placement of stiletted postpyloric tubes** must be done cautiously and by experienced clinicians. When inserted in sedated, patients who are on mechanical ventilation, these soft and sharp-tipped tubes may enter the airway instead of the GI tract.
3. Complications of feeding tube placement include pneumothorax, bowel perforations, and lung infection/abscess secondary to infusion of tube feeds into the airway.

C. Confirmatory radiographs must *always* be performed prior to initiation of EN through a newly inserted feeding tube, as other methods of confirmation, such as aspiration of gastric contents and auscultation are insufficiently accurate.

D. Surgical placement of a gastric or jejunal feeding tube is indicated for long-term nutritional support (>1 month) and may be achieved endoscopically, fluoroscopically, or surgically.

E. A recent ESPEN meta-analysis found that continuous infusion of EN is associated with a significantly lower rate of diarrhea compared to bolus feeds, whereas there was no significant difference for other clinical outcomes.

VIII. DOSE OF ENTERAL NUTRITION

A. Full caloric intake should be aimed in patients at high nutritional risk (NRS 2002 ≥3 or NUTRIC ≥5). These patients represent the population that is most likely to benefit from intensive nutritional support. To maximize the benefits of early EN, caloric intake should be advanced as tolerated with the aim of achieving >80% of the calculated caloric goal within 48 to 72 hours of admission, while remaining vigilant for signs of refeeding syndrome.

B. In patients with acute respiratory distress syndrome (ARDS) or those expected to receive mechanical ventilation for longer than 72 hours, trophic feeding (10-20 kcal/h, or up to 500 kcal/d) may be a viable alternative that is associated with comparable clinical outcomes (eg, survival, ventilator-free days, ICU-free days), although with a lower rate of gastrointestinal intolerance. The benefits of trophic feeding in other critically ill populations are less studied.

C. Full dose of daily protein requirements should be aimed with attention to clinical conditions increasing the need for daily protein (eg, polytrauma, burns).

IX. ENTERAL FORMULAS

Common enteral formulas used at the Massachusetts General Hospital are shown in Table 11.4. They vary by the proportion of carbohydrates, protein, and fat, as well as caloric concentration, osmolality, elemental components, and various additives. Several formulas are particularly designed for certain patient populations (ie, pulmonary or renal disease). Routine use of disease-specific formulas is not recommended. A standard isotonic polymeric formula is the most convenient choice and is usually well tolerated by most patients in the ICU.

X. PARENTERAL NUTRITION

PN is indicated in patients who require aggressive nutritional support but cannot tolerate EN.

A. Initiation and Discontinuation of PN:

1. In patients without high nutritional risk (NRS 2002 <3 or NUTRIC score <5) who cannot receive voluntary intake and in whom EN is unfeasible, initiating PN within 48 hours of ICU has not been found to be beneficial and may be associated with increased morbidity.
2. In patients at high nutritional risk of (NRS 2002 ≥3 or NUTRIC score ≥5) or significant malnutrition at baseline benefits of early initiation of PN are likely to outweigh its risks. In these patients, PN should be initiated without delay following ICU admission if voluntary intake or EN is not feasible.

TABLE 11.4 Enteral Formulas Used at the Massachusetts General Hospital

	Enteral formulas — Massachusetts General Hospital enteral formulas							
	Osmolite	**Osmolite HN**	**Jevity Plus**	**Ensure Plus HN**	**Twocal HN**	**Glucerna**	**Promote with fiber**	
Calories/mL	1.06	1.06	1.2	1.5	2.0	1.0	1.0	
Protein (g/L) (% cal)	37.1 (14.0%)	44.3 (16.7%)	55.5 (18.5%)	62.6 (16.7%)	83.7 (16.7%)	41.8 (16.7%)	62.5 (25%)	
Fat (g/L) (% cal)	34.7 (29%)	34.7 (29%)	39.3 (29.0%)	50 (30%)	89.1 (40.1%)	54.4 (49%)	28.2 (25%)	
Carbohydrate (g/L) (% cal)	151.1 (57%)	143.9 (54.3%)	172.7 (52.5%)	199.9 (53.3%)	216.1 (43.2%)	95.6 (34.3%)	138.3 (50%)	
Osmolality (mOsm)	300	300	450	650	690	355	380	
Comments	Isotonic	Isotonic	Moderate protein, 12 g/L fiber	High calorie, high protein	Hypermetabolic fluid-restricted patients	Low carbohydrates, 14.4 g/L fiber	High protein, low fat, 14.4 g/L fiber	
	Pulmocare	**Suplena**	**Nepro**	**Peptamen**	**Alitraq**	**Tolerex**	**Vital HN**	**Vivonex Plus**
Calories/mL	1.5	2.0	2.0	1.0	1.0	1.0	1.0	1.0
Protein (g/L) (% cal)	62.6 (16.7%)	30.0 (6%)	69.9 (14%)	40.0 (16%)	52.5 (21%)	21 (8.0%)	41.7 (16.7%)	45 (18%)
Fat (g/L) (% cal)	93.3 (55.1%)	95.6 (43%)	95.6 (43%)	39 (33%)	15.5 (13%)	1.5 (1.0%)	10.8 (9.5%)	6.7 (6%)
Carbohydrate (g/L) (% cal)	105.7 (28.2%)	255.2 (51%)	222.3 (43%)	127 (51%)	165 (66%)	230 (91%)	185.0 (73.8%)	190 (76%)
Osmolality (mOsm)	475	600	665	380	575	550	500	650
Comments	High protein, high fat, low carbohydrate (to minimize CO_2 production)	Renal failure—predialysis (low protein, low electrolyte), high calorie	Renal failure—on dialysis (moderate protein, low electrolyte)	Peptide-based, gluten free, glutamine (3 g/L)	Elemental, glutamine (14.2 g/L)	Elemental, low protein	Elemental, higher protein	Elemental, glutamine (10 g/L)

3. Regardless of baseline nutritional risk, if >60% of caloric or protein requirements cannot be delivered via EN by 7 to 10 days, supplemental PN should be considered to reach the calorie and protein goals.
4. Initiation of EN should be attempted as feasible in patients receiving PN. PN can be discontinued when more than 60% of caloric goal is achieved via the enteral route.

B. Peripheral parenteral nutrition (PPN) defines the delivery of nutrients through a peripheral vein, rather than central venous access. The primary concern in PPN is the risk of thrombophlebitis due to the high osmolarity of nutritional solutions. Dextrose and amino acids are significant contributors to osmolarity, whereas larger molecules such as lipids have a lower osmotic load. The ASPEN guidelines suggest that solutions with an osmolarity of less than 900 mOsm/L can be safely administered from a peripheral vein. The use of PPN is limited by the lack of evidence supporting superiority to PN delivered via central route, and the high infusion volume required to keep osmolarity low. PN longer than 7 days is usually delivered via the central route and not as PPN because of the high risk of thrombophlebitis and the difficulty to reach daily goals with lower osmotic solutions.

C. Components of total parenteral nutrition (TPN) include the following:

1. D-glucose (dextrose) is the major source of nonprotein calories (3.4 kcal/g). Maximum daily administration is 5 to 7 g/kg/d. Exceeding this maximum rate of glucose oxidation may result in lipid synthesis with CO_2 accumulation and hepatic steatosis.
2. Lipid emulsion is another source of nonprotein calories (9 kcal/g) and also provides essential fatty acids (Ω6 and Ω3 polyunsaturated fats). Lipid emulsions provide 1.1 kcal/mL (for 10% IV emulsion), 2.0 kcal/mL (for 20% IV emulsion), and 3.0 kcal/mL (for 30% IV emulsion). Current guidelines recommend that daily lipid administration (including nonnutritional lipid sources such as propofol) should be less than 1.5 g/kg/d and total weekly lipid emulsions should not exceed 100 g/wk. Avoid infusion rates greater than 110 mg/kg/h because of neutrophil and monocyte impairment and worsening gas exchange.
3. Amino acids (essential and nonessential) are needed to build muscle and maintain a positive nitrogen balance, but also are a source of calories (4 kcal/g). As in EN, protein requirements should be calculated on the basis of stress level and monitored with weekly urine urea nitrogen (UUN) and nitrogen balance.

D. Calculation of TPN Formulation (Table 11.5)

1. Calculate total calorie requirements.
2. Estimate protein requirements.
3. Calculate maximum carbohydrate and lipid amounts and provide these "nonprotein calories" in a ratio of 70:30 (ideal).
4. Fluid/volume requirements average 30 mL/kg/d, but daily weight and strict measurement of fluid losses (urine, stool, insensible losses) help monitor fluid status.
5. Electrolytes, minerals, vitamins, and trace elements should be added according to usual or recommended doses (Table 11.6). Unlike enteral formulas, most PN formulations do not include micronutrients for stability reasons, and these should be supplemented daily. Adjustments may be needed in critical illness, or with certain disease states (ie, renal failure or high-output fistula), and serum levels should be monitored routinely.
6. Insulin can be added directly to the TPN solution (up to half of the daily sliding scale insulin requirement).

TABLE 11.5 Calculation of TPN Contents

Calculation of total TPN				
Component	**Calorie conversion**	**RQ**	**Maximum daily administration**	**% Total calories**
Amino acids	4 kcal/g	0.8	0.8-1.0 g/kg (normal) 1.25-1.5 g/kg (postsurgery, mild trauma) 1.5-2.0 g/kg (severe trauma, sepsis, organ failure) >2.0 g/kg (>20% TBSA burn, severe head injury)	15%-25%
Dextrose	3.4 kcal/g	1.0	5-7 g/kg (350-500 g or 1190-1700 kcal in 70 kg)	40%-60%
Lipids	9 kcal/g	0.7	2.5 g/kg[a] (175 g or 1575 kcal in 70 kg)	20%-30%[b]
Total calories			25 kcal/kg plus stress factor (1750 + kcal in 70 kg)	
Fluid/volume			25 kcal/kg plus stress factor	

RQ, respiratory quotient; TBSA, total body surface area; TPN, total parenteral nutrition.
[a]Patients who are critically ill may not be able to oxidize more than 1-1.5 g/kg/d.
[b]70:30 ratio of nonprotein calories (carbohydrate:lipid).

TABLE 11.6 Recommended Daily Doses of Electrolytes, Vitamins, and Trace Elements

Additive	**Recommended or usual daily dose**
Electrolytes	
Sodium	100-150 mEq/d
Potassium	60-120 mEq/d
Calcium gluconate	10-20 mEq/d
Phosphate	15-30 mm/d
Magnesium	8-24 mEq/d
Chloride or acetate[a]	Anion for sodium and potassium
Vitamins	
Vitamin C (ascorbic acid)	75-70 mg/d
Vitamin A	3300 IU/d
Vitamin D	400 IU/d
Thiamine (B_1)	1.1-1.2 mg/d
Pyridoxine (B_6)	1.3-1.7 mg/d
Riboflavin (B_2)	1.1-1.3 mg/d
Niacin	14-16 mg/d
Pantothenic acid	5 mg/d
Vitamin E	15 mg/d
Biotin	30 g/d
Folic acid	400 g/d
Vitamin B_{12}	2.4 g/d
Vitamin K	90-120 g/d

(*continued*)

TABLE 11.6 Recommended Daily Doses of Electrolytes, Vitamins, and Trace Elements (*continued*)

Additive	Recommended or usual daily dose
Trace elements	
Zinc	8-11 mg/d
Copper	900 g/d
Manganese	1.8-2.3 mg/d
Chromium	20-35 g/d
Selenium	55 g/d

[a]Chloride can produce metabolic acidosis; use acetate for patients with metabolic acidosis (converted to bicarbonate in the liver).

XI. COMPLICATIONS OF PARENTERAL NUTRITION

A. Catheter-Placement Complications (Pneumothorax, Hemothorax, or Arrhythmia)

B. Catheter Infection

C. Other Infections (Immune Suppression from TPN)

D. Metabolic Derangements (Refeeding Syndrome, Hyperglycemia, Hypoglycemia, Electrolyte Imbalances, Fluid Overload)

XII. SUPPLEMENTAL NUTRITION THERAPY

Trace elements and antioxidants are essential components of nutrition and should be considered in nutrition support therapy. Immunonutrition is the modulation of the immune system through the supplementation of select nutrients. Several nutrients have been studied; however, data have been conflicting regarding the use of immune-enhancing formulas in patients who are critically ill. There is some evidence that immunomodulating formulas may be beneficial in some subpopulations of patients in ICU (also see **Section XIII**).

A. Glutamine: The most abundant nonessential amino acid. It is synthesized predominantly in skeletal muscle and is involved in numerous essential functions such as gluconeogenesis, nitrogen transport, neutrophil function, acid-base balance and is the preferred fuel source for rapidly dividing cells in the intestinal tract and the immune system. In a randomized trial (reducing deaths due to oxidative stress [REDOX] study), early provision of glutamine was associated with an increase in mortality in patients with multiorgan failure. For this reason, glutamine supplementation in the general ICU population is not recommended.

B. Arginine: A conditionally essential amino acid in periods of stress and has important roles in nitrogen metabolism and the formation of nitric oxide. Arginine-containing formulas may have a role in perioperative surgical intensive care unit (SICU) populations or patients with traumatic brain injury, but overwhelming evidence is still lacking.

C. Fatty Acids: There is evidence for the benefit of combined immunomodulating formulas containing arginine and fish oil in patients who are postoperatively critically ill in the SICU, and ASPEN recommends their use (as a combination formula) in this population.

D. Micronutrients: Administration of trace elements (selenium, copper, manganese, zinc, iron, and vitamins E and C) has been proposed to reduce oxidative cellular damage. A 2016 ASPEN & SCCM meta-analysis and a randomized controlled trial suggest that antioxidant and trace element supplementation in safe doses (5-10 times reference daily intake) and for a limited amount of time is associated with improved survival in patients who are critically ill requiring nutritional therapy. Most standard enteral formulas usually include some amount of micronutrients. Whereas standard PN solutions usually do not include micronutrients for stability, and these should be separately supplemented if the patient is receiving PN.

XIII. NUTRITIONAL MODIFICATIONS IN DISEASE

Routine use of disease-specific formulas has not been shown to improve outcomes. However, there are nutrition-specific considerations in certain disease states.

A. Diabetes: Low simple sugar, high fiber, and high fat are recommended to minimize hyperglycemia.

B. Renal Failure: High concentration, low volume (to prevent volume overload), and low electrolytes (phosphorus, potassium) are recommended.

C. Acute Kidney Injury (AKI): Deliberate underprovision of protein to a patient with AKI in order to avoid renal replacement therapy (RRT) is inappropriate. Contrarily, both AKI and RRT are associated with increased protein loss and catabolism; patients with AKI have increased protein requirements. Up to 20% of serum amino acids are lost across the dialysate membrane and thus must be compensated for. For this reason, patients on continuous RRT should be given standard enteral formulas and not renal failure-specific formulas. Daily protein delivery may be increased up to 2.5 g/kg in patients requiring frequent RRT.

D. Liver Failure: The use of standard enteral formulas is recommended in liver failure. Low-protein, high-branched chain amino acids have been developed to prevent encephalopathy, though their efficacy in patients receiving first-line therapies (luminal antibiotics and lactulose) is questionable. Protein restriction for fear of precipitating hepatic encephalopathy may paradoxically result in less ammonia removal and should be avoided. Dry weight should be used in patients with significant portal hypertension and ascites.

E. Respiratory Failure. Care should be given to avoid exceeding the daily calorie requirements. Overfeeding can lead to increased CO_2 production and difficulty with ventilator weaning. High-fat and low-carbohydrate formulas have been developed to reduce CO_2 production and decrease the RQ, though their routine use is not recommended. Concentrated formulas may be considered to limit total infusion volume in patients at risk for pulmonary edema. Patients in ICU receiving EN or PN should be monitored for electrolyte abnormalities (particularly hypophosphatemia), which are associated with impaired respiratory muscle function and consequentially delayed weaning from mechanical ventilation.

F. Pancreatitis. Early EN (within <24-48 hours of admission) is the recommended form of nutrition therapy in moderate to severe acute pancreatitis. Currently, there is no strong evidence supporting the routine use of a specialized enteral formula in acute pancreatitis. Though most patients will tolerate gastric feeding, patients with moderate to severe pancreatitis who have signs of EN intolerance may benefit from postpyloric feeding (or even feeding at a more distal point in the GI tract) and continuous EN infusion (rather than bolus feeds). In the setting of exocrine insufficiency, some patients may better tolerate iso-osmolar, nearly fat-free elemental tube feeds, or formulas containing hydrolyzed peptides. Pancreatic enzyme replacement (eg, Creon, Pancrease, Relizorb) may be required to assist in digestion.

G. Trauma: Trauma is associated with significantly increased energy and protein requirements. If feasible, nutritional therapy should be initiated in the form of EN as soon as the initial resuscitation is completed, and hemodynamic stability is achieved (preferably within 24-48 hours). After the early resuscitative phase, slightly higher energy (20-35 kcal/kg/d) and protein (higher end of 1.2-2 g/kg/d) delivery should be aimed if weight-based formulas are used to estimate daily requirements.

H. Open Abdomen: Akin to the general ICU population, patients managed with an open abdomen should be initiated on EN within 24 to 48 hours if there is no contraindication (ie, intestinal discontinuity, intestinal injury, etc). Evidence suggests that early EN with an open abdomen is associated with higher rates of facial closure and decreased infectious complications. Protein loss associated with exudative fluid loss should be accounted for in the open abdomen patient.

I. Burns: If adequate voluntary intake cannot be achieved, early EN is the nutritional therapy of choice. "Very early" (within 4-6 hours) initiation of EN may have additional benefits in patients with burn. There is markedly elevated protein loss; daily 1.5 to 2 g/kg of protein delivery is recommended. Predictive equations for daily energy requirement have been shown to be unreliable in patients with burn; IC should be used as the most reliable method to calculate REE, if available. Trace elements should be provided in higher-than-standard doses. ESPEN recommends the routine supplementation of glutamine in patients with more than 20% of body surface area.

J. Obesity. Obesity and malnutrition can and often coexist (eg, obesity-related sarcopenia). Early EN (24-48 hours) should be initiated as in the general ICU population. A high protein and hypocaloric (<70% of daily energy requirements) or isocaloric feeding strategy is recommended in patients with obesity admitted to the ICU. Predictive equations are inaccurate in patients with obesity. When available, IC and urinary nitrogen loss should be prioritized for the calculation of REE and protein requirement, respectively. If weight-based equations will be used, actual body weight should be used for patients with BMI between 30 and 50 with the weight-based equation of 11 to 14 kcal/kg. In the super obese (BMI >50), IBW should be used with the weight-based equation of 22 to 25 kcal/kg. Patients with obesity are at higher risk for metabolic complications of nutritional therapy (eg, hyperglycemia, hyperlipidemia) and should be monitored closely.

K. Postoperative Patients: Early EN is safe and beneficial in postoperative patients who require SICU admission and should be administered when feasible. The presence of fresh intestinal anastomosis does not require withholding EN, provided there is no anastomotic leakage. There is some evidence supporting the benefit of combined immune-modulating formulas containing arginine and fish oil (eicosapentaenoic acid [EPA], docosahexaenoic acid [DHA]).

XIV. MONITORING OF NUTRITION

After initiation of nutritional support, basic laboratory values should be monitored to assess the adequacy of nutrition and detect potential complications.

A. Baseline laboratory data should include the following:

1. Glucose, electrolytes, liver function tests, albumin, prealbumin, transferrin, CRP
2. UUN: To ensure the adequacy of protein intake and prevent catabolic state (muscle breakdown)
3. Triglyceride levels in patients receiving fat in emulsions. Levels greater than 500 mg/dL should prompt a decrease in the rate of infusion due to the risk of pancreatitis.
4. Low phosphate is usually indicative of benign refeeding hypophosphatemia but may indicate refeeding syndrome. In malnourished patients, initiation of nutrition can lead to increased utilization and depletion of phosphate, potassium, and magnesium, which in extreme cases can lead to arrhythmias, heart failure, and neurologic disturbances. In the absence of clinical signs of refeeding syndrome, nutrition therapy should continue with frequent monitoring (at least once daily for the first week) and replacement of electrolytes. In patients with refeeding syndrome, daily energy delivery should be restricted for 48 hours.

B. Intolerance should be evaluated holistically by physical examination findings such as abdominal distention, in combination with high GRV (>500), signs of aspiration, signs of transit (flatus and stool), and radiologic evaluations as indicated. Nil per os (NPO) status for interventional procedures is one of the main reasons for EN interruption in patients who are critically ill and should be minimized if possible.

C. Diarrhea should not prompt the immediate withholding of EN. The etiology of diarrhea should be evaluated while EN is continued. Formulas rich in fermentable oligosaccharides, disaccharides, and monosaccharides, and polyols (FODMAPS) have been associated with a higher risk of diarrhea due to their poor absorption and high osmotic load. The addition of fermentable soluble fiber (eg, fructose oligosaccharides, inulin, pectin) to the EN solution has been shown to reduce the rate of diarrhea and should be considered in patients who are hemodynamically stable.

XV. GASTRIC RESIDUAL VOLUME (GRV) AND RISK OF ASPIRATION

GRV measurements are technique dependent and may not reliably measure gastric contents. Data on the association between high residuals and increased risk of aspiration pneumonia are conflicting. Allowing high GRV, or even eliminating GRV measurements altogether, has not been associated with worse outcomes in medical patients on mechanical ventilation. GRV was found to be a poor marker of aspiration at volumes less than 400 mL. ASPEN does not recommend the routine use of GRVs for the monitorization of EN tolerance. In cases when GRVs are measured, holding EN for GRV <500 mL is not recommended.

Major risk factors for aspiration in patients who are critically ill include history of documented episode of aspiration, impaired airway protection (decreased consciousness, neuromuscular dysfunction, anatomical abnormalities of the aerodigestive apparatus), endotracheal intubation, presence of a nasoenteric tube, age >70 years, poor oral care, supine position, gastroesophageal reflux, inadequate nursing availability, and bolus administration of EN. Several precautions may be taken in patients at high risk for aspiration such as postpyloric delivery of EN (rather than gastric), continuous EN infusion (rather than bolus), use of promotility agents as clinically viable, and nursing precautions such as semi-recumbent positioning (head of the bed elevated 30-45°) and chlorhexidine mouthwash. The use of dyes or any other sort of marker is not recommended to monitor aspiration.

Selected Readings

al Saif N, Hammodi A, Al-Azem MA, Al-Hubail R. Tension pneumothorax and subcutaneous emphysema complicating insertion of nasogastric tube. *Case Rep Crit Care.* 2015;2015:1-4. doi:10.1155/2015/690742

Allingstrup MJ, Esmailzadeh N, Wilkens Knudsen A, et al. Provision of protein and energy in relation to measured requirements in intensive care patients. *Clin Nutr.* 2011;31(4):462-468. doi:10.1016/j.clnu.2011.12.006

Bémeur C, Desjardins P, Butterworth RF. Role of nutrition in the management of hepatic encephalopathy in end-stage liver failure. *J Nutr Metab.* 2010;2010. doi:10.1155/2010/489823

Berger MM, Soguel L, Shenkin A, et al. Influence of early antioxidant supplements on clinical evolution and organ function in critically ill cardiac surgery, major trauma, and subarachnoid hemorrhage patients. *Crit Care.* 2008;12(4):1-13. doi:10.1186/CC6981

Blaser AR, Starkopf J, Alhazzani W, et al. Early enteral nutrition in critically ill patients: ESICM clinical practice guidelines. *Intensive Care Med.* 2017;43(3):380-398. doi:10.1007/s00134-016-4665-0

Boullata JI, Gilbert K, Sacks G, et al. A.S.P.E.N. clinical guidelines: parenteral nutrition ordering, order review, compounding, labeling, and dispensing. *JPEN J Parenter Enteral Nutr.* 2014;38(3):334-377. doi:10.1177/0148607114521833

Casaer MP, Mesotten D, Hermans G, et al. Early versus late parenteral nutrition in critically ill adults. *N Engl J Med.* 2011;365(6):506-517. doi:10.1056/NEJMoa1102662

Compher C, Chittams J, Sammarco T, Nicolo M, Heyland DK. Greater protein and energy intake may be associated with improved mortality in higher risk critically ill patients: a multicenter, multinational observational study. *Crit Care Med.* 2017;45(2):156-163. doi:10.1097/CCM.0000000000002083

Doig GS, Simpson F, Heighes PT, et al. Restricted versus continued standard caloric intake during the management of refeeding syndrome in critically ill adults: a randomised, parallel-group, multicentre, single-blind controlled trial. *Lancet Respir Med.* 2015;3(12):943-952. doi:10.1016/S2213-2600(15)00418-X

Dorken Gallastegi A, Gebran A, Gaitanidis A, et al. Early versus late enteral nutrition in critically ill patients receiving vasopressor support. *JPEN J Parenter Enteral Nutr.* 2022;46(1):130-140. doi:10.1002/jpen.2266

Fiaccadori E, Sabatino A, Barazzoni R, et al. ESPEN guideline on clinical nutrition in hospitalized patients with acute or chronic kidney disease. *Clin Nutr.* 2021;40(4):1644-1668. doi:10.1016/j.clnu.2021.01.028

Frankenfield D, Smith JS, Cooney RN. Validation of 2 approaches to predicting resting metabolic rate in critically ill patients. *JPEN J Parenter Enteral Nutr.* 2004;28(4):259-264. doi:10.1177/0148607104028004259

Grant JP, Davey-Mccrae J, Snyder PJ. Effect of enteral nutrition on human pancreatic secretions. *JPEN J Parenter Enteral Nutr.* 1987;11(3):302-304. doi:10.1177/0148607187011003302

Harris JA, Benedict FG. A biometric study of human basal metabolism. *Proc Natl Acad Sci U S A.* 1918;4(12):370-373. doi:10.1073/pnas.4.12.370

Heyland D, Muscedere J, Wischmeyer PE, et al. A randomized trial of glutamine and antioxidants in critically ill patients. *N Engl J Med.* 2013;368(16):1489-1497. doi:10.1056/NEJMoa1212722

Heyland DK, Dhaliwal R, Jiang X, Day AG. Identifying critically ill patients who benefit the most from nutrition therapy: the development and initial validation of a novel risk assessment tool. *Crit Care.* 2011;15(6):1-11. doi:10.1186/CC10546

Kerwin AJ, Nussbaum MS. Adjuvant nutrition management of patients with liver failure, including transplant. *Surg Clin N Am.* 2011;91:565-578. doi:10.1016/j.suc.2011.02.010

Khalid I, Doshi P, DiGiovine B. Early enteral nutrition and outcomes of critically ill patients treated with vasopressors and mechanical ventilation. *Am J Crit Care.* 2010;19(3):261-268. doi:10.4037/ajcc2010197

Kohlhardt SR, Smith RC, Wright CR. Peripheral versus central intravenous nutrition: comparison of two delivery systems. *Br J Surg.* 1994;81(1):66-70. doi:10.1002/bjs.1800810122

Kondrup J, Ramussen HH, Hamberg O, et al. Nutritional risk screening (NRS 2002): a new method based on an analysis of controlled clinical trials. *Clin Nutr.* 2003;22(3):321-336. doi:10.1016/S0261-5614(02)00214-5

Liang T, Liu S, Chou N. Small bowel perforation by nasogastric tube. *Clin Gastroenterol Hepatol.* 2011;9(7):A34-A34. doi:10.1016/j.cgh.2011.02.024

Liggett SB, John RES, Lefrak SS. Determination of resting energy expenditure utilizing the thermodilution pulmonary artery catheter. *Chest.* 1987;91(4):562-566. doi:10.1378/chest.91.4.562

Heather DJ, Howell L, Montana M, et al. Effect of a bulk-forming cathartic on diarrhea in tube-fed patients. *Heart Lung.* 1991;20(4):409-413.

McClave SA, DeMeo MT, DeLegge MH, et al. North American Summit on aspiration in the critically ill patient: consensus statement. *JPEN J Parenter Enteral Nutr.* 2002;26(6 suppl):S80-S85. doi:10.1177/014860710202600613

McClave SA, Lukan JK, Stefater JA, et al. Poor validity of residual volumes as a marker for risk of aspiration in critically ill patients. *Crit Care Med.* 2005;33(2):324-330. doi:10.1097/01.CCM.0000153413.46627.3A

McClave SA, Taylor BE, Martindale RG, et al. Guidelines for the provision and assessment of nutrition support therapy in the adult critically ill patient: Society of Critical Care Medicine (SCCM) and American Society for Parenteral and Enteral Nutrition (A.S.P.E.N.). *JPEN J Parenter Enteral Nutr.* 2016;40(2):159-211. doi:10.1177/0148607115621863

Metheny NA, Meert KL, Clouse RE. Complications related to feeding tube placement. *Curr Opin Gastroenterol.* 2007;23(2):178-182. doi:10.1097/MOG.0b013e3280287a0f

Nicolo M, Heyland DK, Chittams J, Sammarco T, Compher C. Clinical outcomes related to protein delivery in a critically ill population: a multicenter, multinational observation study. *JPEN J Parenter Enteral Nutr.* 2016;40(1):45-51. doi:10.1177/0148607115583675

Ohbe H, Jo T, Matsui H, Fushimi K, Yasunaga H. Differences in effect of early enteral nutrition on mortality among ventilated adults with shock requiring low-, medium-, and high-dose noradrenaline: a propensity-matched analysis. *Clin Nutr.* 2020;39(2):460-467. doi:10.1016/j.clnu.2019.02.020

Parekh D, Lawson HH, Segal I. The role of total enteral nutrition in pancreatic disease. *S Afr J Surg*. 1993;31(2):57-61.

Pertkiewicz M, Dudrick SJ. Basics in clinical nutrition: parenteral nutrition, ways of delivering parenteral nutrition and peripheral parenteral nutrition (PPN). *ESPEN*. 2009;4(3):e125-e127. doi:10.1016/j.eclnm.2009.01.006

Rahman A, Hasan RM, Agarwala R, Martin C, Day AG, Heyland DK. Identifying critically-ill patients who will benefit most from nutritional therapy: further validation of the "modified NUTRIC" nutritional risk assessment tool. *Clin Nutr*. 2016;35(1):158-162. doi:10.1016/J.CLNU.2015.01.015

Reignier J, Mercier E, le Gouge A, et al. Effect of not monitoring residual gastric volume on risk of ventilator-associated pneumonia in adults receiving mechanical ventilation and early enteral feeding: a randomized controlled trial. *JAMA*. 2013;309(3):249-256. doi:10.1001/jama.2012.196377

Rice TW, Mogan S, Hays MA, Bernard GR, Jensen GL, Wheeler AP. Randomized trial of initial trophic versus full-energy enteral nutrition in mechanically ventilated patients with acute respiratory failure. *Crit Care Med*. 2011;39(5):967-974. doi:10.1097/CCM.0B013E31820A905A

Rice TW, Wheeler AP, Thompson BT, et al. Initial trophic vs full enteral feeding in patients with acute lung injury: the EDEN randomized trial. *JAMA*. 2012;307(8):795-803. doi:10.1001/jama.2012.137

Rushdi TA, Pichard C, Khater YH. Control of diarrhea by fiber-enriched diet in ICU patients on enteral nutrition: a prospective randomized controlled trial. *Clin Nutr*. 2004;23(6):1344-1352. doi:10.1016/j.clnu.2004.04.008

Singer P, Anbar R, Cohen J, et al. The tight calorie control study (TICACOS): a prospective, randomized, controlled pilot study of nutritional support in critically ill patients. *Intensive Care Med*. 2011;37(4):601-609. doi:10.1007/s00134-011-2146-z

Singer P, Blaser AR, Berger MM, et al. ESPEN guideline on clinical nutrition in the intensive care unit. *Clin Nutr*. 2019;38(1):48-79. doi:10.1016/j.clnu.2018.08.037

Spapen H, Diltoer M, van Malderen C, Opdenacker G, Suys E, Huyghens L. Soluble fiber reduces the incidence of diarrhea in septic patients receiving total enteral nutrition: a prospective, double-blind, randomized, and controlled trial. *Clin Nutr*. 2001;20(4):301-305. doi:10.1054/clnu.2001.0399

Stapel SN, de Grooth HJS, Alimohamad H, et al. Ventilator-derived carbon dioxide production to assess energy expenditure in critically ill patients: proof of concept. *Crit Care*. 2015;19(1):370. doi:10.1186/s13054-015-1087-2

Weijs PJM, Stapel SN, de Groot SDW, et al. Optimal protein and energy nutrition decreases mortality in mechanically ventilated, critically ill patients: a prospective observational cohort study. *JPEN J Parenter Enteral Nutr*. 2012;36(1):60-68. doi:10.1177/0148607111415109

12

Infectious Disease

Joanne C. Huang and Lisa M. Bebell

I. INTRODUCTION

A. The management of **infectious disease** is a crucial skill for the intensivist. Epidemiologic studies suggest that more than 70% of adult patients in the intensive care unit (ICU) receive antibiotics and about 50% demonstrate overt signs of infection during their stay. Infection is a major contributor to mortality among the most critically ill, especially following trauma, burns, and extensive surgical insults (see Video 12.1: Blood Cultures).

B. Patients who are critically ill have numerous potential **sources** of infection, as outlined in Table 12.1. Tables 12.2 to 12.4 summarize the common bacterial pathogens referred to herein.

C. A broad overview of β-lactam antimicrobial spectra is given in Tables 12.5 and 12.6. More detailed treatment recommendations can be found under **Section IV**.

D. See Video 12.1 regarding how to obtain blood cultures.

II. HOSPITAL-ACQUIRED INFECTIONS

Hospital-acquired infections (HAIs) include the following infections as defined by the Centers for Disease Control and Prevention (CDC): catheter-associated urinary tract infections (CAUTIs), central line–associated bloodstream infection (CLABSI), ventilator-associated events (VAEs), *Clostridioides difficile* infections (CDIs), surgical site infections (SSIs), and methicillin-resistant *Staphylococcus aureus* bloodstream infections (MRSA BSIs). HAIs increase health care costs, extend hospital stays, and contribute to excess mortality. A large proportion of these infections are preventable through multifaceted measures; accordingly, HAI has become the focus of worldwide surveillance and practice improvement measures. Each year, the CDC estimates at least one HAI diagnosis per 25 patients in U.S. hospitals. Reassuringly, a significant decrease in device-associated infections (CAUTI, CLABSI, and VAE) has been observed in acute care hospitals, notably ICUs.

TABLE 12.1 Potential Sites of Infection in Patients in the Intensive Care Unit

Central nervous system	Epidural or brain abscess, encephalitis, meningitis
Head and neck	Sinusitis, pharyngitis, parotitis
Chest	Pneumonia, tracheobronchitis, endocarditis, empyema, mediastinitis, pericarditis
Abdomen	Peritonitis, cholecystitis, cholangitis, appendicitis, diverticulitis, *Clostridioides difficile* colitis
Genitourinary	Pyelonephritis, cystitis, prostatitis
Musculoskeletal and vascular	Cellulitis, abscess, pressure ulcers, osteomyelitis, deep venous thrombosis
Surgical	Wound, implanted hardware, anastomotic failure, abscess
Device-associated infections	Intravascular catheter, urinary catheter, epidural or spinal catheter, intracranial pressure monitor, any drain site or tract

TABLE 12.2 Classification of Common Pathogenic Bacterial Genera and Species

Gram-positive aerobic cocci, clusters	*Staphylococcus*
Gram-positive aerobic cocci, chains	*Streptococcus, Enterococcus*
Gram-positive aerobic bacilli	*Bacillus, Corynebacterium, Listeria*
Gram-negative non-enteric bacilli	*Acinetobacter, Pseudomonas, Burkholderia, Stenotrophomonas*
Gram-negative enteric bacilli	(Enterobacterales family) *Escherichia coli, Klebsiella, Enterobacter, Proteus, Citrobacter, Serratia,*
Gram-positive anaerobic cocci	*Peptostreptococcus*
Gram-positive anaerobic bacilli	*Clostridium* (sporulating), *Actinomyces, Lactobacillus*
Gram-negative anaerobic bacilli	*Bacteroides*

TABLE 12.3 Susceptibility of ICU and Non-ICU Ward Subsets of Lower Respiratory Tract Infection Isolates of *Pseudomonas aeruginosa* and Enterobacterales to C/T and Comparator Agents[a]—SMART 2018-2019, United States

		% Susceptible										% MDR
Species/ward type	***N***	**C/T**	**P/T**	**FEP**	**CAZ**	**CRO**	**ATM**	**MEM**	**IMI**	**LVX**	**AMK**	
P. aeruginosa												
ICU	495	96.0	**72.3**	**78.0**	**76.7**	NA	68.1	**72.9**	64.4	66.7	96.2	**17.8**
Non-ICU	583	96.7	**79.4**	**83.0**	**82.9**	NA	72.2	**79.8**	69.0	61.9	96.6	**10.5**
Enterobacterales												
ICU	1005	91.3	87.4	89.4	83.2	80.5	83.3	97.5	87.5	81.7	99.0	13.0
Non-ICU	726	92.6	89.3	89.4	83.3	79.6	85.1	98.5	85.1	83.0	98.6	11.7
P. aeruginosa + *Enterobacterales*												
ICU	1500	92.9	82.4	85.6	81.0	NA	78.3	89.4	79.9	76.7	98.1	**14.6**
Non-ICU	1309	94.4	84.9	86.6	83.1	NA	79.4	90.1	77.9	73.6	97.7	**11.2**

AMK, amikacin; ATM, aztreonam; C/T, ceftolozane/tazobactam; CAZ, ceftazidime; CRO, ceftriaxone; FEP, cefepime; ICU, intensive care unit; IMI, imipenem; LVX, levofloxacin; MEM, meropenem; NA, not available; P/T, piperacillin/tazobactam.

[a]Statistically significant differences between intensive care unit (ICU) and non-ICU are shown in bold font.

Data from: Karlowsky JA, Lob SH, Young K, et al. Activity of ceftolozane/tazobactam against Gram-negative isolates from patients with lower respiratory tract infections—SMART United States 2018-2019. *BMC Microbiol.* 2021;21:74.

III. ANTIBIOTIC RESISTANCE AND INFECTION PREVENTION

A. Antibiotic Resistance is a growing global challenge. The critically ill are highly susceptible to HAI owing to environmental colonization, immunosuppression, malnutrition, and the use of invasive devices. Coupled with higher rates of resistant organisms in critical care settings (Table 12.4), it is unsurprising that intensivists and their patients frequently encounter infections caused by antibiotic-resistant organisms.

1. The **etiologies** of bacterial resistance are diverse and differ widely depending on the organism; however, they are the result of selective pressures that favor survival of robust organisms. Widespread antibiotic use, ineffective or inappropriate treatment, environmental contamination, incomplete patient isolation, and inadvertent transmission all contribute to the development and spread of resistant organisms.

TABLE 12.4 Common Pathogens and Sites of Infection in Patients Who Are Critically Ill

Site	Pathogen
CNS	*Streptococcus pneumoniae* *Neisseria meningitidis* *Haemophilus influenzae* Group B Streptococcus *Listeria* spp.
Oral	Peptostreptococcus Actinomyces Anaerobic GNR (*Prevotella* spp., etc) Viridans group Streptococcus
Upper respiratory	*Streptococcus pyogenes* *Streptococcus pneumoniae* *Haemophilus influenzae* *Moraxella catarrhalis*
Lower respiratory	*Streptococcus pneumoniae* *Haemophilus influenzae* Atypicals (*Legionella* spp., *Mycoplasma* spp.) *Staphylococcus aureus* Enteric and non-enteric GNR
Intra-abdominal	Enteric GNR *Enterococcus* spp. *Streptococcus* spp. *Bacteroides* spp.
Skin and soft tissue	*Staphylococcus aureus* Coagulase-negative staphylococci *Streptococcus pyogenes*
Bone and joint	*Staphylococcus aureus* Coagulase-negative staphylococci *Streptococcus* spp. Enteric and non-enteric GNR
Genitourinary	Enteric GNR *Staphylococcus saprophyticus*

GNR, gram-negative rods.

2. Epidemiologic studies suggest that **more than 50%** of nosocomial pathogens demonstrate some degree of resistance. The CDC estimates that the worldwide impact of antibiotic resistance in the United States alone exceeds $20 billion in addition to excess mortality and the societal impact of prolonged treatment among affected patients.

B. Attention to **basic principles of antimicrobial therapy** is a key component of reducing antibiotic resistance and improving clinical outcomes.

1. The **diagnosis** of infection in the ICU is a nontrivial task. Fever, leukocytosis, respiratory disturbances, hemodynamic perturbations, and other markers of inflammation are nonspecific. Patients demonstrating these symptoms should also be evaluated for noninfectious sources of inflammation. In short, not all patients with fever or leukocytosis are infected.
2. **Testing** for suspected infection should be directed toward the identification of the **source** and obtaining high-quality specimens for **culture** and **susceptibility** testing. Ideally, specimens should be collected before starting antibiotic therapy to improve their yield. Colonizing organisms often

TABLE 12.5 Review of Selected β-Lactam Antibiotics

β-lactam class	β-lactam (and β-lactamase inhibitor)	Gram Pos[a]	Gram Neg	*Pseudomonas*	Covered organisms
Natural	Penicillin G	±	−	−	*Treponema pallidum*, meningococcal meningitis
Penicillinase resistant	(Methicillin) Nafcillin Oxacillin	++	−	−	penicillin-resistant MSSA, streptococci
Aminopenicillins	Ampicillin, Amoxicillin	+	±	−	Streptococci, enterococci
	with Sulbactam or Clavulanate	++	+	−	Above and penicillin-resistant MSSA, anaerobes, some Enterobacterales
Ureidopenicillins	Piperacillin	+	+	+	Streptococci, enterococci
	with Tazobactam	++	++	+	Above and penicillin-resistant MSSA, anaerobes, some Enterobacterales

++, highly active; +, active; ±, limited activity; −, not active; MSSA, methicillin-sensitive *Staphylococcus aureus*; Neg, negative; Pos, positive.
[a]Therapy with β-lactams in the setting of gram-positive nosocomial infections should be guided by culture data owing to variable rates and patterns of resistance.

TABLE 12.6 Review of Selected Cephalosporin Antibiotics

Gen	Agent	Gram Pos	Gram Neg	Anaerobes	PsA[a]	MRSA	CNS	Covered Organisms
1	Cefazolin	+	±	−	−	−	−	MSSA, streptococci
2	Cefuroxime	+	+	−	−	−	−	MSSA, streptococci, *Haemophilus influenzae*
	Cefoxitin, Cefotetan	±	+	+	−	−	−	Some Enterobacterales and *Bacteroides fragilis*
3	Ceftriaxone, Cefotaxime	+	+	−	−	−	+	± MSSA, streptococci, Enterobacterales
	Ceftazidime	±	+	−	+	−	+	Enterobacterales, *Pseudomonas*
4[b]	Cefepime	+	+	−	+	−	+	MSSA, Streptococci, Enterobacterales *Pseudomonas*
5	Ceftaroline	+	+	+	−	+	?	MRSA, Streptococci, Enterobacterales

+, active; ±, limited activity; −, not active; ?, unknown; MRSA, methicillin-resistant *Staphylococcus aureus*; MSSA, methicillin-sensitive *Staphylococcus aureus*; Neg, negative; Pos, positive.
[a]*Pseudomonas aeruginosa*.
[b]First- through fourth-generation cephalosporins demonstrate no activity against methicillin-resistant staphylococci or enterococci.

complicate culture results. Quantitative analysis and consultation with the microbiology lab can be useful adjuncts. Commonly, the source of infection and associated pathogens are never identified.

3. **Empiric** antibiotic selection should be based on the suspected site of infection (see Table 12.4), likely pathogens at that site, local resistance patterns, prior antibiotic therapy, and comorbidities that may increase the risk of toxicity.
   a. Initiating empiric antibiotic therapy should **not be delayed** on account of diagnostic testing when there is high clinical suspicion for sepsis, meningitis, or pneumonia. Increased latency from diagnosis to treatment leads to higher mortality in these serious infections.
4. **Documentation** of suspected infection, rationale for drug selection, and duration of proposed treatment is critical and reduces confusion during the course of treatment.
5. **Continuous reassessment** of antibiotic therapy is complicated by the fact that many patients who are critically ill will be slow to improve despite treatment with appropriate therapy.
   a. **Antibiotic de-escalation** (Figure 12.1) can be accomplished in one of three ways:
      i. Transitioning from a broad-spectrum to a narrower-spectrum agent based on specimen culture and sensitivity data
      ii. Shortening or limiting the duration of therapy based on clinical improvement when the location of infection is identified
      iii. When an infection is strongly suspected but culture data are unhelpful, antimicrobials can be discontinued in a stepwise manner based on the likely anatomic site and causative pathogen, relying on local patterns, clinical experience, and patient response.
   b. **Persistent fever** despite other signs of resolving infection should prompt reevaluation of other causes rather than unnecessary escalation or continuation of therapy (Table 12.7).

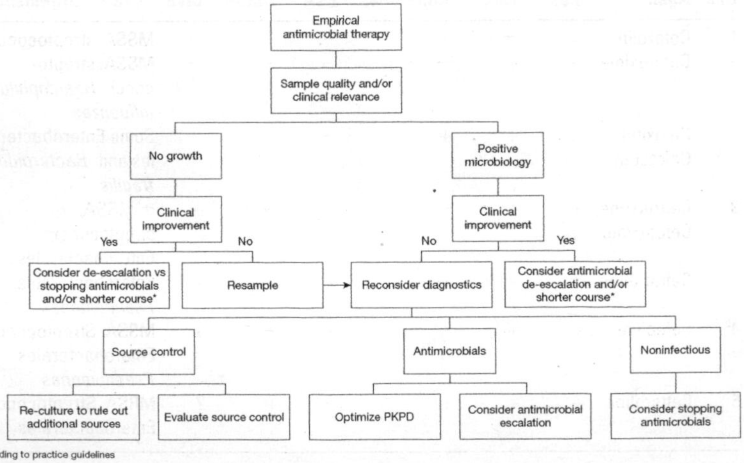

FIGURE 12.1 Antimicrobial de-escalation management strategies. PKPD, pharmacokinetic pharmacodynamics. (Derived from De Waele JJ, Schouten J, Beovic B, et al. Antimicrobial de-escalation as part of antimicrobial stewardship in intensive care: no simple answers to simple questions—a viewpoint of experts. *Intensive Care Med.* 2020;45:236-244.)

TABLE 12.7 Common Causes of Persistent Fever

Site	Infectious	Noninfectious
Head and neck	Meningitis	CVA
	Otitis media	Seizure
	Sinusitis	TBI
Chest	Infective endocarditis	Myocardial infarction
	Ventilator-associated tracheobronchitis	Pericarditis
	Ventilator-associated pneumonia	Pulmonary embolism
	Empyema	ARDS
Abdomen and pelvis	IAI	Pancreatitis
	CDI	Acalculous cholecystitis
	Pyelonephritis	Ischemic colitis
	CAUTI	
	Perineal or perianal abscess	
Extremities	CLABSI	Gout
	Septic arthritis	DVT
Skin and back	Cellulitis	Drug eruptions
	Sacral decubitis ulcer	
	Surgical site infection	
Miscellaneous	N/A	Drugs
		Transfusion reactions
		Endocrine disorders
		Malignancy
		Inflammatory disorders

ARDS, acute respiratory distress syndrome; CAUTI, catheter-associated urinary tract infection; CDI, *Clostridioides difficile* infection; CLABSI, central line–associated bloodstream infection; CVA, cerebrovascular accident; DVT, deep vein thrombosis; IAI, intra-abdominal infection; N/A, not applicable; TBI, traumatic brain injury. Adapted from Rehman T, deBoisblanc B. Persistent fever in the ICU. *Chest.* 2014;145(1):158-165, with permission from Elsevier.

IV. EMPIRIC AND EMERGENCY TREATMENT

Infectious disease specialists are often consulted for infections in the critically ill because of their diagnostic and therapeutic complexity. However, critical care providers need to familiarize themselves with the fundamental management principles emphasized here, including infection presentation, microbiology, and diagnostic and therapeutic approaches. Unless otherwise indicated, antibiotic regimens mentioned here indicate initial empiric therapy. Subsequent therapy should be tailored to culture and susceptibility data, when available.

V. ADVANCES AND CHALLENGES IN SEPSIS

Sepsis and its complications continue to have vast public health consequences. Although there has been significant progress in combating sepsis, major impediments remain, including a relatively poor understanding of sepsis pathophysiology, inadequate diagnostics, and lack of a therapeutic molecular target. Here, we focus on clinical management of sepsis and its complications.

A. Diagnosis and Management

1. **Definitions:** The International Sepsis Forum (2010) defined sepsis as "a life-threatening condition that arises when the body's response to an infection injures its own tissues and organs." A 1991 consensus conference introduced criteria for sepsis phenotypes, including systemic inflammatory

response syndrome (SIRS). These criteria are now outdated, replaced with new definitions in the most recent 2016 iteration, SEPSIS-3, summarized in Table 12.8.

2. **Diagnosis:** Conventional culture-based systems for the detection of bacteremia or fungemia remain the gold standard but are not sensitive. Blood culture results are positive in only 30% to 40% of patients with septic shock. Ninety percent of positive blood culture results are detected within 24 hours of incubation, 95% after 48 hours, and 99% after 72 hours.

B. Treatment: In 2002, the Society of Critical Care Medicine, the International Sepsis Forum, and the European Society of Intensive Care Medicine started the **Surviving Sepsis Campaign** (SSC) to improve the diagnosis, treatment, and outcomes of sepsis. Compliance with the SSC "bundles" is associated with improved patient outcomes. The three consistent foundations of sepsis management are (i) fluid resuscitation; (ii) early, appropriate antibiotic therapy; and (iii) elimination ("control") of the septic source. The recommendations given here follow the latest iterative SSC guidelines (2016), modified by the authors to take into account more recent evidence. The 2020 recommendations including care for patients who are critically ill with COVID-19 are beyond the scope of this chapter but are listed under Selected Readings.

1. **Initial resuscitation:** The landmark Early Goal-Directed Therapy (EGDT) trial established the importance of early, aggressive, and protocolized resuscitation in the management of patients with severe sepsis. Although the principles underlying EGDT remain valid (ie, fluid-resuscitate patients in septic shock), a number of trials cast doubts on the specific metrics derived from the EGDT trial (ie, the use of central venous pressure [CVP], $Scvo_2$, and lactate levels as end points) and the use of blood transfusions and dobutamine to increase $Scvo_2$. Several trials have demonstrated that "usual" non-protocolized care is equivalent to EGDT protocols.
2. **Cultures and broad-spectrum antibiotics:** Administering effective intravenous (IV) antibiotics within 1 hour of recognizing sepsis is one cornerstone of management. Typical empiric therapy uses a combination of antibiotics expected to be active against all likely pathogens in a specific clinical situation. Adequate dosing is equally important, particularly for frequently underdosed antibiotics such as vancomycin. Every hour of delay in appropriate antibiotic initiation increases mortality in patients with septic shock. Blood and other body site cultures should ideally be drawn before starting antibiotics but should not delay initiation of antibiotic therapy.

TABLE 12.8 The Third International Consensus Definitions for Sepsis and Septic Shock (Sepsis-3)

Sepsis: Life-threatening organ dysfunction caused by a dysregulated host response to infection. Clinical criteria include a suspected/documented infection and an acute increase in ≥2 qSOFA points:

- Respiratory rate >22 breaths/min
- Altered mental status
- Systolic blood pressure ≤100 mm Hg

Septic shock: Sepsis with persistent hypotension despite adequate fluid resuscitation, requiring vasopressors to maintain a MAP ≥65 mm Hg in addition to serum lactate >2 mmol/L.
Hypotension: MAP <65 mm Hg
Adapted from Singer M, Deutschman CS, Seymour CW, et al. The Third International Consensus definitions for sepsis and septic shock (sepsis-3). *JAMA.* 2016;315(8):801-810.

MAP, mean arterial pressure; qSOFA, Quick Sequential Organ Failure Assessment.

Need for antibiotics should be reassessed within 24 to 48 hours of initial sepsis presentation to facilitate de-escalation, if appropriate.

3. **Source control:** If a *nidus* of infection is identified, surgical or percutaneous intervention should be considered as soon as possible. The choice of intervention is based on patient stability, resources available, and the source of the infection and should target the least invasive option that will provide adequate source control.
4. **Hemodynamic support**
   a. **Fluids**
      i. **Volume:** We generally prefer **not** to give a predetermined amount of fluid but to titrate volume resuscitation with fluid boluses of 500 to 1000 mL, followed by frequent reassessment of volume status. Because no assessment method of volume status is foolproof, we often combine information from two or more complementary methods (such as bedside echocardiography and a passive leg raise test) to determine ongoing fluid requirements. Recent data suggest an association between increasingly positive fluid balance and mortality, further underlining the need to individualize fluid therapy.
      ii. **Type of fluid: Crystalloids** are the initial fluids of choice in most patients. Of note, fluids with high **chloride** content, including **normal saline,** may worsen renal function. Large-volume normal saline resuscitation can also cause hyperchloremic acidosis and is usually an inferior choice compared with Ringer's lactate in patients with impaired renal function. **Hydroxyethyl starch solutions** should **not be used** in patients with septic shock because multiple trials demonstrated increased mortality when used in patients with septic shock. **Albumin** is safe (and perhaps beneficial) in select patient populations with septic shock, although it does not appear to have a mortality benefit. It is reasonable to use albumin in patients with septic shock who are hypoalbuminemic, although the high cost of albumin should limit indiscriminate use.

   b. **Vasopressors and inotropes: Norepinephrine** is the initial vasopressor agent of choice in septic shock. **Vasopressin** is often added to norepinephrine in an effort to limit norepinephrine dosage. **Epinephrine** can be used if additional hemodynamic support is required, especially chronotropy. **Dobutamine** can be added to increase cardiac output, although there is no benefit in raising cardiac output to supranormal levels.
   c. **Corticosteroids:** There is wide variability in the use of steroids in refractory septic shock. If steroids are used, hydrocortisone should generally be started at a dose of 200 mg/d (as a continuous infusion or repeated boluses). Higher doses are not indicated, and there is no need to add fludrocortisone. Steroids should be used for the shortest time possible—it is unclear whether the dose needs to be tapered.
   d. **Blood transfusion:** Multiple large randomized controlled trials have shown no advantage of liberal transfusion goals (usually defined as a target Hb >10 g%) over more restrictive approaches (targeting Hb between 7 and 9 g%). In the absence of ongoing bleeding or **active** myocardial ischemia (during current admission), it seems safer to adopt restrictive transfusion practices.
5. **Other supportive therapies**
   a. **Mechanical ventilation:** Overall, 20% to 40% of patients with severe sepsis will develop acute respiratory distress syndrome (ARDS). They should be ventilated with the principles of lung-protective ventilation described in **Chapter 5**.
   b. **Glycemic control:** Hyperglycemia in septic shock is associated with worse outcomes, as are large swings in blood glucose. Glucose should be maintained between 140 and 180 mg/dL for patients with severe sepsis.

Patients who are on a regular insulin infusion should have hourly glucose checks and be on a glucose source to avoid hypoglycemia.

VI. THORACIC INFECTIONS

Thoracic infections include infections of the lungs, pleura, and thoracic cavity, either as the presenting diagnosis or discovered during the ICU stay.

A. Community-Acquired Pneumonia (CAP) is an infection of the lower respiratory tract acquired in the community. Although most cases can be managed in the outpatient setting with oral antibiotics, severe cases require critical care, including mechanical ventilation. Severe CAP is associated with advanced age, multiple comorbidities, immune compromise, organism virulence, and high infectious burden. Fever, chills, cough, sputum expectoration, and chest pain are common symptoms. Air hunger, confusion, tachypnea, accessory muscle use, hypoxemia despite oxygen supplementation, hypotension, high leukocytosis, bandemia, and lactic acidosis should increase concern for severe CAP and possible need for ICU admission.

1. **Microbiology:** The distribution of organisms varies slightly between CAP and severe CAP, although *Streptococcus pneumoniae* is the most common in both categories. Other common cases of CAP leading to ICU care are nontypable *Haemophilus influenzae, S. aureus* (including community-acquired methicillin-resistant strains), *Legionella pneumophila, Chlamydia pneumoniae*, and respiratory viruses, including SARS-CoV-2, the pathogen causing COVID-19 disease, and influenza. *Moraxella catarrhalis* and *Pseudomonas aeruginosa* usually cause CAP in patients with bronchiectasis or chronic bronchitis. Certain fungi, including *Histoplasma capsulatum* and *Coccidioides immitis*, and *Mycobacteria (M. tuberculosis)* may cause CAP in endemic regions. *Pneumocystis jirovecii* can cause CAP in the immunocompromised.
2. **Diagnosis:** Chest radiography (CXR) findings vary depending on the pathogen and host. Infiltrates may be interstitial or parenchymal, unilobar or multilobar, and unilateral or bilateral. Infiltrates not apparent on initial CXR in the setting of hypovolemia may "blossom" on subsequent films after rehydration. Despite all efforts, the causative microorganism will not be identified in nearly 40% cases of severe CAP. However, determining the microbial etiology facilitates targeted treatment. Depending on the host local microbiology, it is wise to pursue sputum sampling or bronchoalveolar lavage (BAL) for culture and/or viral polymerase chain reaction (PCR) testing, serologic testing (eg, for *Mycoplasma pneumoniae, C. immitis*), and urine antigen testing (for *S. pneumoniae, L. pneumophila*, and Histoplasma). Gram stain of sputum or BAL fluid may provide important clues regarding the potential causative organism early on depending on the presence of neutrophils and organism presence, abundance, and morphology, which can then be confirmed with culture. Blood culture results may also be positive in severe bacterial CAP. If there is a significant pleural effusion, pleural fluid Gram stain and culture, pH, lactate dehydrogenase, glucose, and protein concentration should be obtained to evaluate for empyema, which warrants drainage or decortication.
3. **Triage:** Several well-validated severity scores have been developed to supplement clinical judgment and help triage patients in the outpatient setting with CAP, including the CURB-65 score (confusion, uremia, respiratory rate, blood pressure, age 65 years and older). However, their utility in triaging patients who are already hospitalized with CAP is limited and mortality rates may be higher. In these settings, the 2007 Infectious Diseases Society of America/American Thoracic Society (IDSA/ATS) severe CAP criteria may be preferred (Table 12.9). One major or three (or more) minor criteria should prompt ICU admission in most cases.
4. **Treatment:** Initial CAP management is based on established guidelines coupled with host and epidemiologic factors and available Gram stain results.

TABLE 12.9 Criteria for Defining Severe Community-Acquired Pneumonia

Severe community-acquired pneumonia includes one major criterion or three (or more) minor criteria

Minor criteria	**Major criteria**
Respiratory rate ≥30 breaths/min	Septic shock with need for vasopressors
PaO_2/FIO_2 ratio ≤250	Respiratory failure requiring mechanical ventilation
Multilobar infiltrates	
Confusion/disorientation	
Uremia (blood urea nitrogen level ≥20 mg/dL)	
Leukopenia[a] (white blood cell count <4000 cells/µL)	
Thrombocytopenia (platelet count <100 000/µL)	
Hypothermia (core temperature <36 °C)	
Hypotension requiring aggressive fluid resuscitation	

[a]Due to infection alone (ie, not chemotherapy induced).

Adapted from Metlay JP, Waterer GW, Long AC, et al. Diagnosis and treatment of adults with community-acquired pneumonia. an official clinical practice guideline of the American Thoracic Society and Infectious Diseases Society of America. *Am J Respir Crit Care Med.* 2019;200(7):e45-e67.

Outcomes are better with early antibiotic administration, especially in severe CAP. Clinical presentation does not reliably predict the pathogens involved. The potential for antibiotic resistance should influence the choice of antibiotics. Early empiric antibiotic regimens should include coverage of the so-called "typical" (eg, *S. pneumoniae*) as well as "atypical" (eg, *Mycoplasma*) microorganisms. Patient-specific risk factors for Pseudomonas infection, including structural lung disease, frequent severe chronic obstructive pulmonary disease (COPD) exacerbations, and recent hospitalization with recent intravenous antibiotics within the last 90 days, should prompt anti-pseudomonal therapy. Antibiotics should be subsequently tailored depending on culture and susceptibility results and serology where applicable. Potential empiric regimens for severe CAP (in the ICU) include the following:

a. A β-lactam such as ceftriaxone, ampicillin/sulbactam, cefotaxime, plus doxycycline, azithromycin, or fluoroquinolone.

b. If Pseudomonas infection is a possibility, an antipseudomonal β-lactam such as cefepime and an antipseudomonal β-lactam/β-lactamase inhibitor such as piperacillin/tazobactam, or a carbapenem such as imipenem or meropenem should be used along with doxycycline, azithromycin, or fluoroquinolone.

c. Ciprofloxacin should not be used as empiric monotherapy because it does not have *S. pneumoniae* coverage.

d. If MRSA is a possibility, add vancomycin or linezolid. Note that MRSA can be community acquired.

B. Hospital-Acquired Pneumonia (HAP) is defined as pneumonia that is recognized at least 48 hours after hospital admission and was not incubating at the time of admission. HAP carries the highest mortality risk among nosocomial infections. Ventilator-associated pneumonia (VAP) is a subset of HAP occurring more than 48 hours after intubation. VAP affects 9% to 27% of patients who are intubated and has a high attributable mortality.

1. **Microbiology:** The microbiology of HAP and VAP is substantially different from that of CAP. Infections can be polymicrobial. Common pathogens include gram-positive cocci such as *S. aureus* and gram-negative bacilli, such as *P. aeruginosa, Escherichia coli, Klebsiella pneumoniae, Acinetobacter baumannii, Serratia marcescens, Enterobacter cloacae, Stenotrophomonas maltophilia*, and *Burkholderia cepacia*. Antimicrobial resistance is becoming more common in these organisms including both preexisting and de novo resistance emerging from selective antibiotic pressure. MRSA is a common cause of HAP, particularly in patients who are MRSA colonized.
2. **VAP diagnosis** can be difficult because many conditions (eg, sepsis, ARDS, congestive heart failure [CHF], atelectasis, thromboembolic disease, pulmonary hemorrhage, etc) common in the critically ill demonstrate similar clinical signs. The clinical criteria to diagnose VAP include *both* the presence of new or progressive radiographic infiltrates *and* one or more of the following: fever, purulent secretions, leukocytosis, tachypnea, decreased tidal volume, and worsening hypoxemia. Radiographic signs alone are nonspecific (see Figure 12.2). Owing to the difficulty in diagnosing VAP, the CDC proposed a new three-tier approach of ventilator-associated condition (VAC), infection-related ventilator-associated complication (IVAC), and possible or probable VAP, but this is not commonly used in clinical practice (Centers for Disease Control and Prevention, 2013).

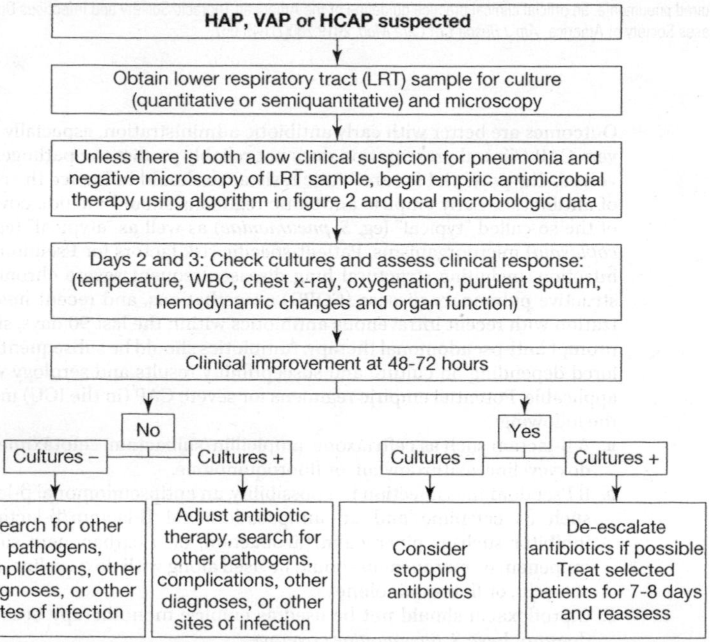

FIGURE 12.2 Summary of the management strategies for a patient with suspected hospital-acquired pneumonia (HAP) or ventilator-associated pneumonia (VAP). The decision about antibiotic discontinuation may differ depending on the type of sample collected (protected specimen brush [PSB], bronchoalveolar lavage [BAL], or endotracheal aspirate), and whether the results are reported in quantitative or semiquantitative terms (see text for details). HCAP, health care–associated pneumonia; WBC, white blood cell. (From American Thoracic Society; Infectious Diseases Society of America. Guidelines for the management of adults with hospital-acquired, ventilator-associated, and healthcare-associated pneumonia. *Am J Respir Crit Care Med.* 2005;171:388-416.)

3. The cornerstone of **VAP management** is lower respiratory tract sampling through the following:

a. Deep tracheal aspiration: Deep suction using a catheter introduced through the endotracheal (ET) tube or tracheostomy

b. Bronchoalveolar lavage: Wedging the tip of the bronchoscope in a segmental bronchus and infusion of sterile saline followed by aspiration of the infusate-secretion mixture. Protected specimen brush (PSB) is a lesser used yet similar technique.

i. BAL and PSB sampling do not provide a survival benefit over deep tracheal aspiration but do provide greater microbiologic specificity. BAL may potentiate early antibiotic de-escalation and diminish de novo resistance development and should be attempted when the risk is low and trained personnel are available.

c. Sampling results must be interpreted depending on whether and which antibiotics were administered before sampling. When possible, empiric antibiotics should be administered post the sampling to maximize culture yield. Severely ill cases may warrant treatment even if they do not meet VAP cutoffs.

i. Gram stain is a valuable tool, especially if empiric antibiotics may have sterilized respiratory samples. Morphologic identification of bacterial "carcasses" may help guide therapy. Abundant neutrophils increase the likelihood of VAP.

ii. Semiquantitative cultures are reported as none, mild, moderate, or abundant bacterial growth. Moderate or abundant growth of a pathogen suggests VAP but distinguishing colonization from infection remains challenging.

iii. Quantitative cultures reporting bacterial growth of more than 100 000 colony-forming unit (CFU)/mL in deep tracheal aspirate cultures, more than 10 000 CFU/mL from BAL cultures, and more than 1000 CFU/mL from PSB cultures make VAP more likely than colonization. Quantitative cultures have not been shown to improve clinical outcomes.

4. Treatment: VAP management principles include early, appropriate, adequately dosed empiric antibiotics, initial antibiotic therapy de-escalation based on lower respiratory tract culture data and patient response, and avoiding overly long treatment.

a. Monotherapy with a single antibiotic such as a third- or fourth-generation cephalosporin, carbapenem, or levofloxacin (in patients allergic to penicillin) is safe and effective when used properly and may decrease the likelihood of de novo antibiotic resistance. Empiric double-coverage of Pseudomonas is unnecessary for most patients. Anaerobic coverage is not recommended for empiric treatment of aspiration pneumonia but should be included when there is empyema, lung abscess, or necrotizing pneumonia. Monotherapy β-lactam/β-lactamase inhibitor combinations such as ampicillin/sulbactam and piperacillin/tazobactam can be used. Alternatively, metronidazole may be added to a β-lactam or fluoroquinolone for adequate anaerobic coverage. Linezolid or vancomycin should be added if MRSA pneumonia is possible. Daptomycin is inactivated by surfactant and should not be used.

C. Mediastinitis: Currently, the commonest presentation of mediastinitis is as a postoperative complication of cardiac or thoracic surgery. Other cases are associated with bacteremia, penetrating chest trauma, retropharyngeal abscess extension, and viscus rupture.

1. Microbiology: Mediastinitis following cardiothoracic surgery that does not involve the esophagus is generally monomicrobial and most often due to *S. aureus*. Mediastinitis from esophageal disruption is usually polymicrobial, caused by mixed anaerobes (*Peptococcus, Peptostreptococcus, Fusobacterium*, and *Bacteroides* spp.), gram-positive, enteric and non-enteric gram-negative bacteria, and yeast (*C. albicans, C. glabrata*). Rare etiologies include *Legionella, Mycoplasma, Histoplasma,* and *M. tuberculosis.*

2. **Diagnosis:** Clinical signs and symptoms commonly include fever, leukocytosis, and chest pain. It is often difficult to differentiate superficial postoperative wound infection from wound infection with mediastinitis, although mediastinitis is usually accompanied by signs of toxicity, including wound crepitus and sternal dehiscence, which are more specific but universal. Chest computed tomography (CT) may reveal mediastinal widening, complicated pleural effusions, and subcutaneous or mediastinal emphysema. However, most findings are difficult to distinguish from early postoperative changes and must be interpreted in the clinical context.
3. **Treatment** in most cases is a combination of rapid surgical intervention (drainage, debridement, and removal or repair of the infected material and tissue) and antibiotics. In some situations, contained esophageal rupture or small perforations can be treated without surgical intervention. Broad empiric antibiotic coverage should be started initially and adjusted depending on intraoperative cultures. Antibiotic coverage should target gram-positive and gram-negative aerobes and obligate and facultative anaerobes. Antipseudomonal β-lactams including piperacillin/tazobactam or cefepime plus metronidazole are reasonable. Empiric coverage for postsurgical mediastinitis should include an antistaphylococcal agent such as nafcillin, oxacillin, or cefazolin. Vancomycin can be used for possible MRSA or patients allergic to β-lactams.

VII. INTRA-ABDOMINAL INFECTIONS

These infections arise endogenously from the gastrointestinal (GI) tract, via contiguous spread from the urogenital/reproductive tract, through hematogenous or lymphatic seeding, or are exogenously introduced (through trauma or surgery). Infections are generally polymicrobial, including enteric gram-negative rods (*E. coli, Klebsiella, Enterobacter,* and *Proteus* spp.), aerobic gram-positive cocci (*Enterococcus* and *Streptococcus* spp.), anaerobes (*Clostridium, Bacteroides, Fusobacterium,* and *Peptostreptococcus* spp.), and sometimes *P. aeruginosa.* Management of intra-abdominal infections depends on the source of the infection, severity, and extent.

A. Microflora of Abdomen and Pelvis

1. **Gastrointestinal tract:** Bacterial concentrations normally increase progressively from the stomach through the small bowel to the colon. Stomach and proximal small bowel bacteria include *Streptococcus, Lactobacillus,* and *Peptostreptococcus* spp. Concentrations of enteric gram-negative rods such as *E. coli* and anaerobic gram-negatives such as *Bacteroides* spp. increase progressively toward the colon. Factors influencing GI microflora include the following:
   a. pH (antacids, histamine-2 blockers, proton-pump inhibitors)
   b. Antimicrobial use
   c. GI dysmotility
   d. Small-bowel obstruction, ileus, or regional enteritis
   e. Bowel resection or intestinal diversion
   f. Prior hospitalization or residence in a chronic care facility
2. Genital tract bacteria include gram-positive aerobes such as *Streptococcus, Lactobacillus,* and *Staphylococcus* spp. and anaerobes *Peptostreptococcus, Clostridium,* and *Bacteroides* spp.

B. Peritonitis: Peritoneal infections can occur following abdominal trauma, contamination of peritoneal dialysis catheters, perforation of abdominal viscus, or spontaneously.

1. **Spontaneous bacterial peritonitis** (SBP) is defined as peritonitis due to bacteria without a surgically correctable cause. It almost exclusively occurs

in patients with end-stage liver disease (ESLD) from cirrhosis. The likely pathogenesis is translocation of gut bacteria across edematous intestinal mucosa and lymphatics or hematogenous seeding into the peritoneal cavity under high portal pressures. Infection of ascites fluid from congestive heart failure, malignancy, or hypoproteinemia in the absence of liver disease is exceedingly rare. Fever, abdominal pain, and confusion are the commonest symptoms. However, patients with SBP may be asymptomatic or have only minor symptoms.

a. Microorganisms: SBP is predominantly monomicrobial, caused most commonly by enteric gram-negatives followed by streptococci. Anaerobes rarely cause SBP. The presence of anaerobes or mixed flora suggests secondary peritonitis.

b. Diagnosis: Early diagnosis is key. Without treatment, most cases will progress to septic shock, which carries a dismal prognosis in patients with ESLD. If SBP is suspected, diagnostic paracentesis should be performed before giving antibiotics. Ascites fluid should be sent for cell counts, Gram stain, and culture. A neutrophil count of more than 250 cells/mm^3 or a positive ascitic fluid culture result is highly suggestive of SBP. However, culture results of ascites fluid are often negative despite a cell count that is consistent with SBP. Use of blood culture bottles (anaerobic and aerobic) to culture ascites fluid may increase the likelihood of detecting the bacteria. Blood cultures should also be obtained.

c. Treatment: Empiric antibiotic therapy should be initiated before obtaining culture results if the ascites fluid neutrophil count is greater than 250 cells/mm^3. Potential empiric regimens include the following:

i. Ceftriaxone or cefotaxime are primary agents for SBP. High doses are used for life-threatening SBP.

ii. A β-lactam/β-lactamase inhibitor combination, such as piperacillin/tazobactam

iii. Fluoroquinolone (use an alternative agent in patients taking fluoroquinolones for SBP prophylaxis or at high risk for fluoroquinolone resistance)

iv. If resistant enteric gram-negatives are a possibility, consider carbapenem therapy.

Antibiotics should be tailored to culture and sensitivity data, when available.

2. Secondary peritonitis usually results from perforation or necrosis of a solid viscus (ruptured appendix, diverticulitis, duodenal ulcer), anastomotic leak following bowel surgery, or suppurative infections of the biliary and female reproductive tracts.

a. Diagnosis can be assisted by upright plain abdominal radiograph, which may show free air under the diaphragm. A CT scan with oral contrast usually identifies the perforated viscus. Exploratory laparotomy may be needed to diagnose and treat the source.

b. Treatment usually involves a combination of surgical/interventional radiology (IR) intervention with drainage catheter placement and broad-spectrum antibiotics active against gram-negative and gram-positive bacteria, including anaerobes. Noninterventional management may be attempted for small walled-off perforations or when operative mortality outweighs potential benefit. Mild to moderate community-acquired peritonitis occurs early in hospitalization in patients who are not chronic care facility residents and who have not had antibiotics recently, resulting in a low risk of antibiotic-resistant bacteria. Patients not meeting these criteria have a higher risk of antibiotic resistance. Local resistance patterns and prior patient colonization by drug-resistant microorganisms should influence empiric antibiotic choices. Antibiotic choices differ depending on infection severity and setting. Potential regimens include the following:

- **i.** A third-generation cephalosporin (ceftriaxone, cefotaxime) or fluoroquinolone plus anaerobic coverage (metronidazole) for community-acquired infections. Ampicillin-sulbactam is not recommended for empiric treatment because of high rates of community-acquired *E. coli* resistance.
- **ii.** A third- or fourth-generation cephalosporin (ceftazidime or cefepime) or fluoroquinolone plus metronidazole. If using ceftazidime, consider adding another agent with greater gram-positive coverage.
- **iii.** For health care–associated infections, consider including an agent effective against enterococci such as ampicillin or vancomycin (in the setting of β-lactam allergy or high rates of penicillin resistance). Linezolid or daptomycin should be used if infection with vancomycin-resistant enterococci (VRE) is likely. Cephalosporins and carbapenems (with the exception of imipenem/cilastatin) provide little to no enterococcus coverage.
- **iv.** If multidrug-resistant or polymicrobial cultures result, consider monotherapy with a carbapenem or tigecycline.

C. Intra-abdominal Abscesses occur by local extension from the GI, upper urinary, or female genital tract, as bacterial persistence after secondary peritonitis, or through hematogenous spread of extra-abdominal infection. Abscess should be suspected in the setting of focal abdominal pain and tenderness, fevers, chills, and/or persistent leukocytosis despite empiric antibiotics. Untreated, they may rupture and cause peritonitis, bacteremia, and septic shock.

1. Microorganisms commonly cultured from abscesses include *Bacteroides* spp. (especially *B. fragilis*), enteric gram-negative bacteria, gram-positive bacteria such as *Enterococcus* spp. and *S. aureus*, and Candida.
2. **Diagnosis:** CT (ideally, with oral and IV contrast) is useful for diagnosing and localizing abscesses. Ultrasonography can be done at the bedside and can be particularly useful in the diagnosis of right upper quadrant (RUQ), renal, and pelvic abscesses. Indium-labeled white blood cell (WBC) and gallium scans have low specificity and limited utility. Magnetic resonance imaging (MRI) is an alternative.
3. **Treatment** includes drainage and antibiotics. The method of drainage (percutaneous under CT or ultrasound guidance vs operative) depends on abscess location, whether the abscess is associated with perforation or gangrene, the presence of loculations that may limit the success of percutaneous drainage, and host factors including surgical candidacy. Abscesses should be sampled for culture data to guide antibiotic selection. Reasonable empiric coverage includes the abovementioned regimens for secondary peritonitis in patients who are hospitalized. *Enterococcus* spp. discovered in abscesses as part of a polymicrobial process are usually low virulence in immunocompetent individuals and often do not require targeted treatment. Serial imaging and abscessogram (imaging following retrograde instillation of contrast into an indwelling drain) can be used to monitor treatment progress.

D. Hepatobiliary System Infections

1. **Acute cholecystitis** results from cystic duct obstruction, called calculous cholecystitis when caused by stone disease. Cholecystitis can lead to severe sepsis and septic shock, and gangrene or perforation can occur. Acalculous cholecystitis (10% of all acute cholecystitis cases, but more common in the ICU) occurs in the setting of critical illness, endothelial injury, gall bladder hypoperfusion, stasis edema, and cystic duct luminal narrowing. Complications and untreated mortality are higher in acalculous cholecystitis.

a. **Microbiology:** Common bacteria include enteric gram-negatives such as *E. coli*, *Klebsiella*, *Proteus*, and *Enterobacter* spp. Anaerobic gram-negatives and facultative anaerobic gram-positives, such as streptococci, enterococci, and staphylococci, can be seen in patients with instrumented/disrupted hepatobiliary tracts or upper GI tract anomalies.

b. **Diagnosis:** Acute cholecystitis is often associated with continuous pain and peritoneal signs such as rebound tenderness and Murphy sign. However, these classic signs are less common in the critically ill, especially those with acalculous cholecystitis, in whom fever or leukocytosis may be the only signs of infection. However, both abdominal ultrasonography and CT have good diagnostic sensitivity and specificity. CT may be more sensitive for acalculous cholecystitis. Cholescintigraphy (hepatobiliary iminodiacetic acid [HIDA] scan) may be useful in equivocal cases, demonstrating gallbladder nonfilling.

c. **Treatment** of acute calculous cholecystitis includes antibiotics and drainage. Imaging-guided percutaneous drainage is commonly performed for patients in the ICU to achieve source control. Surgical management is rare in acute cholecystitis but may be required in severe cases or may be necessary after recovery from the acute phase. Community-acquired biliary infections can be treated with ceftriaxone. Anaerobic coverage (eg, with metronidazole) should be added when a biliary-enteric anastomosis is present. Uncommonly, hospital-associated cases may require pseudomonas and enterococcus coverage. Clinical and laboratory parameters usually improve rapidly after drainage and antibiotics. If the patient fails to improve or the condition worsens, suspect gangrene and/or perforation, which may require urgent cholecystectomy.

2. **Acute cholangitis** is usually caused by partial or complete common bile duct (CBD) obstruction. This obstruction may be due to stone disease, strictures, or neoplasms obstructing or compressing the biliary tract or pancreas.

a. **Diagnosis:** The classic presentation is the Charcot triad of jaundice, fevers, chills, and RUQ pain. Blood culture results are often positive. No further diagnostic tests are needed if this triad is present. In the absence of all classic features, RUQ ultrasound may reveal biliary duct dilatation and CBD stone. CT can also be used but is less sensitive. Magnetic resonance cholangiopancreatography (MRCP) may be helpful for early cases, to visualize small stones, or when ultrasound or CT imaging is equivocal.

b. Nonsuppurative cholangitis resulting from partial CBD obstruction will often respond to antibiotic therapy alone. Suppurative cholangitis due to complete CBD obstruction must be treated urgently with a combined decompression and antibiotics to prevent bacteremia and septic shock. Reasonable antibiotic regimens for cholangitis are the same as those for secondary peritonitis in patients who are hospitalized. Decompression may be achieved endoscopically via endoscopic retrograde cholangiopancreatography (ERCP), or percutaneously using a T-tube, especially for poor surgical candidates.

3. **Liver abscess:** Abscesses can be solitary or multiple. Manifestations range from fever, leukocytosis, and RUQ pain to sepsis. Liver abscesses can result from seeding from the bloodstream and portal pyemia or from local extension of biliary tract infection.

a. **Microbiology:** There is a wide spectrum of difficult-to-predict monomicrobial and polymicrobial etiologies that underscore the importance of sampling. Abscesses may include mixed aerobic and anaerobic bacteria and Candida. Multiple monomicrobial abscesses with *S. aureus* or *S. anginosus* indicate hematogenous spread and potential sources must be investigated. Blood cultures should be drawn before empiric antibiotics are administered because many patients are bacteremic. Amoebic liver abscess should be considered depending on host epidemiology, including travel to endemic regions.

b. **Diagnosis** is made by CT scan or RUQ ultrasound. Microbiologic diagnosis is made by percutaneous aspiration or concurrent positive blood culture results.

c. **Treatment** includes drainage and antibiotics. Smaller abscesses can be drained with needle aspiration but larger ones require drain placement. Abscesses arising from the biliary tract or peritoneum should be treated with antibiotics directed against organisms from the initial infection. Empiric antibiotics for presumed hematogenous abscesses should include regimens active against gram-positive bacteria, or directed at the specific organism, when known. In most other cases, empiric broad-spectrum therapy, as described previously for peritonitis, is appropriate. Because anaerobes are difficult to grow and are highly prevalent in liver abscesses, presumptive anaerobic coverage is often recommended, even when no anaerobes are cultured.

E. **Splenic Abscess** is rare and highly morbid if untreated. It usually results from hematogenous spread (including endocarditis) but can result from splenic trauma or contiguous spread.

1. **Microbiology:** The most common causative organisms are *Streptococcus* spp. followed by *S. aureus* and *Salmonella* spp. and, rarely, anaerobic bacteria.
2. **Signs and symptoms** include left upper quadrant pain, fever, leukocytosis, and left-sided pleural effusion. Splenic abscess can often be mistaken for, or coexist with, splenic infarcts.
3. **Treatment:** Antibiotics and with splenectomy rather than with percutaneous drainage

F. ***Clostridioides difficile*–Associated Diarrhea:** One in every five patients admitted to a U.S. hospital acquires *C. difficile*, a toxigenic spore-forming, gram-positive bacillus, as part of their colonic flora. Although only a fraction develops clinical disease, they form a sizable reservoir and contribute to *Clostridioides difficile*–associated diarrhea (CDAD) propagation. Although most cases are acquired in the health care setting, severe CDAD cases acquired in the community are on the rise. The commonest modifiable risk factor is antibiotic exposure, although CDAD can occur without prior antibiotics. Antibiotics alter normal bowel flora, allowing *C. difficile* spores to convert to vegetative forms that rapidly replicate and produce toxin. Advanced age, comorbidities, immunodeficiency, gastric acid suppression, and health care exposure are other important risk factors.

1. **Clinical features**—diarrhea (up to 15 watery stools daily): Other features may include bloody diarrhea, abdominal cramps and tenderness, toxic megacolon, bowel perforation, and peritonitis. Leukocytosis can be marked, sometimes in excess of 50 000 cells/μL.
2. **Diagnosis:** Enzyme immunoassay (EIA) to detect toxin in liquid/semisolid stool is highly sensitive and specific. Stool sample PCR is becoming common, but controversy exists on diagnosis and management when EIA and PCR tests yield discordant results. CT imaging may show varying degrees of focal to diffuse colonic thickening and pericolic stranding.
3. **Treatment:** Where possible, discontinue causative antibiotics. Other therapeutic options vary with disease severity and frequency. Severe disease may exist in the setting of WBC count greater than 15 000, shock, severe lactic acidosis, acute kidney injury, and toxic mega colon.

a. Fidaxomicin (200 mg twice daily) or oral vancomycin (125 mg every 6 hours) is recommended for 10 days as initial therapy for nonsevere disease. Fidaxomicin is associated with fewer recurrences and higher rates of sustained response and is preferred for initial therapy.

b. Disease recurrence after initial episode of CDI occurs in 20% to 25% of patients. The window for highest risk of recurrence is within 8 weeks of a previous episode. Patients with a first recurrence of CDI should receive a different therapeutic regimen than the one received for previous episodes.

c. Patients with fulminant CDIs should receive high-dose oral vancomycin (500 mg every 6 hours) with or without IV metronidazole.

d. Oral antibiotics concentrate well in the colon, but vancomycin 500 mg enema 4 times daily can be given when there is profound ileus or inability to tolerate oral medication. Surgical consultation for colectomy is indicated in patients with shock, organ failure, or lack of improvement after 24 to 72 hours on treatment. Fecal microbiota transplant (FMT) as well as newer therapies such as bezlotoxumab (anti-*C. difficile* toxin B antibody) should be considered in consultation with local infectious diseases providers, pharmacists, and antimicrobial stewardship teams in fulminant and recurrent cases.

VIII. SKIN AND SOFT TISSUE INFECTIONS

A. Infected Burns and Postoperative Wound Infections: Multiple factors influence the development and severity of wound infections. The incidence of postoperative wound infection due to antibiotic-resistant bacteria increases with the length of hospitalization.

1. Microbiology: Microorganisms often reflect the site of origin of contamination and are altered by recent treatment with antibiotics, prolonged preoperative hospitalization, and coexisting diseases. Infections may be monomicrobial or polymicrobial, and common pathogens include *S. aureus,* coagulase-negative *Staphylococcus,* and *Streptococcus* spp. Severe wound infections that occur in the first 48 hours after surgery may be caused by Clostridium or group A streptococcus (*S. pyogenes*). Gram-negative pathogens, including increasingly resistant organisms, are common in patients with prolonged hospitalization and/or prolonged antimicrobial pressure.

2. Clinical presentation and diagnosis: Erythema, warmth, and swelling are common in superficial wound infections, sometimes with fever and purulence. Surface wound swabs are often not helpful and usually result with polymicrobial growth that may not reflect the true pathogen. Many organisms cultured from superficial swabs do not require treatment. Deeper samples from operative debridement are more specific for the true pathogen.

3. Prevention: Limiting antibiotic use, using narrow-spectrum antibiotics, and good surgical technique are important measures. Single-dose or short-course periprocedural prophylactic antibiotics should be administered according to local and institutional guidelines.

4. Treatment

a. Mild superficial wound infections may be treated with removal of sutures or staples and opening of the wound to drain fluid collections.

b. Severe wound infections are usually treated with parenteral antibiotics and surgical debridement. Superficial swab culture results should not dictate antibiotic choice. Deep, operative cultures from sterile sites should guide antimicrobial therapy. For empiric therapy, first-generation cephalosporins can be used for uncomplicated postoperative wound infections (clindamycin for patients allergic to β-lactams). Vancomycin, linezolid, or daptomycin should be used when MRSA is likely. Additional gram-negative coverage should be given for infections originating in the GI, genitourinary (GU), and respiratory tracts.

B. Necrotizing Soft Tissue Infections: Type 1 (polymicrobial) and type 2 (monomicrobial) are further classified depending on the tissues involved as necrotizing fasciitis, myonecrosis, or both. These life-threatening infections can spread rapidly and cause severe systemic toxicity with mortality approaching 100% without timely surgical control. Appropriate antimicrobial therapy is essential, but not sufficient, because of poor antibiotic delivery to necrotic tissue.

1. **Microbiology**
   a. **Necrotizing fasciitis:** *Streptococcus* spp. are the most common monomicrobial agents. Polymicrobial infections also include anaerobes and enteric gram-negatives.
   b. **Myonecrosis:** Clostridial myonecrosis (gas gangrene) is a severe, fulminant skeletal muscle infection caused by bacterial exotoxins released by *Clostridium* spp. The microbiology of non-clostridial myonecrosis is similar to that of necrotizing fasciitis.
2. **Diagnosis:** Early features include pain out of proportion to the local external findings and systemic toxicity. Crepitus may be present because of soft tissue gas.
3. **Treatment**
   a. **Debridement:** Immediate diagnosis and prompt surgical debridement are critical. Close wound monitoring is essential and repeated surgical debridement is often necessary.
   b. **Antibiotics** are chosen depending on the presentation and likely source of infection. Gram stain of intraoperative wound samples can guide initial therapy. Empiric therapy should be broad and include coverage of *Streptococcus* spp. and *Staphylococcus* spp., enteric gram-negative bacteria, and anaerobes. Clindamycin or linezolid is included in regimens to limit exotoxin production by inhibiting bacterial protein synthesis. Optimal duration of exotoxin coverage is unknown but can consider narrowing following final debridement.

IX. URINARY TRACT INFECTIONS

Urinary tract infections (UTIs) in the ICU can present as community- or hospital-acquired urosepsis or as a CAUTI. CAUTIs comprise 40% of nosocomial infections and up to 30% of gram-negative bacteremia cases in patients who are hospitalized.

A. **Predisposing Factors:** Indwelling urinary catheters remain the leading cause of UTIs in the ICU. Other factors include neurologic or structural abnormalities of the urinary tract and nephrolithiasis.

B. **Microbiology:** Most are ascending infections caused by gram-negative rods including *E. coli*, *Klebsiella*, *Proteus*, and *Enterobacter* spp. Enterococci can cause UTIs but can also be colonizers. *S. saprophyticus*, *Serratia*, and *Pseudomonas* spp. are less common causes. *S. aureus* bacteriuria should raise suspicion of *S. aureus* bacteremia. Contiguous peritoneal infection can cause perinephric and renal abscesses.

C. **Diagnosis:** Urinalysis of the urinary sediment for leukocytes is critical, along with urine culture and clinical features to help distinguish colonization from true infection.

D. **Urinary Tract Infection Subtypes**

1. Cystitis is infection of the bladder characterized by dysuria and frequency, tenderness of the urethra and suprapubic regions, and, sometimes, hematuria. Appearance and odor of urine have little clinical utility diagnosing cystitis and can lead to overtreating asymptomatic bacteriuria.
2. Acute pyelonephritis is a pyogenic infection of the renal parenchyma and pelvis characterized by costophrenic angle tenderness, high fevers, shaking chills, nausea, vomiting, and diarrhea. Risk factors include nephrolithiasis, structural urinary tract abnormalities, urologic trauma or surgery, and diabetes mellitus. Leukocytosis and pyuria are common. Most urinary

tract abscesses are bacterial but may rarely be caused by *Candida* spp. Bacteria are often seen on urine Gram stain, but urine culture results may be negative in the setting of prior appropriate antibiotic treatment, walled-off abscess, or fully obstructing stone disease. Treatment includes antibiotics and investigation and correction of structural urinary tract abnormalities (when present). Complications include sepsis, urinary obstruction causing hydro- or pyonephrosis, and renal or perinephric abscess. Diagnosis can be confirmed by abdominal ultrasound or CT scan.

3. Prostatitis is infrequent in the ICU but can be a complication of CAUTI marked by fevers, chills, dysuria, pyuria, and an enlarged, tender, and boggy prostate on rectal examination.

E. Treatment: Empiric broad therapy should cover likely organisms, including third- or fourth-generation cephalosporins or fluoroquinolones. Fluoroquinolones should be avoided in patients admitted from long-term care facilities, those with recent fluoroquinolone use, or where local resistance rates are high. Antimicrobial therapy must be tailored to culture data when they become available. Treatment duration is controversial, but 3 to 14 days is an accepted range, with uncomplicated cystitis treated for 3 to 7 days in most hosts, and pyelonephritis treated for 7 to 14 days regardless of resistance phenotype. Duration is dependent on class of antimicrobial chosen.

X. INTRAVASCULAR CATHETER-RELATED INFECTIONS

These infections can be localized to the site of insertion (exit-site infections) or can be systemic (catheter-related bloodstream infections or CRBSI). CRBSI risk factors include total parenteral nutrition (TPN), prolonged central line use, and femoral location. Fever is the most common presenting feature, and localized signs of infection at the insertion site are often absent. Inflamed exit site or unexplained fever among patients with central lines should prompt assessment for CRBSI.

A. Microbiology: The most common pathogens are coagulase-negative Staphylococcus (CoNS) and *S. aureus*. Because CoNS are also the commonest blood culture contaminants, CRBSIs caused by CoNS are often difficult to diagnose. *Candida* spp. cause nearly 10% of CRBSI, commonly in patients receiving TPN. Other bacteria are less frequent causes.

B. Management

1. Treatment options vary by type and extent of infection and microorganism involved.
2. Indications for catheter removal:
   a. Septic shock
   b. CRBSI due to *S. aureus, P. aeruginosa, Candida*, or *Mycobacterium* spp.
   c. CRBSI with persistent bacteremia despite 3 days of appropriate antibiotic therapy
3. Lower threshold for removing temporary catheters. A new catheter (including peripherally inserted central catheter [PICC], tunneled) can be placed 72 hours after catheter removal if blood culture results remain negative.
4. Antibiotic choice is dictated by the clinical situation and culture data. Empiric therapy is often started with vancomycin if there are systemic signs of infection or if preliminary blood culture results indicate gram-positive bacteremia. Sometimes an additional agent is added to cover gram-negatives or *Candida* spp. when suspicion for these is high. Further therapy should be tailored to the specific organism identified.
5. Duration of systemic antibiotics upon removal of catheter: 7 to 10 days (14 days minimum for *S. aureus*). Longer antibiotic duration may be necessary if there is endocarditis, venous thrombosis, or an implanted device is present.
6. When catheter salvage is attempted, antibiotics may be administered systemically for 1 to 2 weeks with or without antibiotic lock therapy. Lock

therapy targets microorganisms within the biofilm by allowing the antibiotic to dwell within a long-term catheter.

7. Catheter exchange over a guide wire in response to CRBSI is not routinely recommended.

XI. INFECTIVE ENDOCARDITIS

Infective endocarditis (IE) is caused by microbial invasion of the endocardium, most commonly involving the cardiac valves, but can also occur in the septal or mural myocardium. IE is classified as acute or subacute and as native valve endocarditis (NVE) or prosthetic valve endocarditis (PVE). PVE occurring within 2 months of valve replacement (early PVE) results from microbial colonization of the valve at the time of surgery, most commonly by *Staphylococcus* spp. Late PVE is similar to NVE, where microorganisms enter the bloodstream via direct percutaneous inoculation during airway, GU, GI, and dental procedures, or from an existing infection such as pneumonia or dental abscess.

A. **Predisposing Factors** for IE include IV drug use, previous IE, and rheumatic and congenital heart disease. Intravascular devices such as central venous catheters, pacemaker wires, hemodialysis shunts, and prosthetic valves are additional risk factors. However, endocarditis can also occur in previously normal hearts.

B. **Microbiology:** Most commonly caused by bacteria but also by fungi, viruses, and rickettsiae.

1. **Gram-positive bacteria:** *Streptococcus* spp. are common, particularly the viridans group. *Enterococcus* spp. are common in older patients who have undergone GU procedures. *S. aureus* is a common cause of NVE in people who inject drugs, is usually severe, and is commonly complicated by inflammatory damage to valvular and perivalvular structures, myocardial and valve ring abscesses, emboli, and metastatic lesions (eg, lung, central nervous system [CNS], and splenic abscess). Identification of *S. bovis* as the causative organism should prompt a workup for a GI source such as colon cancer. CoNS often cause PVE accompanied by significant valvular destruction. Evaluate for PVE in patients with CoNS bacteremia who have prosthetic valves, pacer wires, and hardware.

2. **Gram-negative bacteria infrequently cause infective endocarditis:** It is often severe, with an abrupt onset. Often, there is delayed growth in blood cultures, large vegetations, and frequent embolic events. *Pseudomonas* and *Serratia* spp. have been reported. *Brucella* spp. is a common cause in endemic areas.

C. **Diagnosis:** Severe systemic illness with high fevers and chills and new heart murmur is a classic presentation of acute IE. Subacute IE is more difficult to diagnose.

1. **Findings on physical examination** can include heart murmur, petechiae, and nail bed splinter hemorrhages. More specific but less common findings include retinal hemorrhages (Roth spots), painful red or purple nodules on digital pads (Osler nodes), and painless red macules on palms or soles (Janeway lesions). Patients may present with complications such as stroke, osteomyelitis, or metastatic abscesses before the IE diagnosis is made.

2. **Blood cultures:** Three or more sets of blood cultures should be obtained within the first 24 hours if IE is suspected. Blood cultures may be negative when IE is due to intracellular organisms such as rickettsiae, anaerobic bacteria, the HACEK (*Haemophilus* species, *Aggregatibacter* species, *Cardiobacterium hominis*, *Eikenella corrodens*, and *Kingella* species) group of bacteria, and fungi. Inform the laboratory when these pathogens are suspected.

3. **Echocardiography** is an important tool for diagnosing and managing IE. Transthoracic echocardiography (TTE) is less sensitive than is transesophageal echocardiography (TEE) for detecting vegetations but is a reasonable

TABLE 12.10 Definition of Infective Endocarditis According to the Proposed Modified Duke Criteria[a]

Definite infective endocarditis pathologic criteria
1. Microorganisms demonstrated by culture or histologic examination of a vegetation, a vegetation that has embolized, or an intracardiac abscess specimen; or
2. Pathologic lesions; vegetation or intracardiac abscess confirmed by histologic examination showing active endocarditis
Clinical criteria[b]
1. Two major criteria; or
2. One major criterion and three minor criteria; or
3. Five minor criteria
Possible infective endocarditis
1. **One major criterion and one minor criterion**; or
2. **Three minor criteria**
Rejected
1. Firm alternate diagnosis explaining evidence of infective endocarditis; or
2. Resolution of infective endocarditis syndrome with antibiotic therapy for >4 d; or
3. No pathologic evidence of infective endocarditis at surgery or autopsy, with antibiotic therapy for >4 d; or
4. Does not meet criteria for possible infective endocarditis, as mentioned

[a]Modifications shown in boldface.
[b]See Table 12.11 for definitions of major and minor criteria.
From Li JS, Sexton DJ, Mick N, et al. Proposed modifications to the Duke criteria for the diagnosis of infective endocarditis. *Clin Infect Dis.* 2000;30(4):633-638, by permission of Oxford University Press.

first diagnostic test. TEE may be required for diagnosis in some patients, especially when TTE quality is poor. Serial echocardiography can follow the progression of vegetations, identify, and follow complications such as valvular insufficiency, valvular/myocardial abscess, pericardial effusion, and heart failure. The modified Duke criteria is a helpful guide to make a diagnosis in less obvious IE cases (Tables 12.10 and 12.11).

D. Treatment: Patients with acute IE are often critically ill. In addition to supportive care, early empiric antibiotics and prompt management of complications are crucial. Initial blood cultures must be obtained before the first dose of antibiotics. β-lactams should be used when possible, with vancomycin for MRSA or patients allergic/intolerant to β-lactams. Patients with endocarditis complicated by metastatic infection may require duration of therapies longer than the recommended durations. For treatment overview, see Table 12.12.

1. **Surgery:** Most cases of PVE and some cases of NVE require valve replacement or repair. Indications for surgery vary depending on the valve location, host factors, and metastatic sites of infection. Severe and refractory heart failure, acute severe valvular regurgitation or valve obstruction, IE due to fungi or resistant bacteria, multiple embolic events, and failure to clear bacteremia despite appropriate antibiotic therapy are common indications.

E. Complications of Infective Endocarditis

1. **Cardiac**
   - **a.** Valvular insufficiency and heart failure, the most common cause of death in IE
   - **b.** Myocardial and paravalvular abscess with heart block from paravalvular abscess
   - **c.** Obstruction. Rarely, large vegetations (usually caused by fungi) may cause obstruction.

TABLE 12.11 Definition of Terms Used in the Proposed Modified Duke Criteria for the Diagnosis of Infective Endocarditis (IE)[a]

Major criteria

Blood culture positive for IE

Typical microorganisms consistent with IE from two separate blood cultures:

- Viridans streptococci. *Streptococcus bovis,* **HACEK** group, *Staphylococcus aureus*; or
- Community-acquired enterococci, in the absence of a primary focus; or
- Microorganisms consistent with IE from persistently positive blood cultures, defined as follows:
  - At least two positive cultures of blood samples drawn >12 h apart; or
  - All of three or a majority of ≥4 separate cultures of blood (with first and last sample drawn at least 1 h apart)

Single positive blood culture for *Coxiella burnetii* or antiphase I IgG antibody titer >1:800

Evidence of endocardial involvement

- Oscillating intracardiac mass on valve or supporting structures, in the path of regurgitant jets, or on implanted material in the absence of an alternative anatomic explanation; or
- Abscess; or
- New partial dehiscence of prosthetic valve

New valvular regurgitation (worsening or changing of preexisting murmur not sufficient)

Minor criteria

Predisposition, predisposing heart condition, or injection drug use

Fever, temperature >100.4 °F (38 °C)

Vascular phenomena, major arterial emboli, septic pulmonary infarcts, mycotic aneurysm, intracranial hemorrhage, conjunctival hemorrhages, and Janeway lesions Immunologic phenomena: glomerulonephritis, Osler nodes, Roth spots, and rheumatoid factor

Microbiologic evidence: positive blood culture but does not meet a major criterion as noted earlier[b] or serologic evidence of active infection with organism consistent with IE

Echocardiographic minor criteria eliminated

HACEK, *Haemophilus* species, *Aggregatibacter* species, *Cardiobacterium hominis, Eikenella corrodens,* and *Kingella* species; IgG, immunoglobulin G; TEE, transesophageal echocardiography; TTE, transthoracic echocardiography.

[a]Modifications shown in boldface.

[b]Excludes single positive cultures for coagulase-negative staphylococci and organisms that do not cause endocarditis.

From Li JS, Sexton DJ, Mick N, et al. Proposed modifications to the Duke criteria for the diagnosis of infective endocarditis. *Clin Infect Dis.* 2000;30(4):633-638, by permission of Oxford University Press.

d. Purulent pericarditis, most commonly with IE due to *Staphylococcus* spp.

2. Extracardiac

a. Sepsis

b. Embolization causing ischemia, infarction, and abscess formation is common. Left-sided vegetations can embolize to the kidneys, brain, spleen, and heart. Right-sided vegetations embolize to the lungs, causing septic pulmonary emboli and abscess.

c. Mycotic aneurysms are friable and result from focal inflammatory blood vessel dilatation. CNS mycotic aneurysms can result in catastrophic hemorrhage.

d. Neurologic complications include meningitis, cerebritis, brain abscess, infarction, or hemorrhage.

e. Immune complex disease such as glomerulonephritis

f. Osteomyelitis and epidural abscess

TABLE 12.12 Treatment Recommendations for Native Valve and Prosthetic Valve Infective Endocarditis (IE)

Pathogens	Native valve IE Duration: 2-6 wk	Prosthetic valve IE Duration: 6 wk
Streptococci (PCN MIC) ≤0.12 μg/mL)	• **Penicillin G, ceftriaxone**, or vancomycin • *2 wk: gentamicin WITH penicillin G or ceftriaxone*	• **Penicillin G**[a], **ceftriaxone**[a], or vancomycin
Streptococci (PCN MIC >0.12 to <0.5 μg/mL)	• **Ceftriaxone** or vancomycin • *2 wk: gentamicin WITH penicillin G*	• **Gentamicin WITH penicillin G, ceftriaxone**, or vancomycin monotherapy
Streptococci (PCN MIC ≥0.5 μg/mL)[b,c]	• **Gentamicin WITH penicillin G or ceftriaxone**, or vancomycin monotherapy	
MSSA[d]	• **Nafcillin, oxacillin, or cefazolin**	• **High-dose rifampin po**[e] **WITH gentamicin**[j,k] **WITH nafcillin or oxacillin**
MRSA	• **Vancomycin or high-dose daptomycin**[f]	• **High-dose rifampin po**[e] **WITH gentamicin**[j,k] **WITH vancomycin**
Enterococci	• **High-dose ampicillin**[g] **WITH high-dose ceftriaxone**[h] • Gentamicin WITH ampicillin or penicillin G • Gentamicin WITH vancomycin[l]	
HACEK	• **Ceftriaxone, ciprofloxacin**, or high-dose ampicillin (confirm susceptibility)	
GNR	• **Gentamicin WITH β-lactam or high-dose ciprofloxacin**[i]	

Bolded, preferred therapies; *italicized*, 2-week treatment options; penicillin G dose is dependent on pathogen and minimum inhibitory concentration; consult pharmacy for appropriate gentamicin and vancomycin dosing per institution policies; all therapy options are intravenous (IV) unless specified as oral (po).

GNR, gram-negative rods; HACEK, *Haemophilus* species, *Aggregatibacter* species, *Cardiobacterium hominis*, *Eikenella corrodens*, and *Kingella* species; MIC, minimum inhibitory concentration; MRSA, methicillin-resistant *Staphylococcus aureus*; MSSA, methicillin-sensitive *Staphylococcus aureus*; PCN, penicillin.

[a]Adding gentamicin to penicillin G or ceftriaxone is optional.
[b]Duration determined by infectious disease (ID) consultant.
[c]Same treatment as native valve IE.
[d]Two weeks can be considered for uncomplicated right-sided native valve infections.
[e]High-dose rifampin po = 300 mg tid.
[f]High-dose daptomycin = 8-12 mg/kg/d
[g]High-dose ampicillin = 2 g q4h
[h]High-dose ceftriaxone = 2 g q12h
[i]High-dose ciprofloxacin = 400 mg IV q8h or 750 mg PO q12h
[j]Gentamicin for 2 weeks.
[k]If the organism is resistant to gentamicin, then an aminoglycoside to which it is susceptible to should be substituted for gentamicin. If the organism is resistant to all available aminoglycosides, a fluoroquinolone may be considered.
[l]Potential increased risk of toxicities with vancomycin-gentamicin combination. Consider combination for Enterococcus strains that are resistant to penicillin.

XII. MISCELLANEOUS INFECTIONS

A. Sinusitis: Sinusitis is a cause of fever in the ICU that is often overlooked and commonly occurs with prolonged use of nasogastric or nasotracheal tubes. Invasive fungal sinusitis may be seen in patients with prolonged neutropenia or poorly controlled diabetes.

1. **Microbiology:** *S. aureus* or gram-negative bacteria are most common. Invasive fungal sinusitis can be caused by *Mucor, Rhizopus, Aspergillus*, and *Fusarium* spp.
2. **Diagnosis** can be difficult and is often made by CT of the face and sinuses.
3. **Treatment** includes removal of nasal tubes to allow drainage of the obstructed sinus outflow tract, nasal humidification and decongestants, and antibacterial or antifungal agents to target likely pathogens. Invasive fungal sinusitis requires urgent surgical debridement.

B. Central Nervous System Infections

1. **Meningitis:** Most acute bacterial meningitis (ABM) is community acquired, although nosocomial meningitis can occur after neurosurgical intervention or skull base fracture. The meninges are infected by contiguous or hematogenous seeding, direct invasion, or extension following rupture of an abscess into the subarachnoid space.
   a. **Microbiology:** Many organisms cause meningitis and risk can be stratified by age. Community-acquired pathogens infecting all ages include *S. pneumoniae, H. influenzae*, and *Neisseria meningitidis. Listeria monocytogenes* is most common for those aged younger than 1 month or older than 50 years. Enteric and non-enteric gram-negative bacteria and *S. aureus* cause meningitis in patients undergoing trauma, neurosurgery, or are bacteremic. Meningitis associated with cerebrospinal fluid (CSF) shunts is most often caused by *S. epidermidis*.
   b. **Diagnosis:** Although the classic triad of fever, neck stiffness, and altered mental status is present in less than 50% of all ABM cases, if none are present, ABM can be ruled out with 99% certainty. Stroke, cranial nerve palsies, papilledema, seizures, and palpable purpura (in meningococcal ABM) may be accompanying clinical features. Physical exam signs, although specific, are highly insensitive. CSF must be tested for cell counts, glucose, protein, Gram stain, bacterial culture, acid-fast bacillus (AFB) smear, and mycobacterial and fungal cultures. Other CSF tests including cryptococcal antigen, the Venereal Disease Research Laboratory (VDRL), and herpes simplex virus PCR may be indicated depending on the clinical presentation, cell counts and chemistry results, and host factors. In patients suspected of having cerebral edema, a CT scan of the brain should be performed before the lumbar puncture. Blood cultures should be obtained before starting antibiotics, although the lumbar puncture must not delay the timely administration of antibiotics. Presence of high opening pressures, low glucose, raised protein, and high WBC count should raise suspicion for ABM.
   c. **Treatment:** Empiric IV antibiotics covering the broad spectrum of expected microbial etiologies must be administered within 1 hour of presentation with suspected ABM. Emergence of penicillin-resistant community-acquired pathogens has resulted in a shift in treatment to third-generation cephalosporins such as ceftriaxone. Vancomycin is often added to cover resistant pneumococci. When meningitis from *Listeria* spp. is a possibility, ampicillin (or trimethoprim/sulfamethoxazole or meropenem in patients allergic to penicillin) must be added. If nosocomial pathogens are suspected, ceftazidime, cefepime, or meropenem should be added to vancomycin to replace ceftriaxone, covering pseudomonas and resistant gram-negative bacteria. ABM is treated for 2 to 3 weeks. Dexamethasone should be administered before or at the time of administration of antibiotics only when the CSF Gram stain shows lancet-shaped diplococci indicating pneumococcal meningitis. Close contacts of patients with meningococcal meningitis must receive chemoprophylaxis (ciprofloxacin single dose or rifampin four doses over 2 days). Chemoprophylaxis should ideally be administered within 24 hours after onset of illness in an index patient. Chemoprophylaxis administered more than 14 days after initial onset is of limited value.

XIII. FUNGAL INFECTIONS

Fungi cause a wide spectrum of clinical disease in the critically ill; the severity and extent of infection is highly dependent on host immune factors. Infections range from minor skin and mucosal involvement to disseminated and invasive disease causing multi-organ failure.

A. Candida

1. *Candida* spp. are the most common cause of opportunistic fungal infections in ICUs. The incidence of candidal infections is increasing because of greater use of indwelling catheters, TPN, a higher proportion of patients who are immunocompromised, and high antibiotic use, eliminating normal bacterial flora and resulting in candidal overgrowth.
2. **Clinical manifestations**
   a. **Candiduria** is more often due to colonization of the urinary tract than infection. Pyuria can be a helpful indicator of infection. Persistent candiduria in the asymptomatic may be ignored but ultrasound or CT evaluation is recommended for those with diabetes, structural urinary tract abnormalities, and, in some cases, recipients of renal allografts. Candiduria should prompt indwelling urethral catheter replacement.
   b. **Mucocutaneous infections** include oropharyngeal candidiasis, esophagitis, GI candidiasis, vulvovaginitis, and intertrigo.
   c. **Candidemia** is serious and may disseminate to visceral organs including the eyes, cardiac valves, and indwelling devices. All indwelling urinary and vascular catheters in patients with candidemia should be removed.
   d. **Disseminated or invasive deep-organ infections** can result from hematogenous spread, direct extension, or local inoculation in patients with the risk factors described earlier. Diagnosis can be difficult because blood culture results are frequently negative and positive urine, sputum, and wound culture results may represent colonization or contamination. Definitive diagnosis of disseminated infection includes positive culture results from sterile sites, histologically demonstrated invasion, and endophthalmitis.
      i. Hepatosplenic candidiasis is rare, occurring almost exclusively in patients with currently or recently neutropenic hematologic malignancies. This difficult diagnosis is suggested by RUQ pain, fever, and elevated alkaline phosphatase, with or without characteristic CT or MRI findings. Diagnosis can also be made by liver biopsy.
      ii. Candidal peritonitis results from perforation of the intestines or stomach or infection via peritoneal dialysis catheter.
      iii. Cardiac candidiasis includes myocarditis, pericarditis, and endocarditis. Valvular vegetations can be quite large, with frequent and devastating major embolic events.
      iv. Renal candidiasis is an infection that ascends from the bladder, resulting in fungus balls and papillary necrosis, or from hematogenous seeding (usually bilateral).
      v. Disseminated candidiasis can also include the CNS and musculoskeletal systems.
3. **Treatment:** The choice of the antifungal agent is dependent on candida species, penetration, and concentration at infection site and relative toxicity.
   a. Candiduria is treated only in the presence of neutropenia, upper tract involvement, or periprocedurally for urinary tract interventions. Treatment consists of several days of oral or IV fluconazole or IV amphotericin deoxycholate. Echinocandins and liposomal amphotericin do not penetrate the urinary tract. Replacement of indwelling urinary catheters is always recommended.

b. Mucocutaneous candidiasis is treated with topical agents such as nystatin, clotrimazole, or miconazole. Systemic therapy with oral fluconazole may be needed when there is no response to topical therapy or mucosal involvement is deep and not easily accessible.
c. Candidemia is treated with systemic antifungal therapy. All blood isolates should be treated and not considered contaminants. Venous and arterial catheters should be replaced at new sites. Tunneled central venous lines may be preserved in the setting of uncomplicated infection unless the line is the source of candidemia and fails to clear with antifungals. Patients who are nonneutropenic and are clinically well may be treated with fluconazole or echinocandins (caspofungin, micafungin, or anidulafungin). Patients who are neutropenic are usually treated with liposomal amphotericin or an echinocandin. *Candida glabrata* and *C. krusei* are often resistant to fluconazole.
d. Disseminated candidiasis requires a combination of systemic antifungal therapy, drainage or debridement of infected areas, removal of intravascular catheters, and, sometimes, removal and replacement of infected foreign bodies. *Candida* spp. grown from the peritoneal cavity (ie, not just peritoneal drains) should be treated. Patients with candidemia should be evaluated for chorioretinitis, which is treated with parenteral fluconazole, voriconazole, or amphotericin but may require adjunctive intravitreal antifungal therapy and, sometimes, vitrectomy, if there is significant vitreal involvement.

B. Aspergillus-Related Illness in the ICU is usually invasive (often pulmonary or sinus) or disseminated infection in the immunocompromised. Angioinvasion and hemorrhage in cavitary disease are important causes of major hemoptysis requiring ICU support. Distinguishing colonization, indolent infection, and invasive aspergillosis can be difficult. Sputum culture results are neither sensitive nor specific for invasive aspergillosis. Histopathology or a combination of radiologic, culture, and serum or BAL galactomannan assay is needed to establish a high probability of invasive disease. Galactomannan from serum is more specific than that from sputum, and higher galactomannan levels indicate a higher probability of invasion.

1. Clinical manifestations

a. Invasive pulmonary disease presents with fever and pulmonary infiltrates in an immunocompromised host. Pathology reveals infarction, hemorrhage, and direct invasion of vessel walls by acute angle (45°) branching septate hyphae.
b. Dissemination to a variety of organs occurs because of vascular invasion and carries a very poor prognosis. Abscesses occur in the CNS, lung, liver, and myocardium.
c. Aspergillomas are fungus balls that occur in cavities usually in the upper lobes of the lungs, especially in bullae and occasionally in preexisting cavities. Patients present with cough, hemoptysis (which can be life-threatening), fever, and dyspnea and can occur in patients who are asymptomatic or immunocompetent. The symptomatic or immunocompromised may require surgical resection in conjunction with antifungal therapy.

2. Treatment

a. Voriconazole is the treatment of choice in confirmed invasive aspergillosis; however, posaconazole has been shown to be noninferior. Amphotericin may be used when there is azole intolerance or failure. Radiologic embolization may be necessary for massive hemoptysis. Surgical resection may be indicated when embolization fails or if systemic antifungal therapy fails to cure invasive disease.

XIV. VIRAL INFECTIONS

A. Cytomegalovirus (CMV) infection and disease are not synonymous. Positive serologies indicate infection, histopathologic inclusion bodies or immunohistochemical evidence of CMV in an end organ indicates disease. CMV infection can either be primary or more frequently secondary, often a reactivation of latent infection, which is common in the critically ill. The significance of CMV reactivation is unclear. True CMV infection is common in patients who are immunocompromised and is the commonest infection among recipients of solid-organ and hematopoietic cell transplants. High titers of viral DNA in CSF, blood, or BAL fluid may indicate end-organ disease, especially in patients undergoing a transplant.

1. CMV disease in the immunocompromised may manifest as pneumonitis, hepatitis, colitis, or retinitis (sometimes with CNS involvement).
2. **Treatment**: Viremia in patients undergoing transplants is preemptively treated with oral valganciclovir or IV ganciclovir to prevent transformation to CMV disease, which can be devastating. Ganciclovir is the treatment of choice for CMV disease in recipients of organ transplant. Foscarnet is used when there is ganciclovir intolerance or resistance. IV CMV immunoglobulin may be added for life-threatening CMV infection (such as pneumonitis). Ganciclovir and foscarnet are both used to treat CMV retinitis. Neutropenia is common with ganciclovir and valganciclovir; however, it is not dose-dependent. Lowering doses to minimize toxicities is discouraged due to concern for developing resistance. Foscarnet is associated with dose-dependent toxicities including renal failure. Adequate hydration should be encouraged if able to tolerate.

B. Herpes Simplex Virus I and II

1. **Manifestations** of herpes simplex virus (HSV) infection include the following:
   - **a.** Mucocutaneous and genital disease
   - **b.** Esophagitis
   - **c.** Respiratory tract infection including tracheobronchitis and pneumonia
   - **d.** Ocular infection such as blepharitis, conjunctivitis, keratitis, corneal ulceration, and blindness
   - **e.** Encephalitis and meningitis
2. **Disseminated HSV infection** occurs in patients who are highly immunocompromised, manifesting as necrotizing hepatitis, pneumonitis, hematogenously spread cutaneous lesions, fever, hypotension, disseminated intravascular coagulation, and CNS involvement.
3. **Diagnosis:** Tzanck smear of lesion scrapings is insensitive. Viral culture, histology, and DNA or immunostaining of viral antigens from lesions or tissue are other diagnostic tests. HSV DNA testing on CSF is sensitive and specific for HSV meningoencephalitis.
4. **Treatment**
   - **a.** Severe HSV infections, including encephalitis, pneumonitis, and disseminated HSV, are treated with IV acyclovir. Foscarnet may be used to treat acyclovir-resistant HSV.
   - **b.** Mucosal, cutaneous, and genital infections may be treated with acyclovir, famciclovir, or valacyclovir. Normal hosts do not always require treatment, but antivirals should be considered for the critically ill even when not classically immunocompromised.
   - **c.** Ocular infections should be managed with topical antivirals in consultation with an ophthalmologist.

C. Varicella Zoster Virus (VZV) can manifest as primary (chicken pox) or reactivation (herpes zoster or shingles) infection and causes mild to life-threatening disease.

1. Primary VZV infection in adults may have severe systemic effects and pulmonary involvement causing respiratory failure. Patients who are immunocompromised are prone to severe systemic disease with lungs, kidneys, CNS, and liver involvement.
2. Herpes zoster usually manifests as a dermatomal cutaneous infection from reactivation of VZV that has been dormant in the sensory ganglia. Multidermatomal or midline-crossing infection is considered disseminated and occurs in patients who are immunocompromised. Rarely, reactivated herpes zoster causes CNS diseases such as encephalitis and cerebral vasculitis.
3. **Treatment:** IV acyclovir is used for serious VZV infection (pneumonia, encephalitis).

D. **Severe Influenza:** Influenza A and B viruses are responsible for a spectrum of respiratory illnesses that manifest as large pandemics or seasonal outbreaks, especially in the Northern Hemisphere winter months. Antigenic shifts and human-swine-avian strains (eg, hemagglutinin type 1 and neuraminidase type 1 [H1N1]) have caused several pandemics. Sporadic cases may be seen year-round.

1. The virus can cause primary viral pneumonia with a high incidence of ARDS. Secondary bacterial CAP can also occur. *S. pneumoniae* is the commonest cause of postinfluenza CAP but there is an increasing proportion caused by *S. aureus*. Nonpulmonary manifestations are rare and include encephalitis, transverse myelitis, Guillain-Barré syndrome, rhabdomyolysis, and myopericarditis.
2. **Risk factors for influenza complications** include age 65 years and older, pregnancy, asthma, heart disease, stroke, diabetes, HIV/AIDS, and cancer.
3. **Diagnosis:** PCR or rapid antigen detection in nasal swabs. Enzyme-linked immune assay (EIA) has a low sensitivity and is an acceptable initial screening modality but cannot be used to rule out disease. PCR has the highest sensitivity and specificity and should be used for diagnosis whenever possible. BAL sampling may be necessary when there is a strong suspicion of influenza but PCR testing is negative on nasal swab.
4. **Treatment:** The general principles of treatment of acute respiratory failure and ARDS apply. Refer to **Chapter 20** for ARDS management.
   a. **Antiviral therapy:** Severe and complicated confirmed or suspected influenza cases (including patients in the ICU) should be treated with antiviral therapy regardless of symptom duration. Treatment options include oral oseltamivir 75 mg twice a day for 5 days, a one-time dose of inhaled zanamivir 10 mg, or a one-time dose of IV peramivir 600 mg. Inhaled zanamivir may be considered in oseltamivir-resistant cases. Patients who are immunocompromised and severely ill may benefit from a longer duration though optimal duration remains uncertain.

E. **SARS-CoV-2** causes COVID-19 disease. SARS-CoV-2 emerged in late 2019 and rapidly spread, leading to a pandemic. It commonly manifests as primary viral pneumonia with a high incidence of ARDS.

1. **Risk factors for severe disease** include older age; diabetes; immunocompromise; cancer; chronic lung, heart, or liver disease; overweight and obesity; pregnancy; and stroke; among others.
2. Secondary bacterial infection is less common than with influenza but can occur.
3. **Diagnosis:** PCR or rapid antigen detection in nasal swabs. BAL sampling may be necessary when there is a strong suspicion of influenza but PCR test result is negative on nasal swab.
4. **Treatment:** The general principles of treatment of acute respiratory failure and ARDS apply. Refer to **Chapter 20** for ARDS management.

a. **Targeted therapy:** Clinical trials are ongoing and clinical practice is evolving rapidly. Currently recommended treatment is dexamethasone for 10 days and remdesivir for 5 days in patients requiring supplemental oxygen. Some patients in the ICU may also benefit from tocilizumab. Convalescent plasma may be given to those who are immunocompromised. Vaccination is strongly recommended once the patient is clinically stable.

XV. MISCELLANEOUS INFECTIONS

A. **Multidrug-Resistant Bacterial Infections:** Multidrug-resistant (MDR) infections are a global crisis resulting from widespread antimicrobial use with insufficient stewardship. Bacterial isolates are labeled MDR based on susceptibility to key antimicrobial agents using prespecified minimum inhibitory concentration (MIC) or disk-diffusion diameter cutoffs. Molecular testing may identify genes coding for enzymes that confer resistance. Most MDR infections are caused by enteric gram-negatives (*E. coli, Klebsiella* and *Proteus* spp., etc), non-enteric gram-negatives (*P. aeruginosa, Stenotrophomonas, Acinetobacter*), and VRE.

a. **Treatment** options vary depending on available resources and include prolonged β-lactam infusions as monotherapy or in combination with aminoglycosides. Newer β-lactam/β-lactam inhibitor combinations and cephalosporins including ceftolozane/tazobactam, ceftazidime/avibactam, imipenem/relebactam, meropenem/vaborbactam, and cefiderocol can also be used in consultation with local infectious disease providers, pharmacists, and antimicrobial stewardship teams.

b. **VRE treatment** options include daptomycin, linezolid, tigecycline, and oritavancin. Tetracyclines have inadequate serum and urine concentrations and are not recommended as monotherapy when treating active infections at these noted sites.

c. **Bacteriophage therapy** is a remodernized treatment option originally developed in the 1920s. "Phage" therapy may be considered in select cases of pan-resistant infections. This novel therapy utilizes viruses to target specific bacterial hosts, disrupting their replication cycle and lysing bacterial cells. Theoretical benefits include lack of cross-resistance with antimicrobial therapy and less collateral damage to the host microbiome given highly specific bacterial targets. Limitations to consider include the need for multiple phages to target polymicrobial infections and development of phage-resistant infections. Phage therapy is currently experimental and requires U.S. Food and Drug Administration (FDA) approval through compassionate use. Expanded use is limited by the long lead time to obtain targeted therapy, high cost, and undetermined long-term benefits.

Selected Readings

Alhazzani W, Møller MH, Arabi YM, et al. Surviving sepsis campaign: guidelines on the management of critically ill adults with coronavirus disease 2019 (COVID-19). *Crit Care Med.* 2020;48(6):e440-e469.

Angus DC, van der Poll T. Severe sepsis and septic shock. *N Engl J Med.* 2013;369:2063.

Baddour LM, Wilson WR, Bayer AS, et al. Infective endocarditis in adults: diagnosis, antimicrobial therapy, and management of complications: a scientific statement for healthcare professionals from the American Heart Association. *Circulation.* 2015;132(15):1435-1486.

Baddour LM, Wilson WR, Bayer AS, et al. Infective endocarditis: diagnosis, antimicrobial therapy, and management of complications: a statement for healthcare professionals from the Committee on Rheumatic Fever, Endocarditis, and Kawasaki Disease, Council on Cardiovascular Disease in the Young, and the Councils on Clinical Cardiology, Stroke, and Cardiovascular Surgery and Anesthesia, American Heart Association: endorsed by the Infectious Diseases Society of America. *Circulation.* 2005;111(23):e394-e434.

Caironi P, Tognoni G, Masson S, et al. Albumin replacement in patients with severe sepsis or septic shock. *N Engl J Med.* 2014;370:1412-1421.

Centers for Disease Control and Prevention. 2014 HAI progress report. Accessed June 27, 2021. https://www.cdc.gov/hai/data/archive/2014-progress-report.html

Centers for Disease Control and Prevention. Current HAI progress report. Accessed June 27, 2021. https://www.cdc.gov/hai/data/portal/progress-report.html

Centers for Disease Control and Prevention. Meningococcal disease. https://www.cdc.gov/infectioncontrol/guidelines/healthcare-personnel/selected-infections/meningococcal-disease.html#:~:text=Chemoprophylaxis%20is%20administered%20as%20soon,identification%20of%20an%20index%20patient.&text=Chemoprophylaxis%20administered%20more%20than%2014,of%20limited%20or%20no%20value.

Christie A, Mbaeyi SA, Walensky RP. CDC interim recommendations for fully vaccinated people: an important first step. *JAMA.* 2021;325(15):1501-1502.

Cohen J, Vincent JL, Adhikari NK, et al. Sepsis: a roadmap for future research. *Lancet Infect Dis.* 2015;15:581-614.

De Backer D, Biston P, Devriendt J, et al. Comparison of dopamine and norepinephrine in the treatment of shock. *N Engl J Med.* 2010;362:779-789.

Evans LE, Rhodes A, Alhazzani W, et al. Surviving sepsis campaign: international guidelines for management of sepsis and septic shock 2021. *Crit Care Med.* 2021;49(11):e1063-e1143.

Holst LB, Haase N, Wetterslev J, et al. Lower versus higher hemoglobin threshold for transfusion in septic shock. *N Engl J Med.* 2014;371:1381-1391.

Honein MA, Christie A, Rose DA, et al. Summary of guidance for public health strategies to address high levels of community transmission of SARS-CoV-2 and related deaths, December 2020. *MMWR Morb Mortal Wkly Rep.* 2020;69(49):1860-1867.

Johnson S, Lavergne V, Skinner AM, et al. Clinical practice guidelines by the Infectious Diseases Society of America (IDSA) and Society for Healthcare Epidemiology of America (SHEA): 2021 focused update guidelines on management of *Clostridioides difficile* infection in adults. *Clin Infect Dis* 2021;73(5):e1029-e1044.

Kalil A, Metersky M, Klompas M, et al. Management of adults with hospital-acquired and ventilator-associated pneumonia: 2016 clinical practice guidelines by the Infectious Diseases Society of America and the American Thoracic Society. *Clin Infect Dis.* 63(5):e51-e111.

Kaukonen KM, Bailey M, Pilcher D, et al. Systemic inflammatory response syndrome criteria in defining severe sepsis. *N Engl J Med.* 2015;372:1629-1638.

Kelly CR, Fischer M, Allegretti JR, et al. ACG Clinical guidelines: prevention, diagnosis, and treatment of *Clostridioides difficile* infections. *Am J Gastroenterol.* 2021;116(6):1124-1147.

Maertens JA, Rahav G, Lee DG, et al. Posaconazole versus voriconazole for primary treatment of invasive aspergillosis: a phase 3, randomised, controlled, non-inferiority trial. *The Lancet.* 2021;397(10273):499-509.

Martin GS, Mannino DM, Eaton S, et al. The epidemiology of sepsis in the United States from 1979 through 2000. *N Engl J Med.* 2003;348:1546-1554.

Metlay JP, Waterer GW, Long AC, et al. Diagnosis and treatment of adults with community-acquired pneumonia. An official clinical practice guideline of the American Thoracic Society and Infectious Diseases Society of America. *Am J Respir Crit Care Med.* 2019;200(7):e45-e67.

Mouncey PR, Osborn TM, Power GS, et al. Trial of early, goal-directed resuscitation for septic shock. *N Engl J Med.* 2015;372:1301-1311.

Peake SL, Delaney A, Bailey M, et al. Goal-directed resuscitation for patients with early septic shock. *N Engl J Med.* 2014;371:1496-1506.

Russell JA, Walley KR, Singer J, et al. Vasopressin versus norepinephrine infusion in patients with septic shock. *N Engl J Med* 2008;358:877–887.

Solomkin JS, Mazuski JE, Bradley JS, et al. Diagnosis and management of complicated intra-abdominal infection in adults and children: guidelines by the Surgical Infection Society and the Infectious Diseases Society of America. *Clin Infect Dis.* 2010;50(2):133-164.

Tamma PD, Aitken SL, Bonomo RA, et al. Infectious Diseases Society of America guidance on the treatment of extended-spectrum β-lactamase producing Enterobacterales (ESBL-E), Carbapenem-Resistant Enterobacterales (CRE), and *Pseudomonas aeruginosa* with Difficult-to-Treat Resistance (DTR-*P. aeruginosa*). *Clin Infect Dis.* 2021;72(7):e169-e183.

Yealy DM, Kellum JA, Huang DT, et al. A randomized trial of protocol-based care for early septic shock. *N Engl J Med.* 2014;370:1683-1693.

13 Critical Care Management of COVID-19

Rachel C. Frank and Dusan Hanidziar

I. BACKGROUND

A subset of patients with COVID-19 become critically ill and need intensive care unit (ICU) care for close monitoring and physiologic support (eg, mechanical ventilation, hemodynamic support, renal replacement therapy [RRT]). Although the primary reason for admission to the ICU is typically acute hypoxemic respiratory failure due to severe pneumonia or acute respiratory distress syndrome (ARDS), patients may also develop hypotension; shock; new neurologic, cardiac, hepatic, gastrointestinal, or renal dysfunction; thromboembolic complications; and superimposed bacterial infections. Multiorgan dysfunction is the result of direct cytopathic effects of the SARS-CoV-2 virus, dysregulated inflammatory responses, dysregulated coagulation, and endothelial dysfunction. Patients older than 65 and patients with certain comorbidities (obesity, diabetes, hypertension, chronic kidney disease, cancer) are at the highest risk for becoming critically ill from COVID-19. Those critically ill with COVID-19 ARDS commonly have prolonged ICU and hospital stays, and survivors may experience long-term sequelae (eg, chronic lung disease, neuromuscular weakness, cognitive dysfunction).

II. MULTIORGAN INVOLVEMENT

A. Neurologic: Encephalopathy, delirium, and coma are common findings in patients with COVID-19 ARDS who are mechanically ventilated. Abnormal electroencephalogram (EEG) patterns (eg, diffuse slowing, burst suppression, discontinuous EEG) were reported in such patients in the ICU and attributed to critical illness itself as well as to the exposure to high doses of sedatives. Acute stroke, seizures, and Guillain–Barré syndrome are less common. However, the broad spectrum of neurologic complications highlights the need to perform awakening trials and neurologic exams in patients who are mechanically ventilated every day when clinically appropriate to allow for prompt detection and treatment of these complications.

B. Respiratory: Pneumonia is the most common manifestation in patients with severe COVID-19, progressing further into ARDS in a subset of patients. Hypoxemic respiratory failure is caused by impaired ventilation-perfusion matching due to inflammatory infiltrates, edema, and microvascular thromboses in the lung. Increased dead-space fraction, inflammation, and metabolic acidosis (due to renal and/or liver failure) increase respiratory drive and patients commonly present with tachypnea. The progression to ARDS worsens lung compliance, increases work of breathing, and ultimately produces respiratory muscle fatigue. Patients presenting with both severe hypoxemia and excessive respiratory effort need prompt institution of mechanical ventilation.

C. Cardiovascular: Cardiac complications in severe COVID-19 include myocardial injury, heart failure, arrhythmias, and cardiogenic shock. Acute myocardial injury (defined as the rise of the troponin level above the 99th percentile followed by a subsequent fall) is common and has been associated with higher age, comorbidities, and multisystem organ failure. The most common cause of acute myocardial injury is Type 2 myocardial infarction (MI; related to supply-demand mismatch in the setting of infection and critical illness).

Tachyarrhythmias (sinus tachycardia, atrial arrhythmias, ventricular tachycardia) are more common than bradyarrhythmias; however, both have been described in patients with COVID-19. Electrocardiographic (ECG) abnormalities occur frequently, including prolongation of QT intervals and ST-segment changes (T-wave inversions, elevations). Findings on ECG indicative of right ventricular (RV) strain may occur in the setting of hypoxemic respiratory failure and acute rise in pulmonary vascular resistance; however, diagnostic testing for pulmonary embolism should also be considered. ST-segment elevations in a vascular distribution (eg, left anterior descending [LAD]) are suggestive of ST-segment elevation myocardial infarction (STEMI; with differential diagnosis including vasospasm), whereas more diffuse elevations can be seen in myocarditis or stress cardiomyopathy. Myocarditis and new-onset heart failure were also described in COVID-19 infection and sometimes can lead to cardiogenic shock. Urgent echocardiography in the ICU can be helpful to distinguish the different clinical entities in patients who are hemodynamically unstable.

D. Hepatobiliary: Aminotransferase (aspartate aminotransferase [AST], alanine aminotransferase [ALT]) elevation is a common finding in severe COVID-19 and the etiology is most often multifactorial (medications, inflammation, hepatic congestion with RV failure). Gallbladder distension and inflammation were reported in patients who were mechanically ventilated.

E. Gastrointestinal: Ileus and tube feed intolerance are common in patients with COVID-19 who are mechanically ventilated. Mesenteric ischemia and bowel necrosis need to be suspected in patients with acute clinical deterioration (eg, worsening hypotension, leukocytosis, metabolic acidosis).

F. Renal: Acute kidney injury in COVID-19 is typically multifactorial and can be a result of hypovolemia and aggressive diuresis, hypotension, nephrotoxic drugs, intravenous contrast, endothelial dysfunction, and inflammation and is associated with increased mortality. A proportion of patients require RRT.

G. Hematologic: Severe COVID-19 has been associated with several hematologic abnormalities including lymphopenia, thrombocytopenia, fibrinogen elevation, and D-dimer elevation. Prothrombotic state in severe COVID-19 manifests as increased rates of deep vein thrombosis (DVT), pulmonary embolism, and arterial thrombosis.

III. INTENSIVE CARE UNIT MANAGEMENT

A. Criteria for Admission to the Intensive Care Unit: Major criteria for ICU admission are the need for invasive mechanical ventilation and need for vasopressor support. Patients considered at high risk for needing intubation, for example, those with tachypnea (respiratory rate [RR] >30/min), receiving oxygen via high-flow nasal cannula (HFNC), or undergoing a trial of noninvasive positive pressure ventilation (NIPPV), should also be treated in the ICU.

B. Sedation and Analgesia: Sedation and analgesia are administered in patients with COVID-19 who are mechanically ventilated to alleviate anxiety, potential discomfort, and pain. The 2018 PADIS (*P*ain, *A*gitation/Sedation, *D*elirium, *I*mmobility, and *S*leep Disruption) guidelines by the Society of Critical Care Medicine recommended that light levels of sedation are maintained whenever feasible. Such a practice facilitates ventilator weaning, extubation, and early mobilization. However, multiple studies during the COVID-19 pandemic documented that the doses of sedatives in patients with COVID-19 ARDS were excessive, leading to high rates of coma and delirium. The excessive sedation may have been administered in an effort to suppress respiratory drive, because of concerns about patient safety (prone positioning) or staff safety (potential virus exposure with inadvertent extubations). In a subset of patients who also receive neuromuscular blockade, deep levels of sedation need to be administered to prevent awareness.

C. Respiratory Support

1. **High-flow nasal cannula (HFNC):** HFNC should be trialed in patients with hypoxemic respiratory failure due to COVID-19 when conventional oxygen supplementation is not sufficient to maintain adequate oxygenation (Spo_2 >90%). HFNC may reduce the need for intubation in a subset of patients by improving respiratory mechanics and gas exchange. When patients treated with HFNC oxygen continue to have tachypnea, respiratory distress, and recurrent episodes of desaturations, mechanical ventilation should be initiated.
2. **Noninvasive positive pressure ventilation (NIPPV):** A trial of continuous positive airway pressure (CPAP) or bilevel positive pressure ventilation (BiPAP) should be considered when conventional oxygen delivery is not sufficient to maintain target Spo_2 and when patients are thought to benefit from enhanced respiratory support with higher levels of positive end-expiratory pressure (PEEP; eg, chronic obstructive pulmonary disease [COPD], congestive heart failure [CHF], obstructive sleep apnea [OSA]). There is a need for close monitoring to recognize dyssynchrony, leaks, excessive tidal volumes, and NIPPV intolerance.
3. **Invasive mechanical ventilation:** The indication for invasive mechanical ventilation is to decrease the work of breathing and to ensure adequate oxygenation and ventilation when noninvasive support (eg, HFNC, BiPAP) is inadequate. In all patients with COVID-19 ARDS, lung-protective ventilation should be delivered and can be typically achieved by targeting low tidal volumes (6 mL or less per kg of predicted body weight [PBW]), plateau pressures less than or equal to 30 cm H_2O, and driving pressures less than 15 cm H_2O. Individualized adjustments of inspiratory flow and inspiratory time on mechanical ventilator may be needed to match the patient's respiratory drive and thereby minimize ventilator dyssynchrony. In patients with severely impaired oxygenation (Pao_2/Fio_2 <150), an individualized PEEP titration should be performed and additional interventions such as proning, neuromuscular blockade, and inhaled pulmonary vasodilators considered.

D. Hemodynamic Monitoring and Support

Patients with severe COVID-19 who are mechanically ventilated may require invasive hemodynamic monitoring and hemodynamic support with vasopressors/inotropes because of hypotension or shock.

1. **Arterial line:** Placement is helpful for frequent arterial blood gas analysis in patients with ARDS and precise blood pressure monitoring in patients receiving vasoactive infusions.
2. **Central venous catheter (CVC):** CVC placement is needed in patients requiring prolonged infusions of vasopressors/inotropes.
3. **Pulmonary artery catheter (PAC):** PAC placement should be considered in patients with undifferentiated shock and worsening markers of perfusion (lactate, base deficit).
4. **Vasopressors:** Norepinephrine is the first-line vasopressor of choice for patients with septic shock due to COVID-19. Once moderate doses of norepinephrine are reached, addition of vasopressin as a second-line vasopressor can be considered. In the setting of acute RV failure, inotropic support with epinephrine may be required.
5. **Vasodilators:** Inhaled nitric oxide is a selective pulmonary artery vasodilator and remains an option for refractory hypoxemia to improve ventilation/perfusion (V/Q) matching and reduce pulmonary vascular resistance in patients with RV failure.

E. Extracorporeal Membrane Oxygenation

1. **Venovenous (V-V) extracorporeal membrane oxygenation (ECMO):** V-V ECMO is utilized in patients with refractory hypoxemia and/or hypercapnia that persists despite mechanical ventilator optimization and utilization of rescue therapies. The initiation criteria and availability are institution dependent.

A typical approach is the prioritization of patients with the best chance of long-term survival. Consideration for ECMO initiation includes factors such as age, duration of COVID-19 infection (and mechanical ventilation), body mass index (BMI), concomitant renal dysfunction, and bleeding risk. Current Extracorporeal Life Support Organization (ELSO) recommendations for initiation of V-V ECMO in COVID-19 include the following:

- Pa_{O_2}/F_{IO_2} less than 60 mm Hg for more than 6 hours or less than 50 mm Hg for more than 3 hours.
- pH less than 7.2 with CO_2 greater than 80 mm Hg for more than 6 hours (aiming for plateau pressure <30 cm H_2O).

In a multicenter study, in-hospital mortality in patients with COVID-19 requiring V-V ECMO was 37%.

2. **Venoarterial (V-A) ECMO**: V-A ECMO can be considered in patients with COVID-19 having severe cardiac (RV, LV, or biventricular) dysfunction. The ELSO recommends consideration of V-A ECMO in patients with hypotension (systolic blood pressure [SBP] <90 mm Hg) or cardiac index less than 2.2 L/min/m^2 while receiving norepinephrine greater than 0.5 μg/kg/min, dobutamine greater than 20 μg/kg/min, or an equivalent. However, there is institutional variability in criteria for V-A ECMO initiation and familiarity with institutional protocols is necessary.

F. Renal Replacement Therapy

Continuous venovenous hemofiltration (CVVH) is the preferred method of RRT in patients with COVID-19 ARDS and hypotension requiring vasopressors. The indications are similar to that of other patients who are critically ill and include volume overload, uremia, metabolic acidosis, or hyperkalemia.

G. Antivirals

1. Remdesivir

Remdesivir is indicated in patients who are hospitalized early in the course of the disease (eg, in patients who receive supplemental oxygen via nasal cannula or HFNC). Once patients require mechanical ventilation (later stages of the disease), immunomodulatory agents play a more important role in improving outcomes.

H. Immunomodulatory Agents

1. Corticosteroids

In patients with severe COVID-19, a 10-day course of dexamethasone at 6 mg daily was shown to reduce mortality.

2. Interleukin 6 (IL-6) inhibitors

A single intravenous dose of tocilizumab (anti–IL-6 receptor monoclonal antibody) can be used as an adjunct to dexamethasone in patients with severe COVID-19 and preferably administered early in their ICU admission (first 24-48 hours).

3. Janus kinase (JAK) inhibitors

Oral baricitinib (JAK 1 and JAK 2 inhibitor) modulates downstream inflammatory cellular signaling and can be used as an alternative to IL-6 antagonists.

I. Drugs Targeting Coagulation

1. Heparin
   a. Patients in the ICU should receive appropriate anticoagulation for DVT prophylaxis, with either unfractionated heparin or low-molecular-weight heparin.
   b. In the critically ill, therapeutic anticoagulation was not associated with survival to hospital discharge or avoidance of cardiovascular or pulmonary organ support and was associated with an increased risk of bleeding events. Therapeutic anticoagulation may need to be administered for other indications (eg, for atrial fibrillation, pulmonary embolism, or DVT).

IV. LONG-TERM SEQUELAE OF SEVERE COVID-19

A. Pulmonary: Prolonged pulmonary dysfunction and pulmonary structural abnormalities have been identified in a subset of survivors of severe COVID-19. The most common functional changes include impaired diffusing lung capacity for carbon monoxide (DLCO) and restrictive pulmonary impairment. The most common computed tomography (CT) imaging abnormalities at 1 year after severe infection are ground-glass opacities, fibrotic-like changes, bronchiectasis, interlobular septal thickening, and air trapping; and these changes are estimated to be present in at least one-third of survivors. The most common associated symptom is dyspnea.

B. Extrapulmonary: Similar to survivors of ARDS from other causes, survivors of COVID-19 ARDS commonly experience neuromuscular weakness, fatigue, abnormal sleep, pain (myalgias, arthralgias), and neuropsychiatric problems.

V. PREVENTING INFECTION IN THE INTENSIVE CARE UNIT

A. Personal Protective Equipment (PPE): ICU staff members caring for patients with confirmed or suspected COVID-19 are required to use PPE, which includes an N95 respirator, protective eyewear (face shield, goggles), gloves, and a disposable gown. A proper technique of donning and doffing of PPE is critical to prevent the infection of ICU staff.

B. Enhanced Respiratory Isolation (ERI): COVID-19 polymerase chain reaction (PCR) testing in patients with COVID-19 in the ICU is performed every 3 days with nasopharyngeal swab samples. After the first negative result, an additional negative result obtained at least 24 hours later is required to discontinue ERI. In patients who are intubated, one of these two tests must be performed on a lower respiratory tract sample (endotracheal aspirate or bronchoalveolar lavage). National and institutional guidelines for discontinuation of precautions may vary.

Selected Readings

Alhazzani W, Evans L, Alshamsi F, et al. Surviving sepsis campaign guidelines on the management of adults with coronavirus disease 2019 (COVID-19) in the ICU: first update. *Crit Care Med.* 2021;49(3):e219-e234.

Attaway AH, Scheraga RG, Bhimraj A, Biehl M, Hatipoğlu U. Severe covid-19 pneumonia: pathogenesis and clinical management. *BMJ.* 2021;372:n436.

Barbaro RP, MacLaren G, Boonstra PS, et al.; Extracorporeal Life Support Organization. Extracorporeal membrane oxygenation support in COVID-19: an international cohort study of the Extracorporeal Life Support Organization registry [published correction appears in *Lancet.* 2020 Oct 10;396(10257):1070]. *Lancet.* 2020;396(10257):1071-1078. doi:10.1016/S0140-6736(20)32008-0

Beigel JH, Tomashek KM, Dodd LE, et al.; ACTT-1 Study Group Members. Remdesivir for the treatment of Covid-19—final report. *N Engl J Med.* 2020;383(19):1813-1826.

Chanques G, Constantin JM, Devlin JW, et al. Analgesia and sedation in patients with ARDS. *Intensive Care Med.* 2020;46(12):2342-2356.

Conway EM, Mackman N, Warren RQ, et al. Understanding COVID-19-associated coagulopathy. *Nat Rev Immunol.* 2022;22(10):639-649.

Dangayach NS, Newcombe V, Sonnenville R. Acute neurologic complications of COVID-19 and postacute sequelae of COVID-19. *Crit Care Clin.* 2022;38(3):553-570.

Farshidfar F, Koleini N, Ardehali H. Cardiovascular complications of COVID-19. *JCI Insight.* 2021;6(13):e148980.

Gorman EA, O'Kane CM, McAuley DF. Acute respiratory distress syndrome in adults: diagnosis, outcomes, long-term sequelae, and management. *Lancet.* 2022;400(10358):1157-1170.

Grasselli G, Scaravilli V, Mangioni D, et al. Hospital-acquired infections in critically ill patients with COVID-19. *Chest.* 2021:160(2):454-465.

Hanidziar D, Bittner EA. Sedation of Mechanically Ventilated COVID-19 Patients: Challenges and Special Considerations. *Anesth Analg.* 2020;131(1):e40-e41.

INSPIRATION Investigators; Sadeghipour P, Talasaz AH, Rashidi F, et al. Effect of intermediate-dose vs standard-dose prophylactic anticoagulation on thrombotic events, extracorporeal membrane oxygenation treatment, or mortality among patients with

COVID-19 admitted to the intensive care unit: the INSPIRATION randomized clinical trial. *JAMA*. 2021;325(16):1620-1630.

Kaafarani HMA, El Moheb M, Hwabejire JO, et al. Gastrointestinal complications in critically ill patients with COVID-19. *Ann Surg*. 2020;272(2):e61-e62.

Kalil AC, Patterson TF, Mehta AK, et al.; ACTT-2 Study Group Members. Baricitinib plus remdesivir for hospitalized adults with Covid-19. *N Engl J Med*. 2021;384(9):795-807.

Kanne JP, Little BP, Schulte JJ, Haramati A, Haramati LB. Long-term lung abnormalities associated with COVID-19 pneumonia. *Radiology*. 2022;221806.

Lamers MM, Haagmans BL. SARS-CoV-2 pathogenesis. *Nat Rev Microbiol*. 2022;20(5):270-284.

Long B, Brady WJ, Bridwell RE, et al. Electrocardiographic manifestations of COVID-19. *Am J Emerg Med*. 2021;41:96-103.

Metkus TS, Sokoll LJ, Barth AS, et al. Myocardial Injury in severe COVID-19 compared with non-COVID-19 acute respiratory distress syndrome. *Circulation*. 2021;143(6):553-565.

NIH—COVID-19 Treatment Guidelines. Critical care for adults. https://www.covid19treatmentguidelines.nih.gov/management/critical-care-for-adults/

Pun BT, Badenes R, Heras La Calle G, et al. Prevalence and risk factors for delirium in critically ill patients with COVID-19 (COVID-D): a multicentre cohort study. *Lancet Respir Med*. 2021;9(3):239-250.

RECOVERY Collaborative Group; Horby P, Lim WS, Emberson JR, et al. Dexamethasone in hospitalized patients with Covid-19. *N Engl J Med*. 2021;384(8):693-704.

The REMAP-CAP, ACTIV-4a, ATTACC Investigators. Therapeutic anticoagulation with heparin in critically ill patients with Covid-19. *N Engl J Med*. 2021;385:777-789.

The REMAP-CAP Investigators; Gordon AC, Mouncey PR, Al-Beidh F, et al. Interleukin-6 receptor antagonists in critically ill patients with Covid-19. *N Engl J Med*. 2021;384(16):1491-1502.

Sullivan ZP, Zazzeron L, Berra L, Hess DR, Bittner EA, Chang MG. Noninvasive respiratory support for COVID-19 patients: when, for whom, and how? *J Intensive Care*. 2022;10(1):3.

Tisminetzky M, Ferreyro BL, Fan E. Extracorporeal membrane oxygenation in COVID-19. *Crit Care Clin*. 2022;38(3):535-552.

Weeks LD, Sylvester KW, Connors JM, Connell NT. Management of therapeutic unfractionated heparin in COVID-19 patients: a retrospective cohort study. *Res Pract Thromb Haemost*. 2021;5:e12521.

14 Transporting the Patient Who Is Critically Ill

Zachary P. Sullivan and Ilan Mizrahi

I. INTRODUCTION

Critically ill patients often require transfer between or within hospitals when advanced levels of care, diagnostics, and/or procedures are required. The anticipated benefits of relocating a critically ill patient must be weighed against the potential risks involved with the transfer. When conducted in a stepwise, protocolized, and thoughtful fashion, transport of critically ill patients can be done safely. Oras et al found no difference in 90-day mortality between critically ill patients who required interhospital transport due to intensive care unit (ICU) bed shortage compared to those who did not require transport. Generally speaking, there are two types of patient transport.

A. Interhospital Transport refers to the relocation of a patient from one health care institution to another in order to provide more timely or additional specialized care. Issues associated with air transport and specialized teams are covered later in this chapter. Many of the principles of interhospital transfer may be applied to intrahospital transport.

1. **Stages of Transport:** Bourn et al outline six pertinent stages of the interhospital transport process:
   - **a.** Identify the need for patient transport
   - **b.** Agreement between referring and accepting attending physicians
   - **c.** Hand-off from critical care team to transfer team
   - **d.** Transfer of patient between facilities
   - **e.** Hand-off from transfer team to accepting team
   - **f.** Return of transfer team and equipment to referring hospital
2. **Verbal Handoff:** See Table 14.1 for an example of verbal handoff between sending and receiving providers.

B. Intrahospital Transport is the movement of a patient to various sites *within* a health care facility for diagnostic or therapeutic procedures that cannot be performed at the primary location. For example, patients may be transported to the interventional radiology suite, operating room, or gastroenterology suite.

II. RISKS ASSOCIATED WITH TRANSPORT

Regardless of the destination, the benefit of transporting a patient must be balanced with the associated risks. These risks range from minor to major complications. Hemodynamic and respiratory problems are the most common. Patients who require transport out of the ICU have an increased rate of mortality likely related to the severity of illness as opposed to being causally related to transport.

A. Risks of patient transport can be categorized as either *system* or *patient* based (Tables 14.2 and 14.3). System errors may arise from equipment problems or human factors, such as poor provider communication or poor planning. Any deterioration of a patient's condition may increase the risk of adverse events during transport. Sicker patients already have low physiologic reserves and are exposed to more frequent intrahospital transport for procedures or diagnostics. Compared with elective transport, emergent transport is associated with an increase in adverse events.

TABLE 14.1 Verbal Hand-off Between Sending and Receiving Providers

Patient demographics
Reason for transport
History of present illness
Active medical issues
Current vital signs
Airway management
Hemodynamic support
Critical medications
Access and monitoring
Critical laboratory and diagnostic studies
Pending information
Code status
Emergency family contact/health care proxy
Referring physician name
Accepting physician name
Exchange of contact information between care providers

TABLE 14.2 Systems-Based Complications

Equipment
Battery failure of portable equipment
Monitor malfunction
Depletion of portable oxygen supplies
Ventilator failure/disconnect
Disruption in portable medication infusions/pumps
Disconnection or loss of intravenous access
Chest tube failure/disconnect
Inaccurate calibration of hemodynamic monitors
Human
Inadequate training or experience
Poor planning and anticipation
Failure in hand-off and communication
Lack of vigilance and monitoring
Unintended/unrecognized extubation or loss of airway
Under-/overventilation
Under-/overresuscitation
Failure to secure or protect patient extremities

TABLE 14.3 Patient-Based Complications

Neurologic—depth of sedation, analgesia, increased ICP, seizure
Respiratory—secretions, aspiration, derecruitment, increased oxygen consumption
Cardiac—hypertension, hypotension, arrhythmia, ischemia, hemorrhage
Temperature—hypothermia resulting in shivering, hypercarbia, and/or inadequate ventilation

ICP, intracranial pressure.

B. Schwebel et al reviewed 3000 intrahospital transports in 1700 ventilated ICU patients. They matched transported patients with controls who had a similar likelihood of being transported. Intrahospital transport was associated with an increased risk of several complications (Table 14.4).

C. Min et al studied intrahospital transport of critically ill patients and found the incidence of cardiopulmonary arrest to be 1.5%. Independent risk factors for cardiopulmonary arrest during intrahospital transport include previous history of myocardial infarction, manual ventilation with a bag-valve mask, and the use of three or more vasopressors.

TABLE 14.4 Complications Associated With Transport

Deep venous thrombosis
Pneumothorax
Ventilator-associated pneumonia
Atelectasis
Hypoglycemia/hyperglycemia
Hyponatremia/hypernatremia
Increased hospital length of stay

From Schwebel C, Clec'h C, Magne S, et al. Safety of intrahospital transport in ventilated critically ill patients: a multicenter cohort study. *Crit Care Med.* 2013;41:1919-1928.

D. Gimenez et al evaluated intrahospital transport of critically ill patients and found adverse events occurred 40% of the time, with the most likely cause being physiologic alterations, followed by equipment failures and team failures. There were no recorded deaths or serious injury, and half of the adverse events were categorized as moderate. Patients who suffered an adverse event during transport had higher Sequential Organ Failure Assessment (SOFA) scores and longer mean time in the ICU.

III. MINIMIZING RISKS OF TRANSPORT

Various international specialty societies have established essential components for safe patient transport (Table 14.5). The American Society of Critical Care Medicine 2004 guidelines include the following equipment for patient transport: pulse oximeter, capnograph, noninvasive blood pressure monitor, electrocardiogram monitor, vascular pressure monitor, and stethoscope. The Australian

TABLE 14.5 Essential Components of Safe Patient Transport

Stabilization of patient prior to transport
Risk assessment prior to patient transfer
Coordination and detailed communication between clinicians
Training and experience in managing patient condition and support mechanisms
Equipment adapted for transport and monitoring
Documentation—indication for transport and status pre-, during, and posttransport
Continuous patient and equipment checks
Establishing protocols and regular evaluation of transport processes
Minimize transport time
Close proximity of diagnostic and therapeutic units to ICU and emergency room
Adequate number of personnel

New Zealand College of Anesthetists 2015 guidelines also include temperature monitoring. The American Association for Respiratory Care 2002 guidelines include monitoring of pressure, flow, and volume from the transport ventilator, pulse oximeter, electrocardiogram monitor, vascular pressure monitor, stethoscope, and hand-held spirometer. Regardless of the specific approach taken, each institution should have written protocols for transporting patients within and between health care facilities.

Prior to patient transport, pertinent organ systems must be assessed with specific plans for potential complications. Implementation of a pretransport checklist improves compliance with transport safety guidelines (**Appendices 1 and 2, supplemental material**).

A. Airway: The patient's airway must be assessed prior to transport. If intubated, the position, function, stability, and security of an endotracheal tube (ETT) must be confirmed and, if necessary, resecured. Should intubation become emergently necessary, studies show that intubation can be safely accomplished during transport. However, certain patients may benefit from elective intubation prior to transport (Table 14.6). For both intubated and nonintubated patients, backup airway equipment such as a bag-valve mask, oral airway, intubation kit, and full oxygen tank are essential.

B. Breathing and Ventilation: Adequate oxygenation and ventilation must be confirmed prior to transport. An arterial blood gas should reflect a reasonable partial pressure of arterial oxygen ($Pa{O_2}$), alveolar-to-arterial gradient (A-a), and partial pressure of arterial carbon dioxide ($Pa{CO_2}$). Patients with a low $Pa{O_2}$ or high A-a gradient may benefit from increased positive end-expiratory pressure (PEEP), increased fraction of inspired oxygen ($F{IO_2}$), suctioning, or bronchoscopy prior to transport. Elevated $Pa{CO_2}$ can be addressed by optimizing minute ventilation or inspiratory-to-expiratory time. Paralysis may improve ventilator synchrony and prevent auto-PEEP. Compared with manual ventilation, mechanical ventilation may be more appropriate in patients with multiple comorbidities, long transport distances, or specialized modes of ventilation. A chest tube for pneumothorax may be warranted, especially for air transport in which a small pneumothorax has the potential to develop into a tension pneumothorax. Droogh et al place the incidence of respiratory complications between 0% and 15%, with the most common being inadequate oxygenation or ventilation.

C. Circulation and Cardiovascular Support: Adequate and functioning intravenous access must be established, and IV sites should be evaluated for infiltration prior to

TABLE 14.6 Indications for Elective Intubation Prior to Transport

Glasgow Coma Score <9
Respiratory acidosis and impending failure
Status asthmaticus
Shock (septic, hemorrhagic, cardiogenic, neurogenic)
Polytrauma
Recurrent seizures or status epilepticus
Facial or extensive burns
Acute epiglottitis
Angioedema
Anaphylaxis
Laryngeal-tracheal trauma
Combative patients

transport. Actively infusing medications for hemodynamic support must be noted with an appropriate discussion of prior and anticipated trends in hemodynamics. Transporting staff should bring additional medications in case of patient deterioration. All infusion pumps and monitors should be accurately calibrated, reliably functioning, and have sufficient battery life. Droogh et al estimate the incidence of cardiovascular complications between 6% and 24%, with the most common being acute changes in blood pressure, heart rate, or rhythm.

D. **Neurologic Status, Sedation, and Pain Management**: Neurologic status and preexisting deficits should be evaluated and documented before and after transport. Providers must anticipate the potential for a decline in mental status. Adequate sedation and analgesia should be provided to ensure patient comfort and to prevent self-extubation or self-injury; restraints may be warranted. Often critically ill patients require additional ventilator support as they lack the muscle strength to generate sufficient respiratory effort due to myopathy of critical illness or injury. If neuromuscular blocking drugs have been administered, sedation is required to prevent awareness.

E. **Temperature Regulation:** Patient transport from a temperature-controlled operating room or ICU through hospital corridors or diagnostic suites may lead to hypothermia and complications such as coagulopathy or increased $PaCO_2$ secondary to shivering. Forced air warming devices are cost-effective methods to prevent heat loss during transport.

F. **Patient Position:** Patient repositioning, such as from the OR table to the transport bed, may lead to hemodynamic instability, particularly in hypovolemic patients. Ensure all patient extremities are within the confines of the transport vehicle to avoid incidental injury when moving through narrow walkways. Advance the patient bed in a "feet-first direction." A provider should be positioned at the head of the bed, directing the movement and speed of transport, with a clear and constant vision of monitors. There must be sufficient personnel during transport to allow for appropriate division of tasks (pushing the bed, airway management, medication administration, etc). Staff must be able to immediately call for help.

G. **Consent and Legal Issues:** Disclosure of risks and consent to transport is usually implied but should be delineated as separate from the risks associated with a planned procedure. Current guidelines require consent from either the patient or authorized health care proxy agent (if the patient cannot consent for themselves) prior to interhospital, but not intrahospital, transport.

IV. USE OF CHECKLISTS

Implementation of checklists that emphasize safety guidelines pretransport, intratransport, and posttransport is recommended. Protocols developed for intrahospital transfer are often *hospital specific*, but generally strive to achieve a balance between being too vague or too detailed. Our institution uses a practical and focused checklist from the onset to conclusion of patient transport (see supplemental material).

V. SPECIAL PATIENT POPULATIONS

In all patients, the airway, ventilation, and circulation should be prioritized, assessed, and stabilized. Disease progression, decompensation, or complicating comorbidities may dictate preemptive endotracheal intubation and invasive monitoring prior to transfer.

A. **Pediatric Patient:** Adverse events during interhospital transport of critically ill pediatric patients are reduced with the use of specialized pediatric transport teams. Orr et al found that transport with a nonspecialized team was associated with increased unplanned events during transport and higher 28-day mortality. In this study, airway-related events were most common, followed by cardiopulmonary arrest, sustained hypotension, and loss of crucial intravenous access. Previously, the notion of the "golden hour" supported the early transfer of critically ill pediatric patients to centers of specialized care. Bellini et al found a significant difference between ground and helicopter transport times for newborns and suggested utilization of the golden hour as one criterion for the activation of helicopter transport. However, other studies support physiologic stabilization with specialized pediatric critical care teams prior to transfer as adverse events during transport were reduced compared with early transfer. The benefit of physiologic stabilization should be weighed against the risk of delaying definitive treatment at a specialized pediatric care center. Chaichotjinda et al found that adverse events occurred during 22% of pediatric interhospital transports, with physiologic deterioration (hypotension, desaturation, altered mentation, seizure, and hypoglycemia) being the most frequent. Patients accompanied by a physician were less likely to experience a complication (92% vs 76% physician accompaniment). Intrahospital transport of medically complex patients, such as those with congenital heart disease, or patients receiving specialized therapy such as extracorporeal membrane oxygenation or high-frequency oscillatory ventilation can be performed safely with the use of specialized teams and checklists.

B. Obstetric Patient: Maternal morbidity and mortality may be related to pregnancy-related complications, preexisting illness, or fetal delivery. The most common obstetric causes of maternal morbidity, mortality, and ICU admission are obstetric hemorrhage and hypertensive disorders such as eclampsia. Trauma is the most common nonobstetric cause. Interhospital transport is advisable if the primary location of delivery does not have the resources to adequately care for the maternal or neonatal condition. Neonatal outcomes are improved when the mother is transported to a tertiary care center prior to delivery, as opposed to transport of a distressed neonate. Air transport is generally regarded as safe for the obstetric patient and fetus.

C. Viral Respiratory Illness Patient: The COVID-19 pandemic has highlighted the importance of transport protocols for patients with highly virulent infections. The Transport Medicine Society released consensus guidelines for the transport of suspected or patients confirmed with COVID-19, which included both interhospital and intrahospital transport (Table 14.7).

VI. MODES OF TRANSPORT

A. Air-Based Interhospital Transport: Air transport may be accomplished via airplane or helicopter. Helicopter transport is generally more efficient than ground transport for distances more than 45 miles and operates at an altitude below 5000 feet. Airplane transport is best utilized for distances more than 250 miles, with cabins pressurized between 5000 and 7000 feet despite true altitude often greater than 20 000 feet. Teams should be specially trained to deal with the unique potential complications associated with air transport. Air-based in-transit critical events are as high as 5%, with hemodynamic deterioration being the most common. See Table 14.8 for medical conditions potentially worsened by altitude and air transport.

1. **Land-Based Interhospital Transport:** The advantages of ground transport include lower cost, better monitoring, and faster mobilization. The transferring physician should consider the scope of practice of the transporting personnel. Land-based in-transit critical events are as high as 6.5%, with new-onset hypotension being the most common. Patients on mechanical ventilation, with baseline hemodynamic instability, and longer transport duration are associated with the highest rates of critical events. Ground transport is typically faster than air transport for distances less than 10 miles.

TABLE 14.7 Transport Medicine Society Recommendations for COVID-19

Intrahospital transport of suspected or confirmed COVID-19 patient
Confirm intervention/investigation/procedure is necessary, minimize unnecessary interventions
Plan the schedule and route
Transport with nurse or doctor (as dictated by acuity of critical illness)
Transport bed equipped with oxygen, ventilator, monitors, equipment, and emergency medications
If extubated: Administer nasal oxygen, and patient wears a surgical face mask
If intubated: Use heat and moisture exchange (HME) filter and closed suction
PPE for providers: Gloves, N-95, face shield/goggles, water impervious coverall with head hood
Interhospital transport of suspected or confirmed COVID-19 patient
Decide feasibility and definitive need to transfer
Discuss with receiving physician
Plan the schedule and route
Decide on the mode of transfer
Transport with doctor and nurse
Transport bed equipped with oxygen, ventilator, monitors, equipment, and emergency medications
If extubated: Administer nasal oxygen and avoid aerosol-generating procedures, consider intubation prior to transport
If intubated: Use HME filter and closed suction
PPE for providers: gloves, N-95, face shield/goggles, water impervious coverall with head hood
Complete checklist prior to transport
Monitor and recognize signs of deterioration
Be prepared to treat emergencies
Inform receiving facility to be prepared
Hand-off patient and patient record
Decontaminate transport vehicle and monitors

From Munjal M, Ahmed SM, Garg R, et al. The Transport Medicine Society consensus guidelines for the transport of suspected or confirmed COVID-19 patients. *Indian J Crit Care Med.* 2020;24(9):763-770.

TABLE 14.8 Medical Conditions Potentially Worsened by Altitude and Air Transport

Pneumothorax
Pneumopericardium
Subcutaneous emphysema
Gas gangrene
Decompression sickness
Systemic air emboli
Gastric distention or pneumoperitoneum
Pneumocephalus
Ocular or tympanic injury

APPENDIX 1. ICU PATIENT HOSPITAL TRANSPORT CHECKLIST

1. **Patient**
   a. Identify patient (name, date of birth, medical record number)
   b. Stable/appropriate for transport?
2. **Care Team**
   a. Identify team members planning to travel
   b. At least one team member familiar with patient history
   c. Identify receiving care team members and hospital
3. **Medications/Transfusions**
   a. Current infusions (eg, vasopressors, sedative-analgesics, blood products)
   b. Anticipated or scheduled medications
   c. Backup emergency medications
4. **Airway**
   a. Airway status appropriate for travel and planned procedure
   b. Planned mode of ventilation during travel and at receiving site
   c. Is there paralysis or insufficient respiratory effort?
   d. Backup airway equipment (eg, bag-valve mask, backup tracheostomy kit)
5. **Monitoring**
   a. Standard monitor check (eg, SpO_2, $EtCO_2$, blood pressure, telemetry, temperature)
   b. Other monitor checks (eg, intracranial pressure, arterial line, CVP/PA line)
6. **Tubes/Line/Drains**
   a. Chest tube check (eg, leak/no leak, remain on suction)
   b. Spinal drain and/or external ventricular drain check (eg, open/close, height)
   c. Other drain checks (eg, urinary catheter, surgical drains, NG tube)
7. **Additional Safety Checks**
   a. Sufficient oxygen and electrical reserves (eg, full oxygen tank, pump battery)
   b. If mechanically ventilated, pressure alarm active
   c. Sufficient intravenous access
   d. Patient extremities in safe position to avoid trauma or pressure point injury

APPENDIX 2. ICU PATIENT HOSPITAL TRANSPORT STATUS CHECKLIST

1. **Airway**—secure ventilation system
2. **Breathing**—bilateral chest rise and auscultation, insufflation pressure, SpO_2, end-tidal CO_2
3. **Circulation**—vital signs on a portable monitor, noninvasive BP cuff or arterial line, palpable pulse
4. **Disconnect**—airway, oxygen supply, IV lines, infusions, drains, electrical supply
5. **Ergonomics**—patient positioning and support

Selected Readings

American College of Emergency Physicians. Interfacility Transportation of the Critical Care Patient and Its Medical Direction. *Ann Emerg Med.* 2012;60:677.

Australian College for Emergency Medicine, Australian and New Zealand College of Anaesthetists, Joint Faculty of Intensive Care Medicine. Minimum standards for intrahospital transport of critically ill patients. *Emerg Med (Fremantle).* 2003;15(2):202-204.

Bellini C, De Angelis LC, Secchi S, et al. Helicopter neonatal transport: first golden hour at birth is useful tool guiding activation of appropriate resources. *Air Med J.* 2020;39(6):454-457.

Bourn S, Wijesingha S, Nordmann G. Transfer of the critically ill adult patient. *BJA Educ.* 2018;18(3):63-68.

Branson RD, Rodriquez D Jr. Monitoring during transport. *Respir Care.* 2020;65(6):882-893.

Brunsveld-Reinders AH, Arbous MS, Kuiper SG, de Jonge E. A comprehensive method to develop a checklist to increase safety of intra-hospital transport of critically ill patients. *Crit Care.* 2015;19(1):214.

Chaichotjinda K, Chantra M, Pandee U. Assessment of interhospital transport care for pediatric patients. *Clin Exp Pediatr.* 2020;63(5):184-188.

Day D. Keeping patients safe during intrahospital transport. *Crit Care Nurse.* 2010;30:18-32.

Droogh JM, Smit M, Absalom AR, Ligtenberg JJ, Zijlstra JG. Transferring the critically ill patient: are we there yet? *Crit Care.* 2015;19(1):62.

Fanara B, Manzon C, Barbot O, et al. Recommendations for the intra-hospital transport of critically ill patients. *Crit Care.* 2010;14:R87.

Gimenez FMP, de Camargo WHB, Gomes ACB, et al. Analysis of adverse events during intrahospital transportation of critically ill patients. *Crit Care Res Pract.* 2017;2017:6847124.

Intensive Care Society, The Faculty of Intensive Care Medicine. *Guidance On: The Transfer of the Critically Ill Adult.* Intensive Care Society; 2019.

Johnson D, Luscombe M. Aeromedical transfer of the critically ill patient. *JICS.* 2011;12:307-312.

Lahner D, Nikolic A, Marhofer P, et al. Incidence of complications in intrahospital transport of critically ill patients: experience in an Austrian university hospital. *Wein Klin Wochenschr.* 2007;119:412-416.

Low RB, Martin D, Brown C. Emergency air transport of pregnant patients: the national experience. *J Emerg Med.* 1988;6:41-48.

Min HJ, Kim HJ, Lee DS, et al. Intra-hospital transport of critically ill patients with rapid response team and risk factors for cardiopulmonary arrest: a retrospective cohort study. *PLoS One.* 2019;14(3):e0213146.

Munjal M, Ahmed SM, Garg R, et al. The Transport Medicine Society consensus guidelines for the transport of suspected or confirmed COVID-19 patients. *Indian J Crit Care Med.* 2020;24(9):763-770.

Oras J, Strube M, Rylander C. The mortality of critically ill patients was not associated with inter-hospital transfer due to a shortage of ICU beds—a single-centre retrospective analysis. *J Intensive Care.* 2020;8(1):82.

Orr RA, Felmet KA, Han Y, et al. Pediatric specialized transport teams are associated with improved outcomes. *Pediatrics.* 2009;124:40-48.

Parmentier-Decrucq E, Poissy J, Favory R, et al. Adverse events during intrahospital transport of critically ill patients: incidence and risk factors. *Ann Intensive Care.* 2013;3(1):10.

Schwebel C, Clec'h C, Magne S, et al. Safety of intrahospital transport in ventilated critically ill patients: a multicenter cohort study. *Crit Care Med.* 2013;41:1919-1928.

Singh JM, MacDonald RD, Ahghari M. Critical events during land-based interfacility transport. *Ann Emerg Med.* 2014;64:9-15.e2.

Singh JM, MacDonald RD, Bronskill SE, et al. Incidence and predictors of critical events during urgent air-medical transport. *CMAJ.* 2009;181:579-584.

Warren J, Fromm RE, Orr RA, et al. Guidelines for the inter- and intra-hospital transport of critically ill patients. *Crit Care Med.* 2004;32:256-262.

Williams P, Karuppiah S, Greentree K, Darvall J. A checklist for intrahospital transport of critically ill patients improves compliance with transportation safety guidelines. *Aust Crit Care.* 2020;33(1):20-24.

15 Coronary Artery Disease

Ying Hui Low and Michael G. Fitzsimons

Coronary artery disease (CAD) is a leading cause of adult morbidity and mortality in the United States and is responsible for about a third of all deaths in those older than 35 years of age. Although about a third of patients with acute myocardial infarction (MI) die immediately, most deaths are due to early prehospital dysrhythmias. Medical treatment focuses on identifying at-risk patients and preventing sequelae through risk modification. The major risk factors for CAD are hypertension (HTN), diabetes mellitus (DM), smoking, dyslipidemia (high low-density lipoprotein [LDL] or low high-density lipoprotein [HDL]), male sex older than age 45, female sex older than age 55, obesity, elevated homocysteine levels, and physical inactivity. Specific ethnic groups and a family history of CAD are also predisposing factors.

I. DEFINITIONS: Chest discomfort is the most common symptom of myocardial ischemia, and the initial evaluation of chest pain or classic cardiac symptoms (eg, radiation to neck, jaw, or arm; diaphoresis; nausea) should differentiate angina, acute coronary syndrome (ACS), or noncardiac chest pain. Electrocardiographic (ECG) changes can help differentiate cardiac from noncardiac origins. ECG changes without typical anginal symptoms ("silent" ischemia) are common, especially in patients with diabetes, are older adults, or postoperative. Typical angina may be blunted by postoperative pain medications including epidural analgesia or postoperative sedation.

A. Angina Pectoris is retrosternal tightness, pressure, or pain that occurs at rest or with physical or emotional stress, lasting up to 10 minutes. It can radiate to the back, jaw, arm, or shoulder, usually on the left. Angina usually reflects compromise of at least one epicardial artery and implies ischemia but not necessarily myocardial necrosis. Symptoms also include nausea, vomiting, diaphoresis, and shortness of breath. Angina may present in valvular heart disease, hypertrophic cardiomyopathy, or uncontrolled HTN. The Canadian Cardiovascular Society Classification System grades angina severity from Class I (ordinary physical exertion does not cause angina) to Class IV (angina with minimal exertion or at rest).

1. **Stable angina** demonstrates a pattern that has not changed in frequency, duration, or ease of relief for several months. Predictable symptoms present with exertion and abate with rest. A fixed coronary atheroma with a fibrous cap is generally to blame.
2. **Variant (Prinzmetal) angina** occurs at rest, is often worse in the morning, lasts several minutes, and is accompanied by transient ST-segment elevation and/or ventricular dysrhythmias. It can be induced by exercise, stemming from vasospasm in a coronary artery that may not have significant atheromatous disease. Smoking is a major risk factor. Hyperventilation, hypocalcemia, cocaine, pseudoephedrine, and ephedrine have also been implicated.

B. Acute Coronary Syndromes (ACSs) are three conditions associated with acute myocardial ischemia secondary to poor myocardial blood supply: unstable angina (UA), non–ST-segment elevation myocardial infarction (NSTEMI), and ST-segment elevation myocardial infarction (STEMI).

1. **UA** has a recent onset (2 months) with increasing frequency and intensity, and recurs at progressively lower levels of stress, or even at rest. Ten percent of patients have significant disease of the left main coronary artery, and approximately 20% of patients will suffer an acute MI within 3 months. Plaque rupture, platelet aggregation, thrombosis, and vasospasm are the underlying causes.
2. **NSTEMI** presents with ST-segment depressions or prominent T waves and may be associated with a rise in cardiac biomarkers. The management of NSTEMI focuses on improving oxygen (O_2) supply and reducing demand in at-risk myocardium, thus preventing progression of damage. It must always be borne in mind that a nondiagnostic ECG does not rule out MI.
3. **STEMI** reflects severe, possibly irreversible, damage to the myocardium. The joint 2018 European Society of Cardiology/American College of Cardiology Foundation/American Heart Association/World Heart Federation (ESC/ACCF/AHA/WHF) ECG criteria for diagnosis of STEMI are as follows:
   - **a.** New horizontal or downsloping ST depression greater than 0.5 mm in two contiguous leads, and/or:
   - **b.** T inversion greater than 1 mm in two contiguous leads with prominent R wave or R/S ratio greater than 1
   - **c.** The appearance of a new ST-segment elevation at the J point in two contiguous leads greater than 0.1 mV in all leads other than leads V_2 to V_3
   - **d.** For leads V_2 to V_3: greater than or equal to 2 mm in men 40 years or older, or greater than or equal to 1.5 mm in women regardless of age
   - **e.** Left bundle branch block (BBB), left ventricular (LV) hypertrophy, hyperkalemia, pericarditis, early repolarization, or paced rhythms complicate the diagnosis. Treatment focuses on timely reperfusion.
4. **Noncardiac chest pain** is not related to coronary ischemia, but life-threatening causes such as aortic dissection, pulmonary embolism, and pneumothorax should be ruled out immediately.
5. **Perioperative MI** is one of the major adverse cardiac events in major noncardiac surgery. Patients that suffer MI after surgery have a 15% to 25% risk of in-hospital death and a significant increase in 6-month morbidity and mortality. Although there is controversy over accepted definitions of perioperative MI, its incidence may be up to 6% in patients with CAD. Although MI is normally diagnosed on the basis of three criteria (chest pain, biomarker levels, and ECG changes), a perioperative MI may be obscured by pain or pain control techniques to the point of being "silent." A high index of suspicion is critical and increased consideration should be given to the ECG and cardiac enzymes.
6. **Acute MI** is the term used when there is an acute myocardial injury with clinical evidence of acute myocardial ischemia and detection of a rise and/or fall of cardiac troponin (cTn) values, with at least one value greater than the 99th percentile and at least one of the following:
   - **a.** Symptoms of myocardial ischemia
   - **b.** New ischemic ECG changes
   - **c.** Development of pathologic Q waves
   - **d.** Imaging evidence of new loss of viable myocardium or new regional wall motion abnormality in a pattern consistent with ischemic etiology
   - **e.** Identification of a coronary thrombus by angiography or autopsy

C. Pathophysiology

1. **Myocardial O_2 supply-demand balance:** Even at rest, the myocardium extracts O_2 maximally. During exertion, O_2 delivery must increase to meet demand. Myocardial ischemia and infarction occur when O_2 demand exceeds delivery.
   - **a. Myocardial O_2 supply** is determined by the following:
     1. **Coronary blood flow** is determined by the difference between transmural pressure and the aortic root pressure at the beginning of diastole. Because transmural resistance is low in diastole, myocardial blood flow is higher during this period. Tachycardia, which minimizes diastolic time, can thus induce ischemia. Normal coronaries compensate

by dilating to increase blood flow 4- to 5-fold during exercise or stress. However, stenoses can reduce the coronaries' ability to dilate and thus limit O_2 supply downstream. Polycythemia, hyperviscosity, and sickle cell disease may further compromise coronary flow.

2. **O_2 content** is dependent on hemoglobin (Hgb) concentration and its saturation with O_2 (SaO_2), and to a lesser extent on dissolved O_2 concentration (see **Chapter 2**). An ideal Hgb level is not known but compensation through increased cardiac output (CO) occurs with anemia.

b. **Myocardial O_2 demand** is influenced by the following:

1. **Ventricular wall tension (T)**, which according to LaPlace's Law is

$$T = PR/2h$$

where P is transmural pressure, R is ventricular radius, and h is wall thickness. Increase in pressure or radius will increase O_2 demand.

2. **Heart rate (HR)**, which increases O_2 demand by increasing contractility. Tachycardia shortens diastole and maximal coronary perfusion in atherosclerotic vessels, also limiting O_2 supply. Hyperthyroidism, sympathomimetics (eg, cocaine), or anxiety can increase HR and O_2 demand.

3. **Contractility**, which is the intrinsic property of the myocyte to contract against a load, is proportional to O_2 demand. Positive inotropes (eg, digoxin, norepinephrine) increase O_2 demands of myocardium that might already be at risk.

D. **Etiologies of myocardial O_2 demand imbalance:** Over 90% of myocardial ischemia and infarction result from atherosclerosis. Most perioperative MIs stem from abrupt, unpredictable partial or complete occlusion secondary to acute atherosclerotic plaque rupture. Other causes include coronary vasospasm or thromboembolism, vasculitis, trauma, valvular heart disease (eg, aortic stenosis), hypertrophic or dilated cardiomyopathies, and thyrotoxicosis.

II. ANGINA

A. **History** should ascertain whether risk factors (DM, smoking, HTN, family history of early coronary disease) exist. Pain is characterized by character, location, duration, radiation, and exacerbating (emotional stress, eating, cold weather) or alleviating (rest, medications) factors. Pain is often described as a "pressure," "heavy," or "grip-like," with radiation to the arm or jaw. An unstable, changing constellation of symptoms must be differentiated from a stable anginal pattern. Severe angina of recent onset, angina at rest, or angina of increasing duration, frequency, or intensity is classified as unstable and considered a part of the spectrum of ACS.

B. **Physical Examination** may be normal or nonspecific. Findings of distress, anxiety, tachycardia, HTN, an S_4 gallop, pulmonary rales, xanthomas, or peripheral atherosclerosis may be evident. Pulmonary edema, a new or worsening murmur of mitral regurgitation (MR), and angina with hypotension are associated with a high risk of progression to nonfatal MI or death.

C. **Noninvasive Studies**

1. The **resting ECG** is normal in many patients with ischemia. ECG changes indicative of myocardial ischemia that may progress to MI include new ST-segment elevations at the J point in two or more contiguous leads that are greater than or equal to 0.2 mV in leads V_1 to V_3 and greater than 0.1 mV in all other leads. ST-segment elevation at rest is suggestive of transmural ischemia and can occur with coronary artery vasospasm, or severe and, often, multivessel coronary disease, and the affected leads help localize the associated coronary artery. Table 15.1 outlines the ECG changes associated with specific regions of ischemic myocardium. However, isolated J-point elevation may occur as a normal variant in young, healthy adults. A left BBB or pacing can interfere with the ECG diagnosis of coronary ischemia.

TABLE 15.1 Location of Acute Ischemia or Infarct by Electrocardiograph

Region	Leads	Reciprocal ST depression	Vessel
Anterior	V_1-V_6	II, III, aVF	Left anterior descending
Apical	V_1-V_3	II, III, aVF	Left anterior descending
Anterolateral	V_4-V_6	II, III, aVF	Left anterior descending
Lateral	I and aVL	III, III, aVF or V_1-V_2	Left circumflex
Inferior	II, III and aVF There may also be ST elevation in precordial leads V_1-V_2 Obtain right-sided leads to evaluate for RV infarct, confirmed by ST elevation in V_3R-V_4R	I and aVL	Right coronary or left circumflex, depending on which provides the PDA Proximal RCA occlusion may lead to RV infarct
Lateral (previously known as posterior or posterolateral)	ST elevation in V_7-V_9 on a posterior lead ECG Large, broad R wave in V_1, V_2	ST changes in V_1 and V_2 may represent reciprocal change or posterior/ posterolateral involvement	Suggestive of left circumflex involvement
Anteroseptal	V_1-V_2	II, III, aVF	Left anterior descending
Antero-Apical	V_3-V_4	II, III, aVF	Left anterior descending
Anterolateral	V_5-V_6 Often in association with changes in leads I and aVL	II, III, aVF, and sometimes V_1-V_2	
Pericarditis	Diffuse ST segment elevation		
Ischemia in more than one region of the heart	Diffuse ST segment depression		

PDA, patent ductus arteriosus; RCA, right coronary artery; RV, right ventricle.

Significant Q waves are suggestive of a prior MI. Serial ECGs in 15- to 20-minute intervals can determine whether ischemia is evolving. In general, reversibility of ECG changes after therapeutic interventions is highly suggestive of ischemia.

2. **Exercise ECG:** Exercise stress testing involves monitoring blood pressure (BP) and ECG while the patient exercises on a treadmill or bicycle. Indications for exercise testing include diagnosis of obstructive CAD, risk assessment and prognosis in suspected or known CAD, patients with multiple risk factors who are asymptomatic, and certain postrevascularization situations. Most protocols have a warm-up period followed by progressive workload increase. Each level of exercise reflects increased O_2 uptake or metabolic equivalents (METs). A single MET is 3.5 mL O_2/kg/min. The test is discontinued when a patient reaches 85% to 90% of maximal predicted HR, the patient requests its termination, or when angina, serious arrhythmias,

central nervous system (CNS) symptoms, decreased BP, or evidence of poor peripheral perfusion occurs. Subendocardial ischemia during exercise results in ST-segment depression and/or elevation. Upsloping ST depression usually appears first and is less specific for ischemia than is horizontal ST depression. Horizontal or downsloping ST depression is more specific for ischemia and is often associated with T-wave inversion and may be seen during exercise but is more often seen during recovery from exercise. ST-segment depression during exercise testing is one of the most identifiable ECG signs of myocardial ischemia and this is considered positive when there is greater than or equal to 1 mm horizontal or downsloping ST-segment depression in one or more leads that persists at 80 msec after the J point. Leads V_4, V_5, and V_6 are the most sensitive leads for detecting ST depression of subendocardial ischemia; however, unlike with ST elevations, these may not reliably localize the coronary artery responsible for ischemic change. A positive test (ie, one that demonstrates ST-segment elevation or depression, a fall in BP with exercise, development of serious arrhythmias, or the development of anginal chest pain with exercise) indicates a high likelihood of significant CAD. Sensitivity for obstructive CAD increases with the severity of stenotic disease. For CAD involving the left main or for three-vessel disease, sensitivity is 86% and specificity is 53%. Positive tests should prompt consideration of cardiac catheterization and potential revascularization. Absolute contraindications to exercise stress testing include recent MI (within 2 days), severe aortic stenosis, symptomatic heart failure (HF), arrhythmias causing hemodynamic compromise, acute pulmonary embolus, pulmonary infarction, and aortic dissection. Relative contraindications include uncontrolled HTN (systolic BP >200 mm Hg or diastolic BP >110 mm Hg), tachy- or bradyarrhythmias, hypertrophic cardiomyopathy, high-grade atrioventricular block, and a physical or mental limitation to exercise. ECG changes occurring at lower workloads are generally more significant than are those at higher workloads.

3. **Myocardial injury biomarkers:** Myocardial enzyme analysis is often initiated immediately to help determine whether angina is stable or unstable. When damaged (eg, by trauma or infarction), cardiac myocytes release various proteins such as creatine kinase-MB (CK-MB) fraction, troponin, and myoglobin into the blood. cTnI and cTnT are the most specific and sensitive biomarkers of cardiac injury and values greater than or equal to 99th percentile of the upper reference limit are considered abnormal. The history and clinical context should be taken into account when interpreting an elevated cTn, and when ischemia is not present, the term "cardiac injury" should be used. With highly sensitive troponin assays, most patients can be diagnosed within 2 to 3 hours of presentation. When negative at the time of presentation, however, it does not exclude myocardial injury and serial testing is indicated. Because chronic elevations in troponin can occur, a rise and fall should be documented in an acute MI. Troponin levels are also important for risk stratification after STEMI or NSTEMI. Troponin levels may be especially valuable in the perioperative period where CK-MB may be elevated for other reasons and may not reflect myocardial necrosis. If laboratory measurement of troponin is not available, CK-MB is an acceptable alternative; again, a level over the 99th percentile is considered positive for myocardial injury.
4. **Radionuclide perfusion imaging** assesses both myocardial perfusion and function in a patient with stable angina.
   a. **Exercise myocardial perfusion imaging:** Thallium-201 is a radioactive potassium analog that is avidly extracted by viable myocardium in proportion to regional myocardial blood flow during exercise. Regions of decreased uptake correlate with the severity of coronary stenosis supplying the regions. During rest after exercise, a "fixed defect" that takes up no tracer at all represents an area of prior infarct, whereas

a "reversible defect," a region that regains uptake, is considered to be myocardium at risk for ischemia. This test has a sensitivity of 85% and a specificity of 90% for detecting myocardium at risk for ischemia.

b. Exercise radionuclide ventriculography: Intravenous (IV) technetium-99m sestamibi accumulates in the myocardium in proportion to blood flow, and multiple ventricular images that are synchronized to the cardiac cycle are acquired at rest and during exercise. Ischemia is suggested by regional wall motion abnormalities and the inability to increase left ventricular ejection fraction (LVEF) during exercise.

c. Pharmacologic stress perfusion imaging: Adenosine and dipyridamole are coronary vasodilators commonly used in stress imaging. Adenosine is direct-acting, increasing flow in disease-free coronary vessels. Dipyridamole inhibits cellular uptake and degradation of adenosine, indirectly increasing coronary flow in nonstenotic vessels. Because stenotic areas are already maximally dilated, the dilation of disease-free vessels creates differential flow patterns upon coronary imaging. Both drugs may cause angina, headache, or bronchospasm, and must be used with caution in patients with obstructive pulmonary disease. Dobutamine, an inotrope, increases HR, systolic BP, and contractility, causing increased blood flow secondarily. Imaging after dobutamine administration may show heterogeneous flow due to nondilating stenotic areas.

D. Invasive Studies: Coronary angiography remains the gold standard for quantifying the extent of CAD and guiding percutaneous coronary intervention (PCI; eg, angioplasty, stenting, atherectomy) or coronary artery bypass grafting (CABG). Coronary angiography will reveal hemodynamic parameters, as well as cardiac and coronary anatomy. A coronary obstruction is clinically significant when more than 70% of the luminal diameter is narrowed. Coronary angiography is not without risk; the mortality rate related to the procedure has been estimated between 0.1% and 0.25%.

E. Medical Management: Once it has been determined that angina is stable, appropriate management should be initiated.

1. **Smoking cessation**
2. **BP control** to a goal of 140/90 mm Hg (130/80 if DM or renal disease coexists)
3. **Dietary modification**
4. **Medically supervised physical activity and weight reduction**
5. **Aspirin (ASA)** inhibits platelets by irreversibly acetylating cyclooxygenase and decreasing thromboxane levels. If no contraindications exist, it should be started at 81 to 325 mg per day.
6. **Angiotensin-converting enzyme (ACE) inhibitors** reduce sympathetic tone and help stabilize fibrous caps of atherosclerotic plaques and have a survival benefit in HF. They should be started in all patients with no contraindications and an ejection fraction of less than 40%, especially if HTN, DM, or renal disease coexists.
7. **β-Blockers** should be initiated in all patients with a history of MI or ACS unless contraindicated.
8. **β-Hydroxy β-methylglutaryl-CoA (HMG-CoA) reductase inhibitors ("statins")** improve lipid profiles, limiting progression of atherosclerotic disease and coronary calcium deposition while stabilizing existing plaques.

F. Invasive Management for UA includes PCI. Occasionally, CABG may be urgently indicated.

III. ACUTE CORONARY SYNDROMES: Regardless of whether ACS is due to UA, NSTEMI, or STEMI, the goal is to minimize ischemic time and, when appropriate, initiate reperfusion therapy with thrombolysis, PCI, or CABG.

A. The **history** should attempt to differentiate between UA and MI. Symptoms are often indistinguishable (see **Section II.A**). Primary presentations that distinguish ACS from stable or exertional angina are rest angina (often >20 minutes in duration), new-onset angina that markedly limits physical activity, or angina that is more frequent, longer in duration, or occurs with less exertion than before. However, among patients with acute MI, one-third may not have any chest pain on presentation. They are likely to be older, diabetic, and female.

B. The **physical examination** is unlikely to distinguish UA from an acute MI (see **Section II.B**).

C. As for angina, noninvasive studies include the ECG and cardiac enzymes.

1. A **12-lead ECG** should be obtained as soon as possible to determine whether a STEMI is occurring and whether immediate revascularization is needed. Although not often captured, the earliest change in a STEMI is hyperacute or peaked T waves reflecting localized hyperkalemia. The ECG evolves through a typical sequence: initial elevation of the J point with preservation of a concave ST segment, followed by a more pronounced ST elevation where it becomes convex, and eventually the ST segment may become indistinguishable from the T wave. Transient ST-segment elevations (>0.05 mV) that resolve with rest likely indicate true ischemia and severe underlying CAD. Elevation of less than 0.05 mV, ST-segment depression, or T-wave inversion is more often associated with NSTEMI or UA. A normal ECG does *not* rule out MI because up to 6% of patients later confirmed to have had MIs may present as such. Serial ECGs are more accurate than an isolated study. The ECG continues to evolve over the next 2 weeks: the ST segment returns to isoelectric baseline, the R-wave amplitude is reduced, the Q wave deepens and the T wave inverts. In patients with an NSTEMI, ST-segment depressions often do not form pathologic Q waves. In patients with UA, ST-segment and T-wave changes usually resolve completely.
2. The best **biomarker** confirmation is a rise in cTnI or cTnT (>99th percentile. If not initially elevated, these should be repeated at 3 to 6 hours, and if still negative but clinical suspicion for MI is high, serial troponins should be drawn again up to 12 to 24 hours. With a high clinical suspicion, appropriate care should not be delayed even if the cTn is not elevated. cTnI and cTnT are highly specific for myocardial damage but do not indicate the mechanism of damage. CK-MB is less sensitive but may be substituted if troponin measurement is not available.
3. The **chest x-ray** can detect MI complications such as pulmonary venous congestion and can rule out aortic dissection, pneumonia, pleural effusion, and pneumothorax.
4. **Transthoracic echocardiography (TTE)** is not an initial diagnostic study in most presentations of ACS. If biomarkers and ECG analysis are equivocal, TTE may help identify new regional wall motion abnormalities or elucidate complications of ischemia or MI such as thromboembolic events, valve morphologies, and changes in global ventricular function. If TTE is available and the echocardiographer is experienced, this modality offers a convenient method by which a more complete clinical picture of myocardial function can be gained while awaiting the return of biomarker labs.

D. Management of Acute Myocardial Infarction

1. The **general approach** to acute MI focuses on minimizing total ischemic time, which is the time between onset of symptoms and start of **reperfusion therapy**. Ideally, this time should be less than 120 minutes. Initiation of thrombolysis in less than 30 minutes is the system goal for STEMI when PCI is not available.
2. **Supportive measures:** Supplemental O_2, IV access, routine vitals, and continuous ECG monitoring should be initiated. Supplemental O_2 is most useful in patients with an arterial saturation less than 90%, patients in respiratory distress, HF, or high-risk features for hypoxia. In patients without hypoxia, supplemental oxygen has not been associated with benefit or harm. Patients with severe HF or cardiogenic shock may need intubation and mechanical ventilation. Laboratory studies include electrolytes with

magnesium, lipid profile, and complete blood count to detect anemia. Continuous pulse oximetry is critical to evaluate oxygenation, especially in patients with HF or cardiogenic shock.

3. **Medical treatment:** Unless contraindicated, a β-blocker, ASA, anticoagulation, a glycoprotein IIb/IIIa inhibitor, and a thienopyridine (ticlopidine, clopidogrel) should be administered.
   a. **β-Blockers: If no contraindications (significant heart block, bradycardia, reactive airway disease, HF, evidence of low output state, high risk for cardiogenic shock, refer to** Table 15.2) **exist, β-blockers should be administered to all patients with an acute STEMI. β-Blockade** appears to reduce myocardial O_2 consumption by slowing the HR and reducing cardiac contractility. By slowing the HR and lengthening diastole, β-blockade increases the period of reduced wall pressures, augmenting myocardial O_2 delivery. Initially, **metoprolol** 5 mg IV every 5 minutes to a total of 15 mg may be given. If tolerated, metoprolol 25 to 50 mg orally every 6 hours can be administered for 2 days and then increased up to 100 mg orally twice daily. **Carvedilol** 6.25 mg administered orally tid, titrated up to a maximum of 25 mg tid, may reduce mortality in patients with an acute MI and LV dysfunction.
   b. **Nitrates:** Nitrates dilate epicardial coronary arteries and collateral circulation and also inhibit platelet function. They may also increase venous capacitance, thus decreasing preload and cardiac work. Evidence does not support routine long-term nitrate therapy in MI unless pain persists. Patients with acute MI or HF, large anterior infarcts, persistent pain after 3 sublingual nitroglycerin (NTG) tablets, or HTN may benefit from IV NTG for the first 24 to 48 hours. IV NTG is started at 10 μg per minute and titrated until symptom relief or BP response. Those with continuing pulmonary edema or recurrent ischemia or angina may benefit from even more prolonged use of NTG. NTG should be avoided in hypotension, or when hypotension could lead to hemodynamic decompensation such as in severe aortic stenosis or a right ventricular infarct.
   c. **Statin therapy:** Intensive statin therapy should be initiated as early as possible in all patients with a STEMI.
   d. **Analgesia:** Morphine sulfate (1-5 mg IV) for analgesia and anxiolysis is reasonable if there is an unacceptable level of pain but should otherwise be avoided because of an association with adverse outcomes. It is also contraindicated in the presence of hypotension or in patients with a history of morphine intolerance. Modest reductions in HR and BP decrease O_2 consumption. Side effects include hypotension, respiratory depression, bradycardia, or nausea. Recently, concerns have been raised about an increased risk of death in patients receiving morphine but data from a large clinical trial is lacking.
   e. **Antiplatelet therapy** should be considered in any patient presenting with ACS. Agents are chosen depending on whether the proposed management will be conservative or invasive (eg, CABG or PCI, which yields an increased risk of hemorrhage).

TABLE 15.2 Contraindications to β-Blockers in Acute Coronary Syndrome

Marked first-degree AV block, or any form of second or third-degree block
Bradycardia
Reactive airway disease
Heart failure or low cardiac output state
High risk for cardiogenic shock (eg, time delay to presentation, lower blood pressure)

AV, atrioventricular.

1. **Aspirin** 325 mg po should be given to all patients, unless contraindicated by hypersensitivity or a history of major gastrointestinal (GI) bleeding. By irreversibly inhibiting cyclooxygenase-1 in platelets, ASA prevents the formation of thromboxane A_2 and decreases platelet aggregation.
2. If a contraindication exists to aspirin, a 300-mg oral loading dose of **clopidogrel** followed by 75 mg once a day can be started. Clopidogrel and ASA are given together if invasive management is planned.
3. **Glycoprotein IIb/IIIa inhibitors** improve outcomes in patients undergoing a primary PCI.

f. Further **anticoagulation** depends on the choice of reperfusion strategy. Unfractionated heparin (UFH), low-molecular-weight heparin (LMWH), a direct thrombin inhibitor (bivalirudin), or a factor Xa inhibitor (fondaparinux) may be chosen.

1. **UFH** is most commonly used and readily reversible by protamine but has the risk of heparin-induced thrombocytopenia (HIT). Initial dosing is to target an activated partial thromboplastin time (APTT) of 1.5 to 2 times normal. A normal dose is 60 U/kg as a bolus followed by 12 U/kg per hour.
2. **LMWH** has a lower risk of HIT and is easier to administer. Concerns about the ability to monitor the effectiveness of LMWH compared to UFH and less effective reversal with protamine have limited its use when PCI is planned.
3. **Direct thrombin inhibitors** have no risk of HIT but are associated with more bleeding complications and cannot be reversed with protamine or fresh frozen plasma (FFP). **Bivalirudin** is a direct-acting synthetic antithrombin that acts against clot-bound thrombin with a very short half-life (25 minutes). Its major advantages may be a lower rate of bleeding when compared to UFH plus a GP IIb/IIIa inhibitor.
4. **Fondaparinux** is a **factor Xa inhibitor** that confers a lower risk of bleeding when compared to UFH and GP IIb/IIIa inhibitors.

g. **Potassium and magnesium: Although there is a lack of evidence documenting the effects of electrolyte repletion in acute MI, AHA guidelines recommend maintaining serum K above 4.0 mEq/L and Mg above 2.0 mEq/L. Magnesium** dilates coronary arteries, inhibits platelet activity, suppresses automaticity, and may protect against reperfusion injury. Supplemental magnesium is indicated for hypomagnesemia and torsades de pointes. Hypomagnesemia is corrected with magnesium sulfate 2 g IV over 30 to 60 minutes, whereas torsades de pointes is treated with 1 to 2 g IV over 5 minutes. Because most magnesium in the body is intracellular, patients with hypomagnesemia may require multiple replacement doses to achieve normal levels. Prophylactic administration in acute MI is not indicated.

h. **The utility of a glucose-insulin-potassium** infusion, which was thought to limit the extent of myocardial injury and decrease potentially lethal arrhythmias after MI has been recently called into question. Although frank hyperglycemia should be treated with insulin, the use of glucose-insulin-potassium has not been found to confer a benefit in recent trials.

i. **Transfusions:** Evolving thresholds for red blood cell transfusion in MI ultimately take into account balancing the risks of transfusions (transfusion reactions, transfusion-transmitted infections, costs) with a clinical judgment of whether transfusion is likely to improve oxygen delivery (in severe or symptomatic anemia such as Hgb <8 g/dL, or 8-10 g/dL with hemodynamic instability or ongoing ischemia) or if there are other considerations such as active bleeding or trauma.

j. Prompt pharmacologic or mechanical **reperfusion therapy** is critical to optimize the salvage of viable myocardium. Reperfusion reduces infarct size, improves function, and decreases mortality. Temporary myocardial impairment ("stunned myocardium") may exist even after perfusion is restored. Factors to consider when selecting a reperfusion strategy include (i) the timing of presentation and (ii) anticipated PCI availability. Primary PCI is preferred when it can be performed within 120 minutes of first medical contact, and ideally within 90 minutes. It is also preferred over fibrinolytic therapy in some patients even when delayed beyond this time window: those at high bleeding risk and those at high risk of death such as ongoing cardiogenic shock. Otherwise, fibrinolytic therapy should be considered and may be appropriate in patients with up to 12 hours of symptoms. Reperfusion is assessed noninvasively through relief of symptoms, restoration of hemodynamic or respiratory stability, or a 50% or better reduction in initial ST-segment elevation.

1. **Thrombolysis** is only indicated in the presence of ST-segment elevation greater than 0.1 mV in at least two contiguous leads. Thrombolysis yields the greatest benefit when initiated within 6 hours of symptom onset, although definite benefit exists even at 12 hours. Patients presenting within 12 to 24 hours but with continuing symptoms may also benefit. Response to therapy results in improvement in ST-segment elevation and resolution of chest discomfort. Persistent symptoms and ST-segment elevation 60 to 90 minutes after thrombolysis are indications for urgent angiography and possible PCI. Thrombolysis offers no benefit in patients without ST-segment elevation or new BBB, or in those with MI complicated by HF or cardiogenic shock. Table 15.3 compares the commonly used thrombolytic agents. **Absolute contraindications** are any prior intracranial hemorrhage, a cerebral vascular malformation or neoplasm, suspected aortic dissection, active bleeding, or significant head trauma or ischemic stroke within 3 months (except an acute cerebrovascular accident [CVA] within 3 hours). **Relative contraindications** include known bleeding diathesis, concurrent anticoagulation, recent trauma (2-4 weeks), prolonged cardiopulmonary resuscitation (>10 minutes), recent major surgery (<3 weeks), recent internal bleeding (2-4 weeks), severe HTN (systolic BP >180/110 mm Hg), other intracranial pathology, noncompressible vascular puncture sites, pregnancy, active peptic ulcer disease, or prior exposure (5 days to 2 years) to streptokinase or anisoylated plasminogen streptokinase activator complex (APSAC). **Patients requiring retreatment**, having failed streptokinase or APSAC, should receive tissue plasminogen activator (tPA). Those with contraindications to thrombolysis should be considered for PCI.

   a. **Streptokinase** is a bacterial protein produced by α-hemolytic streptococci. It induces activation of free and clot-associated plasminogen, eliciting a nonspecific systemic fibrinolytic state. It may decrease mortality by 18%. Side effects are hypotension and allergic-type reactions.

   b. **Tissue plasminogen activator (tPA)** is a recombinant natural protein. By increasing plasmin binding to fibrin, it provides relative clot-selective fibrinolysis without inducing a systemic lytic state. When given with heparin, its early reperfusion rate is slightly better than that of other agents. Compared to streptokinase, it is less likely to cause hemorrhage requiring transfusion and has greater survival benefit (10 additional lives in 1000 treated). It has

TABLE 15.3 Comparison of Thrombolytic Drugs

	tPA	Streptokinase	APSAC
Half-life	6 min	20 min	100 min
Dosage	100 mg[a]	1.5 million units	30 units
Administration	90 min	30-60 min	5 min
Fibrin selective	Yes	No	Partial
Artery patency rate[b]	79%	40%	63%
ICH	0.6%	0.3%	0.6%
Lives saved/1000 treated	35	25	25
Antigenic	No	Yes	Yes
Hypotension	No	Yes	Yes
Heparin required	Yes	No	No
Cost per dose	$2750	$537	$2368

APSAC, anisoylated plasminogen streptokinase activator complex; ICH, intracranial hemorrhage; tPA, tissue plasminogen activator.
[a]15 mg bolus, then 0.75 mg/kg over 30 minutes (maximum 50 mg), then 0.5 mg/kg over 60 minutes (maximum 35 mg) to provide total of 100 mg over 90 minutes.
[b]Artery patency rate at 90 minutes after treatment.

a modest increase in the incidence of hemorrhagic stroke (0.7% as compared to 0.5%). The global utilization of streptokinase and tPA for occluded arteries (GUSTO) trial showed evidence of higher vessel patency with tPA compared to streptokinase. **Reteplase** is a deletion mutein of tPA but does not appear to have any benefits over tPA. **Tenecteplase** is a genetically engineered tPA mutant with a higher specificity for fibrin and a similar mortality rate.

c. **Anisoylated plasminogen streptokinase activator complex (APSAC)** (anistreplase) has clinical characteristics between those of tPA and streptokinase (see Table 15.3).

2. **PCI and stenting:** The term PCI has replaced percutaneous transluminal coronary angioplasty (PTCA) because atherectomy and stenting have improved patency rates above that of angioplasty alone. **Primary PCI** refers to PCI without prior administration of thrombolysis. **Facilitated PCI** refers to PCI after administration of a medical regimen to improve coronary patency. **Rescue PCI** refers to PCI within 12 hours of a failed fibrinolysis (continuing or recurrent ischemia) but is no longer recommended. All patients who undergo primary PCI should be pretreated at diagnosis with anticoagulant and antiplatelet therapy. In addition to the absence of a thoracotomy and associated complications, there are fewer neurologic sequelae with PCI compared to CABG. The primary constraint of PCI is the availability of personnel and support facilities that are only available in about 20% of hospitals in the United States. Adjuncts to PCI that reduce coronary reocclusion include **IV heparin, ASA, ticlopidine, and GP IIb/IIIa inhibitors.** The benefit of LMWH compared to UFH in PCI is unclear at this time. A glycoprotein IIb/IIIa inhibitor (eg, abciximab) may decrease mortality, MI recurrence, and the need for urgent revascularization.

3. **Acute surgical reperfusion (CABG)** may be emergently indicated for patients with operable coronary anatomy who have failed medical management but are not candidates for PCI; have failed PCI; have persistent ischemia, hemodynamic instability, or cardiogenic shock; have surgically correctable complications of MI (eg, severe MR or

ventricular septal defect [VSD]); or have life-threatening arrhythmias in the presence of severe left main or three-vessel disease. Mortality from emergent CABG and CABG in the first 3 to 7 days after STEMI is high.

k. **Intra-aortic balloon counterpulsation** with an intra-aortic balloon pump (IABP) may be indicated in patients awaiting PCI or CABG who have low CO unresponsive to inotropic support or who demonstrate refractory pulmonary congestion. The effects of IABP counterpulsation include diastolic BP augmentation, thus increasing coronary perfusion, and systolic BP reduction, thus decreasing the impedance to ejection. Although IABP continues to be widely used in this setting, its overall benefit has been questioned in various studies.

IV. COMPLICATIONS OF MYOCARDIAL INFARCTION

A. Recurrent Ischemia and Infarction: Common causes of chest pain after MI are pericarditis, ischemia, and reinfarction. Up to 58% of patients will show early recurrent angina after successful reperfusion. Reinfarction occurs in approximately 3% to 4% of patients in the first 10 days after treatment with thrombolysis and ASA. Patients with reinfarction are at increased risk for cardiogenic shock, fatal dysrhythmias, or cardiac arrest. The initial approach should be to optimize medical therapies and consider either repeat thrombolysis or PCI. Emergency CABG is considered for those who have failed or are not candidates for medical treatment or PCI. Patients with active ischemia unresponsive to medical therapies may be placed on an IABP while awaiting coronary angiography.

B. Cardiogenic Shock: The incidence of cardiogenic shock after MI is approximately 7.5% and mortality is extremely high. It is defined as inadequate end-organ perfusion caused by cardiac dysfunction, represented by the following hemodynamic parameters despite adequate or elevated filling pressures: systolic blood pressure (SBP) less than 80 to 90 mm Hg or mean arterial pressure (MAP) 30 mm Hg less than baseline, cardiac index less than 1.8 L/min/m^2 without support or less than 2 to 2.2 L/min/m^2 with support. Acute MI with LV failure is the most common cause of cardiogenic shock, which develops when contractility of about 40% of the ventricular myocardium is lost. Other mechanical complications of MI discussed later can also result in cardiogenic shock. Patients should be given hemodynamic and respiratory support as needed and β-blockers should be avoided. Hemodynamic support consists of optimizing volume status and initiating pharmacologic (vasopressors and inotropes such as norepinephrine, epinephrine, dopamine, or dobutamine) or mechanical circulatory support. Short-term mechanical circulatory support options include an IABP and percutaneous ventricular assist devices (Impella 2.5 or Impella CP are transvalvular left ventricular assist devices [LVADs], and the Impella RP system is a percutaneous right ventricular assist device [RVAD]), implanted LVAD or biventricular assist devices, extracorporeal mechanical oxygenator (ECMO) circuits, and percutaneous left atrial-to-femoral arterial ventricular assist device (TandemHeart). These mechanical circulatory support devices are addressed in further detail in **Chapter 19**.

C. Mechanical Complications

1. **Mitral regurgitation (MR)** can occur from papillary muscle rupture, often presenting 3 to 5 days postinfarct, and is commonly associated with an inferior MI and rupture of the posteromedial papillary muscle. Findings may include pulmonary edema, hypotension, cardiogenic shock, and a new apical systolic murmur. The pulmonary artery occlusion pressure waveform may exhibit large V waves. A ruptured papillary muscle and MR may be evident on echocardiography. Treatment includes afterload reduction, inotropes, and, in certain cases, an IABP, Impella device, or ECMO while

awaiting emergent surgical repair. Medical management alone results in a mortality of roughly 75% in the first 24 hours.

2. **Ventricular septal defect (VSD)** most commonly occurs between 3 and 5 days after anterior MI. Clinical signs include a new holosystolic murmur with systolic thrill and cardiogenic shock. A septal defect will be seen on echocardiography. An increased SaO_2 between blood sampled from the right atrium and right ventricle can confirm an interventricular shunt. Treatment includes afterload reduction, inotropy; and in settings of cardiogenic shock refractory to medical management, an IABP, Impella device, or ECMO should be considered. Patients who are hemodynamically stable may not require immediate surgical repair but mortality in patients with cardiogenic shock is up to 90% without surgical intervention.
3. **Ventricular free wall rupture** accounts for about 10% of peri-infarct death. Risk factors include sustained HTN after MI, a large transmural MI, late thrombolysis, female gender, advanced age, and exposure to steroids or nonsteroidal anti-inflammatory agents. It is most common in the first 2 weeks after MI, with peak incidence 3 to 6 days postinfarct. Recurrent chest pain, acute HF, and cardiovascular collapse suggest free wall rupture. Death can occur rapidly and overall mortality is high. Diagnosis is by echocardiography. Volume expansion, tamponade decompression, and IABP may be used to temporize before emergent surgical repair.
4. **Ventricular aneurysm** is usually due to thinning of the infarcted ventricular wall. It is characterized by a protrusion of scar tissue in association with HF, malignant dysrhythmias, and systemic embolism. Persistent ST-segment elevation may be evident, while echocardiography confirms. Anticoagulation is required, especially in patients with documented mural thrombus. Surgical correction of ventricular geometry may be necessary.

D. Pericardial Complications: Pericarditis, due to extension of myocardial necrosis to the epicardium, occurs in about 25% of patients within weeks of MI. Pleuritic chest pain or positional discomfort, radiation to the left shoulder, a pericardial rub, diffuse J-point elevation, concave ST-segment elevation, reciprocal PR depression, and pericardial effusion on echocardiography may be evident. Treatment includes **ASA** 162 to 325 mg daily, increased to 650 mg every 4 to 6 hours if necessary. Indomethacin, ibuprofen, and corticosteroids are avoided because wall thinning in the zone of myocardial necrosis may predispose to ventricular wall rupture.

E. Conduction Abnormalities

1. **Dysrhythmias,** including premature ventricular contractions, bradycardia, atrial fibrillation, atrioventricular blocks, ventricular fibrillation, ventricular tachycardia, and idioventricular rhythms are common in the setting of MI. Multiple etiologies may include HF, ischemia, reentrant rhythms, reperfusion, acidosis, electrolyte derangements (eg, hypokalemia, hypomagnesemia, intracellular hypercalcemia), hypoxemia, hypotension, drug effects, and heightened reflex sympathoadrenal and vagal activity. Treatment of any precipitating cause should be undertaken immediately. **Chapter 17** discusses these dysrhythmias and their treatments in detail.

F. Hypertension increases myocardial O_2 demand and may worsen ischemia. Causes of HTN after MI include premorbid HTN, HF, and elevated catecholamines due to pain and anxiety. Treatment includes adequate antianginal therapy, analgesia, anxiolysis, IV NTG, β-blockade, and angiotensin-converting enzyme (ACE) inhibitors. Calcium channel blockers (verapamil or diltiazem) may be indicated in patients who have contraindications to other agents. Nitroprusside may be required if HTN is severe.

V. PERIOPERATIVE MYOCARDIAL ISCHEMIA AND INFARCTION

A. Definition, Incidence, and Risk Factors: An MI in patients undergoing noncardiac surgery is defined as a rise in troponin associated with suggestive symptoms or ECG changes. As medical and surgical therapy for cardiovascular disease continues to improve, more patients with these conditions are living longer, healthier lives. However, as a result, more patients with CAD or related risk factors (advanced age, HTN, DM, HF, decreased exercise tolerance, and renal disease) are presenting for cardiac and noncardiac surgery than ever before and this number is only expected to rise. Normal risks of surgery and anesthesia (pain, tachycardia, HTN, increased sympathetic tone, coronary vasoconstriction, hypoxemia, anemia, shivering, hypercoagulability) place this population at increased risk for ischemia and perioperative MI. Of over 27 million patients undergoing noncardiac surgery each year, approximately 1 million suffer some form of perioperative cardiac complication, contributing to over $20 billion of added health care costs. In patients with preexisting CAD, roughly 6% will experience a perioperative MI. Patients that suffer MI after surgery have a 15% to 25% risk of in-hospital death and a significant increase in 6-month morbidity and mortality. A few scoring systems including the revised cardiac risk index (RCRI) have been created to identify patients at high risk for perioperative cardiac complications including MI.

B. Perioperative Monitoring and Diagnosis: Under normal conditions, MI is diagnosed on the basis of history (see **Sections I.A.1** and **II.A**), increased biomarkers (see **Section III.C.2**), and characteristic ECG changes (see **Section III.C.1**). However, postoperative pain and pain control techniques may render a perioperative MI "silent." Because perioperative MI occurs most often on the day of surgery or postoperative day 1, increased diagnostic weight must be given to ECG changes and cardiac enzymes early in the postoperative course. A high index of suspicion, especially in a population likely to have preexisting ECG abnormalities (eg, arrhythmias, BBBs, LV hypertrophy, pacemakers), should be maintained. Comparison of a daily ECG to baseline is a cost-effective monitoring plan. Biomarkers should be obtained for confirmation rather than surveillance, bearing in mind that these enzymes may be elevated as a direct result of surgery (eg, in CABG). Transthoracic and transesophageal echocardiography (see **Chapter 2**) are excellent investigative modalities when an adverse cardiac event is suspected because regional wall motion abnormalities will precede both ECG changes and biomarker increases.

C. Preventive Strategies: Surgical stress and anesthesia provoke myriad physiologic and biochemical changes that can be influenced to the betterment of postoperative care.

1. **β-Blockade:** There is evidence supporting the use of perioperative β-blockade to decrease cardiovascular complications in patients at risk, including those using tobacco, older than age 65, or with CAD, HTN, DM, hypercholesterolemia, or a family history of CAD. Prescribed β-blockade should be continued up to and including the morning of surgery. Patients not on a regimen can be treated with **metoprolol** 5 mg IV unless HR is less than 60 bpm or systolic BP is less than 110 mm Hg. Metoprolol may also be given in the operating or recovery room to maintain an HR of 50 to 80 bpm. Upon completion of surgery, chronic β-blockade should be resumed and patients at risk may be started on metoprolol 25 mg po tid for at least 2 weeks. Contraindications include bronchospasm, symptomatic HF, third-degree heart block, or prior adverse reaction to β-blockers.
2. **Pain control:** The patient may have postoperative or ischemic pain, but owing to sedation, intubation, or pain control modalities, may not be able to report it. Surgical pain may cause tachycardia, HTN, sympathetic discharge, and coronary vasoconstriction, all of which can raise myocardial

O_2 consumption while compromising supply. Adequate sedation and analgesia (using opioids, benzodiazepines, propofol, or regional anesthesia) are mainstays of postoperative care that may contribute to improved cardiac outcomes. Nonsteroidal anti-inflammatory drugs (NSAIDs) such as ketorolac have both analgesic and antiplatelet effects. Clonidine, an α-2 agonist, inhibits presynaptic norepinephrine release, and producing beneficial effects on HR, BP, and thrombosis.

3. **O_2 carrying capacity:** A true or dilutional anemia may result from excessive intra- or postoperative blood loss or from aggressive IV hydration, respectively. Either etiology may limit O_2 delivery to myocardium at risk. Treatment should be individualized to patient and procedure and should consider the risk of complications of impaired oxygenation. Although absolute transfusion "triggers" should be avoided, judicious fluid resuscitation and transfusion practice should maintain a hematocrit between 25% and 30%.
4. **Temperature regulation:** Postanesthesia homeothermic derangement may cause shivering and an augmented O_2 demand. Low temperatures may also compromise postsurgical hemostasis. Unless contraindicated, patients should be kept normothermic by means of limiting unnecessary exposure, forced air warmers, and warmed IV fluids and blood products. In a patient who is intubated and ventilated, a nondepolarizing muscle blocker can prevent shivering.
5. **Glucose homeostasis:** Surgical stress can exacerbate preexisting DM or impaired glucose tolerance. High glucose levels can worsen to endothelial dysfunction. An insulin infusion or sliding scale should maintain a goal of 110 to 150 mg/dL.
6. **Coagulation:** Surgery can induce a protective hemostatic state that may be detrimental to the patient with CAD. Decreased fibrinolysis, increased platelet count and function, and increased fibrinogen and coagulation factor levels may cause intracoronary thrombosis. ASA, NSAIDs, and α-2 agonists have a role in preventing untoward thrombotic complications.

D. Management

1. **Consultation** with a cardiologist, the primary surgical team, and when indicated, a cardiac surgeon, should begin the moment a perioperative MI is suspected because emergent reperfusion by PCI or CABG may be warranted (see **Section III.D.3.j**). Owing to the patient's recent surgery, thrombolysis will likely be contraindicated.
2. **Supportive measures** include continued ECG, biomarker, and invasive monitoring as appropriate, as well as intervention in all parameters listed under "Preventive Strategies" (see **Section V.C**) can contribute to improved outcomes after a cardiac complication.
3. Current **medications** (as discussed in **Sections II.E**, **III.D.3**, and **V.C**) should be reviewed in light of the change in clinical status. If not begun already, aspirin, β-blockade, ACE inhibitors, and statins should be started if no contraindications exist. Those who are not at increased bleeding risk should be considered for anticoagulation therapy.
4. As mentioned earlier, reperfusion strategies such as thrombolysis, PCI, or CABG should be considered promptly. The benefits and risks of thrombolysis and primary PCI, particularly the bleeding risk in the postoperative setting, should be considered for each individual patient by all managing health care providers. An IABP may be useful for improving coronary blood flow, although device placement may be complicated in patients with peripheral arterial disease.

Selected Readings

Abuzaid A, Fabrizio C, Felpel K, et al. Oxygen therapy in patients with acute myocardial infarction: a systemic review and meta-analysis. *Am J Med.* 2018;131(6):693-701.

Antman EM, Anbe DT, Armstrong PW, et al. ACC/AHA guidelines for the management of patients with ST-elevation myocardial infarction—executive summary: a report of the American College of Cardiology/American Heart Association Task Force on Practice Guidelines (Writing Committee to revise the 1999 guidelines for the management of patients with acute myocardial infarction). *Circulation.* 2004;110(5):588-636.

Antman EM, Hand M, Armstrong PW, et al. 2007 focused update of the ACC/AHA 2004 guidelines for the management of patients with ST-elevation myocardial infarction. A report of the American College of Cardiology/American Heart Association Task Force on Practice Guidelines. *Circulation.* 2008;117(2):296-329.

Auerbach AD, Goldman L. β-Blockers and reduction of cardiac events in noncardiac surgery scientific review. *JAMA.* 2002;287(11):1435-1444.

Butterworth J, Furberg CD. Improving cardiac outcomes after noncardiac surgery. *Anesth Analg.* 2003;97(3):613-615.

Chareonthaitawee P, Askew JW. Exercise ECG testing: performing the test and interpreting the ECG results. *UpToDate.* Updated January 16, 2020. Accessed June 28, 2021. https://www.uptodate.com/contents/exercise-ecg-testing-performing-the-test-and-interpreting-the-ecg-results#:~:text=The%20exercise%20ECG%20indirectly%20detects,epicardial%20coronary%20artery%20obstruction%22

Devereaux PJ, Goldman L, Yusuf S, et al. Surveillance and prevention of major perioperative ischemic cardiac vents in patients undergoing noncardiac surgery: a review. *CMAJ.* 2005;173(7):779-788.

Eagle KA, Guyton RA, Davidoff R, et al. ACC/AHA 2004 guideline update for coronary artery bypass graft surgery: a report of the American College of Cardiology/American Heart Association Task Force on Practice Guidelines (Committee to update the 1999 guidelines for coronary artery bypass graft surgery). *Circulation.* 2004;110(14):e340-e437.

Fraker TD, Fihn SD, Gibbons RJ, et al. 2007 chronic angina focused update of the ACC/AHA 2002 guidelines for the management of patients with chronic stable angina: a report of the American College of Cardiology/American Heart Association Task Force on Practice Guidelines Writing Group to develop the focused update of the 2002 guidelines for the management of patients with chronic stable angina. *J Am Coll Cardiol.* 2007;50(23):2264-2274.

Jansson K, Fransson SG. Mortality related to coronary angiography. *Clin Radiol.* 1996;51(12):858-860.

Landesberg G. The pathophysiology of perioperative myocardial infarction: facts and perspectives. *J Cardiothorac Vasc Anesth.* 2003;17(1):90-100.

Lubbrook GL, Webb RK, Currie M, Watterson LM. Crisis management during anaesthesia: myocardial ischaemia and infarction. *Qual Saf Health Care.* 2005;14(3):e13.

Mehta SR, Yusuf S, Díaz R, et al. Effect of glucose-insulin-potassium infusion on mortality in patients with acute ST-segment elevation myocardial infarction: the CREATE-ECLA randomized controlled trial. *JAMA.* 2005;293(4):437-446.

Meine TJ, Roe MT, Chen AY, et al. Association of intravenous morphine use and outcomes in acute coronary syndromes: results from the CRUSADE Quality Improvement Initiative. *Am Heart J.* 2005;149(6):1043-1049.

Podgoreanu MV, White WD, Morris RW, et al. Inflammatory gene polymorphisms and risk of perioperative myocardial infarction after cardiac surgery. *Circulation.* 2006;114(1 suppl):I275-I281.

Priebe H-J. Perioperative myocardial infarction-aetiology and prevention. *Br J Anaesth.* 2005;95(1):3-19.

Reyentovich A. Prognosis and treatment of cardiogenic shock complicating acute myocardial infarction. *UpToDate.* Updated June, 2021. Accessed July 7, 2021. https://www.uptodate.com/contents/prognosis-and-treatment-of-cardiogenic-shock-complicating-acute-myocardial-infarction?search=a%20prognosis%20and%20treatment%20of%20cardiogenic%20shock&source=search_result&selectedTitle=1~150&usage_type=default&display_rank=1

Reynolds, HR, Hochman JS. Cardiogenic shock: current concepts and improving outcomes. *Circulation.* 2008;117(5):686-697.

Thygesen K, Alpert JS, Jaffe AS, et al. Fourth universal definition of myocardial infarction. *J Am Coll Cardiol.* 2018;72(18):2231-2264.

16 Valvular Heart Disease

Sameer Lakha and Alexander S. Kuo

The prevalence of valvular heart disease is a common complicating comorbidity in the patient who is critically ill.

I. AORTIC STENOSIS

Aortic stenosis (AS) refers to a narrowing of the valvular orifice, restricting flow from the left ventricle into the ascending aorta during systole. Etiologies of AS include senile degeneration (calcific), congenital bicuspid or unicuspid valves, and, rarely in North America, rheumatic disease.

A. Pathophysiology

1. A narrowing of the aortic valve orifice leads to restriction of flow from the left ventricle into the ascending aorta. This causes increased left ventricular (LV) chamber pressures, resulting in increased LV wall tension, myocardial oxygen demand, and compensatory LV concentric hypertrophy with increased **susceptibility to ischemia and arrhythmias.**
2. Adequate coronary perfusion pressure is vital and dependent on maintenance of diastolic pressure through preservation of systemic vascular resistance.
3. Increasing LV wall thickness subsequently leads to diastolic dysfunction with impairment of active relaxation and passive ventricular filling during diastole.

B. Diagnosis

1. **Physical exam:** Auscultation reveals a loud, late-peaking systolic murmur best heard at the right upper sternal border, radiating to the carotids, with delayed carotid upstroke.
2. **Symptoms:** Patients present with dyspnea on exertion, angina, or presyncope/syncope. The onset of symptoms strongly correlates with disease progression and dramatic increase in risk of sudden cardiac death.
3. **Diagnosis:** Echocardiography is used to diagnose AS but cardiac catheterization may also be used. Pressure gradients from simultaneous measurement obtained via catheterization are typically lower than peak-to-peak echocardiography-derived gradients.

C. Severe AS

Severe AS: Aortic valve area (AVA) **less than 1.0 cm^2**, or 0.6 cm/m^2 when normalized to body surface area (BSA) for extremes in body size. Mean gradients **greater than 40 mm Hg**, or peak flow velocity greater than 4 m/s. Pressure gradients are flow dependent and the severity may be underestimated in patients with low cardiac output or decreased LV systolic or diastolic function.

D. Hemodynamic Management

1. **Heart rate: Reduction is essential** in patients with severe AS. Tachycardia leads to significantly increased myocardial oxygen demand and decreased diastolic filling and perfusion time. Extremes of bradycardia can be deleterious because of fixed stroke volume of the thickened ventricle or when it leads to decreased coronary perfusion.
2. **Rhythm:** Sinus rhythm becomes imperative as the hypertrophied left ventricle becomes dependent on atrial contraction to maintain LV diastolic filling. In the setting of impaired LV relaxation, up to 40% of LV end-diastolic volume is contributed by atrial contraction.
3. **Afterload:** Hypotension is poorly tolerated and should be **treated immediately** because of the high susceptibility of the hypertrophied myocardium

to ischemia. First-line treatment is a **pure vasoconstrictor such as phenylephrine** to avoid tachycardia while improving coronary perfusion. In patients with decompensated heart failure and severe AS, afterload reduction can be very carefully titrated with intensive hemodynamic monitoring to improve forward flow. In moderate or asymptomatic AS, hypertension can be treated following standard medical guidelines.

4. **Preload:** Diastolic dysfunction from concentric hypertrophy may require elevated filling pressure for adequate stroke volume. However, in decompensated AS, aggressive fluid administration may lead to pulmonary edema.
5. **Contractility:** Inotropic support may be needed in decompensated severe AS. However, inodilators such as dobutamine and milrinone can lead to marked reduction in systemic blood pressure and tachyarrhythmias.

E. Treatment

1. For mild to moderate asymptomatic AS, medical therapy aimed at blood pressure and heart rate control following established guidelines is generally sufficient.
2. The definitive treatment for severe AS is aortic valve replacement (AVR). Indications for surgical AVR (SAVR) or transcatheter AVR (TAVR) include symptomatic severe AS or severe AS with heart failure. SAVR is recommended for patients who are younger than age 65 and in those with asymptomatic severe AS with rapid progression. Currently, TAVR is recommended in patients who meet indications for AVR but are age 80 or older or at high-to-prohibitive surgical risk but with an expected survival of greater than 12 months. The choice between SAVR and TAVR in all other patients should be made as part of shared decision-making with a multispecialty team.
3. **Percutaneous balloon dilation:** results in a modest reduction in the severity of AS but is often complicated by severe aortic regurgitation (AR), restenosis, and clinical deterioration. Percutaneous aortic balloon dilation as a bridge to AVR is controversial. Palliative balloon dilation is not recommended because of the associated morbidity and lack of improved mortality.

F. Postoperative AS Treatment Care: Although LV outflow resistance and LV cavity pressures should improve following AVR, LV hypertrophic remodeling may not resolve for months. Persistent LV hypertrophy requires higher filling pressures to maintain cardiac output and the thickened myocardium remains susceptible to ischemia at low coronary perfusion pressures.

G. Hypertrophic Obstructive Cardiomyopathy (HOCM): HOCM is subvalvular dynamic obstruction of the left ventricular outflow tract (LVOT) caused by regional hypertrophy of the myocardium. Patients with HOCM are prone to lethal ventricular arrhythmias. Dynamic LVOT obstruction can lead to refractory hypotension and is exacerbated by ventricular underfilling, increased inotropy, decreased afterload, and tachycardia. Acute management includes **increasing preload**, increasing afterload with pure α-agonists such as **phenylephrine**, and administration of **β-blockers, such as esmolol**, to decrease inotropy and chronotropy.

II. AORTIC REGURGITATION

AR is caused by incompetence of the aortic valve, resulting in retrograde blood flow from the ascending aorta into the left ventricle during diastole.

A. Acute AR: Acute severe or moderate AR can lead to LV volume overload, decreased effective systemic output, and terminal ventricular arrhythmias. It is considered a surgical emergency. Acute AR is often a result of aortic dissection, infective endocarditis, trauma, or as a consequence of surgical or percutaneous intervention.

B. Chronic AR: Chronic AR is generally progressive. It may be the result of degenerative calcification, a bicuspid aortic valve, rheumatic fever, or aortic root dilatation. Chronic LV volume overload leads to LV remodeling. Initial eccentric LV hypertrophy often progresses to LV dilation in end-stage disease. Symptoms of severe disease include angina, congestive heart failure, and dyspnea on exertion.

C. **Diagnosis**
   1. **Physical exam:** decrescendo diastolic murmur along left sternal border, widened pulse pressure, and visible capillary pulsation with nail bed compression
   2. Diagnosis and grading are made by echocardiography or catheterization. Echocardiographic evidence of holodiastolic flow reversal in the descending thoracic aorta by spectral Doppler, an AR vena contracta width of greater than 0.6 cm, and an AR jet width/LVOT diameter ratio of greater than 65% by color M-mode are consistent with severe AR by echocardiography.

D. **Hemodynamic Management**
   1. **Afterload: Reduction is critical** and improves forward cardiac output when the patient is acutely decompensated. In chronic AR, treatment of chronic hypertension is recommended; however, it does not alter the natural disease progression.
   2. **Heart rate: Elevation is beneficial** to the acute management of decompensated AR. An elevated heart rate decreases regurgitant time, promotes forward flow, and may reduce diastolic volume overload. However, judicious β-blocker use may be indicated in the setting of aortic dissection to minimize propagation of the dissection.
   3. **Contractility:** Inotropic support is often necessary to support heart failure in AR. Dobutamine and milrinone are often used for afterload reduction and for their positive chronotropic effect.
   4. **Preload:** Fluid administration should be carefully regulated to prevent volume overload.

E. **Treatment**
   1. Acute AR is often poorly tolerated and is considered a surgical emergency. AVR may be indicated for treatment of chronic severe AR when patients are symptomatic or have indications of LV systolic dysfunction or severe LV dilatation.

III. MITRAL STENOSIS

Mitral stenosis (MS) results from obstruction of LV inflow through the mitral valve (MV) during diastole. Common etiologies of MS include rheumatic heart disease and senile calcific stenosis. MS commonly leads to elevated left atrial and pulmonary arterial pressures, which may lead to pulmonary edema and right ventricular (RV) dysfunction.

A. **Diagnosis**
   1. **Physical exam:** loud S1, opening snap after the S2, with a diastolic murmur best heard at the apex
   2. MS may present with atrial fibrillation from left atrial distension, orthopnea, dyspnea on exertion, or heart failure. Hemoptysis can also occur at presentation because of pulmonary hypertension. The appearance of symptoms is an indicator of significantly increased mortality in untreated disease.
   3. Assessment with echocardiography is recommended. Transesophageal echocardiography is frequently a valuable adjunct. Angiography and exercise testing can be performed when symptoms are discrepant with echocardiographic findings because transvalvular pressures are highly dependent on heart rate and hemodynamic loading. RV and LV performance and assessment for left atrial thrombus is also important. Severe MS is defined as a valve area less than 1.5 cm^2 and very severe as less than 1.0 cm^2.

B. **Hemodynamic Management**
   1. **Heart rate: Lowering the heart rate** facilitates diastolic filling of the left ventricle. This improves forward flow and reduces pulmonary congestion. If pacing is needed, a longer PR interval (0.2 seconds) may allow for better filling across the MV.
   2. **Preload:** Maintenance of adequate preload is critical for adequate filling through the stenotic MV. Pulmonary artery occlusion pressures will be elevated but **will not accurately reflect LV end-diastolic filling pressure.** However, the pulmonary vascular congestion resulting from the MS predisposes the patient to pulmonary edema, so preload must be titrated carefully.
   3. **Contractility:** If inotropic support for RV or LV failure is needed, use of drugs without increased chronotropy, such as digoxin, is advantageous.

4. **Arrhythmia:** Atrial fibrillation is common in MS and may be difficult to control. Unfortunately, ventricular filling may be highly dependent on atrial contraction in these patients. Rapid ventricular rates should be avoided and **if rapid rates are associated with hemodynamic instability, it should be treated aggressively.**

C. Treatment

1. Percutaneous mitral balloon commissurotomy can be considered for patients with severe rheumatic MS and favorable anatomy. MV replacement or repair (MVR) is considered for patients who have failed or are not candidates for percutaneous mitral balloon commissurotomy. Calcific MS is associated with worse outcomes than rheumatic MS, even after successful valve intervention or surgery.

D. Anticoagulation With Mitral Stenosis

1. Because of the high risk of embolic events, long-term anticoagulation with a vitamin K antagonist to a goal international normalized ratio (INR) of 2.5 is recommended in patients with MS and one of the following: atrial fibrillation, prior embolism, or left atrial thrombus.

IV. MITRAL REGURGITATION

Mitral regurgitation (MR) is insufficiency of the MV resulting in backflow into the left atrium during systolic ejection of the left ventricle. This progresses to pulmonary hypertension and ultimately right heart failure. The compensatory response of the left ventricle results in dilation and eventually systolic dysfunction.

A. Acute Mitral Regurgitation is poorly tolerated and often presents with sudden hemodynamic decompensation. The sudden regurgitant flow of blood into the pulmonary circulation leads to pulmonary edema. The loss of forward flow leads to systemic shock. Acute MR can occur with papillary muscle or chordae tendinae rupture or dysfunction, often in the setting of an inferior myocardial infarction or valvular damage secondary to infective endocarditis. Early surgical repair is often indicated for severe acute MR.

B. Chronic Mitral Regurgitation: results in eccentric hypertrophy of the left ventricle, allowing it to tolerate volume overload without major increases in LV end-diastolic pressure. Chronic MR is characterized as primary if it is the result of dysfunction in the valvular apparatus or secondary if it is due to severe LV dilation and dysfunction. The etiology of disease influences treatment decisions. Because a fraction of the stroke volume is regurgitant, the ejection fraction (EF) is elevated in MR, 70%. When **EF declines to less than 60%** or end-systolic diameter is greater than 40 mm, **LV dysfunction is inferred.**

C. Diagnosis

1. **Physical exam:** Holosystolic murmur is best heard at the apex with radiation to the left axilla. A hyperdynamic point of maximal impulse is often palpable. In severe acute MR, the murmur may be absent because of the rapid equilibration of pressure between the left atrium and left ventricle.
2. Echocardiography is the primary method for diagnosis of acute MR, with transesophageal imaging indicated if transthoracic echocardiography is inadequate.

D. Hemodynamic Management

1. **Afterload: Reduction is essential** for the management of acute or decompensated MR. Reduced afterload promotes forward flow and reduces regurgitant fraction of the stroke volume. Nitroglycerin or calcium channel blockers are often used in acute management. In patients who are severely unstable, intra-aortic balloon pumps (IABPs) can be very effective in reducing effective afterload while preserving coronary perfusion.
2. **Heart rate: Higher heart rates** decrease regurgitant time and reduce end-diastolic volume preventing LV overdistension.
3. **Preload:** Volume status must be carefully balanced between adequate filling and overdistension of the left ventricle that may dilate the MV annulus and worsen the MR.

4. **Contractility:** Inotropic agents that also have chronotropic and afterload-reducing effects, such as milrinone or dobutamine, can improve forward flow in patients with heart failure from LV dysfunction.
5. **Pulmonary hypertension:** often occurs in severe MR and may lead to right heart failure. Avoid factors that elevate pulmonary artery pressures, such as hypoxia, hypercarbia, and acidosis. Use of pulmonary artery dilators such as inhaled nitric oxide or prostaglandin E1 may be considered.

E. Treatment

1. The mitral valve replacement (MVR) is indicated for patients with primary severe MR who are symptomatic or have signs of LV dysfunction. The treatment for secondary MR is less defined. It involves treatment of the underlying heart failure and possible cardiac resynchronization therapy. The role for surgery is more limited.
2. Transcatheter therapies have an emerging role in patients with primary severe MR and high-to-prohibitive surgical risk, as well as in a subset of patients with secondary MR optimized on medical therapy.

F. Postoperative Mitral Valve Replacement Care

1. After repair or replacement of the MV, the entire LV stroke volume ejecting against the aortic systemic pressures results in higher effective afterload. This **may unmask LV dysfunction** and result in heart failure. Inotropic or mechanical circulatory support may be required. Atrial fibrillation is poorly tolerated and antiarrhythmic or atrial overdrive pacing may be needed.

V. TRICUSPID STENOSIS

Tricuspid stenosis is the narrowing of the tricuspid valve impeding the inflow of blood into the right ventricle. It is relatively rare and most often secondary to rheumatic fever but can also be the result of carcinoid syndrome, systemic lupus erythematosus, or endomyocardial fibroelastosis. As the disease progresses, the right atrium (RA) becomes distended from elevated pressures and predisposes the patient to arrhythmias.

A. Diagnosis

1. **Physical exam:** Diastolic murmur may be difficult to detect on exam. Patients may present with venous congestion, jugular distension, hepatomegaly, peripheral edema, and/or ascites.
2. First presenting sign may also be palpitations or decreased exercise tolerance.
3. It is often diagnosed with echocardiography while evaluating coexisting valvular disease. Severe disease is considered when the valve area is less than 1.0 cm^2.

B. Hemodynamic Management

1. **Preload:** Elevated central venous filling pressures may be needed to maintain adequate cardiac output. In patients who are hemodynamically stable, diuresis can help relieve symptoms of peripheral venous congestion.
2. **Heart rate:** Lower heart rates allow adequate filling of the right ventricle.

C. Treatment

1. Severe symptomatic tricuspid stenosis can be corrected by surgical replacement, although isolated tricuspid surgery carries a high risk of morbidity and mortality relative to other valve surgeries.

D. Postoperative Care After Tricuspid Valve Repair or Replacement for Stenosis

1. Increase in RV filling may provoke RV failure. Inotropic support for the right ventricle and pulmonary artery pressure reduction may be required. It is **inadvisable to float a pulmonary artery catheter** blindly after tricuspid valve replacement or repair.

VI. TRICUSPID REGURGITATION

Tricuspid regurgitation (TR) is insufficiency of the tricuspid valve allowing backflow into the RA during systole. It is usually associated with other valvular lesions. Isolated TR can be well tolerated. Primary TR can be caused by chest trauma, endocarditis, or carcinoid syndrome. TR can also be secondary to pulmonary hypertension or ventricular dysfunction and dilation. The resultant volume overload of the RA predisposes to atrial fibrillation.

A. Diagnosis

1. **Physical exam:** systolic murmur accentuated by inspiration; S3 gallop. There may be pulsatile jugular venous flow. Venous congestion, including congestive hepatopathy and peripheral edema, may be present in severe cases.
2. **Echocardiography:** Doppler evidence of systolic flow reversal in the hepatic veins or tricuspid annular diameter greater than 4 cm suggests severe TR.

B. Hemodynamic Management

1. **Afterload:** Reduction in pulmonary vascular resistance decreases regurgitation and facilitates forward flow.
2. **Heart rate:** Higher heart rates decrease diastolic regurgitant time and reduce RV volume overload.
3. **Contractility:** With RV failure, inotropic agents such as dobutamine and milrinone can be used without significant increases in pulmonary vascular resistance.
4. **Preload:** Adequate preload is important to maintaining cardiac output. Diuresis may be needed in patients with severe congestive heart failure.

C. Treatment

1. Severe symptomatic TR can be alleviated by surgical repair or replacement. Outcomes depend on underlying RV function. Tricuspid surgery is most often performed concomitantly with surgery for a left-sided (ie, mitral) lesion.
2. Transcatheter tricuspid valve replacement and repair techniques are currently in late-stage clinical trials.

D. Postoperative Care After Tricuspid Repair or Replacement for Tricuspid Regurgitation

1. After correction of TR, the entire stroke volume is ejected forward, effectively increasing RV afterload. **This may precipitate RV failure** requiring inotropic support and reduction in pulmonary vascular resistance.

VII. PULMONIC VALVE DISEASE

Congenital pulmonic stenosis presents as right heart failure. Acquired pulmonic stenosis is rare and pulmonic regurgitation is usually well tolerated. Surgical intervention on the pulmonic valve may consist of excision of the valve without prosthetic replacement.

VIII. INFECTIVE ENDOCARDITIS

Infective endocarditis can be caused by bacteremia due to oral infections or other infections, including those associated with intravenous drug abuse. Patients with endocarditis may present with acute valvular dysfunction caused by destructive lesions, large vegetations, or papillary muscle dysfunction. Infectious endocarditis is reviewed in more detail in **Chapter 12**.

IX. ANTIBIOTIC PROPHYLAXIS FOR ENDOCARDITIS/RHEUMATIC HEART DISEASE

A. Antibiotic Prophylaxis for Endocarditis Before Dental Procedures is reasonable in patients who are at high risk, including those with prosthetic valves, a past history of endocarditis, cardiac transplants with structural valve abnormalities, unrepaired cyanotic congenital heart disease, repaired congenital heart disease with prosthetic material within 6 months, or with defects near prosthetic site.

B. Antibiotic prophylaxis is **not recommended in patients for nondental procedures** without active infection. Recurrent rheumatic fever can worsen rheumatic heart disease. Patients with prior history of rheumatic heart disease are often prescribed **long-term prophylaxis**, typically with penicillin.

X. PROSTHETIC VALVES

A. Anticoagulation for Mechanical Valve prostheses requires lifelong anticoagulation with a vitamin K antagonist. If interruption is required, heparin bridging is recommended.

1. Mechanical aortic valves without high-risk factors (see subsequent text): INR goal 2.5
2. Mechanical MV, or aortic valve with atrial fibrillation, LV systolic dysfunction, hypercoagulable state, history of embolic event: INR goal 3.0

TABLE 16.1 Qualitative Summary of Acute Hemodynamic Goals of Left-Sided Valvular Lesions

Valvular lesion	Heart rate	Preload	Afterload	Contractility
Aortic stenosis	↓↓	↑	↑	↔
Mitral stenosis	↓	↔	↔	↔
HOCM	↓↓	↑↑	↑	↓
Aortic regurgitation	↑	↔	↓↓	↑
Mitral regurgitation	↑	↓	↓↓	↑

HOCM, hypertrophic obstructive cardiomyopathy.

3. Aspirin 75 to 100 mg can be added if antiplatelet therapy is required for other indications.
4. **Direct oral anticoagulants are contraindicated** for use with mechanical valves because of increased incidence of both thrombotic complication and bleeding.

B. Anticoagulation for Biologic ("Tissue") Valve Prostheses, including TAVR, typically requires lifelong aspirin 75 to 100 mg. For the 3 to 6 months after surgical valve implantation, vitamin K antagonist anticoagulation is added with an INR goal of 2.5.

C. Prosthetic Valve Dysfunction can manifest as stenosis or regurgitation and can arise from chronic degeneration, mechanical complication/failure, valve thrombosis, or endocarditis. Acute severe prosthetic dysfunction is a potentially life-threatening emergency.

1. **Diagnosis:** Echocardiography is the mainstay of prosthetic valve evaluation, although transthoracic images are often limited in diagnostic yield. Transesophageal echocardiography and fluoroscopy may be required, particularly with mechanical valves.
2. **Thrombus on a left-sided mechanical valve is an emergency**, requiring surgery or thrombolysis. In other cases, a trial of vitamin K antagonist anticoagulation may be reasonable in patients who are hemodynamically stable.
3. Severe symptomatic prosthetic valve stenosis not due to thrombus typically requires repeat surgery. Valve-in-valve TAVR may be possible to replace a stenotic aortic bioprosthetic in a patient at high surgical risk.
4. Prosthetic valve regurgitation can manifest as frank regurgitation or with hemolysis from a smaller paravalvular leak. Surgical correction, valve-in-valve transcatheter replacement, and percutaneous paravalvular leak closure can be employed depending on surgical risk and valve characteristics. The acute hemodynamic goals for each type of valvular lesion have been summarized in Table 16.1.

Selected Readings

Gerlach RM, Sweitzer B. Overview of preoperative assessment and management. In: Longnecker DE, Mackey SC, Newman MF, Sandberg WS, Zapol WM, eds. *Anesthesiology*. 3rd ed. McGraw-Hill; 2017.

Holmes K, Gibbison B, Vohra HA. Mitral valve and mitral valve disease. *BJA Educ.* 2017;17(1):1-9.

Otto CM, Nishimura RA, Bonow RO, et al. 2020 ACC/AHA guideline for the management of patients with valvular heart disease: a report of the American College of Cardiology/American Heart Association Joint Committee on Clinical Practice Guidelines. *Circulation.* 2021;143:e72-e227.

Samarendra P, Mangione M. Aortic stenosis and perioperative risk with noncardiac surgery. *J Am Coll Cardiol.* 2015;65(3):295-302.

17 Cardiac Dysrhythmias

Peter O. Ochieng and Kenneth Shelton

I. INTRODUCTION

Arrhythmias and conduction abnormalities occur in 12% to 20% of patients admitted to medical or surgical intensive care units (ICUs), which increase morbidity and mortality. New-onset arrhythmias affect about 7% of patients following major noncardiothoracic surgery and up to 60% of patients post cardiac surgery. Atrial fibrillation (AF) is the most common postoperative arrhythmia occurring in 10% to 15% patients with critical illness, about 10% of patients undergoing noncardiac surgery, and up to 42% patients undergoing cardiac surgery.

In this chapter, we review the classification, etiology, and treatment of the arrhythmias most frequently encountered in critical care medicine.

II. CLASSIFICATION AND MANAGEMENT

A. The cardiac conduction system consists of three main parts: the sinus node, the atrioventricular (AV) node, and the His-Purkinje system.

B. There is not just one pacemaker system; instead, there are multiple mechanisms in cardiac pacing. Pathology of the sinus node and AV conduction system, as well as the right and left AV rings/right ventricular outflow tract, contributes to arrhythmias in the adult heart.

III. BRADYARRHYTHMIA

A. Pulseless Electrical Activity

1. Pulseless electrical activity (PEA) is cardiac arrest with the presence of spontaneous organized cardiac electrical activity in the absence of adequate organ perfusion sufficient to maintain consciousness.
   a. **Management:** Cardiopulmonary resuscitation (CPR) with uninterrupted chest compressions and standard pharmacologic interventions provide the basis of the treatment. Primary management involves treating the underlying cause (significant hypoxia, profound acidosis, severe hypovolemia, tension pneumothorax, electrolyte imbalance, drug overdose, sepsis, large myocardial infarction, massive pulmonary embolism, cardiac tamponade, hypoglycemia, hypothermia, etc). Extracorporeal cardiopulmonary resuscitation (ECPR) should be considered when there is prolonged failure of return to spontaneous circulation.

B. Abnormal Sympathetic Tone and the Cardiovascular Reflexes

Arrhythmias secondary to cardiovascular reflexes that are commonly seen are described subsequently (Table 17.1).

C. Sinoatrial Node Abnormality

1. **Sick sinus syndrome (SSS):** SSS indicates bradyarrhythmias with or without tachyarrhythmias. More than 50% of patients with SSS develop tachy-brady syndrome with AF or atrial flutter, leading to an increased risk of embolic

TABLE 17.1 Cardiovascular Reflexes

Reflex	Trigger	Receptor	Afferent limb	Nucleus	Efferent limb	Response
Arterial baroreceptor reflex	Increased BP	Baroceptors in aortic arch and carotid sinus	Glossopharyngeal (IX, carotid sinus) and vagus (X, aortic arch) nerves	Medulla (nucleaus solitarius)	The autonomic nervous system	Decreased HR, BP, and contractility
Bezold-Jarisch reflex	Hypotension	Mechanical and chemosensitive receptors in ventricular walls	Nonmyelinated vagal (X) C-fiber	Medulla	Inhibition of sympathetic outflow	Triad: decreased HR, decreased BP, and apnea
Bainbridge reflex	Changes in volume in the central thoracic compartment	Stretch receptors at junction of the vena cava and right atrium, junction of the pulmonary vein and left atrium, and vessel wall of carotid sinus and aortic arch	Vagus (X) nerve	Medulla	Inhibition of vagal outflow and enhancement of sympathetic outflow to sinoatrial node	Increased HR
Chemoreceptor reflex	Low O_2 and hydrogen ion, high CO_2	Chemoreceptors in carotid sinus and aortic body	Fibers in glossopharyngeal (IX, carotid sinus) and vagus (X, aortic arch) nerves	Medulla oblongata	Decreased parasympathetic nerve flow (vagal: X), increased sympathetic nerve flow (sympathetic nerve system)	Increased HR and stroke volume
Cushing reflex	Increased ICP	α-1 adrenergic receptors followed by vagus nerve stimulation	Arterioles of cerebrum	N/A	Sympathetic response activates α-1 adrenergic receptors, followed by vagus nerve parasympathetic response	Increased HR, BP, and contractility
Trigeminal reflex	Any stimulus to the trigeminal nerve	Mechanical and chemosensitive receptors in ventricular walls	Trigeminal nerve	Trigeminus nucleus—nucleus ambiguous in the brain stem	Premotor parasympathetic cardioinhibitory neurons of the vagal nerve	Systemic hypotension, cardiac dysrhythmia (bradycardia), apnea, gastric hypermotility, and coronary vasospasm

BP, blood pressure; HR, heart rate; ICP, intracranial pressure.

stroke. The etiology includes intrinsic dysfunction of the sinoatrial (SA) node including degenerative fibrosis, an infiltrative process, or inherited dysfunction of ion channels within the SA node. Extrinsic conditions, that is, metabolic, infectious, autonomic, or pharmacologic conditions, may also cause SSS (for a review, see Selected Readings).

a. **Management:** Chronic bradycardia may lead to ventricular electrical remodeling, and symptomatic SSS is a class I indication for a permanent pacemaker.

D. Conduction Delay and Bundle Branch Block (Congenital, Acquired)

1. **Conduction delay:** First-degree AV block is not an entirely benign condition. Instead, it may indicate worse clinical prognosis, especially among the older population. Second- and third-degree AV block warrants pacemaker implantation.
   a. **Management:** Cardiac pacing/resynchronization therapy for the patients with/without coexisting SSS; but the optimal pacing (as measured using the aortic flow time velocity integral measured on cardiac ultrasound) depends on intrinsic AV interval and desired pacing frequency.
2. **Bundle branch block:** Bundle branch block occurs secondary to a wide range of cardiac pathology. Compared with right bundle branch block (RBBB), left bundle branch block (LBBB) is considered to have high-diffuse disease, underlying ischemia, and dyssynchrony.
   a. **Management:** Both RBBB and LBBB may benefit from biventricular pacing to restore synchrony of right/left ventricular contraction.

IV. TACHYARRHYTHMIAS

A. Sinus Tachycardia

The etiology may include sepsis, hypovolemia, cardiac ischemia/congestive heart failure (CHF), pain, and endocrine pathology (hyperthyroidism) and management include treating the underlying cause.

B. Atrial Fibrillation

1. AF is characterized by a lack of organized P-wave activity and an irregularly irregular ventricular response on the electrocardiogram (ECG). AF is the most common arrhythmia requiring treatment, affecting around 5 million Americans, with the prevalence expected to triple by 2050.
2. AF is a complex molecular process. It may induce rapid atrial rates and promote increased sympathetic nerve activity, which augments β-adrenergic tone. This leads to an increase in protein kinase A–mediated hyperphosphorylation of atrial ryanodine receptors (RyR2). Increased RyR2 phosphorylation promotes sarcoplasmic reticulum calcium release that induces calcium-mediated inhibition of voltage-dependent L-type calcium currents. This leads to shortening of atrial myocyte action potential duration (ADP) and effective refractory periods (ERPs). The electric remodeling promotes further AF and increased sympathetic nerve output, myocyte apoptosis, and fibrosis and also promotes atrial dilatation and structural remodeling.
3. Mechanism of critical illness–related AF is not well understood, although it is more likely to occur in a predisposed individual with susceptible atrial substrate. Triggers include higher severity of critical illness, use of vasoactive agents, and electrolyte abnormalities.
4. **Management**
   a. **Treatment of stable AF** consists of pharmacologic intervention or overdrive pacing. Pharmacologic treatment involves rate control and rhythm control. These medications are described subsequently (Tables 17.2 and 17.3).
   b. **Unstable AF** (altered mental status, hypotension of systolic blood pressure <90 mm Hg, chest pain, shortness of breath) warrants synchronized cardioversion. For maintaining sinus rhythm after cardioversion, several class IA, IC, and III drugs, as well as class II (β-blockers), are moderately effective in maintaining sinus rhythm after conversion of AF.

TABLE 17.2 Current Antiarrhythmic Drug Therapy for Atrial Fibrillation

Class	Examples	Proarrhythmia	Other significant side effects	Contraindications
IC	Flecainide and propafenone	VT/VF; rapid atrial flutter	Rapidly conducting AF	CAD, hypertrophy
III	Sotalol and dofetilide	Torsade des pointes		Prolonged QT (at baseline or QTc >500 on treatment); heart failure (sotalol)
III	Dronedarone	Torsade des pointes (rare), VT/VF	Heart failure exacerbation and death (in those with CHF); hepatic injury (rare)	NYHA class IV CHF or class II/III with recent exacerbation; prolonged AT (QTc >500); and permanent AF
III	Amiodarone	Torsade des pointes (rare)	Lung toxicity, hepatic toxicity, thyroid toxicity, and optic neuritis (rare)	Liver failure and existing lung disease

AF, atrial fibrillation; CAD, coronary artery disease; CHF, congestive heart failure; NYHA, New York Heart Association; VF, ventricular fibrillation; VT, ventricular tachycardia.
Adapted from Woods CE, Olgin J. Atrial fibrillation therapy now and in the future: drugs, biologicals, and ablation. Circ Res. 2014;114(9):1532-1546.

TABLE 17.3 Rate Control Medications for Atrial Fibrillation

Class	Examples	When to use	Side effects	Contraindications
β-blockers	Metoprolol, esmolol	Considered first line for rate control	Bradycardia, heart block, bronchospasm	Decompensated HF, sick sinus syndrome
Nondihydropyridine calcium channel blockers (CCB)	Verapamil, diltiazem	Patients with pulmonary disease	Negative inotropy, avoid in LV systolic dysfunction	Decompensated heart failure
Class III	Amiodarone	When β-blockers or CCBs are contraindicated or ineffective	Hepatic toxicity, lung toxicity, thyroid toxicity, avoid if QTc >500	Cardiogenic shock second- or third-degree heart block
Cardiac glycosides	Digoxin	In patients with HF	AV block, ventricular arrhythmia, requires dose reduction in renal failure and when combined with other drugs (eg, amiodarone)	Ventricular fibrillation

AV, atrioventricular; HF, heart failure; LV, left ventricular.

c. **Pharmacologic interventions**

1. **β-Blockers:** β-blockers (eg, metoprolol) are the most used drug class for rate control. The atrial fibrillation follow-up investigation of rhythm management (AFFIRM) study has shown that they are the most effective drugs for rate control. Perioperative β-blocker usage has also been shown to prevent postoperative AF in patients undergoing cardiac surgery.

2. **Amiodarone:** Amiodarone prophylaxis reduces the incidence of AF after lung resection, transthoracic esophagectomy, and cardiac surgery. Amiodarone may reduce the incidence of AF to 23% (range: 12%-31%), with a number needed to treat of 4.4 (range: 3.1-7.8; **P**rophylaxis for **A**trial fibrilation in patients undergoing **S**urgery for lung **C**ancer: **A** controlled **R**andomized double blinded [PAS-CART] **T**rial). It is considered a reasonable prophylactic alternative to diltiazem; however, it should be avoided in patients undergoing pneumonectomy because of the risk of pulmonary toxicity.
3. **Diltiazem:** In a randomized, double-blinded, placebo-controlled study of 330 patients, diltiazem almost halved the incidence of clinically significant postoperative atrial arrhythmias ($P = .023$) following pneumonectomy. It is the preferred prophylactic medication after thoracic surgery for patients not on a β-blocker.

d. Ablations

1. **Radiofrequency ablation for paroxysmal AF (vs pharmacologic therapy):** The pulmonary vein-left atrial junction and an enlarged atrium harboring fibrosis and inflammation serve as the substrate for sustaining wavelets of AF. In radiofrequency ablation, low-voltage, high-frequency electricity is used to target focal areas thought to be responsible for AF. In a multicenter randomized trial at 24 months' posttreatment, AF was significantly lower in the ablation group compared with the drug-therapy group (9% vs 18%).

e. Anticoagulation

Anticoagulation is recommended for patients with a CHA_2DS_2-VASc score of 2 or more to reduce stroke risk. However, the critically ill, especially patients post an operation, are at a higher risk for major bleeding, precluding them from routine institution of anticoagulation.

C. Reentrant Tachyarrhythmias

These include AV reentrant and AV nodal reentrant tachyarrhythmias. Intravenous (IV) adenosine can help differentiate AF and atrial flutter from reentrant tachyarrhythmias and can be therapeutic in reentrant tachyarrhythmias. Direct current (DC) cardioversion is recommended in patients who are hemodynamically unstable. β-Blockers or calcium channel blockers may be used in the presence of hemodynamic stability.

D. Ventricular Tachyarrhythmias

The key findings that suggest ventricular tachyarrhythmia (VT) are AV dissociation, fusion or capture beats, QRS width (LBBB >160 msec, RBBB >140 msec), northwest axis, concordance, and LBBB morphology with right-axis deviation. Sustained VT is an unstable rhythm and when hemodynamically unstable needs emergent electrical cardioversion.

E. Torsade de Pointes

1. Risk factors for perioperative torsades de pointes are hypokalemia, hypomagnesemia, hypocalcemia, bradycardia, medications, and congenital long QT syndrome.
2. Risk factors for drug-induced torsades de pointes include female sex, hypokalemia, bradycardia, recent conversion from AF (particularly with a QT-prolonging drug), CHF, digitalis therapy, high drug concentrations (with the exception of quinidine), baseline QT prolongation, subclinical long-QT syndrome, ion channel polymorphisms, and severe hypomagnesemia.
3. In addition to reversing the inciting event, IV magnesium is the recommended therapy. As with any hemodynamically unstable rhythm, electrical cardioversion may be warranted.

V. ETIOLOGY

A. Cardiac Etiologies

1. **Abnormal QT syndromes and channelopathies:** Prolonged QTc affects short-term and long-term outcomes in patients with normal left ventricular function undergoing cardiac surgery. Mutations (inherited or acquired) in ion channels or associated proteins are the cause of a variety of cardiac arrhythmias. The genetics of sudden cardiac death caused by arrhythmias has been widely studied.
   a. Cardiac dysrhythmias may also be due to several genetic mutations.
      1. Alteration of slow delayed rectifier potassium current (Iks) leads to life-threatening cardiac arrhythmias, long QT syndrome, short QT syndrome, sinus bradycardia, and AF.
      2. Congenital sodium channelopathies lead to Brugada syndrome.
      3. Increased RyR2 activity has been shown to cause arrhythmias and increased CaMKII activity and phosphorylation of RyR2 at Ser2814. This may play a role in the pathogenesis of AF and ventricular arrhythmias.
2. **Cardiomyopathy**
   a. **Inherited arrhythmogenic diseases**
      1. Cardiomyopathy (hypertrophic cardiomyopathy, arrhythmogenic right ventricular cardiomyopathy, dilated cardiomyopathy)
      2. *Channelopathy* (long QT syndrome, short QT syndrome, Brugada syndrome, and catecholaminergic polymorphic ventricular tachycardia)
   b. **Ischemic cardiomyopathy**
   c. **Tachycardia-induced cardiomyopathy**
   d. **Frequent premature ventricular contractions**
   Premature ventricular contractions (PVCs) are being recognized as a cause of cardiomyopathy and suboptimal response to cardiac resynchronization therapy.
   e. **Extrinsic cardiomyopathy**
   Alcoholic, cirrhotic, metabolic, chemotherapy induced, radiation
   f. **Infiltrative cardiomyopathy**
   Amyloidosis, sarcoidosis, iron (thalassemia, hemochromatosis, hemosiderosis), autoimmune (rheumatic arthritis, systemic lupus erythematosus, systemic sclerosis, polymyositis, dermatomyositis, ankylosing spondylitis, celiac disease), Fabry disease, glucose-6-phosphate dehydrogenase (G6PD) deficiency, idiopathic fibrosis

B. Drug-Induced QT Prolongation (Table 17.4)

Drug-induced QT prolongation due to cardiovascular therapies (especially medications that delay QT interval) or noncardiovascular therapies (ie, anesthetics, psychotropic medications, etc) have been shown to prolong the QT interval and may lead to torsades de pointes. Inhibition of the cardiac K^+ channels may selectively block the rapidly activating delayed rectifier channel Ikr (ie, repolarizing potassium current) and is a common mechanism across drug classes.

C. Metabolic

1. Perioperative torsades de pointes can be fatal and a major risk factor is QT prolongation secondary to metabolic disarray.
   a. **Management:** Treat hypokalemia, hypomagnesemia, hypoxemia, hypothermia, hypoglycemia, and hypothyroidism.

D. Spinal Cord Injury

1. Bradycardia is the most commonly seen arrhythmia in the acute phase of spinal cord injury (SCI; 1-14 days after injury).
   a. This can be managed with anticholinergic agents (eg, atropine) that are considered first-line therapy or sympathomimetics (eg, dopamine and epinephrine). If there is persistent recurrent symptomatic bradycardia or complete heart block despite pharmacologic management, then a permanent pacemaker is considered.

TABLE 17.4 Drug-Induced Arrhythmias

Drug classification	Drugs
Cardiovascular	Amiodarone, arsenic trioxide, bepridil, cisapride, calcium channel blockers, disopyramide, dofetilide, flecainide, ibutilide, procainamide, quinidine, sotalol
Anesthetics	Volatile anesthetics (halothane, isoflurane, sevoflurane, desflurane)
	Intravenous anesthetics (etomidate, ketamine, propofol, thiopental)
	Local anesthetics
	Opioid receptor agonists or antagonists (alfentanil, buprenorphine, fentanyl, meperidine, methadone, morphine, oxycodone, remifentanil, sufentanyl, tramadol)
Neuromuscular blockers	Depolarizing (succinylcholine)
	Nondepolarizing (atracurium, cisatracurium, rocuronium, vecuronium)
Neuromuscular reversal agents	Anticholinesterases plus anticholinergics (neostigmine + atropine/glycopyrrolate, edrophonium + atropine), sugammadex
Perioperative adjuvants	Benzodiazepine (midazolam, etc), dexmedetomidine, domperidone, droperidol, metoclopramide, promethazine, 5HT-3 antagonists (ondansetron, dolasetron, tropisetron)
Psychotropic medications	Antipsychotic drugs (amisulpride, aripiprazole, chlorprothixene, clozapine, flupentixol, haloperidol, levomepromazine, olanzapine, paliperidone, perphenazine, pimozide, quetiapine, risperidone, sertindole, sulpiride, ziprasidone, zuclopenthixol)
	TCA and MAO inhibitors (amitriptyline, clomipramine, doxepin, imipramine, isocarboxazid, moclobemide, nortriptyline)
	Neurotransmitter uptake inhibitors (agomelatine, bupropion, citalopram, duloxetine, escitalopram, fluoxetine, mianserin, mirtazapine, paroxetine, reboxetine, sertraline, venlafaxine)
	Mood stabilizers (lithium)
	Antiseizure (carbamazepine, lamotrigine, valproate)
	Anxiolytic drugs (benzodiazepines, gabapentin, pregabalin)
	Anticholinergic drugs (biperiden, orphenadrine)
Drugs can cause low K	Diuretics (loop diuretics)
Drugs can cause low Mg	PPI (lansoprazole)
Antibiotics and antivirals	Fluoroquinolones
	Macrolides (azithromycin, erythromycin, clarithromycin)
	Chloroquine
	Protease inhibitors
Chemotherapy agents	Anthracycline, capecitabine (5-FU), cisplatin, histone deacetylase inhibitor (vorinostat)
Toxins	Mad honey intoxication (diterpene grayanotoxins), hydrocarbon, alcohol
Energy drinks	Caffeine
Other medications	Albuterol, colchicine, tosylchloramide

5-FU, 5-fluorouracil; MAO, monoamine oxidase; PPI, proton-pump inhibitor; TCA, tricyclic antidepressant.

E. Infection

1. Bacterial, viral, and parasitic infections are known to cause cardiac arrhythmias. Viral (Coxsackie B, HIV), community-acquired pneumonia (up to 5% may develop arrhythmias), Lyme disease, and Chagas disease are known to induce dysrhythmias. After the initial acute phase (<1% of patients will develop acute myocarditis), chronic disease can lead to upward of 33% of patients developing progressive cardiomyopathy-associated arrhythmias.

VI. ANESTHESIA-RELATED TOPICS

A. Inhalational anesthetics predispose the heart to arrhythmias. Classically, this has included halothane and methoxyflurane. However, even more modern anesthetics (sevoflurane, isoflurane) have been reported to prolong the QT interval.

B. The risk of arrhythmias associated with tracheal intubation was significantly reduced with preinduction administration of local anesthetics, calcium channel blockers, β-blockers, and narcotics compared with placebo.

C. Thoracic Epidural Analgesia: The use of thoracic epidural analgesia in patients undergoing coronary artery bypass graft surgery may reduce the risk of postoperative supraventricular arrhythmias and respiratory complications. There were no beneficial effects of thoracic epidural anesthesia (TEA) with general anesthesia on the risk of mortality, myocardial infarction, or neurologic complications compared with general anesthesia alone.

D. Local anesthetic systemic toxicity (LAST): LAST occurs when the local anesthetic reaches the systemic circulation at a supratherapeutic level. It can present with neurologic symptoms (metallic taste, tinnitus, circumoral numbness, altered mental status, and seizures) and cardiovascular symptoms (hypotension, bradycardia, ventricular arrhythmias, and cardiovascular collapse).

1. Management includes standard advanced cardiovascular life support (ACLS) and prompt lipid emulsion bolus of 1.5 mL/kg and subsequent infusion. Low-dose epinephrine (<1 μg/kg) may be used; however, vasopressin should be avoided because it can result in worsening acidosis. Cardiopulmonary bypass has also been used in some cases.

VII. EPILEPSY

Sudden, unexpected death has been reported in patients with epilepsy. Primary etiologies include channelopathies that involve both the brain and the heart (long QT syndrome type 2). Syncope, seizure-induced bradycardia, and asystole may be secondary to an activated sympathetic system, increased compensatory responses (elevated adenosine levels), hypoxemia, hypercarbia, and pulmonary edema.

VIII. CONCLUSION

Arrhythmias predispose patients to increased morbidity and mortality. A thorough preoperative assessment, appropriate monitoring, and perioperative vigilance may reduce the inherent risks associated with these arrhythmias. As perioperative practitioners, we are often the first clinicians to intervene when lethal dysrhythmias occur.

Selected Readings

Bosch NA, Cimini J, Walkey AJ. Atrial fibrillation in the ICU. *Chest.* 2018;154(6):1424-1434. doi:10.1016/j.chest.2018.03.040

El-Boghdadly K, Pawa A, Chin KJ. Local anesthetic systemic toxicity: current perspectives. *Local Reg Anesth.* 2018;11:35-44.

Fleisher LA, Beckman JA, Brown KA, et al. ACC/AHA 2007 guidelines on perioperative cardiovascular evaluation and care for noncardiac surgery: executive summary: a report of the American College of Cardiology/American Heart Association Task Force on Practice Guidelines (Writing committee to revise the 2002 guidelines on perioperative cardiovascular evaluation for noncardiac surgery) developed in collaboration with the American Society of Echocardiography, American Society of Nuclear Cardiology, Heart Rhythm Society, Society of Cardiovascular Anesthesiologists, Society for Cardiovascular Angiography and Interventions, Society for Vascular Medicine and Biology, and Society for Vascular Surgery. *J Am Coll Cardiol.* 2007;50(17):1707-1732.

Frendl G, Sodickson AC, Chung MK, et al. 2014 AATS guidelines for the prevention and management of perioperative atrial fibrillation and flutter for thoracic surgical procedures. *J Thorac Cardiovasc Surg.* 2014;148(3):e153-e193. doi:10.1016/j.jtcvs. 2014.06.036

January CT, Wann LS, Alpert JS, et al. 2014 AHA/ACC/HRS guideline for the management of patients with atrial fibrillation: a report of the American College of Cardiology/American Heart Association Task Force on Practice Guidelines and the Heart Rhythm Society. *J Am Coll Cardiol.* 2014;64(21):e1-e76. doi:10.1016/j.jacc.2014.03.022

Kim SH, Jang MJ, Hwang HY. Perioperative beta-blocker for atrial fibrillation after cardiac surgery: a meta-analysis. *Thorac Cardiovasc Surg.* 2021;69(2):133-140. doi:10.1055/s-0040-1708472

Kornej J, Börschel CS, Benjamin EJ, Schnabel RB. Epidemiology of atrial fibrillation in the 21st century: novel methods and new insights. *Circ Res.* 2020;127(1):4-20.

Lin MH, Kamel H, Singer DE, Wu YL, Lee M, Ovbiagele B. Perioperative/Postoperative atrial fibrillation and risk of subsequent stroke and/or mortality. *Stroke.* 2019;50(6):1364-1371.

Link MS. Clinical practice. Evaluation and initial treatment of supraventricular tachycardia. *N Engl J Med.* 2012;367(15):1438-1448.

Olshansky B, Rosenfeld LE, Warner AL, et al. The Atrial Fibrillation Follow-up Investigation of Rhythm Management (AFFIRM) study: approaches to control rate in atrial fibrillation. *J Am Coll Cardiol.* 2004;43:1201-1208.

Peretto G, Durante A, Limite LR, et al. Postoperative arrhythmias after cardiac surgery: incidence, risk factors, and therapeutic management. *Cardiol Res Pract.* 2014;2014:615987.

Roden DM. Drug-induced prolongation of the QT interval. *N Engl J Med* 2004;350(10):1013-1022.

Szelkowski LA, Puri NK, Singh R, et al. Current trends in preoperative, intraoperative, and postoperative care of the adult cardiac surgery patient. *Curr Probl Surg.* 2015;52(1):531-569. doi:10.1067/j.cpsurg.2014.10.001

Vardas PE, Simantirakis EN, Kanoupakis EM. New developments in cardiac pacemakers. *Circulation* 2013;127(23):2343–2350.

Woods CE, Olgin J. Atrial fibrillation therapy now and in the future: drugs, biologicals, and ablation. *Circ Res.* 2014;114(9):1532-1546.

18 Heart Failure

Rachel C. Frank, Adil Yunis, and David M. Dudzinski

INTRODUCTION

Heart failure (HF) management in the critical care setting includes patients with an acute decompensation of an underlying cardiomyopathy, tailoring therapy for chronic heart failure in the setting of critical illness, or malperfusion and congestion complicating a host of other acute critical illness. Therefore, intensivists of all backgrounds need to understand the etiology, diagnosis, and management of HF.

I. DEFINITION OF HF

Clinical syndrome resulting from a mismatch between the ability to generate cardiac output and metabolic tissue demands (or the ability to meet these demands but only at abnormally elevated cardiac filling pressures). HF may be driven by impairments in stroke volume (SV) (due to impaired systolic function or impaired diastolic filling) or more rarely insufficient heart rate (HR) (significant bradycardia). HF can be univentricular (left ventricle [LV] or right ventricle [RV]) or biventricular. From the perspective of the LV ejection fraction, there are HF syndromes with reduced ejection fraction versus preserved ejection fraction (crudely "systolic" vs "diastolic" HF respectively). HF symptoms may be viewed as secondary to low cardiac output or impaired "forward flow" versus congestion (pulmonary or venous) or "backward fluid build-up". An additional entity known as high-output HF is distinguished from other forms of HF above by having a high cardiac output but low systemic vascular resistance, resulting in low systemic pressure and activation of the renin-angiotensin-aldosterone axis with resultant salt and water retention (seen in arteriovenous fistulae, cirrhosis, sepsis, anemia, hyperthyroidism, beriberi, etc.).

A. Etiologies and Triggers of Acute HF

1. Be aware of potential triggers that may precipitate HF in patients in the ICU (see Table 18.1).
2. There are multiple mimics of the HF syndrome manifesting with low output and/or congestion, of which ICU clinicians need to be cognizant. These include pericardial effusion and tamponade, pulmonary embolism, pneumothorax, SVC syndrome, and anemia.

B. Signs and Symptoms

Signs and symptoms of HF can be organized conceptually based on the affected ventricle and mechanism of HF (see Table 18.2).

C. HF Classifications

1. A syndrome of **low cardiac output (LCOS)** is defined as a cardiac index <2.2 L/min/m^2. This may occur in the absence of hypotension, so should be considered even in normotensive patients and the appropriate clinical context. There is a continuum of LCOS to **cardiogenic shock (CS)**, with the latter including hypotension (with the need for pharmacologic or mechanical circulatory support to maintain normotension and systemic perfusion) coupled with end-organ hypoperfusion and dysfunction.

TABLE 18.1 Triggers of Acute HF

Ischemia or infarction (see **Chapter 15**)
Dietary indiscretion (high salt and/or fluid intake)
Fluid and salt intake intravenously and from medications (Many intravenous antibiotics and medications may provide iatrogenic salt loads due to their formulation or volume loads depending on how concentrated the IV preparation is; see **Chapter 8**)
Medications with direct cardioinhibitory effect that depress cardiac function by decreasing chronotropy and/or inotropy (eg, β antagonists or calcium channel antagonists, sodium channel blockers, etc.)
Worsening or acute valvular disease (see **Chapter 16**)
Tachyarrhythmias (which may impair LV output and/or ventricular filling) and less commonly **bradyarrhythmia** (loss of atrioventricular synchrony or insufficient heart rate) (see **Chapter 17**)
Pacemaker related due to chronic RV pacing, pacemaker-mediated tachycardia, or inadequate biventricular pacing (CRT)
Comorbid renal and/or hepatic failure with impacts on fluid and sodium homeostasis
Endocrinopathy (thyroid dysfunction)
Uncontrolled hypertension
Acute infections
Acute neurologic insults (may provoke secondary cardiomyopathy)
Acute inflammatory conditions with various **cardiomyopathies** and **myocarditis** are discussed below.

CRT, cardiac resynchronization therapy; ICU, intensive care unit; LV, left ventricle.

TABLE 18.2 Signs and Symptoms of HF

Mechanism of HF	LV	RV
Impaired output or perfusion ("Forward" HF)	• Organ ischemia and dysfunctions (altered mentation or somnolence, azotemia, oliguria, hepatic insufficiency) • Low cardiac index, low mixed venous oxygen saturation • Mitral regurgitation • On examination, pallor, cool extremities, impaired capillary refill, hypotension, narrow pulse pressure (<25% of systolic blood pressure), pulsus alternans • Symptoms: fatigue, dyspnea	• Insufficient LV preload, with manifestations of impaired forward LV flow • Tricuspid regurgitation • Elevated CVP:PCWP (>0.6:1) • Low RV pulse pressure • Low PAPI (pulmonary arterial pulsatility index) • Low cardiac index, low mixed venous oxygen saturation
Congestion ("Backward" HF)	• Elevated PCWP • Pulmonary edema, pleural effusion, secondary pulmonary hypertension • RV congestion and dysfunction • On examination, pulmonary rales, S3 heart sound • Symptoms: dyspnea, orthopnea, paroxysmal nocturnal dyspnea	• Elevated CVP • Renal congestion (may manifest as AKI) • Visceral congestion (may impact intestinal medication absorption, liver function) • Hepatic congestion (unconjugated hyperbilirubinemia, prolonged INR) • On exam: ascites, pulsatile liver, leg edema, elevated JVP. • Symptoms: Satiety, anorexia

AKI, acute kidney injury; CVP, central venous pressure; HF, heart failure; LV, left ventricle; PCWP, pulmonary capillary wedge pressure; RV, right ventricle.

2. **Stevenson Matrix:** A clinical assessment of HF, useful for ICU applications, that groups patients into hemodynamic profiles based on perfusion (warm vs cold) and congestion (cold vs dry) axes. These profiles have been shown to predict outcomes, with patients in profiles B and C having higher mortality. These classifications can guide therapy: type B patients have intact perfusion, so their congestion can be treated with fluid removal; type C (cardiogenic shock) and type L patients may require pharmacologic or mechanical circulatory support to augment cardiac output and end-organ perfusion (see Table 18.3).
3. **New York Heart Association (NYHA) Class and American Heart Association (AHA)/ACC Stage:** These are the primary systems used to classify patients with HF (Table 18.4). The AHA/ACC system describes patients based on the stage of their disease whereas the NYHA classification system categorizes patients clinically based on their degree of symptoms or functional limitation.
4. **INTERMACS** (Interagency Registry for Mechanically Assisted Circulatory Support): This seven-tiered system is used to further describe and risk-stratify patients with advanced heart failure, specifically NYHA III–IV class patients, and for guiding consideration for mechanical circulatory support candidacy. The higher INTERMACS profiles have been associated with worse outcomes and mortality.

TABLE 18.3 Stevenson Matrix

		Congestion: No	Congestion: Yes
Malperfusion	No	**Warm and Dry** (not HF; type A)	**Warm and Wet** (type B)
	Yes	**Cold and Dry** (type L)	**Cold and Wet** (type C)

TABLE 18.4 New York Heart Association (NYHA) Class and AHA/ACC Staging

NYHA class		AHA/ACC stage		Overlap between NYHA and AHA/ACC
I	Asymptomatic from HF with physical activity	A	At risk, but without structural heart disease or signs or symptoms of HF	Based on the stage definitions (patients lacking symptoms), stage A and B correlate with NYHA I.
II	Mild symptoms with ordinary physical activity	B	Structural heart disease, without signs or symptoms of HF	
III	Significant symptoms with ordinary physical activity.	C	Structural heart disease, with prior or current signs or symptoms of HF	Stage C can have range of class NYHA II-III.
IV	HF symptoms with any level of physical activity and at rest	D	Refractory HF; requires consideration for advanced HF therapies	Stage D correlates with class IV symptoms.

ACC, American College of Cardiology; AHA, American Heart Association; HF, heart failure.

D. Diagnostic Evaluation of HF

1. Signs, symptoms, and examination findings are outlined in Section III.
2. Laboratory markers to evaluate clinical manifestations of heart failure include these.

a. Volume overload: natriuretic peptides (BNP and NT-proBNP), released by cardiac myocytes in response to volume expansion and myocardial wall stress in HF. May be generated in other ICU conditions (eg, pulmonary embolism).

b. Troponin: to evaluate for coronary ischemia precipitating HF, but can also be elevated in a host of ICU comorbidities including myocarditis and myocardial oxygen supply-demand mismatch.

c. End-organ perfusion: include liver function tests (LFTs), lactate, and renal function (using creatinine or Cystatin C).

d. Laboratory markers of advanced heart failure: Hyponatremia (may be seen in HF due to the secretion of arginine vasopressin in the setting of reduced effective arterial circulating volume and renal hypoperfusion) and blood urea nitrogen.

e. Electrolyte monitoring during diuresis: potassium and magnesium levels fluctuate and require replenishment. Hypernatremia may develop during diuresis prompting use of acetazolamide for natriuresis.

f. Central and mixed venous oxygen saturations can help assess cardiac output.

3. Echocardiography is a key method to assess ventricular function, valvular disease, and other structural heart issues (see **Chapter 3**). Pericardial effusions may also be detected. Thoracic ultrasound is also useful in identifying pleural effusions and B lines reflective of pulmonary edema.

4. Electrocardiogram (EKG) may reflect underlying pathophysiology leading to heart failure. Q waves and ST/T wave changes (reflecting an ischemic process), low voltages (may indicate an infiltrative process), ventricular hypertrophy, or arrhythmias.

5. Chest radiography can show pulmonary edema, pleural effusions, and cardiomegaly.

6. Ischemia evaluation to assess coronary artery disease as etiology if clinically indicated, such as new diagnosis of cardiomyopathy.

7. Many patients in the ICU will have had a CT scan, and this may show coronary calcification, valve calcification, or cardiac chamber enlargement.

8. Other cardiac investigation are sometimes considered including cardiac MRI or endomyocardial biopsy. Cardiac MRI can provide quantitative assessment of biventricular function, valvular disease, shunt hemodynamics, structural heart disease as well as characterizing the myocardium through T2 mapping and late gadolinium enhancement. Endomyocardial biopsy is employed when clinical suspicion is high for particular cardiomyopathy etiologies in which distinct histopathologic findings can aid in the diagnosis.

II. CARDIOMYOPATHIES

A. Dilated Cardiomyopathy: This is a phenotype of ventricular dilatation and reduced systolic function, rather than a distinct pathologic condition. Many of the etiologies of heart failure can lead to dilatation: viral-mediated (may or may not be preceded by symptoms of viral prodrome), genetic mutations (eg, Lamin A/C cardiomyopathy, arrhythmogenic cardiomyopathy), diabetes, hemochromatosis, Chagas disease, HIV-related and idiopathic. Late stages of other HF disease types may also result in LV dilation including ischemic cardiomyopathy, myocarditis, and hypertrophic cardiomyopathies. Specific treatment and prognosis differ by specific etiology.

B. Ischemic Cardiomyopathy: Coronary artery disease leading to ventricular dysfunction either due to infarction (irreversible) or hibernating myocardium (reversible through revascularization). EKG may show chronic or acute ischemic changes.

1. **Diagnostics:** Evaluating for coronary artery disease includes EKG (ST/T wave changes), echocardiography (regional wall motion abnormalities), troponin, and CT or catheterization-based coronary angiogram. Acute coronary

syndrome precipitating decompensated heart failure warrants cardiac catheterization with coronary angiography in addition to appropriate medical management. In the absence of active acute coronary syndrome, evaluate for hibernating myocardium and potential reversibility with stress imaging (echocardiography, MRI, CT).

2. **Management:** Acute coronary syndrome management involves medications (antiplatelets, heparin) and revascularization (see **Chapter 15**). Medications may help reduce myocardial oxygen demand including targeting lower systolic blood pressure and targeting lower heart rate (in the absence of cardiogenic shock).

C. Myocarditis related: Inflammatory disorder of the myocardium caused by either autoimmune disease or infection. Patients may have elevated inflammatory and cardiac biomarkers in the absence of ischemic changes on EKG. EKG may show nonspecific ST/T wave changes, arrhythmias, and conduction disease. Can be subacute or fulminant.

1. Two main causes of fulminant myocarditis with associated heart failure:
   - **a.** Giant cell myocarditis: A rare form of autoimmune myocarditis associated with high mortality if not treated with high-grade immunosuppression and/or cardiac transplant. Thought to be T-cell mediated and characterized by giant cells on endomyocardial biopsy. Suspect in patients with new-onset systolic dysfunction with or without shock, conduction disease, and electrical instability with ventricular arrhythmias. Most common in middle-aged males.
   - **b.** Eosinophilic myocarditis (see Section II. J): characterized by eosinophils on endomyocardial biopsy and often (but not always) peripheral eosinophilia. Several causes including drug-related hypersensitivity, vaccine-related, hypereosinophilic syndrome, and eosinophilic granulomatosis with polyangiitis.
2. **Diagnosis:** cMRI may show edema with T2 enhancement, edema/fibrosis with late gadolinium enhancement. Consideration of endomyocardial biopsy in certain clinical scenarios which have characteristic histopathologic findings that aid in diagnosis including giant cell and eosinophilic myocarditis.
3. **Management:** Early involvement of HF specialists for indication of endomyocardial biopsy and consideration of advanced therapies including mechanical circulatory support and transplant evaluation. Prompt immunosuppression medications are indicated in some etiologies like giant cell myocarditis.

D. Stress Cardiomyopathy (Takotsubo cardiomyopathy): A transient stress-induced cardiomyopathy most commonly involving the left ventricle with regional wall motion abnormalities that may mimic left coronary artery ischemic/infarction, but in the absence of coronary artery involvement on angiography. Triggers include emotional stress or physiologic stress such as severe illness, postoperative state, asthma exacerbation, or adrenergic medications. Thought to be mediated by catecholamine excess with associated coronary vasospasm and myocardial dysfunction. Classical Takotsubo pattern (apical LV hypokinesis with apical ballooning, but hyperkinesis of the basal segment) is most common. Other variants include: Mid apical variant which occurs with hypokinesis of apex and basal segment with hyperdynamic mid ventricular cavity, and rarer forms include reverse Takotsubo cardiomyopathy (apical hyperkinesis with basal hypokinesis) and an isolated RV stress cardiomyopathy.

1. **Diagnosis:** EKG and cardiac biomarkers to exclude ischemia (ST elevations, ST depression, or T wave inversion may be seen and mimic ACS). Transthoracic echocardiography (TTE) shows characteristic wall motion abnormalities. Note that ischemia or infarction in a large left anterior descending artery territory can also cause wall motion abnormalities that appear to be similar to classic stress cardiomyopathy. For that reason, Takotsubo cardiomyopathy is a diagnosis of exclusion, and ischemia must be ruled out. In classical

Takotsubo, dynamic left ventricular outflow tract (LVOT) obstruction may occur due to the hyperdynamic LV base.

2. **Management:** Treat for mixed shock/CS (depending on clinical scenario), with caveat to be careful with β-adrenergic agonism as it can worsen basal hyperkinesis and cause LVOT obstruction (see section II.I). For this reason, IABP is contraindicated (deflation during systole encourages decreased systemic vascular resistance, which can worsen LVOT obstruction). Avoid hypovolemia and inadequate LV preload as well as low afterload, both of which may worsen LVOT obstruction. Supportive therapy and then initiation of guideline-directed medical therapy (GDMT, see **Section III.F**) following recovery of shock.

E. Septic Cardiomyopathy: Common in patients admitted to the ICU with sepsis and may manifest LV dysfunction and dilatation. Etiology related to cytokines, bacterial endotoxins, and impaired nitric oxide regulation. Literature is unclear on predictors of mortality (some studies suggest RV dysfunction and LV strain as possible predictors of increased mortality).

1. **Diagnosis:** Rule out ischemia. TTE, EKG
2. **Management:** Supportive care, hemodynamic support as needed typically with norepinephrine, treatment of underlying infection (see **Chapter 12**). If volume replete and low central venous oxygen saturations, consideration of inotropes to support cardiac output.

F. Restrictive Cardiomyopathy: Phenotype of markedly impaired ventricular filling due to reduced ventricular compliance; stroke volume is restricted and thus cardiac output is heart rate dependent. Ventricles are not dilated, and many times the noncompliance is due to LV wall infiltration (infiltrative cardiomyopathy) or less commonly endomyocardial fibrosis. Examples include amyloidosis, storage diseases, and sarcoidosis. In early stages, abnormal diastolic function results in impaired stroke volume and CO. In later stages, there is abnormal systolic function, atrial dilatation, arrhythmias, and systemic thromboembolism.

1. **Diagnosis:** Exclude ischemia. Expect S4 on examination due to impaired ventricular filling. TTE shows wall thickening, atrial enlargement, and diastolic impairment. EKG may show discordance between apparently thick LV walls and low EKG voltage; EKG may also show atrioventricular and bundle branch blocks). cMRI, cardiac positron emission tomography (PET) (sarcoid), PYP scan (amyloid). Invasive hemodynamics
2. **Management:** Hemodynamic support as needed. Steroids/immunosuppression/ICD (sarcoid), and Tafamidis (amyloid). Anticoagulation for atrial fibrillation risk. GDMT if not in shock, but since stroke volume is fixed lowering heart rate will impact CO. Consider transplant in late stages (systolic HF, CS, refractory arrhythmias). Nondilated ventricles and overall preserved ejection fraction (EF) may preclude consideration for most types of mechanical circulatory support.

G. Constrictive Pericarditis: Not a myocardial process but rather a pericardial process, however, often mimics syndrome of restrictive cardiomyopathy and thus is on the differential diagnosis. Fibrous thickening or calcification of the pericardium, resulting in impaired and abnormal filling pressures due to rigid pericardium. May occur subacutely or chronically after any cause of pericarditis, including bacterial, connective tissue disorder, radiation, tuberculosis, postcardiac surgery.

1. **Diagnosis:** Physical exam may demonstrate pericardial knock, pulsatile liver, JVP elevation with Kussmaul sign. EKG findings: low QRS voltage, T wave abnormalities. Chest x-ray (CXR) may show pericardial calcifications. Echocardiogram, thickened pericardium ± adherence to myocardium, septal bounce, IVC plethora, increased respirophasic variation of intracardiac Doppler flow. Compared to restrictive cardiomyopathy, echocardiographic diastolic indices are preserved (such as tissue Doppler). CT/MRI evaluation of the pericardium for signs of constriction. Invasive hemodynamics

2. **Management:** Diuresis, treatment of underlying pericardial process (if appropriate), consideration of surgical pericardial pericardiectomy in refractory cases (high mortality)

H. **Hypertrophic Cardiomyopathy (HCM):** Genetic cardiomyopathy (large number of cases are de novo mutations, ie, no family history) resulting from abnormal myocyte organization and hypertrophy. Multiple phenotypes possible with most common being septal predominant LV thickening, and other variants including midcavity, apical, and RV thickening. Approximately 70% of patients will have dynamic LVOT obstruction (LVOTO), which is defined by ≥ 30 mm Hg peak gradient. Gradient is worsened by decreased LV preload (hypovolemia—commonly encountered in ICU such as sepsis, GI bleeding, tamponade, RV failure), decreased diastolic filling time (tachycardia, atrial arrhythmias), and decreased afterload (also commonly encountered in the ICU in various hypotensive states). LVOTO can occur with systolic anterior motion of the mitral valve (SAM), resulting from hypertrophy and abnormal papillary muscle insertion. SAM may result in dynamic mitral regurgitation, which is eccentrically and posteriorly directed. Myocardial scaring and LV apical aneurysm increase risk of sudden cardiac death.

1. **Diagnosis:** EKG (may show left ventricular hypertrophy [LVH] pattern, and subendocardial ischemia, with deep early precordial T wave inversions indicating septal HCM, and apical T wave inversions indicating apical HCM), TTE (with echo enhancing agent to rule out LV apical aneurysm), cardiac MRI, consideration of genetic testing. Broad differential diagnosis includes all secondary causes of LV wall thickening including hypertension, valvular disease, infiltrative cardiomyopathies, and so on.
2. **Management:** Optimization of preload (caution with diuretics), optimization of heart rate. Avoidance of β agonists (vasopressors, inotropes) when LVOTO may be provoked; for hypotensive state, consider pure α agonist like phenylephrine. Long-term, CCB, beta blockers (BB), ICD if risk factors for sudden cardiac death, and consideration of ablative therapies like septal ablation or myectomy. Anticoagulation if atrial fibrillation (most common arrhythmia in HCM)

I. **LVOT Obstruction.** This is a phenotype that may occur in ICU patients. As described earlier, it occurs classically in HCM with systolic anterior motion (SAM) of the mitral valve leading to LVOT obstruction. This may also occur with Takotsubo cardiomyopathy, as the basal segment exhibits hyperkinesis in response to apical ballooning and akinesis. In ICU patients, LVOTO can also occur in patients with combinations of upper septal hypertrophy, small LV cavities, hypovolemia, and exposure to beta agonist vasoactive infusions.

1. **Diagnosis:** Can be made with echo (showing LVOTO) and clinically may continue to have worsening hypotension after induction of anesthesia, and with β adrenergic medications.
2. **Management:** Fluid resuscitation, avoidance of β agonism, consideration of BB to decrease HR (increased diastolic filling time)

J. **Toxin-Mediated Cardiomyopathy:** Chemotherapeutics (anthracycline, trastuzumab, anti-VEGF agents, and immune checkpoint inhibitor myocarditis), methamphetamines, cocaine, alcohol, and radiation. Mechanism varies based on the causative agent but may include free radical formation, induction of apoptosis, impacts on myocyte bioenergetics and changes in intracellular calcium handling. Acute necrotizing eosinophilic myocarditis is one type due to hypersensitivity to an allergen causing acute cardiomyopathy.

1. **Diagnosis:** Comprehensive history including medications and supplements and exposures. Toxicology screen. Complete blood count (CBC) and differential. EKG, TTE, assess other causes of cardiomyopathy
2. **Management:** Steroids if immune checkpoint inhibitor myocarditis (discuss with oncologist prior to initiation), cessation of other toxin exposure, GDMT

K. Tachycardia-Related Cardiomyopathy: Systolic ventricular dysfunction in setting of prolonged tachyarrhythmias. Most frequently seen in atrial fibrillation or atrial flutter with rapid ventricular response. Systolic dysfunction may reverse when tachyarrhythmia has resolved (rate controlled or converted to normal sinus rhythm). PVC-mediated cardiomyopathy can be seen with high burden of ectopic beats, typically greater than 10%-20% of all QRS complexes.

1. **Diagnosis:** EKG, TTE, TSH, telemetry while in the hospital and outpatient HR monitoring, ambulatory electrocardiography.
2. **Management:** Rate control (β blockers), rhythm control (cardioversion, anti-arrhythmic drugs)

L. RV Pacing Cardiomyopathy: Chronic RV pacing leading to mechanical and electrical dyssynchrony resulting in systolic dysfunction.

1. **Diagnosis:** EKG, pacemaker interrogation.
2. **Management:** includes reducing RV pacing by optimizing pacemaker settings to use the native conduction pathway (may include programming longer AV delay) or device upgrade to biventricular pacing

M. Peripartum CM: Occurs in the last month of pregnancy or within 5 months of delivery and in the absence of other causes of HF. Risk factors: maternal age > 30 years, hypertensive disorders of pregnancy, multiparity, and diabetes mellitus. High risk for LV thrombus formation due to systolic dysfunction and hypercoagulable state of pregnancy; screen for using TTE with contrast.

1. **Diagnosis:** EKG, TTE
2. **Management:** If the patient is still pregnant or breast feeding, then GDMT classes that are contraindicated in such states should be avoided (such as ACEi, ARB, and mineralocorticoids when pregnant; and use loop diuretics, hydralazine, nitrates). Interdisciplinary management with maternal–fetal medicine, cardio-obstetrics team to discuss timing of delivery and mechanical/pharmacologic support in the setting of shock. If the patient has given birth and is not breast feeding, then standard GDMT is employed. Contraceptive counseling due to risk of recurrence (long-acting reversible contraception is preferred, ie, IUD)

N. RV Failure: Etiologies include acute PE, right ventricular myocardial infarction (RV MI), ARDS, or any condition that acutely increased RV afterload, which can be commonly encountered in ICU. More subacute causes include pulmonary hypertension (which can itself be due to LV failure) or arrhythmogenic right ventricular dysplasia.

1. **Diagnosis:** TTE, pulmonary artery catheter, cMRI
2. **Management:** Inotropes, inopressors, increased HR (to augment CO, as the LV filling and SV will be somewhat fixed in setting of RV impairment). Optimization of factors that influence RV afterload, including pulmonary vasodilators (see **Chapter 23**)

O. Miscellaneous: Etiologies that are more rarely seen, but should be ruled out in the appropriate clinical scenario: LV noncompaction, infectious cardiomyopathy (HIV, Chagas, Lyme disease), mitochondrial disease, lysosomal storage disease, genetic syndromes, endocrine disease (thyrotoxicosis, etc), nutritional deficiencies (thiamine), high-output HF (related to anemia, arteriovenous malformations, or fistulae).

III. HF MANAGEMENT AND TREATMENT

A. Treatment of HF depends on accurate phenotyping based on the principles in Part 1. First critical inquiry is if malperfusion or CS is present, which requires rapid triage and escalation of medical support, and if appropriate consideration of mechanical circulatory support, with the intent to prevent multisystem organ failure.

1. **Treatment goals in HF**: One can think about treating HF in the ICU based on what physiologic parameters we can adjust and intervene upon (independent variables) (see Table 18.5).

TABLE 18.5 Treatment Goals in HF

			Availability	
		Independent variable	ICU therapy	Outside ICU (eg, hospital floor or outpatient)
Cardiac Output (*=SV × HR*)	Stroke volume	*Preload (CVP and PCWP)*	Intravenous diuretics; continuous renal replacement therapy (Intravenous fluids if "dry")	Intravenous and oral diuretics; Dialysis
		Contractility	Inotropes (Mechanical circulatory support)	No real inotropes outside ICU (consider digoxin) (Durable ventricular assist device or OHT)
		Afterload (SVR, SBP, MAP)	Parenteral vasodilators (Vasopressors)	Oral vasodilators
	HR	*Heart rate*	Intravenous chronotropes Temporary pacing	Permanent pacing
		Atrioventricular and ventriculoventricular synchrony	Typically unavailable acutely	Pacer and CRT

CRT, cardiac resynchronization therapy; CVP, central venous pressure; HR, heart rate; ICU, intensive care unit; MAP, mean arterial pressure; OHT, orthotopic heart transplant; PCWP, pulmonary capillary wedge pressure; SBP, systolic blood pressure; SV, stroke volume; SVR, systemic vascular resistance.

2. **Acute decompensated HF (ADHF)**, without malperfusion ("warm and wet" phenotype), typically treatment relies on:
   a. **Adjusting preload:** Intravenous diuretics targeting filling pressure goals, urine output, pulmonary edema, and clinical signs of congestion including JVP. Serial assessment of NT-proBNP may also guide diuresis when approaching euvolemia. The amount of daily diuresis tolerated will vary based on the patient and degree of congestion, but most clinicians consider net 1 to 2 L negative per day adequate for routine ADHF, and the average weight loss across HF hospitalizations is about 4 kg. Careful attention to avoid overdiuresis on a day-to-day basis; meaning patients may remain total volume up but do not tolerate rapid shifts in intravascular volume due to rapid diuresis and become intravascularly hypovolemic. This may manifest as hypotension or AKI. If this occurs, then provide a "diuresis holiday" where diuretics are typically held for 24 hours to allow the patient's intravascular and extravascular volume to equilibrate before resuming diuretics.
      1. Agents like nitrates may also reduce venous return (as well as provide modest LV afterload reduction and coronary vasodilatation).
      2. Morphine is used in myocardial infarction in part for reduction of symptoms but also impacts preload and myocardial oxygen demand. Caution as opiates can impair absorption of enteral P2Y12 agents.
   b. **Adjusting afterload**: A ventricle that has difficulty ejecting against a high afterload will be encouraged to eject blood antegrade by reducing the

force against which it has to pump. As a result, by reducing LV afterload, systemic vasodilators may increase blood pressure by increasing cardiac output in a patient with LV systolic HF. Analogously, RV afterload reduction can be achieved with pulmonary vasodilators.

c. Pay attention to offending medications: Beta blockers and calcium channel blockers, with negative inotrope effects, for example, may precipitate ADHF and need to be dose adjusted or held in the acute setting.

3. Advanced HF (ADHF), including LCOS and CS: More advanced strategies are required when malperfusion is an issue. Some of these patients will not respond to diuresis without support of perfusion and/or may be unable to tolerate a trial of vasodilators.

a. Various tools assist the ICU clinician in treating advanced HF:

1. Central line: transduce central venous pressure (CVP) to assess venous congestion, as a surrogate for volume status and RV filling pressures. Trend central venous oxygen saturation (proxy for cardiac output)

2. Pulmonary arterial line: (also called right heart catheter, or Swan-Ganz catheter; see **Chapters 1** and **6**): can assess LV filling pressures, measure mixed venous oxygen saturation (thereby also used to calculate Fick cardiac output), and thermodilution cardiac output. Hemodynamic data obtained from PA lines is helpful in cases of isolated cardiogenic and mixed shock including cases of complex biventricular disease, severe valvular disease, pericardial disease, uncertain volume status, pulmonary hypertension, or when pharmacologic or mechanical circulatory support are needed.

3. Venous oxygen saturation: Central venous and mixed venous oxygen saturations differ in that the first is measured from the superior vena cava (or central vein) whereas that the latter is measured from the proximal pulmonary artery and includes blood return mixing from the inferior vena cavae and the coronary sinus, which is the most deoxygenated blood in the body after the heart extracts oxygen. Mixed venous saturation will therefore typically be lower than central venous saturation by 5% to 10%.

4. Arterial line: for invasive hemodynamic monitoring while titrating vasoactive medications

5. POCUS/critical care echo: Evaluation of biventricular function, valvular disease, LVOT obstruction, pericardial effusion. Particularly helpful if rapid clinical change occurs, as ultrasonography can be repeated quickly at bedside. Be aware of what is not evaluated on bedside ultrasound and the negative and positive predictive values (see **Chapter 3**). Thoracic POCUS to evaluate for B-lines (pulmonary edema), lung sliding (for pneumothorax), and pleural effusions.

b. "Tailored therapy": Describes a targeted approach to optimize the ICU patient with advanced HF, by titrating medications to optimize preload, afterload, and cardiac output through serial hemodynamic measurements; tailored therapy works toward a goal cardiac index >2.2 L/min/m2, SVR 800-1200 dynes/sec/cm−5, MAP typically > 60-65 mm Hg, and specific ventricular filling pressures.

c. Preload optimization: Goal is optimization of LV end-diastolic volume and pressure. Because we cannot measure LVEDP directly at the bedside, we measure the pulmonary capillary wedge pressure (PCWP) which acts as a surrogate for LA pressure which itself approximates left ventricular end-diastolic pressure. These assumptions may be confounded depending on which West lung zone the right heart catheter tip is in, by intrinsic pulmonary disease (fibrosis, veno-occlusive disease, pulmonary vein stenosis), mitral valve disease, ventricular interdependence, and noncompliant LV.

1. Typical **PCWP goal 10-12**, but higher in patients with acute MI or restrictive heart disease where the ventricle compliance is lower. Targeting a higher PCWP is also favored in patients who require higher LV preload to maintain a normal cardiac output, including patients with severe AS and those with severe LV systolic dysfunction. In the ICU, clinicians can utilize pulmonary artery line hemodynamics to assess stroke volume and cardiac output at different filling pressures.
2. Many patients with advanced HF are operating at filling pressures higher than optimal by their Starling curve and may need diuretic drips or renal replacement therapy to achieve euvolemia if diuretic nonresponsive (see **Chapters 3** and **25**).
3. RV filling pressure is assessed by CVP, and patients with noncompliant RV may require CVP goals that are higher.
4. Closely monitor input fluid and output fluid balance in the ICU. Many medications require high infusion rates that may contribute to volume overload; work with the ICU pharmacist to concentrate or change agents to avoid obligate fluid inputs.

d. **Afterload optimization**: Goal is optimization of LV myocardial oxygen demand and reduction in wall stress. Systemic vascular resistance (SVR) is given by the formula (MAP − CVP)/CO × 80. SVR can be useful but must be considered in context of the patient's MAP and also with some caution because estimates of CO may bring their own sources of error to the SVR calculation. A typical SVR goal range is **800 to 1200**, and patients with advanced HF will have calculated SVR much higher. By reducing the SVR, the intent is to allow the ventricle to eject. Various parenteral vasodilators can be used for this purpose. However, in patients who are in shock, the first goal must be maintaining a MAP for adequate end-organ perfusion (MAP > 60-65). Some patients with decompensated advanced HF present with hypotension caused by low cardiac output resulting in compensatory sympathetic activation leading to elevated SVR; despite an elevated SVR, their hypotension must initially be treated with vasopressors. As there is improvement in hemodynamics, a switch from vasopressor to vasodilator can be considered, often guided by PA line hemodynamics.

e. **Contractility optimization**: In the ICU, contractility can be directly augmented with inotrope infusions. Inotropes have a variable effect on MAP and SVR, as some are inopressors and some are inodilators. Inotropes are also generally positive chronotropes, and thus tachyarrhythmia is a common side effect. Contractility is not routinely measured directly in ICU clinical care. Typical goal is improvement in the cardiac index (which summates contributions from all of the aforementioned interventions) to more than 2.2 L/min/m^2. If pharmacologic intervention is insufficient, mechanical circulatory supports are available in contemporary practice; consult with your hospital HF service, at an early stage, before metabolic dysfunction due to CS becomes severe or irreversible.

f. **Mechanical circulatory support**: See **Chapter 19**. Devices in contemporary practice include:
   1. Intra-aortic balloon pump
   2. Percutaneous ventricular assist device (LV, RV, or both)
   3. Paracorporeal ventricular assist device (LV, RV, or both)
   4. Veno-arterial extracorporeal membrane oxygenation
   5. Durable ventricular assist device (primarily LV)

4. **Medications:** Tenets of HF treatment in ICU as well as inpatient and outpatient contexts. Specific classes and their medications include:

a. **Diuretics**
   1. Intravenous loop diuretics (furosemide, bumetanide)

a. DOSE trial found no significant differences in symptoms, weight loss, net diuresis, or renal function with bolus versus continuous infusion diuretic in ADHF. However, intensification of bolus dosing was associated with weight loss, symptom reduction, and net diuresis.

b. In practice, diuretic infusions are often employed as they allow patients to maintain a continuous diuresis without relying on clinicians to reorder or adjust bolus dosing in a timely manner. Some data from ICU literature suggests that continuous infusion may be more effective in patients in the ICU.

2. Diuretic resistance: Loop diuretic alone may be inadequate especially in older patients, advanced HF, and renal dysfunction. Adjunct blockade may be useful and may include thiazide-type diuretics (intravenous chlorothiazide, oral metolazone) that target the distal renal tubule. Newer data suggest acetazolamide may be an adjunct in ADHF.

a. In states of significant renal congestion (elevated visceral and central filling pressures) limiting adequate renal perfusion, or in the setting of severe kidney injury, renal replacement therapy may be needed.

b. Consider whether perfusion must be optimized with inotropes first in order to facilitate renal perfusion and diuresis.

b. Inotropes: Parenteral agents that boost contractility are divided into inodilators and inopressors based on variable effects on blood pressure.

1. Inodilators: May cause hypotension and could need to be used with vasopressors. Pure inodilators are helpful if SVR is high and patient is normotensive.

a. Milrinone: Phosphodiesterase inhibitor. Increases contractility and vasodilation. Half-life 2 to 3 hours, longer with renal impairment as renally cleared (up to 20 hours on renal replacement therapy). Provides pulmonary vasodilation, helpful with RV failure. Watch for ventricular arrhythmia and hypotension.

b. Dobutamine: Beta-1 agonist, increasing contractility and chronotropy, and also β-2 agonist that can cause vasodilatation. Onset 2 minutes, half-life 2 minutes. Increased risk of ventricular arrhythmias

c. DoReMI trial found no difference on composite CS outcomes with dobutamine versus milrinone.

2. Inopressors: Provide vasoconstriction along with inotropy and thus may be needed if there is hypotension.

a. Norepinephrine: Agonist at α-1, α-2, and β-1 receptors. Alpha-1 agonism provides vasoconstriction and β-1 agonism provides inotropy and chronotropy.

b. Epinephrine: Similar pattern to norepinephrine but provides β-2 agonist activity, and with β effects greater than α effects. Epinephrine can be helpful for RV failure.

c. Dopamine: targets dopamine, β-1, and α-1 receptors in a dose-dependent manner, providing inotropy and chronotropy at mid-range doses (>5 μg/kg/min) and vasopressor activity via α receptors at high doses (10 μg/kg/min).

d. SOAP II trial evaluated vasoactive agents across multiple shock phenotypes and found more tachyarrhythmias and increased mortality risk in dopamine group.

e. Wean inotropes first, as fluid and afterload status are optimized; this is because in general inotropes cannot be continued out of the ICU setting, but oral diuretics and oral vasodilators are available.

3. Parenteral vasodilators

a. Nitroprusside: potent arterial vasodilator (NO pathway), caution in renal failure: byproduct cyanide, methemoglobin. Caution with severe unrevascularized CAD, impaired cerebral perfusion (can cause steal).

b. Nitroglycerin: Venous (2/3) > arterial dilation (1/3). Venodilatation reduces RV preload, improves pulmonary edema. Coronary vasodilator activity. Tachyphylaxis if on continuous infusion.

c. Other options include nicardipine and clevidipine.

5. Optimization of ventilator mechanics/positive end-expiratory pressure (PEEP): PEEP decreases LV afterload and preload. Optimal PEEP decreases RV preload and optimizes pulmonary vascular resistance (decreases atelectatic lung, optimizes oxygenation, both of which decrease pulmonary vascular resistance [PVR] and RV afterload), though nonoptimized PEEP can increases RV afterload. Ventilation and correction of hypercarbia decreases PVR and optimizes RV afterload.

a. Maintaining adequate exogenous oxygenation is important to support oxygen delivery. Analogously, maintaining Hb in terms of oxygen-carrying capacity may be a goal.

6. Guideline-directed medical therapy (GDMT): In contemporary practice, HF patients with reduced EF use four "pillars" of medication classes, designed to improve EF and reduce HF events:

a. Renin-angiotensin-aldosterone system (RAAS) In HF patients, low perfusion pressure results in RAAS activation through baroreceptor response and increased sympathetic tone. Initially a compensatory mechanism, RAAS activation progresses to having detrimental effects by increasing both preload and afterload and adverse cardiac remodeling.

1. Renin-angiotensin inhibitors: (ACEI, ARB, and sacubitril-valsartan): Provides afterload reduction in addition to RAAS inhibition. Side effects include hypotension, acute kidney injury (AKI), hyperkalemia, postoperative vasoplegia (particularly cardiac surgery). Typically hold 48 to 72 hours prior to surgery.

2. Aldosterone antagonism (spironolactone, eplerenone): Provides diuretic and antihypertensive effect. Side effects include hyperkalemia and hyponatremia.

b. Beta antagonist: Inhibits the heightened sympathetic tone that is activated in HF patients. Besides hemodynamic effects, these agents impact cardiac remodeling. Typically continued in the perioperative period.

c. SGLT-2i: Some proposed mechanisms of its beneficial effect include optimization of cardiac energy metabolism, inhibition of adverse cardiac remodeling, diuresis and blood pressure lowering. It is a glycosuric that can increase the risk for UTIs. May also trigger euglycemic diabetic ketoacidosis particularly if patients are NPO. Hold this agent if patient NPO or unable to take adequate nutrition, and approximately 72 hours prior to surgery.

d. In general, holding GDMT during acute HF is associated with higher risks of hospital mortality, short-term mortality, and rehospitalization (meta-analysis for β blockers and registry data for ACEI/ARB). Guidelines suggest to not hold GDMT for mild aberrations in blood pressure or renal function; however, shock may preclude use of β blockers and vasodilators. Titration and reinitiation of GDMT agents typically conducted once the patient has left the ICU and is on the inpatient unit.

IV. ORTHOTOPIC HEART TRANSPLANT (OHT)

A. Indications: stage D HF that cannot be addressed by pharmacologic, device, or surgical optimization, including refractory CS or inotrope dependence, repeated HF hospitalizations, severe ischemic heart disease not amenable to revascularization, refractory ventricular arrhythmias

B. Contraindications: fixed pulmonary hypertension (PVR > 3.5 can increase risk of post-OHT RV failure), systemic illnesses, or irreversible multi-organ dysfunction that will impact overall survival, active infection, nonadherence, extreme obesity or cachexia, active substance use, untreated malignancy or recent malignancy, severe diabetes, and severe PAD.

C. Pretransplant evaluation optimization

1. Assess burden of noncardiac organ comorbidities (vascular disease, lung disease, renal disease etc.) and perform routine cancer screening.
2. Assess the need for concomitant transplantation of other organs (lung, kidney, liver); about 1 in 15 heart transplants also involve transplant of a second organ.
3. Broad infectious evaluation including viral hepatitis, HIV, syphilis, CMV, EBV, Toxoplasma, and COVID. Assess need for pre-OHT vaccines as live vaccines cannot be administered after OHT.

D. Posttransplant intensive care unit management

1. **Hemodynamics**
   a. Immediate post-OHT patients in the ICU experience RV systolic dysfunction, and even in the setting of a normal graft LV ejection fraction, the SV may be fixed due to edema and ischemia of the myocardium. RV dysfunction can be due to graft and donor ischemia, reperfusion injury, allograft dysfunction, volume overload, recipient precapillary pulmonary hypertension, and donor-recipient size mismatch.
   b. Atrial pacing to HR > 100 to 110 bpm is used to maintain cardiac output while the SV is impaired in the short term.
   c. Inotropes, commonly dual inotropes, are used to preserve contractility and address RV dysfunction.
   d. Pulmonary vasodilators are also commonly used to unload the RV.
   e. Early extubation is a worthwhile goal to remove the impacts of PEEP on RV afterload.
2. **Immunosuppressive medications**
   a. Induction: early immunosuppression, to combat robust early alloimmune response. Agents include antithymocyte antibodies, interleukin-2 receptor antagonists.
   b. Maintenance: combination therapy targets multiple pathways of immunosuppression, with the goals of limiting risk of rejection while minimizing risks of drug toxicity, opportunistic infections, and malignancy. Standard early maintenance therapy includes corticosteroid, antiproliferative with mycophenolate mofetil (azathioprine less commonly) and calcineurin inhibitor (tacrolimus or cyclosporine).
      1. Specific regimens tailored with transplant cardiologist and transplant pharmacist to minimize rejection, and minimize toxicities and side effects of the various agents. Typically, corticosteroids are downtitrated over months.
   c. Prophylaxis: Infection prophylaxis is given against CMV, PCP, HSV, and oral candidiasis during the first 6 to 12 months after transplantation. Depending on the status of the donor, anti-HCV therapy may be required.
      1. Aspirin and statin will be required to address coronary allograft vasculopathy.
      2. Specific prophylaxis to side effects of immunosuppressive medications include prevention of osteoporosis and gastric ulcers.
   d. Many medications interact with immunosuppression (including calcium channel blockers) and prophylactic medications (fungal prophylaxis). Interdisciplinary management of medications with transplant pharmacists and transplant cardiologists is crucial in and out of the ICU.

e. Post-OHT patients are at high risk for infection including fungal and atypical pathogens. Have a low threshold to culture and engage Infectious Disease consultation.

Selected Readings

Beesley SJ, Weber G, Sarge T, et al. Septic cardiomyopathy. *Crit Care Med.* 2018;46(4):625-634. doi:10.1097/CCM.0000000000002851

Heidenreich PA, Bozkurt B, Aguilar D, et al. 2022 AHA/ACC/HFSA guideline for the management of heart failure: a report of the American College of Cardiology/American Heart Association Joint Committee on Clinical Practice Guidelines [published correction appears in *Circulation.* 2022 May 3;145(18):e1033; *Circulation.* 2022 Sep 27;146(13):e185]. *Circulation.* 2022;145(18):e895-e1032. doi:10.1161/CIR.0000000000001063

Khurshid S, Frankel DS. Pacing-induced cardiomyopathy. *Card Electrophysiol Clin.* 2021;13(4):741-753. doi:10.1016/j.ccep.2021.06.009

Medina de Chazal H, Del Buono MG, Keyser-Marcus L, et al. Stress cardiomyopathy diagnosis and treatment: JACC state-of-the-art review. *J Am Coll Cardiol.* 2018;72(16):1955-1971. doi:10.1016/j.jacc.2018.07.072

Troughton RW, Asher CR, Klein AL. Pericarditis. *Lancet.* 2004;363(9410):717-727. doi:10.1016/S0140-6736(04)15648-1

19 ECMO and Ventricular Assist Devices

Jerome Crowley

I. INTRA-AORTIC BALLOON PUMP

A. The Intra-Aortic Counter pulsation Balloon Pump (IABP) is a device used to support the failing left ventricle. It is inserted (usually percutaneously) via the femoral or axillary artery and serves to augment coronary perfusion and reduce left ventricular afterload.

B. The IABP is most commonly inserted in the setting of high-risk coronary artery disease (CAD) with or without refractory chest pain as a bridge to definitive management (high-risk percutaneous coronary intervention [PCI] or Coronary artery bypass graft [CABG]). It may also be inserted to support a ventricle with severe mitral regurgitation or an infarct-related ventricular septal defect.

C. The IABP is not indicated for the management of right ventricular failure as unloading of the left ventricle may worsen interventricular septal displacement and further worsening of ventricular function.

D. Background

1. No survival benefit to IABPs has been identified in a randomized clinical trial; however, the ease of insertion and familiarity with the device allow for its continued widespread use.
2. The IABP consists of a flexible catheter that contains a flexible balloon that is inflated with helium in specific timing with the cardiac cycle.
3. IABPs come in a variety of sizes (30-50 mL) with appropriate sizing chosen based on patient's height.
4. Placement is most appropriately guided by fluoroscopy but may be done using echocardiographic guidance or anatomic landmarks in an emergency setting.

E. Function

1. The IABP inflates in diastole and deflates in systole. This allows for an increase in diastolic blood pressure and a decrease in cardiac afterload during systole. In clinical practice, however, this leads to a variable effect on coronary blood flow and cardiac output.
2. The IABP is programmed to trigger off of EKG morphology, arterial pressure, fiberoptic sensing, or manual mode. The rate of trigger is a ratio of heart rate; most commonly 1:1 or 1:2. Rates less than 1:1 require anticoagulation, and any ratio less than 1:3 provides no significant support and is only used as part of the weaning.
3. Precise timing is necessary to ensure proper IABP function. An improperly timed IABP can have detrimental effects. Timing is checked periodically by placing the balloon pump in a 1:2 ratio in order to compare the augmented to nonaugmented pressure waveform. Figure 19.1 shows the IABP waveform.

F. Indications

1. IABPs are commonly inserted for the following conditions:
   - **a.** Acute left ventricular failure
   - **b.** Refractory angina
   - **c.** Coronary perfusion support for high-risk CAD (usually left main disease)
   - **d.** Chronic left ventricular failure as a bridge to heart transplant or LVAD
   - **e.** Inability to wean from cardiopulmonary bypass

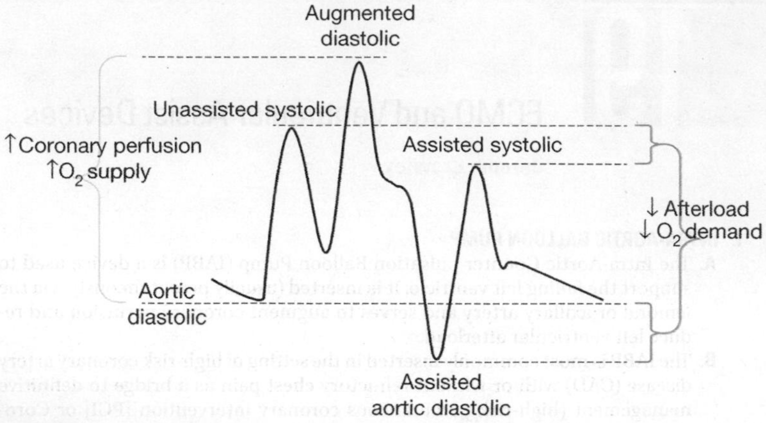

FIGURE 19.1 IABP tracing.

G. Contraindications

1. IABPs have few absolute contraindications, but in many conditions may not have significant benefit.
2. Absolute contraindications
   a. Aortic dissection
   b. Aortic aneurysm
   c. Degree of aortic insufficiency greater than mild (IABP will increase the degree of AI.)
3. Relative contraindications
   a. Significant atherosclerosis or peripheral vascular disease (increase the complication rate)
   b. Left ventricular outflow tract obstruction (IABP will likely worsen this phenomenon.)
   c. Tachydysrhythmias (inability for appropriate timing of IABP)
   d. Young age (Compliant blood vessels reduce the efficacy of IABP.)

H. Complications

1. Vascular compromise to limb
   a. Risks include preexisting vascular disease, small arteries, female gender, older age.
2. Visceral ischemia
   a. Likely due to occlusion from IABP. Daily chest x-rays are indicated to ensure a stable IABP position.
3. Thrombocytopenia
4. Stroke

I. Weaning

1. Once support is no longer deemed necessary, the IABP is weaned by reducing the ratio from 1:1 to 1:2 to 1:4. With each ratio reduction after a period of time (usually 1-2 hours), the patient is assessed with EKGs, markers of perfusion, symptoms, and if applicable pulmonary artery catheter numbers to determine the wean is being tolerated. More patients who are critically ill may require a more prolonged wean; however, it is important that the patient remains therapeutically anticoagulated to reduce the risk of thrombus with a balloon triggering at a low ratio.
2. The IABP is usually removed at the bedside with manual pressure. The standard procedure is as follows:
   a. The IABP is paused and the helium line disconnected.
   b. The helium port is aspirated to ensure balloon deflation.

c. The IABP is removed with the sheath together (the balloon cannot be removed from the sheath), and the arteriotomy is allowed to bleed for 2 to 3 beats to ensure no clot.

d. Manual pressure held for 5 minutes X French size of sheath. Additional pressure may be needed to ensure hemostasis.

II. EXTRACORPOREAL MEMBRANE OXYGENATION (ECMO)

A. Description of ECMO Circuit: See Figure 19.2

1. A modern ECMO circuit consists of several standard components:

a. A drainage cannula that serves to remove blood from the patient

b. A centrifugal pump that actively pumps the blood

c. An oxygenator that allows for gas exchange

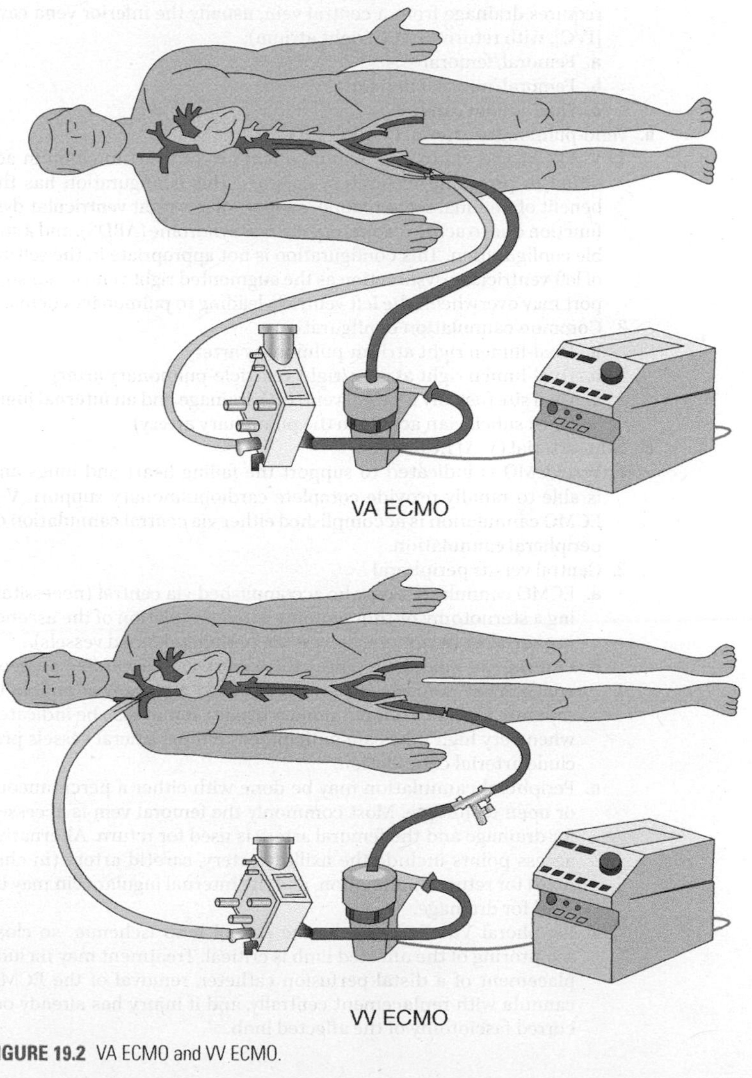

FIGURE 19.2 VA ECMO and VV ECMO.

   d. A return cannula that serves to return the blood to the patient
   e. Optionally there may be a heat exchanger interfacing with the oxygenator to provide thermal control of the patient's temperature.
2. ECMO is defined by the location and type of cannulation. Letters before the hyphen refer to drainage cannula, and letters after the hyphen refer to return cannula.
   a. Veno-venous (V-V) ECMO
      1. V-V ECMO serves to replace a patient's pulmonary function and is indicated for respiratory failure. It does not provide any hemodynamic support although correction of hypoxia and respiratory acidosis may improve cardiovascular function. It is almost always performed via percutaneous peripheral cannulation.
      2. Common cannulation configurations (effective veno-venous ECMO requires drainage from a central vein, usually the inferior vena cava [IVC], with return to SVC/right atrium):
         a. Femoral/femoral
         b. Femoral/internal jugular
         c. Dual-lumen cannula
   b. Veno-pulmonary arterial (V-P) ECMO
      1. V-P ECMO serves to augment a patient's right heart function in addition to providing respiratory support. This configuration has the benefit of minimal recirculation, support of any right ventricular dysfunction due to acute respiratory distress syndrome (ARDS), and a stable configuration. This configuration is not appropriate in the setting of left ventricular dysfunction as the augmented right ventricular support may overwhelm the left ventricle leading to pulmonary edema.
      2. Common cannulation configurations:
         a. Dual-lumen right atrium-pulmonary artery
         b. Dual-lumen right atrium/right ventricle-pulmonary artery
         c. Dual site (usually femoral vein/IVC drainage and an internal jugular or subclavian access to the pulmonary artery)
   c. Veno-arterial (V-A) ECMO
      1. V-A ECMO is indicated to support the failing heart and lungs and is able to rapidly provide complete cardiopulmonary support. V-A ECMO cannulation is accomplished either via central cannulation or peripheral cannulation.
      2. Central versus peripheral
         a. ECMO cannulation may be accomplished via central (necessitating a sternotomy or thoracotomy with cannulation of the ascending aorta) or peripheral (access via peripheral blood vessels).
         b. Central cannulation requires the expertise of a cardiac surgeon and is most commonly performed when a patient is unable to separate from a cardiopulmonary bypass. It may also be indicated when very high flows are anticipated or if peripheral vessels preclude arterial cannulation.
         c. Peripheral cannulation may be done with either a percutaneous or open technique. Most commonly the femoral vein is accessed for drainage and the femoral artery is used for return. Alternative access points include the axillary artery, carotid artery (in children) for return cannulation, and the internal jugular vein may be used for drainage.
         d. Peripheral V-A ECMO runs the risk of limb ischemia, so close monitoring of the affected limb is critical. Treatment may include placement of a distal perfusion catheter, removal of the ECMO cannula with replacement centrally, and if injury has already occurred fasciotomy of the affected limb.

d. Cannula sizing

1. Cannula sizes are selected based on goal flow and the patient's vasculature. Manufacturer tables should be consulted to determine appropriate cannula sizing.

a. Venous cannulas are larger and range in size from 21 to 30F in adults.

b. Arterial cannulas are smaller and are commonly 15 to 21F in adults.

c. For distal limb perfusion, a 5 to 8F cannula may be used.

2. Goal flows are based on the patient's body surface area and desired cardiac index for venoarterial ECMO. For veno-venous ECMO, goal flows are dependent on native lung function and cardiac output. Roughly 60% to 70% of cardiac output must participate in gas exchange to maintain adequate oxygenation.

B. Patient Selection: ECMO is resource intensive and should be offered when there is reasonable hope of recovery. Overutilization of ECMO serves to waste valuable resources as well as cause significant moral distress for providers and families of patients.

1. Indications:

a. For VA ECMO:

1. Cardiogenic shock with evidence of end-organ hypoperfusion refractory to medical management

a. Poor ventricular function noted on echocardiography

b. Cardiac index refractory to inotropic support

c. Worsening acidosis from hypoperfusion

d. Refractory arrhythmias

2. Defined exit strategy

a. Recovery

b. Transplant

c. Durable mechanical assist device

d. Bridge to decision

b. For V-V ECMO

1. Hypoxemic respiratory failure

a. P/F < 80 despite:

i. Prone positioning (unless contraindicated)

ii. Neuromuscular blockade

iii. Positive end expiratory pressure (PEEP) optimization

iv. Lung-protective ventilatory strategy

b. Inability to maintain a driving pressure <15 cm H_2O

2. Hypercapnic respiratory failure

a. pH < 7.2 and Pco_2 > 80 mm Hg despite optimized ventilator settings

b. Auto-PEEP contributing to hemodynamic compromise

3. Bridge to lung transplant

4. Procedure support (high-risk thoracic surgery)

2. Contraindications

a. Absolute contraindications (for all ECMO)

1. Inadequate vascular access

2. Aggressive measures not within patient's goals of care

3. Life expectancy < 6 months

b. Absolute contraindications (for V-V ECMO)

1. Refractory shock

2. Duration of respiratory failure >14 days and lack of candidacy for lung transplantation

c. Absolute contraindications (for V-P ECMO)

1. Left ventricular dysfunction

2. Acute PE with clot in main pulmonary artery

d. Absolute contraindications (for V-A ECMO)
   1. Aortic insufficiency greater than mild
e. Relative contraindications (use of ECMO is favored in patients with a more reversible disease process)
   1. Age >75
   2. Inability to be anticoagulated
   3. Severe underlying comorbidities:
      a. Lung disease requiring home oxygen
      b. End-stage renal disease requiring dialysis
      c. Significant neurologic injury
      d. Cirrhosis

3. Extracorporeal resuscitative ECMO (E-CPR): The use of ECMO in cardiac arrest remains controversial but is a reasonable treatment for refractory arrest, provided the following are met:
   a. Age < 70
   b. Witnessed cardiac arrest with immediate (within 10 minutes, ideally 5) CPR
   c. No sustainable return of spontaneous circulation (ROSC) for more than 10 minutes
   d. Duration of arrest less than 60 minutes (ideally $<$ 30 minutes)
   e. Initial rhythm reported to be shockable
      1. PEA arrest has a much poorer prognosis; however, special populations are exceptions:
         a. Pulmonary emboli
         b. Hypothermia (see hypothermia outcome prediction after extracorporeal life support [HOPE] Protocol)
         c. Arrests under general anesthesia
         d. Known drug intoxication
   f. No significant preexisting medical comorbidities (listed above under relative contraindications)
   g. End tidal $CO_2 > 10$ mm Hg
   h. $Pao_2 > 50$ mm Hg

C. Management of ECMO

1. Parameters
   a. ECMO circuit parameters
      1. Sweep gas flow (LPM)
         a. This reflects the rate of gas flow through the oxygenator and determines the rate of CO_2 removal. Care should be taken to avoid rapid correction of $Paco_2$ as this is associated with an increased risk of intracranial hemorrhage.
      2. Fraction of delivered oxygen (%)
         a. This is the percentage of the sweep gas that is oxygen and is one component of the amount of oxygenation of the blood.
      3. Rotations per minute (RPMs)
         a. This determines the flow on the ECMO circuit. Flow for a given RPM is a function of pre and afterload on a pump. Changes in flow for a given RPM should warrant investigation of the patient's clinical status. Flow is the other determinant of oxygenation on ECMO. On V-A ECMO, flow determines the degree of hemodynamic support.
2. Ventilatory management
   a. Once a patient is on ECMO, ventilator settings should be reduced to lung-protective settings. There remains controversy on what settings are best, but consensus does support avoiding high tidal volumes, minimizing driving pressures, and providing optimized PEEP to reduce driving pressure.
3. Anticoagulation
   a. Although there are emerging data on the safety of ECMO circuits without anticoagulation, the standard of care recommends anticoagulation

for all patients on ECMO. Targets of anticoagulation will vary by institution but are similar to therapeutic levels used in acute coronary syndromes or pulmonary embolism.

b. Heparin is the most common drug utilized due to familiarity although it possesses several drawbacks: unreliable dosing due to consumption of antithrombin III and a risk of heparin-induced thrombocytopenia.

c. Bivalirudin is emerging as an acceptable alternative agent and is recommended if any suspicion for heparin induced thrombocytopenia (HIT) develops.

4. Critical care management

a. Patients on ECMO are susceptible to similar critical illness injury as other patients.

b. Vigilance for infection is critical, a falling fibrinogen on ECMO likely represents either clot formation or sepsis. Due to the difficulty in replacing ECMO cannula, a low index of suspicion for sepsis must be maintained at all times.

c. Monitoring for hemolysis is important and involves following lactate dehydrogenase (LDH) (nonspecific), plasma-free hemoglobin (most specific), and carboxyhemoglobin (surrogate for red cell lysis).

D. Troubleshooting ECMO

1. Inadequate drainage/"Chatter"

a. This results from intermittent occlusion of the drainage limb due to hypovolemia or cannula malposition. Initial treatment is with volume expansion. Cannula position should be checked to ensure appropriate location. If drainage is still inadequate, then consideration should be made to place additional venous drainage cannulation (VV-V or VV-A ECMO).

2. Elevated return pressures

a. Increases in return pressures raise the risk of hemolysis. This may be due to inadequate return cannula positioning, inadequate sizing of return cannula, or in V-A ECMO elevated systemic vascular resistance. Treatment is directed at the underlying cause (addition of a new or upsized cannula, conversion to central ECMO, or administration of vasodilators if blood pressure will tolerate).

3. Recirculation

a. Recirculation is unique to V-V ECMO and refers to the phenomenon where blood cycles through the ECMO circuit rather than through the heart reducing the fraction of systemic blood that is being oxygenated. The most common reason is that the drainage/return cannulas are too close or that the dual-lumen cannula has migrated. Imaging with x-rays and or echocardiography is indicated to reposition the cannula.

4. North/South syndrome

a. Patients placed on peripheral V-A ECMO with both cardiac and pulmonary pathology run the risk of differential hypoxia. Here, native blood ejected from the heart reflects native pulmonary function and meets the blood oxygenated by the ECMO circuit in the aorta. This location of mixing will vary based on the cardiac output of the native heart. If the patient's lungs are poorly functioning, this can lead to hypoxic blood being delivered to the cerebral circulation and the coronary arteries. Monitoring of the patient on peripheral V-A ECMO should always include arterial gas sampling from the right upper extremity to reflect the oxygenation of the brain. Treatment for north/south syndrome involves ventilator optimization and if not possible or severe conversion to V-AV ECMO where some of the return blood is diverted to the venous circulation to "preoxygenate" the blood entering the heart. This is effectively supporting the patient with both V-A and V-V ECMO.

5. Left ventricular distension
   a. In a patient placed on peripheral V-A ECMO for cardiogenic shock, the retrograde flow from the ECMO circuit will increase the loading conditions of the left ventricle leading to left ventricular (LV) distension. This can lead to pulmonary edema as well as impede LV recovery due to increased wall tension. Treatment involves optimizing left ventricular ejection and decompression. Options include:
      1. Medical therapy with inotropes
      2. Surgical LV vent placement via sternotomy or thoracotomy
      3. Septostomy creation in a catheterization laboratory
      4. Intra-aortic balloon pump placement
      5. Placement of percutaneous left ventricular assist device to decompress the left ventricle.
6. Circuit emergencies (inadvertent decannulation, mechanical failure, cardiac arrest on V-V ECMO)
   a. ECMO centers are advised to have protocols in place with appropriate training for patients with emergencies on ECMO.
   b. Pearls
      1. Patients on ECMO are often on rest ventilator settings, during an arrest the degree of vasoactive and ventilatory support needs to be increased.
      2. Inadvertent decannulation leads to massive blood loss, and massive transfusion protocols should be implemented.

E. Weaning from ECMO

1. V-V ECMO weaning should be attempted once a patient has demonstrated some pulmonary recovery. This usually coincides with a reduced need for ECMO fraction of delivered oxygen as well as an improvement in compliance on the ventilator. At this time, the sweep gas should be reduced to 1 LPM and the ventilator set at a reasonable respiratory rate. If the blood gas is acceptable, a cap trial may be undertaken for 8 to 24 hours in which the sweep flow is turned to 0; effectively the patient is off ECMO support (the blood flowing through the circuit undergoes no gas exchange). If after the cap trial the blood gas is acceptable, the patient may be decannulated from ECMO.
2. V-A ECMO is more challenging to wean as capping the sweep flow would lead to a large shunt which is not sustainable. Therefore, V-A ECMO weaning is somewhat more center variable. Once a patient has demonstrated myocardial recovery (usually assessed by echocardiography), the ECMO flows are decremented by 0.5 LPM every 6 to 12 hours until the patient is on 2 LPM of flow. Further reductions are only advised if the patient is able to tolerate anticoagulation. At this point, the ECMO circuit is reduced to 1 LPM, and assessment of the cardiovascular function is undertaken. If there is remaining uncertainty, the patient can be given additional heparin to a goal activated clotting time (ACT) of 250 and the circuit clamped for 15 minutes. This will serve as a final test to see if a patient can be decannulated. If the patient passes, flows are increased to 2 to 2.5 LPM (if a distal perfusor is present, it is advised to maintain a flow of at least 100 mL/min) and the patient is transported to the operating room for decannulation.
   a. Signs of failing a weaning trial include worsening mitral regurgitation, right ventricular dysfunction, and failure of stroke volume augmentation as the patient is weaned from ECMO.

III. VENTRICULAR ASSIST DEVICES

A. Temporary Ventricular Assist Devices

1. Percutaneous left ventricular assist devices (pLVADs) (Impella CP, Impella 5.5; Abiomed) (See Figure 19.3)

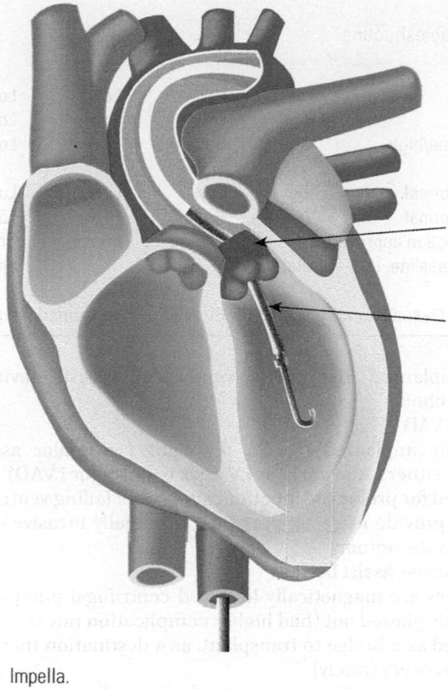

FIGURE 19.3 Impella.

a. The Impella CP is placed percutaneously via femoral artery to provide temporary support of the left ventricle, up to 4 LPM.
   1. Complications include hemolysis, limb ischemia, and stroke.

b. The Impella 5.5 is placed via surgical graft to the axillary artery and provides up to 5.5 LPM of support. This device is more suited to support on the order of weeks to a month to support a patient as a bridge to recovery, transplant, or LVAD.
   1. Complications are similar to the Impella CP, but there is a reduced risk of hemolysis for a given flow.

2. Percutaneous right ventricular assist devices

a. There are two classes of devices: dual-lumen cannulas that are usually inserted via the internal jugular vein and can also serve as V-P ECMO cannula and axial pumps inserted via the femoral or internal jugular vein.
   1. Dual-lumen cannula: Spectrum, Protek Duo (Liva Nova)
      a. Larger, but able to provide oxygenation support if needed
   2. Axial pumps: Impella Flex, Impella RP
      a. Smaller cannula but no oxygenation

3. Transseptal support devices

a. TandemHeart (LivaNova)
   1. A long cannula is placed from the femoral vein to the left atrium via transseptal puncture.
   2. Arterial return cannula
   3. Able to provide oxygenation support if needed
   4. Can be used in the presence of severe aortic insufficiency (left atrial drainage will decompress left circulation.)

TABLE 19.1 LVAD Troubleshooting

LVAD flow	High	Low	Low	Low	Low
MAP	Low	High	Low	Low	Low
Mean PAP	Baseline/high	High	Baseline/high	Low	Low
PCWP	Low/normal	High	Low	Low	Low
CVP	Low/normal	Variable	High	High	Low
Echocardiographic Findings	RV function improved from baseline, LV small	LV dilated	Dilated RV	Effusion	Small RV and LV
Diagnosis	Sepsis/vasodilation	High SVR	RV failure	Tamponade	Hypovolemia

4. Surgically implanted temporary ventricular assist device (VADs) (Centrimag, Abbott)
    a. Centrimag VAD
        1. Surgically implanted (RA-PA for right ventricular assist device [RVAD], either LA to aorta or LV apex to aorta for LVAD)
        2. Indicated for prolonged inpatient support of failing ventricles
        3. Able to provide more support than minimally invasive options but require a sternotomy

B. Durable Left Ventricular Assist Devices

1. Modern devices are magnetically levitated centrifugal pumps. Older devices are mostly phased out (had higher complication rates)
    a. May be used as a bridge to transplant, as a destination therapy, or as a bridge to recovery (rarely)
2. These devices require anticoagulation with coumadin.
    a. Common complications include strokes and gastrointestinal (GI) bleeding.
3. Troubleshooting LVADs
    a. See Table 19.1.

Selected Readings

Baran DA, Jaiswal A, Hennig F, Potapov E. Temporary mechanical circulatory support: devices, outcomes, and future directions. *J Heart Lung Transplant.* 2022;41(6):678-691. doi:10.1016/j.healun.2022.03.018

Combes A, Price S, Slutsky AS, Brodie D. Temporary circulatory support for cardiogenic shock. *Lancet.* 2020;396(10245):199-212.

Munshi L, Walkey A, Goligher E, Pham T, Uleryk EM, Fan E. Venovenous extracorporeal membrane oxygenation for acute respiratory distress syndrome: a systematic review and meta-analysis. *Lancet Respir Med.* 2019;7(2):163-172.

Pratt AK, Shah NS, Boyce SW. Left ventricular assist device management in the ICU. *Crit Care Med.* 2014;42(1):158-168.

Sidebotham D. Troubleshooting adult ECMO. *J Extra Corpor Technol.* 2011;43(1):P27-P32.

Thiele H, de Waha-Thiele S, Freund A, Zeymer U, Desch S, Fitzgerald S. Management of cardiogenic shock. *EuroIntervention.* 2021;17(6):451-465.

van Diepen S, Katz JN, Albert NM, et al; Council on Quality of Care and Outcomes Research; and Mission: Lifeline. Contemporary management of cardiogenic shock: a scientific statement from the American Heart Association. *Circulation.* 2017;136(16):e232-e268.

20 Acute Respiratory Distress Syndrome

Sylvia Ranjeva, Roberta Ribeiro De Santis Santiago, and Lorenzo Berra

I. DEFINITION

Acute respiratory distress syndrome (ARDS) is an inflammatory lung condition characterized by increased vascular permeability, pulmonary edema, consolidation, and hypoxemia. It can be triggered by direct and indirect injuries and is usually combined with other organ dysfunction. Although histopathologically well defined (diffuse alveolar damage [DAD]), the clinical diagnosis of ARDS has relatively poor specificity for the presence of DAD at postmortem. The patients diagnosed with severe ARDS for more than 72 hours more likely presented with postmortem DAD. Recently, great effort has been put into redefining the diagnostic criteria of ARDS (Berlin definition of ARDS). The new ARDS criteria still have relatively low specificity for DAD. In a group of patients diagnosed with severe ARDS for more than 72 hours based on the Berlin definition, 69% presented with postmortem DAD. Finally, it still is unknown whether patients meeting the clinical criteria for ARDS but without DAD behave differently than do patients with clinical ARDS with DAD.

II. ETIOLOGY

ARDS usually develops in patients with underlying risk factors that can induce a systemic inflammatory response. ARDS can be caused by pulmonary conditions (pneumonia, aspiration pneumonitis, and contusions) or, less commonly, by extrapulmonary conditions (abdominal sepsis, acute pancreatitis, and multiple trauma). Pneumonia is by far the most common cause of ARDS, and it is more severe when compared to trauma-associated ARDS. Computed tomography (CT) traditionally helped in distinguishing different patterns of ARDS. ARDS secondary to pneumonia (direct lung injury) shows most of the dense consolidations localized to the lower lung fields, whereas ARDS secondary to acute pancreatitis (indirect lung injury) shows a diffuse, almost homogeneous pattern of consolidation. However, there is substantial overlap in CT findings between ARDS caused by direct and indirect lung injury. Some pathogens causing direct lung injury (such as the hemagglutinin type 1 and neuraminidase type [H1N1] virus and, recently, the novel SARS-CoV-2) may present with diffuse consolidation on CT.

III. EPIDEMIOLOGY

ARDS can be classified as community acquired and nosocomial based on its onset. Nosocomial ARDS may be a "preventable" syndrome. Over the past 20 years, the incidence of nosocomial ARDS has declined remarkably. In a population-based cohort study (from 2001 to 2008) conducted in Olmsted County, Minnesota, Li et al observed a steady decrease in nosocomial ARDS; however, the incidence of community-acquired ARDS was unchanged. These observations corroborate the hypothesis that ARDS can be prevented by improved care of patients who are critically ill. Important elements that might have contributed to a reduced incidence of nosocomial ARDS are lung-protective ventilation for patients at risk for ARDS, ventilator care bundles, goal-directed therapy in sepsis and septic shock, early antimicrobial administration, male donor plasma, and more cautious fluid administration and transfusions of blood products. Despite these encouraging findings, mortality among patients with ARDS remains high, up to 45% for severe disease. In the ongoing SARS-CoV-2 pandemic, a European multicenter study described a 90-day mortality of 31% among 4244 patients with COVID-19-associated ARDS. Recovery from severe ARDS and prolonged ventilation is slow and accompanied by muscle wasting and weakness. Five years from the ARDS episode, exercise limitation, impairment of memory, cognition, and ability to concentrate may persist.

IV. PATHOPHYSIOLOGY

Wide variation in the etiology, physiology, clinical course, and radiographic attributes of ARDS reflects its underlying pathophysiologic complexity. Multiple frameworks that stratify patients with ARDS into distinct subgroups according to clinical, biological, and radiographic discriminants exist.

A. Direct Versus Indirect Lung Injury: One classical framework of ARDS pathophysiology differentiates between insults that cause direct (intrapulmonary) lung injury and indirect (extrapulmonary) lung injury. Direct lung insults include trauma associated with mechanical ventilation (ventilator-induced lung injury [VILI]), massive aspiration, infection (mainly pneumonia), near drowning, and pre–intensive care unit (ICU) chest and lung trauma. Indirect injuries include systemic inflammatory processes, such as sepsis and pancreatitis, that may lead to diffuse inflammatory lung injury. Early studies showed distinct clinical and radiographic characteristics between the two subgroups. For example, direct ARDS was associated with more homogeneous distribution of ground-glass opacification on CT chest imaging and increased lung elastance compared to indirect ARDS. However, it remains debatable whether these observed patterns translate into clinically significant differences in lung recruitability and response to ventilatory management. Therefore, the clinical utility of classification according to direct or indirect ARDS is unclear. Notably, this framework ignores etiology-specific processes that underlie ARDS development. Identifying and treating the underlying cause of ARDS given a pattern of direct or indirect injury remains crucial for patient recovery.

B. Biological Phenotypes: Another framework of ARDS pathophysiology uses clinical and biochemical data to establish biologically derived subpopulations, or phenotypes, of patients with ARDS. The goal of this approach is to highlight underlying processes involved in ARDS pathogenesis, thereby identifying targets for therapeutic interventions. Secondary investigations of landmark ARDS clinical trials established two predominant biological phenotypes—patients with and without a hyperinflammatory response (~30% and 70% of patients with ARDS, respectively). The hyperinflammatory phenotype demonstrated dramatically elevated levels of inflammatory plasma biomarkers (interleukin [IL]-6, IL-8, and soluble tumor necrosis factor receptor [sTNFR-1]), relative metabolic acidosis, and higher prevalence of shock and sepsis compared to the hypoinflammatory phenotype. The hyperinflammatory phenotype was also associated with increased mortality and decreased ventilator-free days. Furthermore, the hyperinflammatory and hypoinflammatory phenotypes have been associated with differences in the response to clinical management strategies, including positive end-expiratory pressure (PEEP) and fluid management.

Tissue-specific biomarkers are being increasingly used to identify more precise ARDS subphenotypes. A range of biomarkers have been associated with poor ARDS outcomes, including proinflammatory markers (as mentioned), markers of endothelial injury (eg, intercellular adhesion molecule 1 [ICAM-1] and apurinic/apyrimidinic endonuclease 3 [APE-3]) and epithelial injury (eg, soluble receptor for advanced glycation end products [sRAGE] and surfactant), and markers of vascular dysregulation (eg, protein C). The movement toward higher resolution subphenotypes can greatly advance a mechanistic understanding of pathogenic pathways that contribute to ARDS progression.

C. COVID-19-Associated ARDS: The COVID-19 pandemic highlights the importance of etiology-specific considerations in ARDS. Early observations during the first 2020 pandemic wave suggested that ARDS secondary to COVID-19 disease exhibits atypical ARDS physiology marked by severe hypoxemia in the setting of preserved respiratory compliance. COVID-19-associated ARDS has also been associated with atypical radiographic features, such as dilated pulmonary vessels on chest CT. Within COVID-19-associated ARDS itself, there appears to be substantial heterogeneity in clinical presentation, radiographic characteristics, and response to treatment maneuvers. It is unclear whether previously established ARDS phenotypes based on degree of inflammation extend to COVID-19-associated ARDS. Recent studies found low prevalence of the classical hyperinflammatory phenotype among COVID-19 ARDS cohorts. Rather, multiple studies have suggested that altered coagulation and endothelial dysfunction are key elements of systemic COVID-19 disease, and therefore may represent important phenotypic axes in COVID-19-associated ARDS. Accordingly, histologic analyses of pulmonary vessels in patients with COVID-19 have shown extensive thrombosis and endothelial injury, and postmortem analysis of patients with COVID-19 ARDS has revealed a high burden of thrombotic disseminated intravascular coagulation. The pathophysiology of COVID-19-associated ARDS remains poorly understood, and research into differences between classical and COVID-19-associated ARDS is ongoing. However, existing work motivates future etiology-specific studies of ARDS and emphasizes the importance of identifying and treating the underlying trigger in patients with ARDS.

V. DEVELOPMENT AND PROGRESSION OF ACUTE RESPIRATORY DISTRESS SYNDROME

After an initial infectious, inflammatory, or traumatic insult, ARDS classically progresses via sequential degrees of alveolar injury and fibrosis.

A. Primary Immune Response: Activation of resident macrophages, release of inflammatory mediators (cytokines and chemokines), and recruitment of neutrophils into the lung with the release of additional inflammatory mediators and toxic products cause lung epithelial and endothelial injury. Activation of coagulation in the microcirculation contributes to additional endothelial injury. A number of inflammatory mediators have been associated with worse outcomes in patients with ARDS. Dysregulated apoptosis and autophagy as well as impaired function of T regulatory lymphocytes contribute to injury and/or delayed resolution. The disruption of the endothelial-epithelial barrier because of inflammation causes the accumulation of protein-rich edema fluid in the airspaces and interstitium as well as impaired lung edema clearance. Inactivation of the existing surfactant and production of abnormal surfactant may occur. Alveolar exudate, lung consolidation, and alveolar collapse produce low lung compliance and right-to-left intrapulmonary shunt, leading to arterial hypoxemia.

B. Secondary Lung Injury: Additional injury, such as from VILI and/or ventilator-associated pneumonia (VAP), may lead to an increased severity of ARDS and prolonged time to recovery. VILI is caused by mechanical stress and strain induced by positive pressure ventilation. Overdistension of the lung when ventilating with an excessively high tidal volume or the recurrent recruitment and derecruitment of alveoli through insufficient application of PEEP can lead to lung damage. VAP may develop during mechanical ventilation because of microaspiration of bacteria-laden secretion into the lungs. Bacterial virulence (ie, *Pseudomonas aeruginosa* and oxacillin-resistant *Staphylococcus aureus*) and inadequate initial antibiotic treatment have been shown to increase morbidity and mortality in patients with ARDS.

C. Physiologic Characteristics and Evolution of ARDS: ARDS evolves in three different phases that do not represent discrete entities but are meant to describe a *continuum* of the same pathologic process. During the **first phase**, alveolar damage is predominant, resulting in loss of surfactant production, atelectasis, and hypoxemia. The main feature of the second phase of ARDS, the **exudative phase**, is the disruption of the endothelial barrier with exudation of protein-rich fluid and blood cellular elements. The last phase of ARDS, the **fibroproliferative phase**, is characterized by an organizing inflammatory process of fibroblast growth. All three phases may be completely reversible.

D. Dead Space and Prognosis: In a landmark study, Nuckton et al showed that dead space is increased from the early stage of ARDS and that it is independently associated with higher mortality. The increased dead space is probably due to pulmonary vascular injury, although hyperinflation may also contribute. Pulmonary capillary microthrombi, inflammation, and obstruction of regional pulmonary blood probably result in areas of ventilated lung with no perfusion (increased dead-space ventilation), which results in hypercapnia for a given minute ventilation.

VI. TREATMENT

Management of ARDS requires an intensive and systematic approach to diagnosing and treating the underlying cause of lung injury, preventing secondary injuries to the lungs and other organs, avoiding complications, and providing overall supportive care.

A. Initial Diagnosis and Management: To prevent progression and severity of ARDS, treatment of the underlying condition is a priority. Important early interventions include **early** and **appropriate** antibiotic administration and drainage and debridement of abscesses and necrotic tissue or burned tissue ("source control").

B. Hemodynamic Management: Conservative fluid management has been advocated in patients with ARDS and has been shown to reduce the duration of mechanical ventilation as well as ICU stay. However, judicious fluid restriction should be balanced against inadequate organ perfusion (most commonly manifesting as prerenal kidney injury). There is no role for the routine use of pulmonary artery catheterization in the management of ARDS, although it may be useful in select populations, such as in the presence of severe pulmonary hypertension and right ventricular dysfunction.

C. Treatment and Prevention of Infections: Early and appropriate antibiotic treatment for sepsis together with de-escalation of antibiotics when no longer needed have been shown to decrease incidence of multidrug-resistant bacterial infection. Decrease in nosocomial ARDS incidence as observed by Li et al can be attributed to the widespread adoption of clinical bundles designed to prevent health care–associated infections.

D. Early Nutrition is recommended. The enteral route is preferred either through nasogastric or jejunal access. Trophic enteral nutrition (providing 20%-40% of caloric needs) for the first 6 days appears to provide similar short- and long-term outcomes with less gastrointestinal intolerances than does early full-calorie nutrition, at least in medical patients with ARDS. A combination of enteral and supplemental parenteral nutrition should be considered if meeting the nutritional target through the enteral route is difficult later in the course. In patients with elevated dead space, special formulation should be administered to optimize V_{CO_2} and V_{O_2} (ie, low carbohydrates, high-lipid formulation). Immune-modulatory formulations (such as ω-3 enriched) should be avoided.

E. Support of Other Organ System Functions is an integral part of the treatment of ARDS. Hemodynamic instability, acute renal failure, gastrointestinal hemorrhage, coagulation abnormalities, and neuromuscular changes may complicate the course of these patients who are critically ill.

VII. MECHANICAL VENTILATION IN PATIENTS WITH ACUTE RESPIRATORY DISTRESS SYNDROME

In ARDS, portions of the lungs are not available for normal gas exchange and ventilation occurs in a small fraction of the lung (the so-called baby lung). The ARDSNet trial showed that a ventilation strategy with a lower tidal volume (4-8 mL/kg of predicted body weight [PBW]) was associated with lower mortality and shorter length of mechanical ventilation. This trial used a combination of volume and pressure limitation. For example, if the plateau airway pressures were higher than 30 cm H_2O, tidal volumes were reduced to 5 or 4 mL/kg PBW. This approach was designed to reduce the mechanical damage on lung tissue and the associated inflammatory response caused by overdistension of the alveolar wall. Permissive hypercapnia is tolerated, if pH is higher than 7.20, to obtain lung-protective ventilation with low tidal volume and low plateau pressure. The optimal approach to patients with severe acidemia (pH < 7.2) is not clear. One strategy for the management of severe, symptomatic acidemia is presented in **Chapter 8**. In case of lung resection, administration of volumetric ventilator support should be carefully adjusted according to the estimated lung volume. A recent multilevel mediation analysis on 3562 patients with ARDS found that the reduced driving pressure (plateau pressure minus PEEP) was associated with increased survival and suggested that driving pressure could be used to titrate tidal volume to the size of the baby lung. Prospective validation of this approach is needed.

A. Lung Recruitment

Recruitment maneuvers are used to open areas of atelectasis and improve lung compliance and oxygenation. Owing to the heterogeneity of the disease, patients show different degrees of response to recruitment. It is important to note that increasing PEEP without lung recruitment may not provide much benefit because the pressures required to reopen atelectatic alveoli are greater than are typical PEEP levels. In fact, increasing PEEP without recruitment may promote overdistension of the expanded portions of the lung and increased mortality. Selection of patients is crucial, and it appears that patients with obesity and ARDS might benefit the most. Recruitment maneuvers can be performed using different methods.

1. A sustained pressure of 30 to 40 cm H_2O is applied to the airways for 40 seconds to 1 minute. If improvement in respiratory system compliance and oxygenation occurs, a higher PEEP approach, such as the higher PEEP/FIO_2 tables used in the assessment of low tidal volume and elevated end-expiratory volume to obviate lung injury (ALVEOLI) or lung open ventilation (LOV) studies, would be applied.
2. **Incremental recruitment:** The lung is incrementally recruited from lower to higher plateau pressure, up to 40 to 50 cm H_2O. This would be followed by a decremental PEEP trial, as noted later.
3. A sigh is a cyclical large breath for about a 3-second period to a plateau pressure of 30 to 40 cm H_2O.

B. PEEP Titration Techniques

The optimal PEEP titration technique is controversial. In general, a higher PEEP strategy seems beneficial for patients with more severe ARDS and for those with improved mechanics or oxygenation on higher PEEP levels.

1. Decremental PEEP trial assesses the oxygenation and respiratory system compliance response after a recruitment maneuver and during a decremental PEEP trial. PEEP is set 2 cm H_2O above the best PEEP identified and the respiratory system recruited again.
2. Positive end-expiratory transpulmonary pressure. The transpulmonary pressure is the difference between the airway pressure and the pleural

pressure. Pleural pressure can be estimated through the positioning of an esophageal balloon. In this approach, PEEP is adjusted to achieve zero to a positive transpulmonary pressure at the end of expiration followed by a recruitment maneuver.

3. PEEP/FIO_2 table
4. A prospective evaluation of four different PEEP titration techniques found, on average, similar levels of PEEP; however, important differences in the volume of recruitable lung were noted for each technique. Hyperinflation by CT was seen at the level of "best PEEP" in all techniques, suggesting a fundamental limitation of low tidal volume ventilation and best PEEP for recruitment (eg, trying to strike the balance between lung recruitment and hyperinflation) when patients are ventilated in the supine or semirecumbent position.

VIII. ADDITIONAL STRATEGIES

A. Sedation and Paralysis: The compromised gas exchange can induce a rise in respiratory rate, leading to patient-ventilator dyssynchrony. One of the possible interventions for reducing the respiratory drive is the administration of opioids. Opioids offer one of the best profiles, and continuous infusion can be titrated until ventilator-patient synchrony is restored, and the optimal respiratory rate reached (up to 35 breaths/min). Although recent studies have shown an immunosuppressing effect of carbon dioxide that could reduce the inflammatory response of ARDS and improve outcome, the overall risk-to-benefit profile of hypercapnia for patients with ARDS is unknown and could be deleterious in the setting of sepsis-related ARDS because an acidotic pH has shown to promote bacterial growth. In addition, hypercapnia should be avoided in subjects with or at risk for increased intracranial pressure. In the setting of severe ARDS ($P/F < 100$), paralysis and controlled mechanical ventilation has been also suggested. However, a recent trial comparing the continuous infusion of neuromuscular blockers and deep sedation for 48 hours after the onset of ARDS in patients with moderate-to-severe presentation was ended earlier because no difference in mortality was observed. The decision about levels of sedation and paralysis may be individualized and should also consider the frequency and type of patient-ventilator dyssynchrony.

B. Prone Positioning: Ventilation in the prone position usually improves gas exchange in patients with ARDS when a better ventilation-perfusion matching is achieved. A randomized clinical trial (RCT) showed survival benefit when early prone ventilation for at least 17 hours daily was applied until the P/F ratio exceeded 150 (on average for 4 days). The maneuver requires team coordination and training. In the current SARS-CoV-2 pandemic, prone ventilation is being broadly applied including in spontaneously breathing patients with COVID-19 pneumonia. Confirmatory studies addressing the impact of prone ventilation and COVID-19-associated ARDS are underway.

C. Pleural Effusion Drainage: Patients with ARDS frequently have pleural effusion due to fluid overload, septic heart failure, or altered pleural hydrostatic pressure due to pneumonia or atelectasis. The presence of a massive pleural effusion can alter the regional transmural pressure of the lung, causing passive atelectasis and, possibly, worsening gas exchange. However, no guideline exists on pleural effusion management in ARDS. In the presence of a normally distensible abdomen, an adequately titrated PEEP level should compensate for the increase in transmural pressure caused by the pleural effusion itself. Placement of a chest tube for drainage of the pleural effusion should be considered on a case-by-case basis and after other interventions (assist-control ventilation, paralysis, pronation) have failed.

D. Extracorporeal Membrane Oxygenation (ECMO): With the epidemic of ARDS secondary to H1N1, venous-venous ECMO was shown to be a valuable therapeutic option in severe ARDS. The use of ECMO allows decreased minute ventilation, smaller tidal volumes, and low airway pressure allowing the lung to rest and recover. Nonetheless, despite the technologic advances and the encouraging results, ECMO is a technique that should be confined to a few, highly specialized centers for limited indications. ECMO has been utilized in patients with severe COVID-19-associated ARDS. The Extracorporeal Life Support Organization (ELSO) guideline recommends similar indications and management for this population.

E. Pharmacologic Adjuncts

1. **Inhaled selective pulmonary vasodilators:** Inhaled nitric oxide (iNO) has been traditionally used as a rescue therapy in ARDS because it improves oxygenation (due to improved ventilation-perfusion matching) and reduces pulmonary artery hypertension secondary to inflammation and thrombosis. iNO might also be a useful adjunct in cases of severe ARDS with pulmonary hypertension to reduce pulmonary vascular resistance and improve oxygenation as a bridge to another intervention such as prone ventilation or ECMO. iNO is administered at a dose of 5 up to 80 parts per million. **Inhaled epoprostenol** also may improve gas exchange and reduce pulmonary artery pressures as iNO does and is substantially less expensive, although there are less data for its use in ARDS compared with iNO. The dose ranges from 10 to 50 ng/kg/min.
2. **Corticosteroids:** After decades of controversies, recent trials on the use of dexamethasone in patients with ARDS and in ARDS due to COVID-19 showed it reduced duration of mechanical ventilation and overall mortality in patients with established moderate-to-severe ARDS. Steroids should be now considered in the treatment of ARDS.
3. β-Hydroxy β-methylglutaryl-CoA (HMG-CoA) reductase inhibitors should not be recommended because a multicenter double-blinded RCT showed no effect on mortality and increased side effects such as hepatic and renal dysfunction.

IX. BEDSIDE IMAGING AND MONITORING

Patients with ARDS require closer imaging and monitoring.

A. Chest X-ray (CXR): It classically shows diffuse, bilateral opacities and has been part of the ARDS diagnosis since the first description of the syndrome. The image is two-dimensional, and it has a poor interobserver agreement; however, at the bedside, it can be used to investigate deterioration of a patient's clinical status as well as the impact of changes in ventilatory settings. Besides, CXR can monitor tube and line positions.

B. Lung Ultrasound: It is considered superior to chest auscultation and x-ray in assessing patients with ARDS; it helps in identifying the origin of the lung edema (ie, whether cardiogenic or inflammatory). The exam can be repeated as many times as necessary, being very helpful in tracking the effect of lung recruitment maneuvers (reaeration of previous collapsed regions) and their potential complication (pneumothorax). It is operator dependent, and therefore the application of standardized protocols can reduce misdiagnoses.

C. Electrical Impedance Tomography (EIT): It is a bedside tool that provides real-time lung imaging. The image is acquired by electrodes placed around the chest. A pair of electrodes inject an alternating current and the remaining electrodes read the difference in voltage (Figure 20.1). Biological tissues can conduct electricity and they can be good or poor conductors; this difference in resistivity allows image reconstruction of distribution of ventilation and

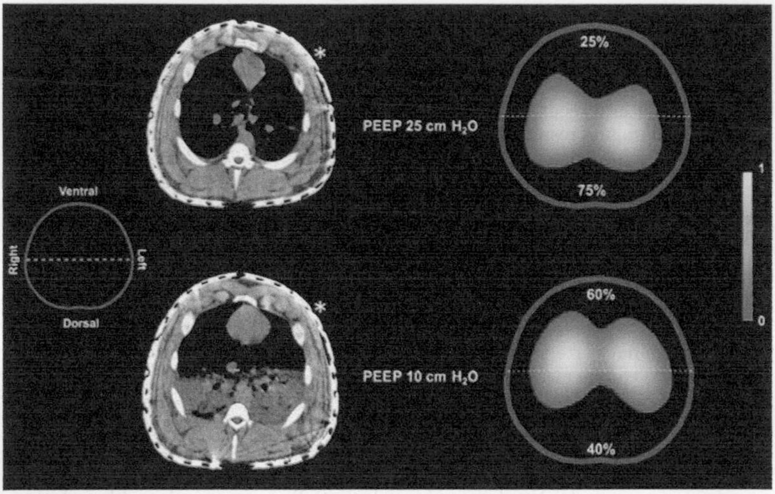

FIGURE 20.1 Electrical impedance tomography (EIT). Simultaneous image acquisition, computed tomography (CT), and EIT, in an experimental model of acute respiratory distress syndrome (ARDS) at positive end-expiratory pressure (PEEP) of 25 and 10 cm H_2O. EIT functional image shows regional changes in ventilation distribution (%) between ventral and dorsal regions of the lungs after the impact of ventilatory settings in the lung parenchyma detected by the CT. *Of note, the EIT electrodes (in this example, 32 electrodes) were connected to the chest during the CT acquisition.

pulmonary blood flow. In addition, it estimates regional collapse and overdistension. The anatomic resolution of the EIT is limited.

D. **Esophageal Manometry:** An air-filled balloon, placed in the distal third segment of the esophagus, is used to measure esophageal pressure, a surrogate for pleural pressure. A reliable measurement depends on adequate esophageal balloon placement and inflation. The proper filling volume needs to be checked before utilization. An underfilled balloon underestimates pleural pressure, whereas if the balloon is overfilled, the esophagus elastance will interfere with the measurement. The esophageal manometry can partition the respiratory system mechanics into lungs and chest wall components. Transpulmonary pressure (airway pressure minus pleural pressure) is calculated with esophageal manometry during inspiratory and expiratory holds. Transpulmonary pressure, by definition, is the pressure across the lungs, and it is a valuable information for lung-protective ventilation in patients with severe ARDS. In addition, the effect of body position (supine vs prone position) on the chest wall shape can be monitored by esophageal manometry.

E. **Computed Tomography:** The image is tridimensional and plays a fundamental role in ARDS, from the identification of anatomic structures, differential diagnosis, and disease severity to determination of responsiveness to ventilatory adjustments (tidal volume, PEEP, lung recruitment maneuvers, and prone ventilation). A CT can influence medical decisions in more than 20% of the cases. The current limitations are the transportation of patients who are critically ill to the dedicated room and exposure to radiation.

F. **Positron Emission Tomography (PET):** It utilizes radioactive isotopes as markers of lung regular function or injury. The type of tracer will depend on what is being investigated and its biological pathway. For instance, inhaled nitrogen $[^{13}N]$-N_2 traces lung volumes and response to recruitment, whereas the neutrophil's activity can be tracked with $[^{18}F]$-fluoro-2-deoxy-D-glucose as a marker.

Selected Readings

Ackermann M, Verleden SE, Kuehnel M, et al. Pulmonary vascular endothelialitis, thrombosis, and angiogenesis in Covid-19. *N Engl J Med.* 2020;383(2):120-128.

Amato MB, Meade MO, Slutsky AS, et al. Driving pressure and survival in the acute respiratory distress syndrome. *N Engl J Med.* 2015;372(8):747-755.

ARDS Definition Task Force; Ranieri VM, Rubenfeld GD, Thompson BT, et al. Acute respiratory distress syndrome: the Berlin Definition. *JAMA.* 2012;307(23):2526-2533.

Bachmann MC, Morais C, Bugedo G, et al. Electrical impedance tomography in acute respiratory distress syndrome. *Crit Care.* 2018;22(1):263.

Bellani G, Messa C, Guerra L, et al. Lungs of patients with acute respiratory distress syndrome show diffuse inflammation in normally aerated regions: a [18F]-fluoro-2-deoxy-D-glucose PET/CT study. *Crit Care Med.* 2009;37(7):2216-2222.

Binnie A, Tsang JL, dos Santos CC. Biomarkers in acute respiratory distress syndrome. *Curr Opin Crit Care.* 2014;20(1):47-55.

Calfee CS, Delucchi K, Parsons PE, et al. Subphenotypes in acute respiratory distress syndrome: latent class analysis of data from two randomised controlled trials. *Lancet Respir Med.* 2014;2(8):611-620.

Cereda M, Xin Y, Goffi A, et al. Imaging the injured lung: mechanisms of action and clinical use [published correction appears in *Anesthesiology.* 2019 Aug;131(2):451]. *Anesthesiology.* 2019;131(3):716-749.

COVID-ICU Group on behalf of the REVA Network and the COVID-ICU Investigators. Clinical characteristics and day-90 outcomes of 4244 critically ill adults with COVID-19: a prospective cohort study. *Intensive Care Med.* 2021;47(1):60-73.

Gattinoni L, Caironi P, Cressoni M, et al. Lung recruitment in patients with the acute respiratory distress syndrome. *N Engl J Med.* 2006;354(17):1775-1786.

Gattinoni L, Pelosi P, Suter PM, et al. Acute respiratory distress syndrome caused by pulmonary and extrapulmonary disease. Different syndromes? *Am J Respir Crit Care Med.* 1998;158(1):3-11.

Gimenez G, Guerin C. Alveolar recruitment assessed by positron emission tomography during experimental acute lung injury. *Intensive Care Med.* 2006;32(11):1889-1894.

Guérin C, Reignier J, Richard JC, et al. Prone positioning in severe acute respiratory distress syndrome. *N Engl J Med.* 2013;368(23):2159-2168.

Li G, Malinchoc M, Cartin-Ceba R, et al. Eight-year trend of acute respiratory distress syndrome: a population-based study in Olmsted County, Minnesota. *Am J Respir Crit Care Med.* 2011;183(1):59-66.

Matthay MA, Ware LB, Zimmerman GA. The acute respiratory distress syndrome. *J Clin Invest.* 2012;122(8):2731-2740.

National Heart, Lung, and Blood Institute Acute Respiratory Distress Syndrome (ARDS) Clinical Trials Network; Rice TW, Wheeler AP, Thompson BT, et al. Initial trophic vs full enteral feeding in patients with acute lung injury: the EDEN randomized trial. *JAMA.* 2012;307(8):795-803.

National Heart, Lung, and Blood Institute Acute Respiratory Distress Syndrome (ARDS) Clinical Trials Network; Wiedemann HP, Wheeler AP, Bernard GR, et al. Comparison of two fluid-management strategies in acute lung injury. *N Engl J Med.* 2006;354(24):2564-2575.

National Heart, Lung, and Blood Institute ARDS Clinical Trials Network; Truwit JD, Bernard GR, Steingrub J, et al. Rosuvastatin for sepsis-associated acute respiratory distress syndrome. *N Engl J Med.* 2014;370(23):2191-2200.

Nuckton TJ, Alonso JA, Kallet RH, et al. Pulmonary dead-space fraction as a risk factor for death in the acute respiratory distress syndrome. *N Engl J Med.* 2002;346(17):1281-1286.

Papazian L, Forel JM, Gacouin A, et al. Neuromuscular blockers in early acute respiratory distress syndrome. *N Engl J Med.* 2010;363(12):1107-1116.

Ranjeva S, Pinciroli R, Hodell E, et al. Identifying clinical and biochemical phenotypes in acute respiratory distress syndrome secondary to coronavirus disease-2019. *EClinicalMedicine.* 2021;34:100829.

Reynolds AS, Lee AG, Renz J, et al. Pulmonary vascular dilatation detected by automated transcranial Doppler in COVID-19 pneumonia. *Am J Respir Crit Care Med.* 2020;202(7):1037-1039.

Talmor D, Sarge T, Malhotra A, et al. Mechanical ventilation guided by esophageal pressure in acute lung injury. *N Engl J Med.* 2008;359(20):2095-2104.

Thille AW, Esteban A, Fernández-Segoviano P, et al. Comparison of the Berlin definition for acute respiratory distress syndrome with autopsy. *Am J Respir Crit Care Med.* 2013;187(7):761-767.

Thille AW, Richard JC, Maggiore SM, et al. Alveolar recruitment in pulmonary and extrapulmonary acute respiratory distress syndrome: comparison using pressure-volume curve or static compliance. *Anesthesiology.* 2007;106(2):212-217.

21

Asthma and Chronic Obstructive Pulmonary Disease

Lauren E. Gibson and Lorenzo Berra

I. INTRODUCTION

Asthma and chronic obstructive pulmonary disease (COPD) are common clinical conditions that are characterized by airflow obstruction measured with spirometry. Obstruction is usually defined by a forced expiratory volume in 1 second (FEV_1) to forced vital capacity (FVC) ratio of less than 0.7 or the lower limit of normal based on a 95% confidence interval in population-based studies of healthy subjects of similar sex, height, age, and race. Asthma and COPD can lead to respiratory failure and intensive care unit (ICU) admission during acute exacerbations of these conditions or they can complicate the ICU care of a patient who is admitted for other reasons. Because the effect of each condition on lung physiology is very similar and they share many treatments, they are discussed together here.

II. DEFINITIONS

A. COPD—Global Initiative for Chronic Obstructive Lung Disease Definition

The Global Initiative for Chronic Obstructive Lung Disease (GOLD) defines COPD as "a common preventable and treatable disease, characterized by persistent airflow limitation that is usually *progressive* and associated with an enhanced chronic inflammatory response in the airways and the lung to noxious particles or gases. Exacerbations and comorbidities contribute to the overall severity in individual patients."

B. Asthma—Global Initiative for Asthma Definition

The Global Initiative for Asthma (GINA) defines asthma as "a chronic inflammatory disorder of the airways in which many cells and cellular elements play a role. The chronic inflammation is associated with airway hyperresponsiveness that leads to recurrent episodes of wheezing, breathlessness, chest tightness, and coughing, particularly at night or in the early morning. These episodes are usually associated with widespread, but variable, airflow obstruction within the lung that is often *reversible* either spontaneously or with treatment."

C. Acute Severe Asthma

Acute severe asthma, formerly known as status asthmaticus, is defined as severe asthma unresponsive to repeated courses of β-agonist therapy such as inhaled albuterol, levalbuterol, or subcutaneous epinephrine. Acute severe asthma is not a distinct condition but rather the most severe manifestation of an asthma exacerbation along a continuous spectrum of severity. These patients often require ventilatory assistance in addition to inhaled bronchodilators and intravenous (IV) corticosteroids. Treatments for acute severe asthma and all asthma exacerbations in general are discussed together because they are essentially the same, except that more treatments are added as the patient's condition worsens.

III. EPIDEMIOLOGY

A. Chronic Obstructive Pulmonary Disease

1. Recent epidemiologic studies report a prevalence of COPD in developed countries of 8% to 10% in adults older than 40 years, with 1.4% having severe COPD. Although the prevalence of COPD has been stable in the United

States in recent years, it is increasing in women and decreasing in men, as is mortality attributable to COPD.

2. Acute COPD exacerbations account for approximately 2.5 hospitalizations per 10 000 people per year and have an in-hospital mortality of approximately 5%. Currently, COPD is the sixth leading cause of death in the United States, where it affects more than 15 million people.

3. A recent large study reported that approximately 9% of patients admitted to the ICU have a diagnosis of COPD and roughly one-third of them, corresponding to 2.5% of all admissions, are due to acute respiratory failure from COPD exacerbation.

4. COPD is an independent risk factor for ICU mortality even when it is a comorbid condition rather than the primary cause for admission.

B. Asthma

a. Asthma affects more than 25 million people in the United States and accounts for approximately 1.25 million hospitalizations per year, corresponding to an annual hospitalization rate of 13.5 per 10 000 individuals.

b. About 10% of asthma hospitalizations result in admission to the ICU and approximately 2% require endotracheal intubation.

c. Both ICU admission and intubation, as well as the presence of comorbidities, increase the odds of in-hospital death. In-hospital asthma mortality is approximately 0.5%.

IV. PHYSIOLOGY

A. Airway Inflammation

Although both asthma and COPD are characterized by airway inflammation, there are important differences in the cause of the inflammation and the inflammatory cell composition in each condition. Asthma is most commonly caused by an allergic reaction to one or more airborne environmental allergens, whereas COPD is the result of chronic inhalation of noxious particles or gases including smoke. The airway inflammation in asthma is dominated by eosinophils, whereas the inflammation in COPD is largely composed of neutrophils. In fact, in atopic asthma, uptake of [^{18}F] fluorodeoxyglucose measured with positron emission tomography in inflamed lung regions, an index of inflammatory cell activation, correlates with eosinophil counts from those regions. In contrast, in COPD, pulmonary [^{18}F] fluorodeoxyglucose uptake is related to neutrophil infiltration. Although both can have airway inflammation, edema, and constriction, COPD very often results in structural changes including enlargement of the airspaces distal to the terminal bronchioles, termed *emphysema*. Thus, for COPD, there has historically been a distinction made between those patients who have primarily upper airway disease from those who have primarily emphysema, although there is great overlap between the two phenotypes. In fact, it is accepted that there are likely many different phenotypes, both in asthma and COPD, and recognition of these phenotypes may lead to important treatment decisions.

B. Phenotypes

There is a growing appreciation that patients with asthma and COPD are very heterogeneous and likely have multiple causes for their intermittent airway obstruction. In asthma, at least five clinical phenotypes have been identified: (i) early-onset allergic, (ii) late-onset eosinophilic, (iii) exercise induced, (iv) obesity related, and (v) neutrophilic. COPD also represents a heterogeneous syndrome with chronic bronchitis and emphysema being recognized early on as distinct phenotypes. *Chronic bronchitis* has classically been associated with cough, obesity, hypoxemia, and hypoventilation, whereas emphysema has been associated with muscle wasting and hyperinflation but preserved gas exchange. COPD can be further characterized by the degree, type, and distribution of emphysematous changes, as well as by nonspirometric physiologic parameters, such as diffusing capacity and hyperinflation. As with asthma, classification schemes of COPD phenotypes based on the frequency of exacerbations, radiologic parameters, and inflammatory biomarkers are being developed. There has also been a more recently identified phenotype termed *asthma-COPD overlap*, or ACO. ACO is characterized by persistent airflow obstruction, a history of asthma or atopy, and evidence of partial bronchodilator reversibility. These patients are prone to frequent exacerbations and lung function decline.

C. Airflow Obstruction

1. The pathophysiologic hallmark of both asthma and COPD is airway narrowing with ensuing increase in respiratory resistance and wheezing.
2. In asthma, airway narrowing is due predominantly to contraction of smooth muscle cells in the airway wall, edema, and mucus plugging. Consequently, airway narrowing is present during both inspiration and expiration. The narrowed airways impair expiratory airflow resulting in *dynamic hyperinflation*, which is an increase in end-expiratory lung volume above functional residual capacity due to lack of equilibration between alveolar pressure and pressure at the airway opening. In fact, bronchoconstriction can be so severe that the airways completely occlude, trapping gas behind them. Interestingly, the size of these gas-trapping areas, termed *ventilation defects*, appears to be less in the prone than in the supine position, suggesting a rationale for the use of prone positioning to treat patients with acute severe asthma.
3. In COPD with emphysema, airway narrowing is due predominantly to intrapulmonary airway collapse during expiration. Because of the destruction of lung tissue, there is a reduction in the tethering forces exerted by the parenchymal septae on the intrapulmonary airway wall. Consequently, during expiration, when the transmural pressure in these airways becomes negative (ie, when the intraluminal airway pressure becomes lower than the surrounding extraluminal airway pressure), the airways collapse and interrupt flow. As flow is interrupted, upstream pressure rises and the airways reopen. As flow restarts, the transmural pressure becomes negative and flow again stops. This "flutter" pattern is responsible for the observed expiratory airflow limitation.
4. *Expiratory airflow limitation* is defined as a state in which expiratory flow is independent of transpulmonary pressure and hence is maximal. In the presence of flow limitation, an increase in upstream pressure, such as by activation of expiratory muscles, will *not* result in a higher expiratory flow. The point in the airway tree in which the transmural airway pressure turns negative is called *equal pressure point*. If this point localizes within the collapsible intrapulmonary airway, it will become a "choke point" that impedes further increases in expiratory flow. In this situation, a negative pressure applied at the opening of the airway during expiration will be ineffective in increasing airflow.
5. Similarly, if pressure at the airway opening is raised, flow will not decrease until the applied pressure is sufficiently high to overcome flutter at the choke point, that is, to render transmural pressure positive along the entire collapsible airway. Levels of applied pressure higher than this critical threshold will decrease expiratory flow, causing further hyperinflation.
6. Consequently, in the presence of expiratory flow limitation, flow is maximal because neither an increase in upstream pressure nor a decrease in downstream pressure will result in higher flows, and an increase in downstream pressure will either not affect flow ("waterfall" effect) or decrease flow if the increase is sufficiently high to overcome the critical threshold.

In the presence of flow limitation, expiratory flow is thus independent of the pressure gradient along the airway and depends only on lung volume, being higher at higher volumes. However, although it is maximal, the absolute flow is quite minuscule, and prolonged expiratory times would be needed to reach functional residual capacity.

D. Risk Factors for Death in the Intensive Care Unit

For patients admitted to the ICU with respiratory failure from an asthma or a COPD exacerbation, the major risk factors for death are need for mechanical ventilation, hyperinflation and auto-PEEP causing hypotension (from decreased venous return), profound acidemia, and barotrauma.

V. ASSESSMENT

A. History

1. A history of poorly controlled asthma as evidenced by nocturnal awakening for asthma symptoms, increased dyspnea and wheezing, increased β-agonist use, increased peak flow variability (>20%), recent or frequent emergency room visits or hospitalizations, a previous history of intubation and mechanical ventilation, and glucocorticoid nonadherence are risk factors for fatal asthma. Active smoking is also a high-risk feature among patients with asthma. Patients with nonallergic asthma, asthma triggered by aspirin, exercise-induced asthma, or patients with asthma who use cocaine or heroin also have a higher risk of mortality, and these factors should be assessed. A history of rapid improvement with intubation can often be a clue to an upper airway cause of respiratory failure, and in particular a condition termed *paroxysmal vocal cord motion*. Patients with paradoxical vocal cord motion often have mild asthma and a history of frequent severe attacks, many times with intubation followed by rapid extubation.
2. For patients with COPD, risk factors for mortality include multiple admissions for exacerbations, intubation and mechanical ventilation, age (both younger and older age groups), lower body mass index (BMI), history of lung cancer, and cardiovascular comorbidity. It is important to establish the baseline arterial $PaCO_2$ (or try to infer it from the patient's baseline bicarbonate level) of a patient with COPD. This serves two purposes—a warning that the patient may be particularly susceptible to the hypercarbic effects of supplemental oxygen (discussed subsequently) and as a target for setting minute ventilation should mechanical ventilation become necessary.

B. Physical Examination

1. Appearance

Patients with severe exacerbations of asthma or COPD are often unable to lie down, so they are often sitting upright or leaning forward slightly. An inability to speak in full sentences can often indicate impending respiratory failure. As with any patient with respiratory failure, it is important to note the patient's color to assess perfusion and oxygenation. A patient with respiratory failure without a previous diagnosis of COPD is likely to have a maximum laryngeal height (the distance from the sternal notch to the thyroid cartilage) of less than 4 cm at end exhalation. This is caused by hyperinflation of the lungs, which pulls the trachea downward.

2. Assess for intubation difficulty

a. Although neither COPD nor asthma per se has been associated with an increased incidence of difficult intubation, the association of obesity with asthma and early COPD can make the intubation of these patients more challenging than in the general population. In contrast, patients with moderate to severe COPD (GOLD stages 3 and 4) have a lower BMI.

b. Irrespective of body mass, a thorough assessment of the airway including Mallampati class, thyromental distance, receding mandible, and protruding upper incisors should be performed in all patients admitted to the ICU even if they do not yet require mechanical ventilation. These patients are at high risk for rapid deterioration and may require emergent intubation.

3. Auscultation

Wheezing may be audible even without a stethoscope and should be expiratory and polyphonic, indicating that it is coming from multiple small airways. A monophonic wheeze might indicate a single large airway obstruction. Stridor indicates obstruction that is extrathoracic, usually at the vocal cords or above. In patients with COPD and asthma who appear to be in respiratory distress, lack of wheezing or vesicular (normal) breath sounds can be a sign of impending respiratory arrest because ventilation becomes so poor that there is very little air movement with each breath. In patients with COPD, it may be difficult to hear breath sounds normally because they may have very little lung tissue left through which to transmit airway sounds.

4. Accessory muscle use

Patients with exacerbations of asthma and COPD are often anxious, sitting upright with arms extended, supporting the upper chest. This position allows the abdominal contents to pull the diaphragm downward and expand the lungs. It also allows the rib cage to be expanded and the accessory muscles of the neck and shoulders to pull upward on the rib cage when inhaling. Accessory muscle use and retraction of the rib cage or of the intercostal muscles is an ominous sign and indicates increased mechanical work to ventilate. Even more ominous is "abdominal paradox" where the usual abdominal protrusion during inhalation is reversed, such that the abdomen pulls inward during inspiration. This indicates that the diaphragm is either not functioning (due to paralysis or paresis) or the lungs are so hyperinflated that the diaphragm is at a mechanical disadvantage and can no longer pull the lungs downward. Once this happens, only the accessory muscles are able to lower intrathoracic pressure, drawing the abdominal contents inward toward the thorax. Hyperinflation of the lungs with a flattened diaphragm can also result in "Hoover sign," where the lower costal margin is drawn inward during the contraction of the diaphragm. Although often a sign of respiratory failure in COPD, it can also be seen in outpatients with severe underlying disease who are stable.

C. Laboratory

1. Arterial blood gas

a. Depending on the severity of disease, patients with COPD may present a chronic respiratory acidosis (ie, increased arterial $Paco_2$) that is partially offset by renal tubular excretion of hydrogen ions (H^+) and reabsorption of bicarbonate (HCO_3^-), resulting in a compensatory metabolic alkalosis. Carbon dioxide (CO_2) retention is a result of both hypoventilation due to airflow obstruction and ventilation-perfusion (V/Q) mismatch due to heterogeneous parenchymal involvement in COPD. To preserve the equilibrium of the Henderson-Hasselbalch equation, these patients will have a largely increased HCO_3^- concentration and base excess. A typical blood gas in this setting would be as follows: $Paco_2 = 60$ mm Hg, pH = 7.36, $HCO_3^- = 33$ mEq/L. Pao_2 and Sao_2 also depend on the severity of disease and whether the patient is on supplemental oxygen therapy, but are often moderately decreased ($Pao_2 = 60$-80 mm Hg and $Sao_2 = 90\%$-95%).

b. An acute on chronic exacerbation of COPD often results in further CO_2 retention and uncompensated respiratory acidosis, in addition to worsening hypoxemia. The presence of hypercapnia and acidosis despite markedly increased bicarbonate and a base excess is indicative of acute decompensation in a patient with COPD.

c. In patients with asthma, blood gases are usually normal at baseline, except in very advanced stages of disease when chronic features of obstructive disease appear. During an acute attack, however, PaO_2 may decrease below 60 mm Hg (SaO_2 <90%) and hypercapnia may also ensue. Importantly, because an asthma attack is accompanied by increased respiratory drive, a $PaCO_2$ that is only mildly elevated (eg, >42 mm Hg) could signify impending respiratory failure because for that level of drive the expected $PaCO_2$ in the absence of significant bronchoconstriction should be much lower.

2. Complete blood count

a. A complete blood count (CBC) is not usually required during asthma exacerbations but may be warranted in patients with a fever or purulent sputum. Even in the absence of superimposed bacterial infection, these patients may show neutrophilia due to the stress response and concomitant therapy (corticosteroids and β_2-agonists). Furthermore, asthma can cause eosinophilia, which is usually mild to moderate (500-1500 eosinophils/μL).

b. During an acute exacerbation of COPD, the patient may present with neutrophilia if the cause of the exacerbation is an acute bacterial infection. However, as for asthma, such leukocytosis could be simply the result of concurrent stress or therapy.

3. Theophylline level

A serum theophylline level should be checked in patients with acute exacerbations who have been on this medication, especially if symptoms of toxicity, such as nausea and vomiting, are present.

4. Electrocardiogram

The electrocardiogram (ECG) may show sinus tachycardia, right ventricular strain that may normalize with the relief of airflow obstruction, and right-axis deviation. Multifocal atrial tachycardia is associated with COPD and its appearance may portend a poor outcome. Calcium channel blockers and amiodarone can be used to treat supraventricular tachycardia. Nonselective β-blockers should be used with caution in patients with asthma because they can increase airway reactivity.

5. Peak Expiratory Flow

Peak expiratory flow (PEF) monitoring can be useful in the acute care setting, where spirometry and FEV_1 measurement are hardly feasible. PEF is usually reduced to 40% to 70% of predicted in moderate obstruction and to 25% to 39% in severe obstruction. PEF can also be useful to monitor response to therapy.

D. Imaging

1. The value of routine chest radiography in both asthma and COPD is controversial. The prevalence of abnormalities on plain chest films in asthma was found to be 9% in one study of patients with acute severe asthma who were admitted to the hospital. These were abnormalities that were felt to affect management and were not predicted on the basis of physical exam findings. In COPD, two studies found opposite results. One large study of 847 emergency room visits found abnormalities in 16% of patients and about 25% of those could not be predicted. A smaller study of 128 patients admitted for COPD exacerbations found that only in those with prespecified "complicated" presentations was management changed by the chest radiograph. In COPD and asthma, the main value of the chest radiograph may be to assess for changes that would alter the likelihood of pulmonary embolus (discussed subsequently), which is a major confounding diagnosis for these patients.

2. If pulmonary embolus is suspected, a protocolled computed tomography (CT) scan can be performed and may even replace plain chest radiography. Epidemiologic studies have shown that the presence of a diagnosis of asthma or COPD increases the risk of pulmonary embolus substantially. In fact, pulmonary embolism is diagnosed in up to 25% of patients who present with a COPD exacerbation. Given the high prevalence of COPD exacerbations, it is reasonable to obtain a pulmonary embolus protocol CT scan in these high-risk patients. For asthma, the need for CT scanning is less clear because there have been no studies evaluating the risk of pulmonary embolus in patients presenting with an asthma exacerbation.

VI. RESPIRATORY SUPPORT

A. Supplemental Oxygen

Supplemental oxygen should be administered to maintain Spo_2 greater than 88% in both asthma and COPD. Asthma rarely leads to severe hypoxemia unless it is associated with another pulmonary condition such as lobar pneumonia or there is significant hypoventilation and hypercarbia. For patients with COPD, the administration of supplemental oxygen can lead to excessive hypercarbia, a condition termed *hyperoxic hypercarbia*. In addition to the well-known decrease in minute ventilation that can occur because of the relief of the patient's hypoxic drive (or inducing sleep), it is thought that supplemental oxygen can cause hypercarbia by releasing CO_2 from hemoglobin (Haldane effect), increasing dead-space fraction by releasing hypoxic pulmonary vasoconstriction in poorly ventilated areas (thus worsening V/Q mismatch) and causing bronchodilation from a direct effect of CO_2 on the airway. When supplemental oxygen is given by face mask, these effects can be magnified because patients decrease their minute ventilation and entrain less air.

B. Helium/Oxygen Gas Mixtures (Heliox)

Helium is less dense than is nitrogen and has nearly the same viscosity; so, theoretically, a mixture of helium and oxygen should reduce turbulence in airways, thus allowing more gas for the same pressure gradient. In both asthma and COPD, helium-oxygen mixtures have been used with varying success. Studies have been inconclusive when using helium-oxygen delivered by face mask or by ventilator, and no definite conclusions can be made regarding its efficacy in either condition. Overall, the evidence appears weaker in COPD than in asthma, either for improving ventilation or when used to drive impact nebulizers. It should be noted that because of the differences in density of helium-oxygen mixtures versus nitrogen-oxygen mixtures, mechanical ventilator flow sensors need to be calibrated for helium-oxygen for proper functioning. A recent meta-analysis of 11 trials in adults and children of driving nebulizers with helium-oxygen mixtures appeared to show benefits in improvement of airflow limitation and hospital admission (number needed to treat to prevent one admission = 9) when given in the emergency room for acute asthma.

C. Noninvasive Positive Pressure Ventilation

1. Patients with COPD and asthma develop respiratory failure most often because of increased airway resistance and inefficient respiratory muscle mechanics from hyperinflation. Therefore, they cannot ventilate effectively. Noninvasive positive pressure ventilation (NPPV), delivered through a tight-fitting nasal or oronasal mask, has become an important tool for the prevention of intubation in many patients with respiratory failure. In

obstructive lung disease, NPPV would be expected to dilate airways with the use of positive expiratory pressure and assist the inspiratory muscles with the use of positive inspiratory pressure.

2. For exacerbations of COPD, the data clearly show efficacy for NPPV on mortality, need for intubation, treatment failure, and hospital stay. Studies have consistently shown that improvements in pH, $Paco_2$, and respiratory rate are seen within the first hour of use. The number needed to treat to save one life with NPPV is 4, and the complications of the therapy are low. The indications for use in COPD exacerbations usually consist of patients with increased respiratory rate and hypercapnic respiratory failure. Contraindications are few, but consist of vomiting, unconsciousness, and inability to fit a mask to the patient's face.

3. NPPV has been used in asthma, but the studies are often small and potentially subject to publication bias. In a recent Cochrane Review, the authors conclude that given the paucity of data, the use of NPPV is controversial in this setting. Mortality from exacerbations of asthma is much lower than from exacerbations of COPD, so very large studies would be required to see any possible effect on mortality. To date, NPPV has not shown definitive efficacy on other important end points such as intubation, ICU length of stay, or hospital stay.

D. Intubation

1. Timing

a. Compared with a few years ago, the availability of adjunct therapies such as helium-oxygen and NPPV has resulted in a postponement, on average, of the decision to intubate a patient with acute exacerbation of obstructive lung disease. Although adjunct therapies have spared patients from avoidable intubations, their increased use has also resulted in patients often having exhausted their respiratory reserve by the time the decision to intubate is taken.

b. Consequently, signs of impending respiratory failure such as intercostal retraction during inspiration, asynchronous movement of the abdomen and rib cage, use of accessory respiratory muscles (eg, sternocleidomastoid and scalene muscles), inability to speak, altered mental status, and worsening hypercapnia or hypoxemia should prompt the decision to intubate. Most studies of NPPV have determined that improvements in signs of respiratory failure should be seen within the first 2 hours of use, and if these are not seen, intubation should be performed without delay.

c. Although the specific intubation technique (eg, asleep direct or video laryngoscopy, awake or asleep fiberoptic intubation) is at the discretion of the individual provider, it is important to have an array of airway equipment readily available and a backup plan should the first intubation attempt fail. This is especially important given the low respiratory reserve of these patients.

2. Hypotension

a. After confirming intubation of the trachea with a CO_2 sensor, the provider should resist the instinct to aggressively ventilate these patients. The presence of dynamic hyperinflation and the consequent impediment to venous return, as well as the abolition of inspiratory efforts that favored venous return and the increase in pulmonary vascular resistance due to positive pressure ventilation in patients who may have underlying pulmonary hypertension can all contribute to systemic hypotension.

b. Vasopressors (eg, phenylephrine) and inotropic agents (eg, norepinephrine or epinephrine) should be readily available at the time of intubation to treat hypotension, as should IV fluids and proper IV access.

E. Bronchoscopy

For asthma, where increased mucus production is part of the pathophysiology of airway obstruction, it might seem that bronchoscopy would be a valuable tool, especially in patients on mechanical ventilation. In fact, there was initial enthusiasm for the use of bronchoscopy in asthma, but this was tempered by reports of bronchoscopy-induced bronchospasm in patients with asthma receiving bronchoscopy for reasons not necessarily related to their asthma. It was postulated that the severe bronchospasm was caused by mechanical stimulation of vagal afferents in the airway by the bronchoscope. A subsequent study found bronchospasm in only 1 of 10 patients with mild asthma undergoing bronchoscopy and no change in FEV_1 after the procedure in any of the subjects. These subjects were pretreated with aminophylline before the procedure, and all had a history of only mild asthma. Subsequently, there have been multiple case reports of successful bronchoscopic lavage, sometimes with acetylcysteine or deoxyribonuclease (DNAse), to improve lung function among patients with asthma who are intubated. Overall, it appears from a limited number of cases that bronchoscopy with lavage in patients with asthma on mechanical ventilation is well tolerated and can result in improvements in lung mechanics. However, data are too limited to make any definitive conclusions about the role of bronchoscopy in the routine care of patients in the ICU with an asthma exacerbation. For respiratory failure caused by COPD, there has not been any study showing benefit with the use of bronchoscopy as a therapeutic tool.

F. Mechanical Ventilation

Mechanical ventilation aims to decrease the patient's work of breathing and support gas exchange. Work of breathing is increased during acute exacerbation of asthma or COPD due to both increased resistive and elastic load. Airway narrowing increases resistive work, whereas air trapping and increased lung volumes increase elastic work. The latter occurs because expiratory flow obstruction and dynamic hyperinflation place the respiratory system on a less compliant part of its pressure-volume curve, thereby increasing the elastic component of the work of breathing. Ventilator management must balance the goal to achieve adequate oxygenation ($SpO_2 = 88\%-92\%$) and ventilation with avoidance of further hyperinflation and barotrauma.

1. Dynamic hyperinflation and auto–positive end-expiratory pressure

Because of the increase in airway resistance and, in COPD, also compliance, the time constant of the respiratory system (equal to the product of resistance and compliance) is increased in patients with obstructive lung disease, especially during acute exacerbations. Consequently, the expiratory time may not be sufficient to allow complete lung emptying, resulting in an increase in end-expiratory lung volume above functional residual capacity (or equilibrium volume if positive end-expiratory pressure [PEEP] is applied). This is known as *dynamic hyperinflation*. Accordingly, alveolar pressure is higher than is the pressure at the airway opening at the end of expiration and this increase is termed "auto" (or "intrinsic") PEEP. Note that although dynamic hyperinflation is always accompanied by auto-PEEP, auto-PEEP can also occur without hyperinflation or even at an end-expiratory volume lower than functional residual capacity in a subject who is actively exhaling. For example, patients with very low respiratory compliance and impending respiratory failure (eg, acute respiratory distress syndrome [ARDS]) may use the expiratory muscles to "push" the respiratory system below functional residual capacity at end exhalation, such that the first phase of the ensuing inspiration is passive because it is driven by the outer recoil of the respiratory system. This "work sharing" is a protective mechanism to partly unload the fatigued inspiratory muscles at the expense of the expiratory muscles.

a. Clinical assessment of auto–positive end-expiratory pressure

Signs of auto-PEEP include the following: (i) Inspiratory efforts by the patient that do not trigger the ventilator (patient-ventilator dyssynchrony) because auto-PEEP essentially acts as an additional pressure trigger; (ii) expiratory flow does not reach zero before the next inspiration. However, in the presence of flow limitation, end-expiratory flow can be minuscule despite significant auto-PEEP; or (iii) a biphasic expiratory flow pattern (sharp spike followed by almost a plateau at a very low flow rate) caused by rapid emptying of a small volume of gas from the large airways followed by a very slow emptying of distal alveoli.

b. Measurement of auto–positive end-expiratory pressure

1. **Controlled mechanical ventilation:** The easiest way to measure auto-PEEP in a patient whose muscles are relaxed is to perform an end-expiratory airway occlusion (Figure 21.1). The occlusion interrupts flow, allowing the pressure at the airway opening to equilibrate with alveolar pressure, so that what is being measured at the airway opening is the auto-PEEP. An occlusion lasting 3 to 5 seconds is usually sufficient to obtain a stable measurement of auto-PEEP. However, this method could underestimate the degree of auto-PEEP in patients with acute severe asthma because of complete closure of airways leading to lung units with the highest alveolar pressure. The alveolar pressure in these units would then not be transmitted to the proximal airway. This interpretation is consistent with the observation that the gas tracer delivered to alveoli through the bloodstream is retained in the alveolar airspace in acute asthma rather than being excreted by ventilatory efforts.
2. **Assisted breathing:** In a patient with spontaneous respiratory efforts, measurement of auto-PEEP requires esophageal manometry. Auto-PEEP corresponds to the deflection in esophageal pressure from the start of the patient's inspiratory effort to the start of inspiratory flow. In the absence of an esophageal balloon, a rough estimate of auto-PEEP can be obtained with an end-expiratory occlusion, provided the patient reaches a fairly relaxed state.

c. Strategies to reduce dynamic hyperinflation

Given that expiration is either passive or flow is not increased by activation of expiratory muscles in the presence of flow limitation, the only strategies to decrease dynamic hyperinflation at a given minute ventilation are (i) relief of bronchoconstriction (eg, β_2-agonists); (ii) reduction of the inspiratory-to-expiratory time ratio, with ensuing prolongation of expiratory time; and (iii) possibly, use of a helium-oxygen gas mixture.

2. Initial settings

a. The fundamental concept in the initiation of mechanical ventilation in patients with acute exacerbation of asthma or COPD is to avoid aggressive ventilation, which can further worsen dynamic hyperinflation and cause barotrauma or cardiovascular collapse. Reasonable initial settings for most patients are a tidal volume of 6 to 8 mL/kg predicted body weight and respiratory rate of 8 to 12 breaths/min with 25% inspiratory time (ie, inspiratory-to-expiratory ratio of 1:3).

b. If pressure-controlled ventilation is chosen, tidal volume should be closely monitored because it can decrease over time if airway resistance worsens and/or auto-PEEP increases. With volume-controlled ventilation, peak and plateau airway pressure should be closely monitored.

3. Setting positive end-expiratory pressure

There is no general agreement as to whether PEEP should be used in airflow obstruction. Part of this lack of consensus stems from the fact that whether PEEP has a beneficial or detrimental effect on respiratory mechanics in this setting depends on the underlying mechanism of auto-PEEP.

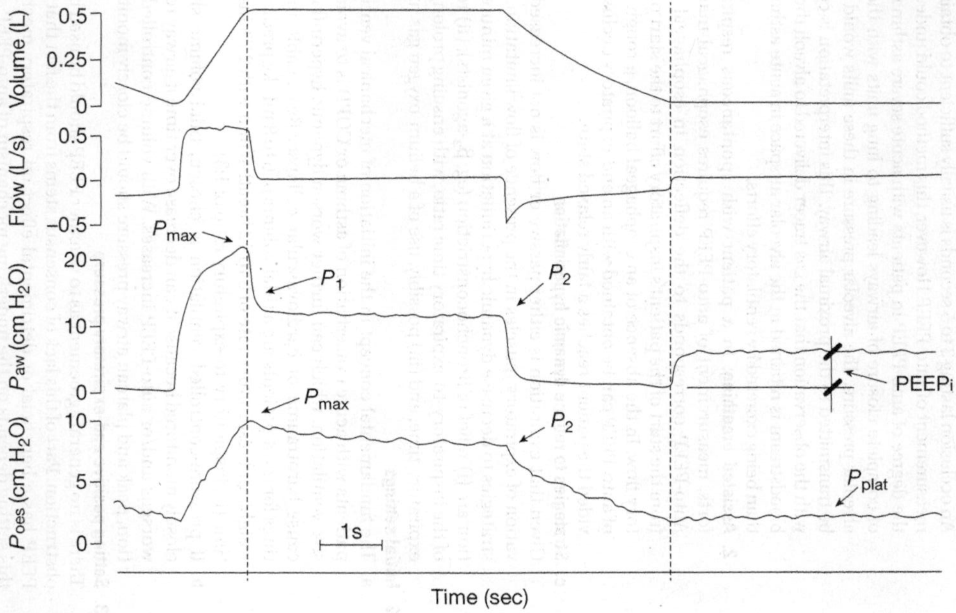

FIGURE 21.1 Tracings of volume (obtained by integration of the flow signal), flow, airway pressure (P_{aw}), and esophageal pressure (P_{oes}) in a representative patient with chronic obstructive pulmonary disease (COPD) during an end-inspiratory occlusion followed by an end-expiratory occlusion. Dashed lines indicate timing of occlusions. P_{max}, maximum value; *P*1, zero flow value; *P*2, plateau value; PEEPi, intrinsic positive end-expiratory pressure is the static end-expiratory recoil pressure of the respiratory system; P_{plat}, plateau value of P_{oes} after end-expiratory occlusion. Values of P_{aw}, P_{max}, used for calculations were corrected for the resistive pressure drop due to the artificial airway. (Reproduced with permission of the © ERS 2022: Musch G, Foti G, Cereda M, Pelosi P, Poppi D, Pesenti A. Lung and chest wall mechanics in normal anaesthetized subjects and in patients with COPD at different PEEP levels. *Eur Respir J.* 1997;10(11):2545-2552.)

a. Auto–positive end-expiratory pressure with airflow limitation

When the underlying pathophysiologic mechanism for auto-PEEP is expiratory flow limitation, PEEP will not impair expiratory flow until the critical pressure at the "choke point" is reached. This pressure has been reported to range from 70% to 85% of auto-PEEP. Consequently, setting PEEP up to 70% of auto-PEEP measured at zero end-expiratory pressure will not cause substantial further hyperinflation and will instead decrease the work of breathing in a patient who is spontaneously breathing and decrease the pressure that the inspiratory muscles must generate to trigger the ventilator. In a patient on controlled, rather than assisted, ventilation, applying PEEP up to 70% of auto-PEEP may still be beneficial because it favors a more uniform distribution of tidal volume. In fact, the value of auto-PEEP measured with an end-expiratory pause is the average of many different values of individual respiratory units. When inspiration starts from zero end-expiratory pressure, units with the lowest auto-PEEP receive proportionally more tidal volume than those with the highest auto-PEEP, which start to inflate only later during inhalation. In this setting, PEEP acts as an "equalizer" of auto-PEEP within individual lung units, promoting more uniform distribution of ventilation and improved (V/Q) matching.

b. Auto–positive end-expiratory pressure without airflow limitation

If, instead, auto-PEEP is due to airflow obstruction without flow limitation (ie, there is no "flutter"/"waterfall" mechanism), then extrinsic PEEP will be transmitted all the way up to the alveoli and will result in further hyperinflation, increased (elastic) work of breathing, and hypotension.

c. Detecting the presence of airflow limitation

From the earlier discussion, it follows that the clinician must determine whether the patient is flow limited to decide whether and how much PEEP to apply. The classical method of obtaining isovolume pressure-flow curves by changing pressure at the airway opening while measuring flow at a given absolute lung volume has been applied in patients with COPD on mechanical ventilation. Signs indicative of expiratory flow limitation include the following: (i) a biphasic expiratory flow-volume curve showing a sharp peak expiratory flow that falls abruptly to a much lower flow (Figure 21.2), which then decreases linearly with exhaled volume at a very slow rate; (ii) the value of end-expiratory flow does not decrease substantially when expiratory time is prolonged, that is, even with very long expiratory times it is hard to reach zero flow; (iii) if PEEP is applied stepwise, inspiratory plateau pressure will not increase until the critical pressure threshold is achieved. This test can also be used to set PEEP at the highest value that will not cause a significant increase in plateau pressure when an end-expiratory hold button is not available; (iv) if an end-expiratory hold can be performed with the ventilator, stepwise application of PEEP will result in a decrease of auto-PEEP of similar magnitude to the increase in PEEP until flow limitation is reversed (usually 70%-85% of auto-PEEP at zero end-expiratory pressure).

4. Permissive hypercapnia

Permissive hypercapnia was originally conceived as a strategy for the ventilation of patients with acute severe asthma, in whom the goal was no longer to restore adequate alveolar ventilation and $PaCO_2$ but to limit airway pressures to avoid barotrauma (eg, pneumothorax) and cardiocirculatory failure. It is implemented by reduction of tidal volume to 4 to 6 mL/kg and reduction of respiratory rate with prolongation of expiratory time. $PaCO_2$ of 60 to 80 mm Hg and pH as low as 7.15 are considered acceptable in the

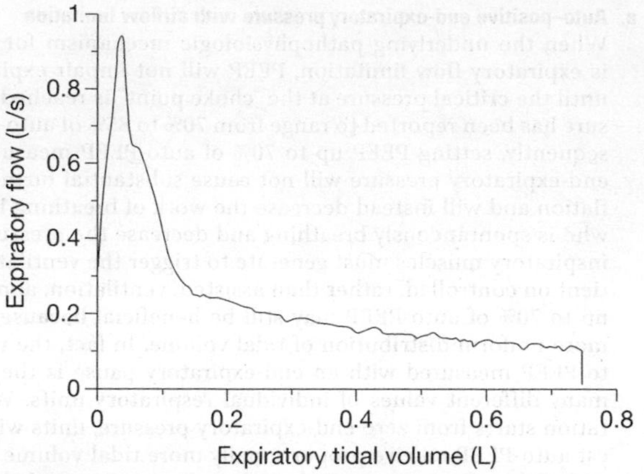

FIGURE 21.2 Expiratory flow volume curve during passive exhalation at zero end-expiratory pressure in a patient with chronic obstructive pulmonary disease. Notice the bowing toward the volume axis (ie, upward concavity) especially during the first part of exhalation, which suggests the presence of flow limitation. (Reproduced with permission of the © ERS 2022: Musch G, Foti G, Cereda M, Pelosi P, Poppi D, Pesenti A. Lung and chest wall mechanics in normal anaesthetized subjects and in patients with COPD at different PEEP levels. *Eur Respir J.* 1997;10(11):2545-2552.)

absence of contraindications such as intracranial hypertension. The main side effects of this strategy are as follows:

a. Need for deep sedation and, possibly, neuromuscular blockade to prevent patient-ventilator dyssynchrony. Propofol is a commonly used sedative with bronchodilating properties. Atracurium is a neuromuscular blocker with predictable pharmacokinetics, a feature than can be helpful because neuromuscular blockers should be titrated carefully in these patients who are usually on high doses of corticosteroids and hence prone to myopathy. Sedatives and paralytics also reduce CO_2 production and hence dampen hypercapnia.

b. Increased intracranial pressure due to cerebral vasodilation. Consequently, permissive hypercapnia is contraindicated in patients with preexisting intracranial lesions. Subarachnoid hemorrhage has been reported after institution of permissive hypercapnia for acute severe asthma.

G. Extracorporeal membrane oxygenation and extracorporeal CO_2 removal

For patients with acute severe asthma and hypoxemia or hypercapnia that is refractory to other therapies, extracorporeal membrane oxygenation (ECMO) or extracorporeal CO_2 removal ($ECCO_2R$) has been used successfully to maintain gas exchange. More recently, extracorporeal techniques have been used to allow early extubation, ambulation, and weaning and to prevent intubation in patients failing NPPV or awaiting lung transplantation.

VII. PHARMACOLOGIC THERAPY

Common (and less common) medications used in asthma and COPD are listed in Table 21.1.

A. Bronchodilators

1. β_2-Agonists

a. Inhaled β_2-agonists are the primary treatment for acute asthma, and in patients who are not intubated, they can be given via metered-dose inhaler (MDI) or nebulizer. Studies have shown equivalence for the use of MDI with a valved holding chamber or nebulizer, provided that patients

TABLE 21.1 Medications Used in Asthma or Chronic Obstructive Pulmonary Disease

Drug	Dose	Interval
Albuterol MDI	108 μg, 2 inhalations	q4-6h
	4 inhalations	q10min for acute severe asthma
Albuterol nebulized	2.5 mg or 5 mg	q4-6h
		q20min or continuous for acute severe asthma
Levalbuterol MDI	45 μg, 2 inhalations	q4-6h
Levalbuterol nebulized	1.25 mg	q20min
Formoterol	12 μg, 2 inhalations	q12h
Arformoterol	15 μg in 2 mL	q12h
Salmeterol	50 μg, 1 inhalation	q12h
Olodaterol	2.5 μg, 2 inhalations	q24h
Indacaterol	75 μg, 1 inhalation	q24h
Ipratropium	MDI 21 μg, 2 inhalations	q4-6h
Ipratropium nebulized	2.5 mL (500 μg)	q6-8h
Aclidinium	400 μg, 1 inhalation	q12h
Tiotropium	18 μg, 1 inhalation	q24h
Albuterol/ipratropium MDI	120 μg albuterol/21 μg ipratropium	q6h
Albuterol/ipratropium nebulized	3 mg albuterol/0.5 mg ipratropium in 3 mL	q4h
Umeclidinium/vilanterol	62.5/25 μg, 1 inhalation	q24h
Theophylline	300-600 mg	q12h
Aminophylline	380-760 mg	q6-8h
Terbutaline	0.25-0.5 mg sc	q15-30min
Epinephrine	0.1-0.5 mg sc	q3-4h
	0.25-2 μg/min IV	Continuous
Beclomethasone	40 or 80 μg, 1-4 inhalations	q12h
Fluticasone	44, 110, 220 μg, 2 inhalations	q12h
Mometasone	220 μg, 1-2 inhalations	q12h
Flunisolide	80 μg, 2-4 inhalations	q12h
Ciclesonide	80 or 160 μg, 1 inhalation	q12h
Budesonide	90 or 180 μg, 1-4 inhalations	q12h
Budesonide nebulized	0.25-1 mg/2 mL	q12h
Salmeterol/fluticasone	100-500/50 μg, 1 inhalation	q12h
Fluticasone/vilanterol	100/25 μg, 1 inhalation	q24h
Mometasone/formoterol	100-200/5 μg, 2 inhalations	q12h
Prednisone	40-60 mg (1 mg/kg)	qd
Methylprednisolone	Up to 125 mg IV	X1, then lower doses q6h
Magnesium sulfate	Pediatric 25-75 mg/kg IV	
	Adult 2 mg IV over 20 min	
Ketamine	bolus dosing 0.5 mg/kg	q20min

IV, intravenous; MDI, metered-dose inhaler.

are able to use the MDI correctly. One Cochrane Review of seven studies found that for nebulized albuterol or salbutamol, continuous nebulization provided greater improvement in PEF and FEV_1 and reduced hospitalization in patients with more severe acute asthma. For patients who are mechanically ventilated, either MDIs or aerosol provided by vibrating mesh nebulizer are efficacious. Levalbuterol, the R-enantiomer of albuterol that is responsible for bronchodilation, has been shown to be effective at half the dose of albuterol, but randomized trials comparing this with racemic albuterol have been mixed.

b. It has been noted that patients with acute asthma often have very elevated lactate levels. The origin of this lactate has been the source of debate, with respiratory muscles and altered metabolism from β_2-agonist therapy being some of the suggested sources. The elevated lactate can be so severe as to cause significant acidemia and prompt an investigation for sources of infection. In a recent study of 175 patients with acute asthma, plasma albuterol was significantly correlated with serum lactate concentration after adjusting for asthma severity. Elevated lactate was not associated with worse FEV_1, increased hospitalization, or relapse at 1 week. These data suggest that the elevated lactate is from treatment with β_2-agonists, but that it has no effect on outcome. Elevated lactate has been reported with other drugs with β_2-agonist activity, such as terbutaline and epinephrine.

c. Inhaled β_2-agonist therapy is also used for acute management of COPD because of its rapid onset of action. As with asthma, MDIs or nebulized β_2-agonist therapy can be utilized, although nebulized therapy is often used in those patients who have difficulty with MDI technique. MDIs or nebulized β_2-agonist via vibrating mesh nebulizer can be used in patients on mechanical ventilation.

2. β_1-Antagonists

a. Many patients with asthma and COPD are either taking or may require β_1-antagonist therapy for heart conditions or for other conditions such as variceal bleeding prevention. In asthma, it has been known for a long time that nonselective β-blockers such as propranolol can precipitate asthma exacerbations, particularly at high doses and some, such as pindolol, can increase airway resistance in small airways. For selective β_1-antagonists, two meta-analyses have demonstrated that most patients have only a modest reduction in FEV_1 (mean drop of 7.5% predicted), but that approximately one in eight could have an acute drop of more than 20% in the absolute FEV_1. Interestingly, however, chronic, regular use of even nonselective β-blockers such as propranolol or nadolol may actually not change FEV_1 appreciably or even improve bronchodilator response to albuterol. Therefore, for acute asthma exacerbations, and certainly for acute severe asthma, the introduction of selective or nonselective β_1-antagonists should be avoided, if possible, but if patients with asthma are on β_1-antagonists chronically, it is not necessary to stop them. Obviously, in some situations (acute myocardial infarction), the benefits of selective β_1-antagonist therapy may outweigh the risks.

b. For COPD, the beneficial effects of cardioselective β_1-antagonists greatly outweigh the risks of worsening lung function. The acute effects of cardioselective β_1-antagonists such as esmolol seem less or nonexistent in COPD compared with those in asthma, but noncardioselective β_1-antagonists such as propranolol have been shown to adversely affect lung function in either condition.

3. Ipratropium bromide

Inhaled ipratropium has a slower onset of action compared with albuterol and therefore is not as effective for acute asthma. However, it can be added to albuterol for a greater bronchodilator action. In patients with severe airflow obstruction, ipratropium and albuterol are superior to albuterol alone in terms of bronchodilation and rates of hospitalization. The results of combined albuterol and ipratropium therapy for acute exacerbations of COPD have been mixed, with some studies showing modest improvement and others showing no difference.

B. Methylxanthines

IV aminophylline has been used for years for exacerbations of asthma and COPD. It is a weak bronchodilator that has been largely replaced by more effective β_2-agonists or ipratropium. Its major drawback is the narrow therapeutic window and risk of side effects such as nausea and vomiting, tachyarrhythmias, and seizures. A Cochrane Review from 2012 demonstrated no additional benefit in peak flow rate or hospital admission. For every 100 patients treated with aminophylline, 20 patients experienced vomiting and 15 experienced arrhythmias. For COPD, there is even less evidence for efficacy in acute exacerbations. Although oral theophylline may have benefits for reduction in exacerbations of COPD through anti-inflammatory effects, there is no evidence that either oral theophylline or IV aminophylline is useful for short-term treatment of exacerbations and, given the high frequency of side effects, its use cannot be recommended.

C. Corticosteroids

1. Treatment of exacerbations of COPD with systemic corticosteroids by the oral or parenteral route has been shown in multiple studies to reduce the likelihood of treatment failure and relapse at 1 month and shorten length of stay in hospital inpatients. There is no evidence for benefit of parenteral treatment over oral treatment when looking at treatment failure, relapse, or mortality. There is an increase in adverse drug effects with corticosteroid treatment, which is greater with parenteral administration compared with oral treatment. Although traditional treatment has been high-dose methylprednisolone (125 mg IV) followed by 60 mg every 6 hours for 3 days and then tapering over 2 weeks, recent data suggest that a short course starting with 40 mg of IV methylprednisolone followed by 5 days of oral prednisone has efficacy equivalent to 2 weeks of steroid therapy.
2. The data are very similar for asthma, with corticosteroids demonstrating improvements in meaningful outcomes and no difference in lower (≤80 mg methylprednisolone) versus higher doses of IV steroids or in oral versus IV route when given in equipotent doses.

D. Neuromuscular Blockade

With the use of permissive hypercapnia in patients with asthma on mechanical ventilation, neuromuscular blockade would seem particularly attractive in addition to deep sedation in the early treatment of status acute severe asthma. However, patients with asthma have been shown to be particularly prone to prolonged neuromuscular weakness when neuromuscular blockade has been used, even for periods as short as 12 hours. It is not entirely clear whether this weakness is the direct effect of neuromuscular blockade or another effect, such as the deep sedation that is often required to achieve low ventilatory goals. The effects of neuromuscular blockade and deep sedation in acute exacerbations of COPD are even less clear, although they might be expected to have even greater effects on prolonged weakness because COPD is often associated with lower BMI and skeletal muscle weakness as part of its systemic effects.

E. Antibiotics

1. The use of antibiotics in acute exacerbations of asthma or COPD in the ICU should be guided by the acuity of the illness and the symptoms and signs of infection. Acute exacerbations of COPD are thought to arise from direct bacterial or viral infection or the immune response to changes in respiratory flora. When antibiotics are chosen, consideration should be given to covering *Haemophilus influenzae* because this organism is often recovered from bronchial secretions of patients with COPD with acute exacerbations who do not have risk factors for hospital-acquired organisms. One small study of 93 patients with acute exacerbation of COPD who are intubated and have clear chest radiographs randomized to a fluoroquinolone versus placebo showed a remarkable clinical benefit to treating with

a fluoroquinolone, with a number needed to treat of 6 patients to save one life. The procalcitonin level at admission is a promising biomarker for deciding who can have antibiotics safely stopped and does not result in increased rates of hospital readmission over a 6-month follow-up period. Predictors of patients with COPD who may have infections with multidrug-resistant organisms are those with antibiotic exposure in the previous 2 weeks or intubation in the past 6 months.

2. For acute exacerbations of asthma, a randomized trial of telithromycin in patients who are hospitalized showed an improvement in symptoms but not in peak flow, and the symptom improvement was not related to the presence of *Chlamydophila pneumoniae* or *Mycoplasma pneumoniae*, two organisms that would be expected to be treated by a macrolide antibiotic. Similar to exacerbations of COPD, the use of procalcitonin for antibiotic management in patients with asthma who are hospitalized reduced the use of antibiotics significantly without any change in length of hospital stay or readmission over a 12-month follow-up period. Patients with asthma admitted to the ICU with respiratory failure should also be tested and treated for influenza because they are a high-risk group for respiratory failure, ARDS, and death from hemagglutinin type 1 and neuraminidase type 1 (H1N1) infection.

F. Mucolytics

Mucolytic therapy may be beneficial for patients with COPD or asthma with copious or retained secretions during acute exacerbations, but there are no data supporting their routine use.

G. Leukotriene-Receptor Antagonists

Leukotriene-receptor antagonists montelukast and zafirlukast are important controller medications for asthma but have not been shown to improve outcomes in the treatment of patients who are hospitalized. Although some case series have reported benefit with IV leukotriene antagonists, currently these medications are only available in oral form in the United States. The 5-lipoxygenase inhibitor zileuton has been tried in a randomized trial for treatment of COPD exacerbations. This trial did not find a difference in length of hospital stay in patients treated with zileuton.

H. Magnesium Sulfate ($MgSO_4$)

IV magnesium sulfate (2 g over 20 minutes), when given early in acute asthma, has been shown to prevent the need for mechanical ventilation in children and to improve spirometry and reduce hospitalizations in adults. In adults, the effect of magnesium seemed to be greatest in those with more severe airflow obstruction. Nebulized magnesium sulfate has also been used in combination with inhaled albuterol, but results have been mixed. Neither IV nor nebulized magnesium has been shown to be effective in acute exacerbations of COPD.

I. Ketamine

Ketamine has both adrenergic and anticholinergic activity through inhibition of vagal pathways, leading to bronchodilation. Despite numerous case reports and case series of improvement when used in acute severe asthma, in two randomized trials, one in children who are not intubated and another in adults who are intubated, ketamine did not prove superior to conventional therapy. Ketamine has not been studied for use in acute exacerbations of COPD.

J. Inhaled Anesthetics

1. Halogenated inhaled anesthetics have both direct bronchodilator properties, by modulating Ca_2^+-dependent contractile mechanisms in airway smooth muscle and indirect bronchodilatory effects by reversing muscarinic receptor–mediated bronchoconstriction.
2. Clinical and experimental evidence suggests that isoflurane and sevoflurane may improve respiratory mechanics in asthma.

3. Several case series have reported on the potential usefulness of halogenated anesthetics in the treatment of status asthmaticus both in adults and children, occasionally used in conjunction with ketamine.
4. Despite these anecdotal reports, one retrospective study has failed to associate improved outcome with the use of inhaled anesthetics in severe asthma. Consequently, in the absence of definitive data from clinical trials, the use of these agents should be reserved for the treatment of severe asthma attacks refractory to maximal conventional treatment.

Selected Readings

Bateman ED, Hurd SS, Barnes PJ, et al. Global strategy for asthma management and prevention: GINA executive summary. *Eur Respir J.* 2008;31:143-178.

Camargo CA, Spooner CH, Rowe BH. Continuous versus intermittent beta-agonists in the treatment of acute asthma. *Cochrane Database Syst Rev.* 2003;(4):CD001115.

Funk G-C, Bauer P, Burghuber OC, et al. Prevalence and prognosis of COPD in critically ill patients between 1998 and 2008. *Eur Respir J.* 2013;41:792-799.

Howton JC, Rose J, Duffy S, et al. Randomized, double-blind, placebo-controlled trial of intravenous ketamine in acute asthma. *Ann Emerg Med.* 1996;27:170-175.

Jat KR, Chawla D. Ketamine for management of acute exacerbations of asthma in children. *Cochrane Database Syst Rev.* 2012;11:CD009293.

Kimball WR, Leith DE, Robins AG. Dynamic hyperinflation and ventilator dependence in chronic obstructive pulmonary disease. *Am Rev Respir Dis.* 1982;126:991-995.

Leatherman JW, Ravenscraft SA. Low measured auto-positive end-expiratory pressure during mechanical ventilation of patients with severe asthma: hidden auto-positive end-expiratory pressure. *Crit Care Med.* 1996;24:541-546.

Leuppi JD, Schuetz P, Bingisser R, et al. Short-term vs conventional glucocorticoid therapy in acute exacerbations of chronic obstructive pulmonary disease: the REDUCE randomized clinical trial. *JAMA.* 2013;309:2223-2231.

Lewis L, Ferguson I, House SL, et al. Albuterol administration is commonly associated with increases in serum lactate in patients with asthma treated for acute exacerbation of asthma. *Chest.* 2014;145:53-59.

Lim WJ, Mohammed Akram R, Carson KV, et al. Non-invasive positive pressure ventilation for treatment of respiratory failure due to severe acute exacerbations of asthma. *Cochrane Database Syst Rev.* 2012;12:CD004360.

Lindenauer PK, Pekow PS, Lahti MC, et al. Association of corticosteroid dose and route of administration with risk of treatment failure in acute exacerbation of chronic obstructive pulmonary disease. *JAMA.* 2010;303:2359-2367.

Malhotra A, Schwartz DR, Ayas N, et al. Treatment of oxygen-induced hypercapnia. *Lancet.* 2001;357:884-885.

Manser R, Reid D, Abramson M. Corticosteroids for acute severe asthma in hospitalised patients. *Cochrane Database Syst Rev.* 2001;(1):CD001740.

Morales DR, Jackson C, Lipworth BJ, et al. Adverse respiratory effect of acute b-blocker exposure in asthma: a systematic review and meta-analysis of randomized controlled trials. *Chest.* 2014;145:779-786.

Musch G, Foti G, Cereda M, et al. Lung and chest wall mechanics in normal anaesthetized subjects and in patients with COPD at different PEEP levels. *Eur Respir J.* 1997;10:2545-2552.

Pendergraft TB, Stanford RH, Beasley R, et al. Rates and characteristics of intensive care unit admissions and intubations among asthma-related hospitalizations. *Ann Allergy Asthma Immunol.* 2004;93:29-35.

Ram FS, Picot J, Lightowler J, et al. Non-invasive positive pressure ventilation for treatment of respiratory failure due to exacerbations of chronic obstructive pulmonary disease. *Cochrane Database Syst Rev.* 2004;(1):CD004104.

Salpeter SR, Ormiston TM, Salpeter EE. Cardioselective beta-blockers in patients with reactive airway disease: a meta-analysis. *Ann Intern Med.* 2002;137:715-725.

Vaschetto R, Bellotti E, Turucz E, et al. Inhalational anesthetics in acute severe asthma. *Curr Drug Targets.* 2009;10:826-832.

Vestbo J, Hurd SS, Agustí AG, et al. Global strategy for the diagnosis, management, and prevention of chronic obstructive pulmonary disease: GOLD executive summary. *Am J Respir Crit Care Med.* 2013;187:347-365.

Wenzel SE. Asthma phenotypes: the evolution from clinical to molecular approaches. *Nat Med.* 2012;18:716-725.

22 Deep Venous Thrombosis and Pulmonary Embolism in the Intensive Care Unit

Manolo Rubio Garcia and Alison S. Witkin

I. INTRODUCTION

Venous thromboembolic event (VTE) refers to both deep venous thrombosis (DVT) and pulmonary embolism (PE). Episodic thrombosis and/or embolism may appear to be discrete events, but increasingly they are considered to be manifestations of the same process.

A. Deep Venous Thrombosis refers to a clot in the deep vessels of the venous circulation. Although local discomfort with limb swelling and postthrombotic syndrome can occur, the majority of morbidity and mortality results from embolization to the pulmonary circulation. Although the proximal veins of the lower extremity are the most common sites of involvement and have a higher risk of embolization, upper extremity DVT can also lead to PE. Without DVT prophylaxis, the incidence of DVT in the intensive care unit (ICU) is quite high with ranges of 10% to 30% in medical patients and up to 60% in trauma patients. This risk can be significantly reduced, but not eliminated, with prophylaxis.

B. Pulmonary Embolism occurs when the pulmonary artery or one of its branches becomes obstructed by material. Although thrombus is the most common, air, fat, or tumor can also cause embolism. The clinical significance of PE is broad and ranges from an incidental finding with no signs or symptoms to catastrophic circulatory collapse leading to death. The incidence of PE is approximately 112 per 100 000 person-years. The mortality from PE approaches 20%, with higher mortality rates in those who are unstable at the time of presentation.

C. Risk Factors: DVT and PE have similar risk factors. Some of the most common risk factors in patients in the ICU include the following:

1. **Recent surgical procedures:** The risk of VTE is highest in patients who have had major orthopedic or general surgery procedures. Specific procedures associated with a high risk of VTE include hip or knee replacement and coronary artery bypass. Major trauma also has a high risk of VTE.
2. **Spinal cord injury:** Risk is highest immediately following injury and decreases with time.
3. **Malignancy:** Risk is highest in patients with advanced solid organ malignancies. Certain chemotherapy regimens may also increase risk.
4. **Central venous lines** can lead to line-associated DVT with potential for embolization to pulmonary vasculature.
5. **Oral contraceptive pills** also increased with hormone replacement therapy for other indications
6. **Pregnancy:** Greatest risk occurs in the postpartum period.
7. **Immobility:** due to injury, travel, or hospitalization
8. **Thrombophilias:** including antiphospholipid antibody syndrome, heparin-induced thrombocytopenia (HIT), as well as hereditary causes, including antithrombin deficiency, protein C and S deficiencies, factor V Leiden mutations, and prothrombin gene mutation
9. **Previous venous thromboembolic event**
10. **Infections:** respiratory (including coronavirus disease 2019), intra-abdominal, and urinary tract or bloodstream infections

D. Venous Thromboembolic Event in the Intensive Care Unit: The incidence of VTE in the ICU is difficult to determine because the diagnosis requires a high degree of suspicion in patients with other ongoing pulmonary processes and obtaining confirmatory testing is not always feasible in a patient who is critically ill. Regardless of the reason for ICU admission, such patients are at increased risk for VTE because most of them are immobile and many receive central venous catheters. The incidence of VTE in the ICU is estimated to be 8% (5% DVT, 2% PE, and 1% both) in patients who are critically ill.

E. Prophylaxis in Patients in the Intensive Care Unit: The use of pharmacologic prophylaxis with either low-dose heparin or low-molecular-weight heparin (LMWH) decreases but does not eliminate the risk of DVT in patients admitted to the ICU and thus should be used in patients without contraindications, such as active bleeding. Patients who cannot receive pharmacologic prophylaxis should receive mechanical prophylaxis. Intermittent pneumatic compression of the lower limbs is the mechanical intervention with the highest quality data. Failure to start thromboprophylaxis within 24 hours of ICU admission increases mortality. Regardless of the strategy used for prophylaxis, it is important to remember that no strategy provides complete protection against VTE.

II. DIAGNOSIS

A. Deep Venous Thrombosis

1. **Exam:** Limb pain, edema, and palpable cord are suggestive of DVT. Sudden severe pain associated with cyanosis or evidence of compartment syndrome or impaired arterial circulation is suggestive of massive proximal thrombosis (phlegmasia cerulea dolens). Exam alone is not sufficient to rule in or rule out DVT.
2. **Ultrasound** utilizes vein compressibility and/or color flow imaging. It has high sensitivity and specificity for DVT, although it may miss clots in pelvic veins. Ultrasound is ideal in patients in the ICU because it can be done at the bedside without radiation exposure.
3. **Computed tomography venogram** can be done at the same time as a computed tomography (CT) for evaluation of PE, eliminating the need for an additional imaging study; however, this test leads to increased radiation exposure and many protocols have higher doses of contrast material. CT-venogram, unlike ultrasound, can evaluate for pelvic thrombosis.
4. **Magnetic resonance venogram** can image the lower extremity veins, including pelvic veins, without use of contrast material or radiation. Disadvantages include availability and time required to obtain study.
5. **D-Dimer:** The main utility of the D-dimer assay is in ruling out DVT in the emergency department setting. Owing to a high degree of false positives in the setting of critical illness, this test has minimal utility in the ICU.

B. Pulmonary Embolism

1. **Clinical exam:** Although findings such as tachycardia, hypoxia, tachypnea, fever, and hypotension may raise clinical suspicion for PE, exam alone is not enough to rule in or rule out PE.
2. **Lab tests:** Although brain natriuretic peptide (BNP), N-terminal pro–brain natriuretic peptide (NT-proBNP), and troponin may be elevated, these tests lack the necessary specificity to be useful in diagnosis. In addition, as in DVT, the D-dimer is often elevated even in patients in the ICU without PE, limiting its utility in diagnosis.
3. **Electrocardiogram:** Although electrocardiogram (ECG) abnormalities, such as sinus tachycardia and evidence of right ventricular (RV) strain, are common, they lack both the specificity and sensitivity to make a diagnosis of PE.

4. **Chest x-ray:** The majority of patients have nonspecific abnormalities on chest x-ray (CXR) and up to 20% have a normal CXR finding. If infarction has occurred, this may appear as a wedge-shaped opacity at the periphery.
5. **CT angiography** has become the diagnostic imaging study of choice because it can be performed in minutes and, in addition, allows for simultaneous evaluation of other pulmonary processes. Addition of venous imaging improves sensitivity. Disadvantages include the requirement that the patient be able to comply with a breath hold, radiation exposure, and need for iodinated contrast. Poor-quality imaging because of either motion artifact or poor timing of contrast bolus may decrease sensitivity (Figure 22.1).
6. **Ventilation/perfusion scan** is useful in patients who cannot tolerate CT angiography (CTA) because it does not require iodinated contrast. However, its interpretation requires clinical correlation because a low-probability scan does not entirely rule out PE and a high-probability scan does not guarantee presence of PE. In addition, in patients with significant underlying pulmonary disease, perfusion scans are difficult to interpret and have a high false-positive rate. Ventilation/perfusion ($\dot{V}/\dot{Q}$) scans are often not feasible in patients in the ICU because ventilation imaging is typically not able to be performed on a patient on mechanical ventilation.
7. **Pulmonary angiography:** Because the quality of CTA has improved, the use of pulmonary angiography has decreased; however, it remains the gold standard for diagnosis of PE. Angiography is generally well tolerated with a low complication rate and has the additional benefit of allowing for direct assessment of pulmonary hemodynamics.
8. **Echocardiogram** is useful in assessing RV function. Findings suggestive of PE include increased RV chamber size with decreased function, although this finding can be seen in a variety of cardiac and pulmonary diseases. More specific findings include presence of RV clot and McConnell sign, in which there is akinesis of the mid-free RV wall with normal apical function. Although none of these findings are diagnostic of PE, because echocardiogram can be performed at the bedside, it can be used to help confirm a clinical diagnosis in a patient too unstable to travel for more definitive testing.

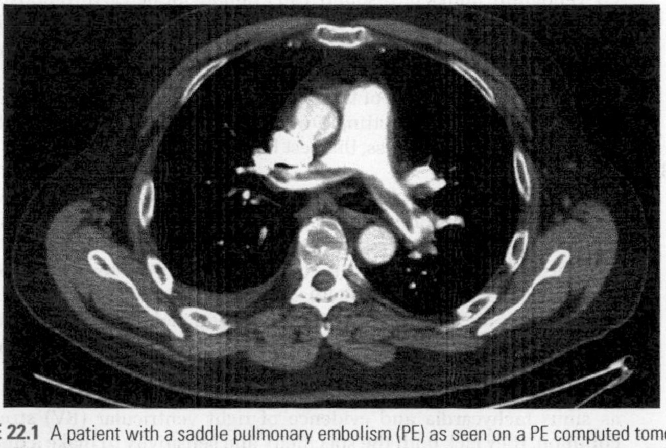

FIGURE 22.1 A patient with a saddle pulmonary embolism (PE) as seen on a PE computed tomography (CT). The filling defect can be seen crossing the saddle and extending into the left and right main pulmonary arteries.

III. INITIAL EVALUATION OF THE PATIENT WITH CONFIRMED OR SUSPECTED PULMONARY EMBOLISM

A. Assess Severity: The initial bedside assessment of a patient with PE is focused on assessing severity. Patients with hypotension and shock without other causes are considered to have massive PE (defined as systolic blood pressure of <90 mm Hg or a drop of at least 40 mm Hg from baseline for at least 15 minutes) and require immediate intervention.

1. The pathophysiology of massive PE is complex. When obstruction occurs by embolism, the right ventricle experiences an acute rise in pressure and volume, causing the interventricular septum to shift toward the left ventricle. In addition, as RV output decreases, the left ventricular (LV) preload also falls. This combination of septal shift and decreased RV output can ultimately lead to decreased cardiac output, shock, and hemodynamic collapse (Figure 22.2).
2. In patients without massive PE, it is important to distinguish between those at higher risk for hemodynamic collapse versus those with lower-risk PE. This is primarily accomplished through either direct or indirect assessment of RV compromise or strain. Those patients with hemodynamic stability but evidence of RV strain are considered to have intermediate-risk PE. Patients with only abnormalities in biomarkers or imaging are considered to have low-intermediate PE and those with abnormalities in both have high-intermediate-risk PE.
3. PE can also be classified according to severity into low, intermediate, or high risk. For this, the pulmonary embolism severity index (PESI) score or its simplified version (sPESI) can be used (Table 22.1).

B. Physical Exam should focus on signs of shock, including hypotension and signs of end-organ hypoperfusion, indicating massive PE. In the patient who is hemodynamically stable, hypoxia and tachycardia, particularly if worsened with activity, may suggest the patient is at risk for decompensation.

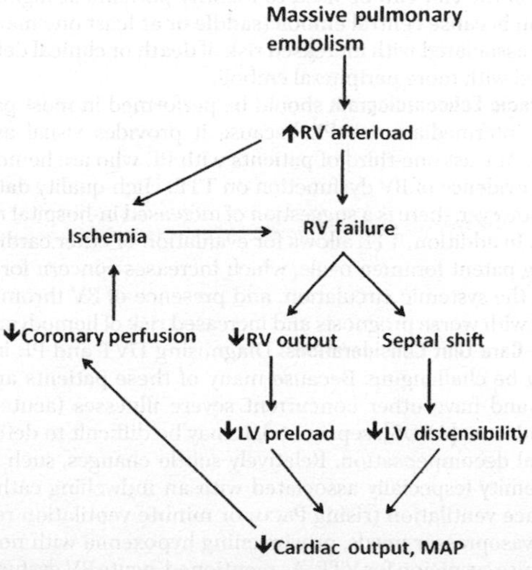

FIGURE 22.2 A schematic of how pulmonary embolism (PE) can lead to death. The PE increases right ventricle (RV) afterload, which impairs the RV cardiac output, and the resultant septal shift also impairs left ventricular (LV) function. This leads to systemic hypotension and impaired coronary perfusion, which further impairs the RV function, perpetuating the cycle. MAP, mean arterial pressure.

TABLE 22.1 This Table Shows the Clinical Features That Are Used to Calculate the sPESI Score in Assessing PE Servility

Simplified PESI (sPESI)
Presence of one or more indicates increased risk
Age older than 80 years
History of cancer
History of cardiopulmonary disease
Heart rate ≥100 beats/min
Systolic blood pressure <100 mm Hg
Oxygen saturation on room air <90%

PE, pulmonary embolism; PESI, pulmonary embolism severity index.

C. **Lab Testing:** Troponin elevation is seen in roughly one-third of patients with PE and is likely due to increased stretch on the right ventricle due to pressure overload in massive or intermediate-risk PE. Troponin elevation is associated with both presence of RV strain on transthoracic echocardiogram (TTE) and increased mortality. BNP or NT-proBNP elevation is seen in approximately one-half of patients with PE, reflecting RV myocyte stretch. As with troponin, an elevation is associated with RV strain on TTE and increased mortality when compared with patients with normal BNP and NT-proBNP levels. Troponin levels typically normalize sooner than when there is a myocardial infarction. The arterial blood gas may reveal hypoxemia, hypocapnia, respiratory alkalosis, and a widened alveolar-arterial oxygen gradient.

D. **Computed Tomography Findings:** In addition to the finding of the PE itself, the CTA chest can demonstrate findings of RV dysfunction and allow for assessment of clot burden. RV enlargement on CT (defined as the ratio of RV to LV diameter > 0.9) is associated with increased 30-day mortality. In addition, the location of the clot can be used to identify patients at higher risk of decompensation because central emboli (saddle or at least one main pulmonary artery) are associated with increased risk of death or clinical deterioration when compared with more peripheral emboli.

E. **Transthoracic Echocardiogram** should be performed in most patients with concern for intermediate-risk PE because it provides visual assessment of RV function. At least one-third of patients with PE who are hemodynamically stable have evidence of RV dysfunction on TTE. High-quality data on mortality is sparse; however, there is a suggestion of increased in-hospital mortality in these patients. In addition, TTE allows for evaluation of other cardiac abnormalities including patent foramen ovale, which increases concern for paradoxical embolus to the systemic circulation, and presence of RV thrombus, which is associated with worse prognosis and increased risk of hemodynamic instability.

F. **Intensive Care Unit Considerations:** Diagnosing DVT and PE in patients in the ICU may be challenging. Because many of these patients are intubated and sedated and have other concurrent severe illnesses (acute respiratory distress syndrome [ARDS], sepsis, etc), it may be difficult to determine the cause of clinical decompensation. Relatively subtle changes, such as a swollen upper extremity (especially associated with an indwelling catheter), increasing dead-space ventilation (rising $Pa{CO_2}$ or minute ventilation requirements), increased vasopressor needs, or worsening hypoxemia with no apparent cause, should raise suspicion for VTE. As mentioned, acute RV dysfunction in patients in the ICU may be due to several processes beside VTE, including sepsis, acute lung injury, intrinsic positive end-expiratory pressure (PEEP), and RV infarct.

IV. TREATMENT

A. Resuscitation: The first priority in treating a patient with PE is ensuring hemodynamic stability. Most patients with PE will have an increased A-a gradient due to V/Q mismatch combined with surfactant dysfunction due to release of inflammatory mediators, atelectasis, and shunt (particularly intracardiac in patients with a patent foramen ovale). Supplemental oxygen can be used to correct hypoxia, and inhaled nitric oxide may decrease shunting and improve pulmonary hemodynamics through pulmonary vasodilation. Caution should be used if a patient requires intubation because severe hypotension may result in the presence of significant RV dysfunction.

1. For patients who are hypotensive, fluid should be given cautiously to correct any volume deficit, with typically no more than 1000 mL of crystalloid given. Aggressive fluid resuscitation may worsen hypotension both by increasing RV stretch and worsening the interventricular shift, further impairing LV function. If a vasopressor is required, there are no randomized controlled trials to guide management; therefore, norepinephrine, dopamine, or epinephrine, plus the consideration of dobutamine, are reasonable selections. If a patient is in refractory shock, the use of extracorporeal membrane oxygenation (ECMO) should be considered. ECMO can provide both ventilatory and hemodynamic support while a patient is treated with more definitive therapy.

B. Systemic Anticoagulation should be promptly initiated when PE or DVT is diagnosed or strongly suspected. Unfractionated LMWH and fondaparinux are all considered first line for the acute treatment of PE and DVT. Owing to less reliable dosing and time to achieve therapeutic range, unfractionated heparin (UFH) should be used only if patients are not candidates for LMWH or fondaparinux because of renal failure or the need for a rapidly reversible agent. Although the direct oral anticoagulants (DOACs) may be used as initial anticoagulation, given the long half-life, this is rarely appropriate for patients in the ICU. Contraindications to anticoagulation include active bleeding, major trauma, acute intracranial hemorrhage, intracranial tumor, and severe bleeding diathesis. Patients with recent bleeding events, invasive procedures, or who are otherwise at increased risk of complications should be evaluated on an individual basis.

1. **Unfractionated heparin** has several advantages over other parenteral agents. Compared with LMWH and fondaparinux, UFH has the shortest half-life and can be reversed with protamine if needed, making it a good choice in patients with increased risks of bleeding. Owing to the short half-life, it should be used in patients who are being considered for thrombolysis. In addition, UFH does not rely on renal clearance, so it is ideal for use in renal failure. The main drawback to UFH use is that it requires frequent laboratory monitoring and can take time to reach therapeutic levels. Such delays have been associated with increased mortality from PE and higher rates of VTE recurrence.
2. **Low-molecular-weight heparins:** Multiple formulations of LMWH exist, with variations in dosing. Compared with UFH, LMWH is associated with decreased complications, lower incidence of bleeding, and decreased mortality. However, because LMWH is cleared renally and can be challenging to reverse, its use should be avoided in patients with decreased creatinine clearance or who are considered to be at increased bleeding risk.
3. **Factor Xa inhibitors:** Fondaparinux is an injectable factor Xa inhibitor that has efficacy similar to that of UFH and does not require drug level monitoring. Rivaroxaban and apixaban are oral factor Xa inhibitors that are approved for treatment of VTE as monotherapy and may be considered for first-line therapy in appropriate patients with a low risk of bleeding and where invasive procedures are not anticipated. Apixaban is approved for use in renal failure.

This class of medication can be safely used in patients with a history of HIT. Andexanet alfa is the reversal agent for factor Xa inhibitors.

4. **Direct thrombin inhibitors:** Argatroban is an intravenous direct thrombin inhibitor approved for treatment of thrombosis when associated with HIT. Some centers may use bivalirudin, a direct thrombin inhibitor approved for anticoagulation for percutaneous coronary intervention, in an off-label manner for treatment of thrombosis with HIT. Dabigatran is an oral direct thrombin inhibitor approved for treatment of VTE. Its use has not been studied in the acute setting and thus is not recommended as initial therapy. Dabigatran should be avoided in patients with impaired renal function. Idarucizumab is the reversal agent for dabigatran.
5. **Warfarin:** Owing to the initial prothrombotic effects of warfarin, it should not be used alone in the acute setting; however, its efficacy in preventing recurrent VTE has been well established. Warfarin requires close monitoring of international normalized ratio (INR) to avoid inadequate treatment while minimizing the risk of bleeding. In the event of overdose or bleeding, fresh frozen plasma, vitamin K, or 4-factor prothrombin complex concentrate can be used to reverse its effects.

C. Systemic Thrombolysis

1. **Overview:** Thrombolytic agents activate plasminogen to form plasmin, leading to increased lysis of thrombus. Owing to increased bleeding risk, including fatal intracranial bleeding, patients must be carefully screened for contraindications. Major and absolute contraindications include intracranial lesions, previous intracranial hemorrhage, ischemic stroke within 3 months, recent head trauma, recent brain or spine surgery, active bleeding, and bleeding diathesis. Notable relative contraindications include systolic or diastolic hypertension, recent invasive procedures, recent bleeding, and history of ischemic stroke more than 3 months prior. Studied thrombolytic agents include tissue plasminogen activator (tPA; eg, alteplase, tenecteplase), streptokinase, and urokinase. The last two are no longer available in the United States for the management of acute VTE.
2. **Indications:** Systemic thrombolysis is recommended for patients with massive PE without contraindications, taking into consideration the mortality risk and the risk of bleeding. Systemic thrombolysis is not recommended for the majority of patients with DVT, although it can be considered in patients with acute, extensive proximal or iliofemoral clot. Systemic thrombolysis is also generally not recommended for patients with intermediate-risk PE. Several studies that examined the use of full-dose thrombolytic therapy in patients with nonmassive PE and evidence of RV dysfunction found decreased rates of hemodynamic decompensation and need for escalation in treatment; however, there was no improvement in mortality and most studies reported increase in major bleeding. The moderate pulmonary embolism treated with thrombolysis (MOPETT) study gave patients with "moderate" PE, as defined by degree of involvement on angiography or $\dot{V}/\dot{Q}$ scan, no more than half-dose tPA and found that this regimen improved pulmonary artery pressures without an increase in bleeding. However, this was a single-center study with much higher than expected rates of pulmonary hypertension in the anticoagulation-only arm, which limits its generalizability. Therefore, the use of reduced or full-dose systemic thrombolysis in this group of patients needs to be individualized.

D. Surgical Embolectomy should be considered in patients with massive PE who either fail or are not candidates for systemic lysis or catheter-directed therapies. One advantage of surgical embolectomy is that it allows for simultaneous intervention on associated abnormalities, such as patent foramen ovale closure or removal of intracardiac clot. This intervention is limited to hospitals with experienced staff and appropriate resources.

E. Catheter-Directed Therapies are emerging tools in the treatment of both massive and submassive PE, particularly when patients have contraindications to systemic lysis or have failed initial interventions. The role in patients with lower-risk PE is an ongoing area of study. Catheter-based interventions fall into catheter-directed thrombolysis and catheter-based thrombectomy.

1. **Catheter-directed thrombolysis** involves local administration of thrombolytics directly into the pulmonary artery. This has the advantage of ensuring high concentration of medication at the clot location and can use lower doses of thrombolytics than is required for systemic thrombolysis. The use of ultrasound-enhanced catheters has been proposed to break up fibrin cross-links and allow for deeper penetration of lytics.
2. **Catheter-directed thrombectomy** involves removal of embolic material through a percutaneous catheter. This has been associated with an improvement in RV/LV ratio. This is primarily used for more proximal emboli and has the advantage over catheter-directed thrombolysis in that no thrombolytic administration is required.

F. Vena Cava Filters should be used in patients who have DVT with contraindications to anticoagulation or who fail anticoagulation. Filters appear to primarily decrease PE in the acute setting and their long-term use is associated with recurrent DVT, often at the filter site. In the prevention of recurrent pulmonary embolism by vena cava interruption (PREPIC2) study, the use of an inferior vena cava (IVC) filter in patients at higher risk who are able to tolerate anticoagulation did not improve outcomes. Removable filters should be considered in those with only temporary indications for placement.

G. Multidisciplinary Approach: Treatment of patients with intermediate-risk and massive PEs often requires a multidisciplinary approach with collaboration between the emergency department, cardiology, surgery, radiology, and ICU teams. In addition, the ideal treatment for a particular patient will depend on available resources and patient-specific information. The use of a multidisciplinary pulmonary embolism response team (PERT) to help coordinate these efforts has been described and may streamline the care for these patients.

V. FOLLOW-UP

A. Duration of Anticoagulation varies depending on the presence of reversible risk factors and whether the patient has a history of VTE. Most patients require a minimum of 3 months of systemic anticoagulation, with prolonged or even lifelong therapy in those with irreversible risk factors or recurrent VTE. The choice of the long-term anticoagulant agent should be tailored to the individual patient's risk factors and comorbidities.

B. Chronic Thromboembolic Pulmonary Hypertension occurs in approximately 3.8% of patients following acute PE. During outpatient follow-up, patients should be assessed for residual symptoms of dyspnea, particularly on exertion. Those who have persistent symptoms or RV dysfunction should be considered for additional screening, including V/Q scan and repeat TTE.

Selected Readings

Anderson FA, Spencer FA. Risk factors for venous thromboembolism. *Circulation.* 2003;107:I-9-I-16.

Attia J, Ray JG, Cook DJ, et al. Deep vein thrombosis and its prevention in critically ill adults. *Arch Intern Med.* 2001;161:1268-1279.

Bilaloglu S, Aphinyanaphongs Y, Jones S, et al. Thrombosis in hospitalized patient with COVID-19 in a New York City Health System. *JAMA.* 2020;324:799-801.

Büller HR, Davidson BL, Decousus H, et al. Subcutaneous fondaparinux versus intravenous unfractionated heparin in the initial treatment of pulmonary embolism. *N Engl J Med.* 2003;349:1695-1702.

Capellier G, Jacques T, Balvay P, et al. Inhaled nitric oxide in patients with pulmonary embolism. *Intensive Care Med.* 1997;23:1089-1092.

Chan CM, Shorr AF. Venous thromboembolic disease in the intensive care unit. *Semin Respir Crit Care Med.* 2010;31:39-46.

Cohoon KP, Ashrani AA, Crusan DJ, et al. Is infection an independent risk factor for venous thromboembolism? A population-based, case-control study. *Am J Med.* 2018;131(3):307-316.e2.

Decousus H, Leizorovicz A, Parent F, et al. A clinical trial of vena caval filters in the prevention of pulmonary embolism in patients with proximal deep-vein thrombosis. *N Engl J Med.* 1998;338:409-415.

Donzé J, Le Gal G, Fine MJ, et al. Prospective validation of the pulmonary embolism severity index. A clinical prognostic model for pulmonary embolism. *Thromb Haemost.* 2008;100(5):943-948.

Eid-Lidt G, Gaspar J, Sandoval J, et al. Combined clot fragmentation and aspiration in patients with acute pulmonary embolism. *Chest.* 2008;134:54-60.

EINSTEIN-PE Investigators; Büller HR, Prins MH, et al. Oral rivaroxaban for the treatment of symptomatic pulmonary embolism. *N Engl J Med.* 2012;366:1287-1297.

Elliott CG, Goldhaber SZ, Visani L, et al. Chest radiographs in acute pulmonary embolism. Results from the International Cooperative Pulmonary Embolism Registry. *Chest.* 2000;118(1):33-38.

Engelberger RP, Kucher N. Catheter-based reperfusion treatment of pulmonary embolism. *Circulation.* 2011;124:2139-2144.

Erkens PM, Prins MH. Fixed dose subcutaneous low-molecular-weight heparins versus adjusted dose unfractionated heparin for venous thromboembolism. *Cochrane Database Syst Rev.* 2010;9:CD001100.

Geerts W, Selby R. Prevention of venous thromboembolism in the ICU. *Chest.* 2003;124: 357S-363S.

Goldhaber SZ, Visani L, De Rosa M. Acute pulmonary embolism: clinical outcomes in the International Cooperative Pulmonary Embolism Registry. *Lancet.* 1999;353:1386-1389.

Ho KM, Chavan S, Pilcher D. Omission of early thromboprophylaxis and mortality in critically ill patients: a multicenter registry study. *Chest.* 2011;140(6):1436-1446.

Ho KM, Tan JA. Stratified meta-analysis of intermittent pneumatic compression of the lower limbs to prevent venous thromboembolism in hospitalized patients. *Circulation.* 2013;2013:1003-1020.

Horlander KT, Leeper KV. Troponin levels as a guide to treatment of pulmonary embolism. *Curr Opin Pulm Med.* 2003;9:374-377.

Jiménez D, Aujesky D, Moores L, et al. Simplification of the pulmonary embolism severity index for prognostication in patients with acute symptomatic pulmonary embolism. *Arch Intern Med.* 2010;170(15):1383-1389.

Kanne JP, Lalani TA. Role of computed tomography and magnetic resonance imaging for deep venous thrombosis and pulmonary embolism. *Circulation.* 2004;109:I-15-I-21.

Kline JA, Nordenholz KE, Courtney DM, et al. Treatment of submassive pulmonary embolism with tenecteplase or placebo: cardiopulmonary outcomes at 3 months: multicenter double-blind, placebo-controlled randomized trial. *J Thromb Haemost.* 2014;12:459-468.

Klock FA, Mos ICM, Huisman MV. Brain-type natriuretic peptide levels in the prediction of adverse outcome in patients with pulmonary embolism. *Am J Respir Crit Care Med.* 2008;178:425-430.

Konstantinides S, Geibel A, Heusel G, et al. Heparin plus alteplase compared with heparin alone in patients with submassive pulmonary embolism. *N Engl J Med.* 2002;347:1143-1150.

Konstantinides SV, Meyer G, Becattini C, et al. 2019 ESC Guidelines for the diagnosis and management of acute pulmonary embolism developed in collaboration with the European Respiratory Society (ERS): the Task Force for the diagnosis and management of acute pulmonary embolism of the European Society of Cardiology (ESC). *Eur Respir J.* 2019;54(3):1901647.

Kucher N. Deep-vein thrombosis of the upper extremities. *N Engl J Med.* 2011;364:861-869.

Kucher N, Boekstegers P, Müller OJ, et al. Randomized, controlled trial of ultrasound-assisted catheter-directed thrombolysis for acute intermediate-risk pulmonary embolism. *Circulation.* 2014;129(4):479-486.

Lensing AW, Prandoni P, Brandjes D, et al. Detection of deep-vein thrombosis by real-time B-mode ultrasonography. *N Engl J Med.* 1989;320:342-345.

Lim W, Meade M, Lauzier F, et al. Failure of anticoagulant thromboprophylaxis: risk factors in medical-surgical critically ill patients*. *Crit Care Med.* 2015;43(2):401-410.

McConnell MV, Solomon SD, Rayan ME, et al. Regional right ventricular dysfunction detected by echocardiography in acute pulmonary embolism. *Am J Cardiol.* 1996;78:469-473.

Meyer G, Vicaut E, Danays T, et al. Fibronolysis for patients with intermediate-risk pulmonary embolism. *N Engl J Med.* 2014;370:1402-1411.

Mismetti P, Laporte S, Pellerin O, et al. Effect of a retrievable inferior vena cava filter plus anticoagulation vs anticoagulation alone on risk of recurrent pulmonary embolism: a randomized clinical trial. *JAMA.* 2015;313(16):1627-1635.

Müller-Bardorff M, Weidtmann B, Giannitsis E, et al. Release kinetics of cardiac troponin T in survivors of confirmed severe pulmonary embolism. *Clin Chem.* 2002;48(4):673-675.

Ogren M, Bergqvist D, Eriksson H, et al. Prevalence and risk of pulmonary embolism in patients with intracardiac thrombosis: a population-based study of 23796 consecutive autopsies. *Eur Heart J.* 2005;26:1108-1114.

Pengo V, Lensing AWA, Prins MH, et al. Incidence of chronic thromboembolic pulmonary hypertension after pulmonary embolism. *N Engl J Med.* 2004;350:2257-2264.

PIOPED Investigators. Value of the ventilation/perfusion scan in acute pulmonary embolism. *JAMA.* 1990;263:2753-2759.

Provias T, Dudzinski DM, Jaff MR, et al. The Massachusetts General Hospital Pulmonary Embolism Response Team (MGH PERT): creation of a multidisciplinary program to improve care of patients with massive and submassive pulmonary embolism. *Hosp Pract (1995).* 2014;42:31-37.

Rodger M, Makropoulos D, Turek M, et al. Diagnostic value of the electrocardiogram in suspected pulmonary embolism. *Am J Cardiol.* 2000;86:807-809.

Schoepf UJ, Kucher N, Kipfmueller F, et al. Right ventricular enlargement on chest computed tomography: a predictor of early death in acute pulmonary embolism. *Circulation.* 2004;110:3276-3280.

Schulman S, Kearon C, Kakkar AK, et al. Dabigatran versus warfarin in the treatment of acute venous thromboembolism. *N Engl J Med.* 2009;361:2342-2352.

Sharifi M, Bay C, Skrocki L, et al. Moderate pulmonary embolism treated with thrombolysis (from the "MOPETT" trial). *Am J Cardiol.* 2013;111:273-277.

Smith SB, Geske JB, Maguire JM, et al. Early anticoagulation is associated with reduced mortality for acute pulmonary embolism. *Chest.* 2010;137:1382-1390.

Stein PD, Athanasoulis C, Alavi A, et al. Complications and validity of pulmonary angiography in acute pulmonary embolism. *Circulation.* 1992;85:462-468.

Stein PD, Fowler SE, Goodman LR, et al. Multidetector computed tomography for acute pulmonary embolism. *N Engl J Med.* 2006;354:2317-2327.

Stein PD, Goldhaber SZ, Henry JW, et al. Arterial blood gas analysis in the assessment of suspected acute pulmonary embolism. *Chest.* 1996;109(1):78-81.

Stein PD, Hull RD, Patel KC, et al. D-dimer for the exclusion of acute venous thrombosis and pulmonary embolism: a systematic review. *Ann Intern Med.* 2004;140:589-602.

Tapson VF, Sterling K, Jones N, et al. A randomized trial of the optimum duration of acoustic pulse thrombolysis procedure in acute intermediate-risk pulmonary embolism: the OPTALYSE PE Trial. *JACC Cardiovasc Interv.* 2018;11(14):1401-1410.

ten Wolde M, Sohne M, Quak E, et al. Prognostic value of echocardiographically assessed right ventricular dysfunction in patients with pulmonary embolism. *Arch Intern Med.* 2004;164:1685-1689.

Torbicki A, Galie N, Covezzoli A, et al. Right heart thrombi in pulmonary embolism results from the International Cooperative Pulmonary Embolism Registry. *J Am Coll Card.* 2003;41:2245-2251.

Tu T, Toma C, Tapson VF, et al. A prospective, single-arm, multicenter trial of catheter-directed mechanical thrombectomy for intermediate-risk acute pulmonary embolism: the FLARE study. *JACC Cardiovasc Interv.* 2019;12(9):859-869.

Vedovati MC, Becattini C, Agnelli G, et al. Multidetector CT scan for acute pulmonary embolism: embolic burden and clinical outcome. *Chest.* 2012;142:1417-1424.

Wiener RS, Schwartz LM, Woloshin S. Time trends in pulmonary embolism in the United States: evidence of overdiagnosis. *Arch Intern Med.* 2011;171:831-837.

Wood KE. Major pulmonary embolism: review of a pathophysiologic approach to the golden hour of hemodynamically significant pulmonary embolism. *Chest.* 2002;121:877-905.

23 Pulmonary Hypertension

Hilary L. Zetlen and Josanna Rodriguez-Lopez

I. DEFINITIONS

A. Pulmonary Hypertension (PH) is broadly defined by a mean pulmonary arterial pressure (mPAP) greater than or equal to 20 mm Hg measured by right heart catheterization (RHC) at rest. This hemodynamic definition was updated in 2018 from the historical threshold of mPAP greater than or equal to 25 mm Hg given accumulating evidence that mPAP greater than or equal to 20 mm Hg is abnormal.

B. Hemodynamic Definitions

Pulmonary vascular resistance (PVR) is calculated by dividing the transpulmonary pressure gradient (TPG) by the cardiac output (CO). The TPG can be calculated using invasive hemodynamic measurements from RHC and is typically defined as the mPAP minus the left heart pressure. Left heart pressure is most commonly estimated by the pulmonary capillary wedge pressure (PCWP) on RHC but can also be measured as the left atrial pressure (LAP) or left ventricular end-diastolic pressure (LVEDP) on left heart catheterization (LHC).

$$\text{TPG} = \text{mPAP} - \text{PCWP}$$

$$\text{PVR} = \text{TPG} / \text{CO}$$

Rearranging this equation shows that mPAP can be elevated because of increased CO (eg, cirrhosis, anemia), elevated PCWP (eg, left heart disease), increased PVR (eg, pulmonary arterial hypertension [PAH], chronic respiratory failure), or a combination of these factors:

$$\text{mPAP} = \text{PVR} \times \text{CO} + \text{PCWP}$$

C. Precapillary Versus Postcapillary Pulmonary Hypertension

A useful framework for categorizing PH is to define it by the involved component of the pulmonary circulation (Table 23.1). PH due to constriction, remodeling, occlusion, or destruction of the pulmonary arteries and arterioles (eg, PAH, chronic thromboembolic PH [CTEPH], chronic lung disease) is defined as **precapillary PH**—that is, arising from the components of the pulmonary circulation proximal to the pulmonary capillary bed. PH due to left heart disease with an elevated PCWP or LAP is defined as **postcapillary PH**. Precapillary and postcapillary PH can, and often do, coexist. Of note, pulmonary veno-occlusive disease (PVOD), although technically a disease of the pulmonary venules (ie, postcapillary), is hemodynamically defined as precapillary PH given PCWP is typically normal.

D. Clinical Classification of Pulmonary Hypertension

The World Health Organization (WHO)/World Symposium on Pulmonary Hypertension (WSPH) clinical classification system categorizes patients with PH into diagnostic groups on the basis of shared clinical, pathophysiologic, and

TABLE 23.1 PH Hemodynamic Definitions

	Hemodynamics
Precapillary PH	mPAP ≥ 20 mm Hg PCWP ≤ 15 mm Hg TPG > 12 mm Hg PVR ≥ 3 Woods units
Postcapillary PH	mPAP ≥ 20 mm Hg PCWP ≥ 15 mm Hg
• **Isolated postcapillary**	TPG < 12 mm Hg
• **Combined pre- and postcapillary**	TPG >12 mm Hg and/or PVR > 3 WU

mPAP, mean pulmonary arterial pressure; PCWP, pulmonary capillary wedge pressure; PH, pulmonary hypotension; PVR, pulmonary vascular resistance; TPG, transpulmonary pressure gradient.

hemodynamic characteristics. This classification system is clinically useful because treatment and management strategies vary by group.

1. **Pulmonary arterial hypertension**
   - **a.** Idiopathic PAH
   - **b.** Heritable PAH
   - **c.** Drug- and toxin-induced PAH
   - **d.** PAH associated with (also called *associated PH*) the following:
     - **1.** Connective tissue disease
     - **2.** HIV infection
     - **3.** Portal hypertension
     - **4.** Congenital heart disease
     - **5.** Schistosomiasis
   - **e.** PAH long-term responders to calcium channel blockers (CCBs)
   - **f.** PAH with overt features of venous/capillaries (PVOD/pulmonary capillary hemangiomatosis [PCH]) involvement
   - **g.** Persistent PH of the newborn syndrome
2. **Pulmonary hypertension due to left heart disease**
   - **a.** PH due to heart failure with preserved left ventricular ejection fraction (LVEF)
   - **b.** PH due to heart failure with reduced LVEF
   - **c.** Valvular heart disease
   - **d.** Congenital/acquired cardiovascular conditions leading to postcapillary PH
3. **Pulmonary hypertension due to lung diseases and/or hypoxia**
   - **a.** Obstructive lung disease
   - **b.** Restrictive lung disease
   - **c.** Other lung disease with mixed restrictive/obstructive pattern
   - **d.** Hypoxia without lung disease
   - **e.** Developmental lung disorders
4. **Pulmonary hypertension due to pulmonary artery obstructions**
   - **a.** Chronic thromboembolic PH
   - **b.** Other pulmonary artery (PA) obstructions (eg, sarcoma, other malignancy, arteritis, congenital, parasitosis)
5. **Pulmonary hypertension with unclear and/or multifactorial mechanisms**
   - **a.** Hematologic disorders
   - **b.** Systemic and metabolic disorders (eg, sarcoidosis, glycogen storage diseases)
   - **c.** Others
   - **d.** Complex congenital heart disease

II. EVALUATION

A. Clinical Presentation

1. **Symptoms** of PH are nonspecific. The most common presenting symptoms are dyspnea and fatigue. In advanced disease, symptoms suggestive of right ventricular (RV) failure, including exertional chest pain and presyncope/syncope, may also be present.
2. **Physical exam** findings of PH include a loud pulmonic component of the second heart sound (P2) on cardiac exam and/or a split second heart sound. Signs of RV failure include peripheral edema, elevated jugular venous pulse (JVP), and other evidence of right-sided volume overload including ascites.

B. Transthoracic Echocardiogram

1. **Right ventricular systolic pressure (RVSP)** is calculated using Doppler measurement of peak **tricuspid regurgitation velocity (TRV)** and estimated right atrial pressure (RAP) on echocardiogram in the modified Bernoulli equation:

$$RVSP = 4(TRV)^2 + RAP$$

RVSP approximates the pulmonary artery systolic pressure (PASP), except when right ventricular outflow tract (RVOT) obstruction is present. RAP is typically estimated from measures of inferior vena cava (IVC) collapsibility and is subject to significant variability. As a result, echocardiographically measured RVSP is frequently inaccurate and correlates with PASP on RHC only about 50% of the time. In more recent guidelines, TRV is preferentially used to determine echocardiographic probability of PH, in combination with other echocardiographic features suggestive of PH.

2. **Echocardiographic features suggestive of PH** must be present from greater than or equal to two of the following categories (a, b, or c) to increase the diagnostic likelihood of PH.
   - **a.** Ventricles
     1. RV:LV basal diameter ratio greater than 1.0
     2. Interventricular septal flattening (Figure 23.1)
   - **b.** Pulmonary artery
     1. PA diameter greater than 25 mm
     2. RV outflow acceleration time less than 105 msec
     3. Early diastolic pulmonary regurgitant velocity greater than 2.2 m/s
   - **c.** IVC and right atrium (RA)
     1. IVC diameter greater than 21 mm with decreased collapse on inspiration (<50% with sniff, <20% with normal inspiration)
     2. RA area greater than 18 cm^2
3. On the basis of TRV and the echocardiographic features already defined, probability of PH can be estimated according to the following criteria:
   - **a.** TRV less than or equal to 2.8 m/s or unmeasurable without other echocardiographic features of PH = **Low probability**
   - **b.** TRV less than or equal to 2.8 m/s or unmeasurable with other echocardiographic features of PH = **Intermediate probability**
   - **c.** TRV 2.9 to 3.4 m/s without other echocardiographic features of PH = **Intermediate probability**
   - **d.** TRV 2.9 to 3.4 m/s with other echocardiographic features of PH = **High probability**
   - **e.** TRV >3.4 m/s = **High probability**

C. Computed Tomography (CT) Chest, Pulmonary Function Testing, and Polysomnogram

are typically performed as part of a diagnostic workup for PH to evaluate for the presence of lung disease and/or sleep disordered breathing.

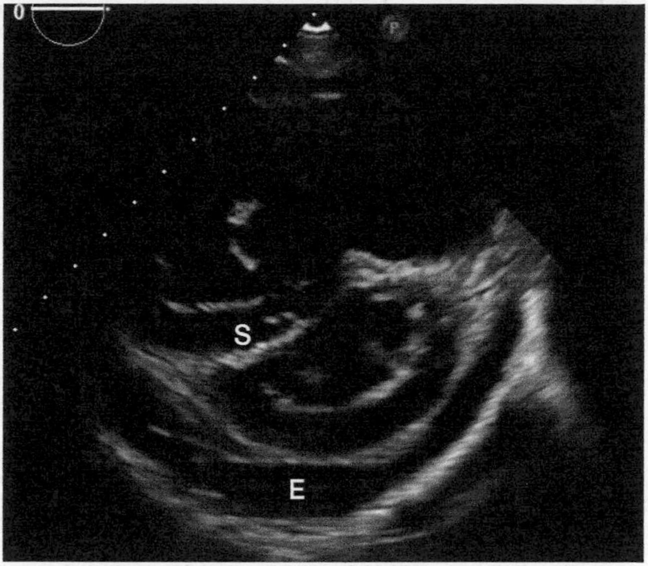

FIGURE 23.1 Diastolic interventricular septal flattening ("D sign"). Note the flattening of the interventricular septum (S), in this case during diastole. A pericardial effusion (E) is also present, which is another finding indicative of right ventricular failure.

D. **Ventilation/Perfusion** ($\dot{V}/\dot{Q}$) **Scan** should be performed as part of the initial diagnostic algorithm for PH. $\dot{V}/\dot{Q}$ scan is the screening test of choice for CTEPH because it is more sensitive than is CT pulmonary angiogram for the detection of chronic pulmonary emboli, which are visualized on $\dot{V}/\dot{Q}$ as (generally large, often numerous) mismatched $\dot{V}/\dot{Q}$ defects.

E. **Right Heart Catheterization (RHC)** is the gold standard diagnostic test for PH. For a patient in whom PH is suspected on the basis of the abovementioned evaluation (and for whom PH-specific therapy may be considered), RHC should be performed. As discussed throughout this section, hemodynamic data from RHC is used to confirm the diagnosis of PH, categorize PH (as pre- or post-capillary and by diagnostic group), and to assess PH severity. In addition to obtaining hemodynamic data, the following maneuvers can be performed during RHC to provide additional clinical information.

1. **Vasoreactivity testing** with inhaled nitric oxide (iNO), prostacyclins, or adenosine should be performed in patients with a higher likelihood of vasoreactive PAH (idiopathic, heritable, and drug- or toxin-induced PAH). A small minority of patients with PAH (10%-20%) will meet the criteria for vasoreactivity (a >10 mm Hg drop in mPAP to <40 mm Hg, without a drop in CO or systemic BP) and are candidates for CCB therapy.
2. A **fluid or exercise challenge** can be performed in patients with PCWP at the upper limit of normal (ie, PCWP 13-15 mm Hg) in whom left heart disease is strongly suspected. There are pitfalls to these approaches given lack of standardization and lack of agreement over what constitutes a "normal" physiologic response to exercise. An increase in PCWP to greater than 18 mm Hg after infusion of 500 mL normal saline over 5 minutes or an increase in PCWP to greater than 20 mm Hg with upright exercise is suggestive of left heart dysfunction.

3. **Pulmonary arteriograms** should be performed in patients with an abnormal $\dot{V}/\dot{Q}$ scan or when there is a high index of clinical suspicion for CTEPH. Pulmonary arteriogram can be used to confirm a diagnosis of CTEPH and to identify potential targets for therapeutic intervention surgical pulmonary thromboendarterectomy (PTE) or balloon pulmonary angioplasty (BPA).

F. **Diagnosis of PH** based on the abovementioned evaluation is further outlined in the diagnostic algorithm shown in Figure 23.2.

III. MANAGEMENT

A. **Treatment of PH** is dependent on etiology. **PH-specific therapy** refers to medications that function as pulmonary vasodilators and remodeling agents. Use of these agents is typically reserved for patients with PAH (group 1 disease) and are currently only U.S. Food and Drug Administration (FDA) approved for use in these patients. There is a limited role for the off-label use of pulmonary vasodilators in groups 2 to 4, which is further discussed subsequently.

1. **PH-specific therapies** include the following classes of medications with pulmonary vasodilatory effects. The most commonly used medications in the United States for PH in each class are also listed.
   a. **CCBs** inhibit L-type calcium channels in vascular smooth muscle. Both dihydropyridine and non-dihydropyridine CCBs are used for the treatment of PH. These agents should only be utilized in patients who meet the criteria for vasoreactive PH on RHC, as described in **Section II.**
      1. Oral: nifedipine, diltiazem
   b. **Phosphodiesterase-5 inhibitors** (PDE5Is) inhibit the degradation of cyclic guanosine monophosphate (cGMP), an enhancer of smooth muscle relaxation via nitric oxide–mediated vasodilatory pathways.
      1. Oral: sildenafil, tadalafil
   c. **Guanylate cyclase stimulators** (sGCs) also induce pulmonary vasodilation through increased production of cGMP. sGCs and PDE5Is cannot be used in combination given their similar mechanisms and their potential to cause significant systemic hypotension when used together.
      1. Oral: riociguat
   d. **Endothelin receptor antagonists** (ERAs) block endothelin receptors on vascular smooth muscle, inhibiting vasoconstriction.
      1. Oral: bosentan, ambrisentan, macitentan
   e. **Prostacyclin receptor agonists** (PCAs) directly induce pulmonary vasodilation and have vascular remodeling effects, including inhibition of inflammation and smooth muscle proliferation.
      1. Oral: selexipag (non-prostanoid, IP receptor agonist), treprostinil
      2. Intravenous (IV): epoprostenol, treprostinil
      3. Subcutaneous (SC): treprostinil
      4. Inhaled: treprostinil, iloprost
2. **Management of group 1 pulmonary arterial hypertension**
   a. **Risk stratification**

      Once the diagnosis of PAH is confirmed, the treatment approach is based on patient risk stratification into low-, medium-, and high-risk groups (on the basis of estimated 1-year mortality). The approach to risk assessment is not standardized and can integrate measures of functional class, assessment of high-risk features, and multivariable risk assessment models.
      1. **WHO functional assessment for PH** is commonly used to risk stratify patients with PH either on its own or as part of a risk model.
         a. Class I: No activity limitation
         b. Class II: Slight activity limitation, comfortable at rest
         c. Class III: Marked activity limitation, comfortable at rest

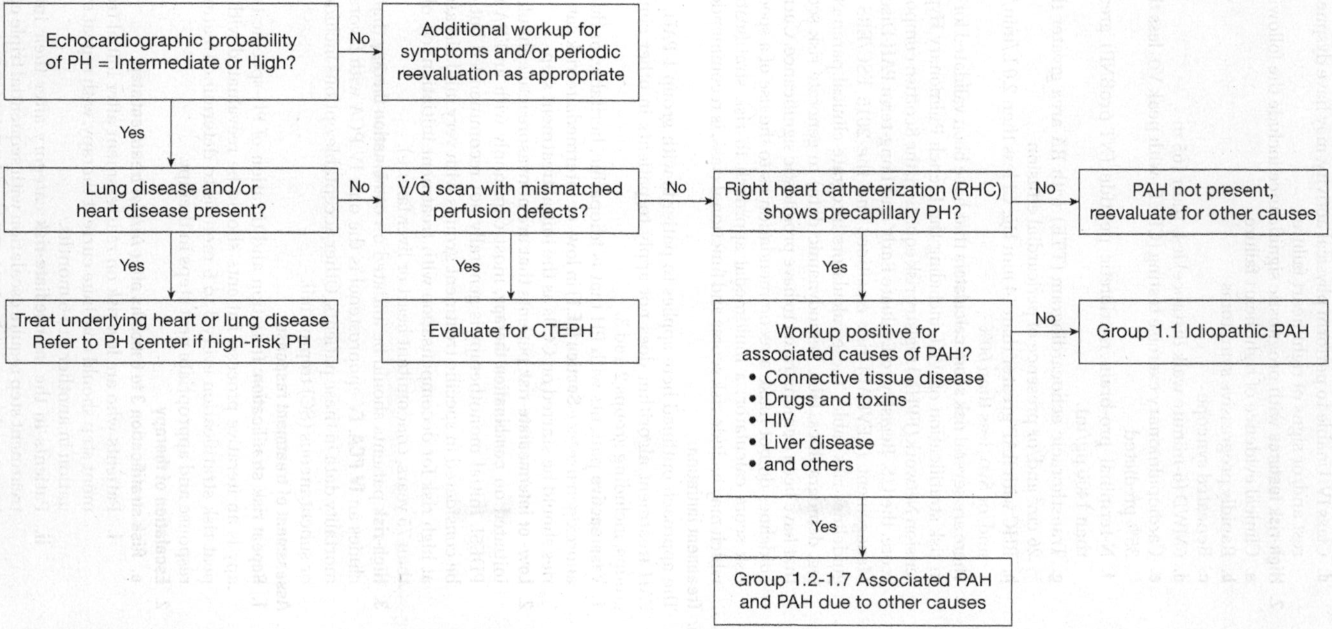

FIGURE 23.2 PH diagnostic algorithm. CTEPH, chronic thromboembolic pulmonary hypotension; PAH, pulmonary arterial hypotension; PH, pulmonary hypotension; V̇/Q̇, ventilation perfusion. (Adapted with permission from Galiè N, Humbert M, Vachiery J-L, et al. 2015 ESC/ERS guidelines for the diagnosis and treatment of pulmonary hypertension. *Eur Heart J*. 2016;37(1):67-119. © 2023 European Society of Cardiology & European Respiratory Society.)

d. Class IV: Unable to perform physical activity, may have dyspnea at rest and/or signs of right heart failure
2. **High-risk features** with prognostic significance include the following:
a. Clinical evidence of right heart failure
b. Rapidly progressive symptoms
c. Repeated syncope
d. 6MWD (6-minute walk distance) less than 165 m
e. Cardiopulmonary exercise testing (CPET) with peak Vo_2 less than 35% predicted
f. N-terminal pro-brain natriuretic peptide (NT-proBNP) greater than 1400 pg/mL
g. Transthoracic echocardiogram (TTE) with RA area greater than 26 cm^2 and/or presence of pericardial effusion
h. RHC with RAP greater than 14 mm Hg, CI less than 2.0 L/min/m^2, and/or Svo_2 less than 60%
3. There are several **risk score calculators** that have been validated for use in risk stratification of PAH, including the French Pulmonary Hypertension Network (FPHN) registry risk equation, the Scottish composite score, the U.S. Registry to Evaluate Early and Long-term PAH Disease Management (REVEAL) risk equation, and the 2015 ESC/ERS PH guidelines risk table. These calculators integrate clinical parameters (eg, demographics, labs, hemodynamic data) to generate risk scores that have been demonstrated to have prognostic significance. Current guidelines do not make a recommendation as to the use of a specific risk score calculator; a multimodal approach to risk stratification, which may include risk scores and functional class, is recommended.

b. Treatment initiation

The approach outlined here applies to patients with group 1 PAH. The PAH treatment algorithm does not apply to patients in other clinical groups, including groups 2 and 3.
1. **Vasoreactive** patients with PH that is idiopathic, heritable, or due to anorexigen use (see **Section II.E.1**) in low- or intermediate-risk categories should be started on CCBs as the initial treatment step.
2. **Low- or intermediate-risk** patients that are nonvasoreactive should be initiated on **combination therapy**, most commonly with an ERA and PDE5I. Initial monotherapy is generally not recommended but can be considered in specific treatment groups with very mild disease or at high risk for decompensation with treatment initiation (eg, older than 75 years, concomitant heart or liver failure).
3. **High-risk** patients should be initiated on **combination therapy** that includes an **IV PCA**. IV epoprostenol is the only IV PCA with favorable mortality data in these patients. Other acceptable options include IV or subcutaneous (SC) treprostinil.

c. Assessment of treatment response
1. **Repeat risk stratification:** Initiation and titration of PH-specific therapy is an iterative process. Patients should be reevaluated with repeat risk stratification every 3 to 6 months to determine treatment response and appropriate next steps in therapy.
2. **Escalation of therapy**
a. **Risk stratification 3 to 6 months after *initial* treatment step**
i. Patients who are **low risk** on reassessment after initial treatment step should continue current therapy, with repeat evaluation in another 3 to 6 months.
ii. Patients in the **intermediate-risk** category after their initial treatment step require escalation with sequential triple combination therapy with a PCA, ERA, and PDE5I/sGC.

iii. Patients who are **high risk** after their initial treatment step should be on **maximal medical therapy**, which typically consists of triple combination therapy including an IV PCA.

b. Risk stratification 3 to 6 months after *second* treatment step

i. Patients in the **low-risk** category after the second treatment step should continue current therapy with ongoing structured follow-up.

ii. Patients in **intermediate-** or **high-risk** categories after the second treatment step should be escalated to **maximal medical therapy** including an IV (preferred for high-risk patients) or SC PCA.

d. Referral for consideration of lung transplantation should be considered in all patients with intermediate- or high-risk disease on subsequent evaluation despite optimal medical treatment.

3. Management considerations for patients in WHO groups 2-5

a. Group 2: Management should be focused on optimization of heart disease. It is unclear whether there is a role for PH-specific therapy in selected patients with combined pre-/postcapillary PH. This is controversial and should be managed at an expert center.

b. Group 3: Management also centers on optimization of lung disease. PH-specific therapies are generally not beneficial in this group given their potential to worsen $\dot{V}/\dot{Q}$ matching. The FDA recently approved the use of inhaled treprostinil in patients with PH and interstitial lung disease (ILD) because it was shown to improve 6MWD in this select patient group.

c. Group 4: All patients with CTEPH should be started on indefinite anticoagulation and evaluated at a CTEPH center for consideration of PTE, which is the only potentially curative therapy available. For patients who are not surgical candidates, BPA and/or PH-specific therapy can be considered. The sGC riociguat is the only PH-specific therapy that is FDA approved for the management of group 4 PH.

d. Group 5: This is a heterogeneous group of patients whose treatment is oriented toward the underlying disease process.

IV. CRITICAL CARE MANAGEMENT OF PULMONARY HYPERTENSION AND RIGHT VENTRICULAR FAILURE

A. Causes of Right Ventricular Failure in the Intensive Care Unit

1. Acute RV failure in the critically ill can be due to a variety of causes, including, but not limited to, pulmonary embolism (PE), acute respiratory distress syndrome (ARDS)/acute respiratory failure, decompensated left heart disease, RV infarction, or preexisting PH.

2. RV failure in patients with preexisting PH can occur due to both disease progression and acute decompensation in the setting of other critical illnesses. RV failure is the most common cause of death in patients with PH.

B. Definition: Right-sided heart failure is characterized by low CO/cardiac index (CI) and/or elevated right-sided filling pressures. When right heart failure is severe, it results in end-organ hypoperfusion, often manifesting as kidney injury, liver injury, or intestinal ischemia.

C. Pathophysiology of Right-Sided Heart Failure: The right ventricle is a thin-walled crescent-shaped structure that is adapted to eject into the low-resistance pulmonary circulation and generates less contractile force than does the left ventricle. Because of these characteristics, the right ventricle is particularly sensitive to volume and pressure loading. Excessive RV preload or afterload results in RV dilation, increased RV wall stress, and impairment in right coronary perfusion. RV hypoperfusion further impairs RV contractility, worsening RV dilation and wall stress and contributing to the development of tricuspid regurgitation. RV dilation and volume overload also lead to displacement of the interventricular septum and impairment of LV diastolic filling, further worsening CO. This cyclical cascade of RV distension, dysfunction, and ischemia is often referred to as the *RV death spiral* and is summarized in Figure 23.3.

D. Management of Right Ventricular Failure

1. Fluid management and optimization of right ventricular preload

The phrase "preload dependent" is often applied to the right ventricle and should be used with caution. RV output is augmented by increases in preload only within a certain range of volumes (as illustrated by the Starling curve). Management of volume status can be challenging in patients with RV failure because both hypovolemia and hypervolemia can have negative effects on blood pressure, organ perfusion, and CO. If hypovolemia is suspected, fluid administration should be done cautiously and with the guidance of objective data—central venous pressure (CVP) monitoring, although of dubious utility in the general population in the ICU, may be useful for guiding fluid management in RV failure, as is monitoring of CO via $ScvO_2$. Most cases of RV failure, particularly in patients with excessive RV afterload (eg, patients with pulmonary vascular disease), are associated with volume overload and high right-sided filling pressures. Volume removal via diuresis or ultrafiltration in this setting is paramount for optimizing RV function. Given the compliant, distensible nature of the right ventricle, significant volume removal may be required to achieve any improvement

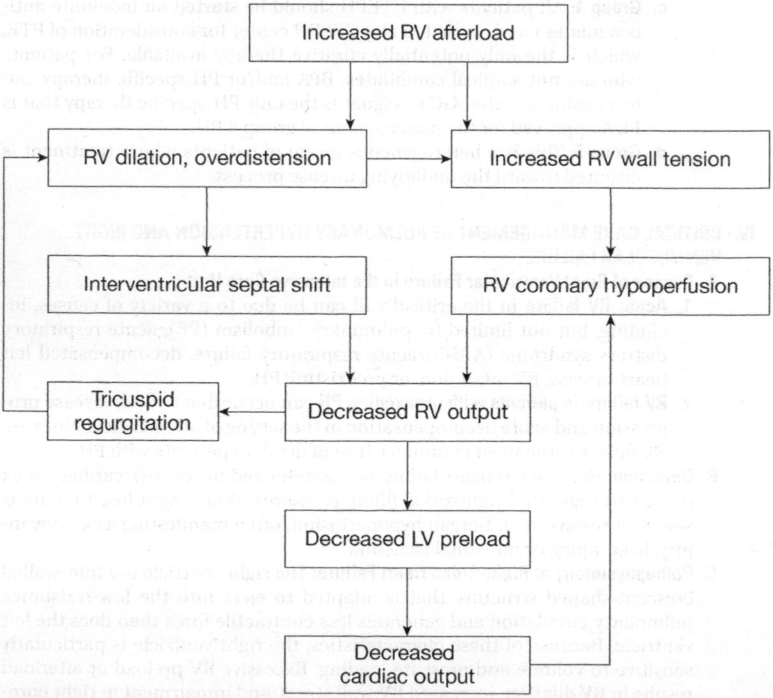

FIGURE 23.3 The "death spiral" of RV failure. LV, left ventricular; RV, right ventricular.

in RV contractility and CO in a patient who is volume overloaded. In some instances, vasopressors may be required to maintain adequate mean arterial pressure (MAP) to facilitate volume removal and maintain coronary perfusion pressure.

2. **Vasopressors and inotropes in RV failure:** There is relatively limited evidence available from clinical trials to guide use of vasoactive and inotropic agents in patients with PH and RV failure. This is a generalized approach based on available evidence and guidelines.
   a. **Vasopressors** should be used for the management of systemic hypotension in patients with RV failure. As discussed earlier, maintaining systemic blood pressure (typically MAP >60 mm Hg) is critical for adequate coronary perfusion of the RV. Norepinephrine is the preferred initial pressor given its balance of vasoconstrictive and inotropic effects. Vasopressin is also a good choice and has been shown to have pulmonary vasodilatory effects at lower doses. Phenylephrine does have favorable effects on coronary perfusion; however, it is typically avoided in RV failure because it can increase PVR and worsen RV afterload.
   b. **Inotropes** can be used in RV failure to optimize CO. Inotropes to choose from include epinephrine, dopamine, dobutamine, and milrinone. The use of inotropes with systemic vasodilatory effects such as dobutamine and milrinone may be limited by systemic hypotension and often need to be utilized in conjunction with vasopressors. Both dobutamine and milrinone increase contractility and are commonly used in RV failure. Milrinone may have the added benefit of lowering PVR, whereas dobutamine has been shown to improve RV/PA coupling. Dopamine does improve CI in patients with RV failure; however, many avoid this agent given the increased risk of tachyarrhythmia. Epinephrine may be favored in cases of refractory shock or low systemic vascular resistance (SVR) state given its vasoconstrictive effects.
3. **Management of pulmonary vasodilators**
   a. **For patients who are already on PH-specific therapy with decompensated PH and RV failure,** consultation with a PH specialist or transfer to a PH specialty center is strongly recommended to assist with management. In general, PH-specific therapies should be continued in an effort to offload the failing RV. However, therapies with greater systemic vasodilatory effects—for example, PDE5Is, sGCs—may need to be withheld in the setting of hypotension and shock. ERAs are less likely to cause systemic hypotension and can often be continued. IV and SC PCAs should be continued at their current doses unless otherwise directed by a PH specialist. If systemic administration of pulmonary vasodilators is not feasible, either due to systemic hypotension or due to technical issues, then substitution with inhaled pulmonary vasodilators (eg, iNO, inhaled PCAs) can be considered.
   b. **For patients with PH and RV failure *not* already on PH-specific therapy**, pulmonary vasodilators can be advanced in the ICU setting. These agents should generally only be considered once patients' RV hemodynamics are otherwise optimized through volume management, ventilator management, and vasoactive medications. Use of systemic PH-specific therapy is often limited by hypotension and the potential for worsening $\dot{V}/\dot{Q}$ mismatch for patients with concomitant respiratory failure. Inhaled pulmonary vasodilators—including iNO and inhaled PCAs—are frequently used given their rapid onset of action, minimal systemic absorption, and theoretically favorable effects on $\dot{V}/\dot{Q}$ matching. For patients with known PAH, combination PH-specific therapy has been

successfully advanced in the patient with RV failure who is critically ill; if pursued, this should be done cautiously and under the supervision of a PH specialist.

4. **Mechanical circulatory support**
   a. **Extracorporeal membrane oxygenation (ECMO)** has been used successfully as a bridge to recovery in the setting of reversible causes of PH (eg, acute PE) and as a bridge to pulmonary or cardiopulmonary transplant (eg, for patients with PAH). Venoarterial (VA) cannulation is typically required in the setting of PH and RV failure to manage concomitant cardiogenic shock and respiratory failure. ECMO is a short-term intervention associated with significant complications and should only be considered in cases refractory to maximal medical management and where there is a reasonable "exit strategy" from ECMO (ie, reversible condition or transplant).
   b. **Right ventricular assist devices (RVADs)** have also been utilized in cases of RV failure related to PH. Both percutaneous and surgically implanted devices are available and are only approved for temporary use. Some RVADs can be combined with an extracorporeal membrane oxygenator for combined cardiopulmonary support.

Selected Readings

Benza RL, Miller DP, Gomberg-Maitland M, et al. Predicting survival in pulmonary arterial hypertension. *Circulation.* 2010;122(2):164-172. doi:10.1161/CIRCULATIONAHA.109.898122

Boucly A, Weatherald J, Savale L, et al. Risk assessment, prognosis and guideline implementation in pulmonary arterial hypertension. *Eur Respir J.* 2017;50(2):1700889. doi:10.1183/13993003.00889-2017

Frost A, Badesch D, Gibbs JSR, et al. Diagnosis of pulmonary hypertension. *Eur Respir J.* 2019;53(1):1801904. doi:10.1183/13993003.01904-2018

Galiè N, Channick RN, Frantz RP, et al. Risk stratification and medical therapy of pulmonary arterial hypertension. *Eur Respir J.* 2019;53(1):1801889. doi:10.1183/13993003.01889

Galiè N, Humbert M, Vachiery J-L, et al. 2015 ESC/ERS guidelines for the diagnosis and treatment of pulmonary hypertension. *Eur Heart J.* 2016;37(1):67-119. doi:10.1093/eurheartj/ehv317

Harjola V-P, Mebazaa A, Čelutkienė J, et al. Contemporary management of acute right ventricular failure: a statement from the Heart Failure Association and the Working Group on Pulmonary Circulation and Right Ventricular Function of the European Society of Cardiology. *Eur J Heart Fail.* 2016;18(3):226-241. doi:10.1002/EJHF.478

Hoeper MM, Benza RL, Corris P, et al. Intensive care, right ventricular support and lung transplantation in patients with pulmonary hypertension. *Eur Respir J.* 2019;53(1):1801906. doi:10.1183/13993003.01906-2018

Hoeper MM, Granton J. Intensive care unit management of patients with severe pulmonary hypertension and right heart failure. *Am J Respir Crit Care Med.* 2011;184(10):1114-1124. doi:10.1164/rccm.201104-0662CI

Hoeper MM, Humbert M. The new haemodynamic definition of pulmonary hypertension: evidence prevails, finally! *Eur Respir J.* 2019;53(3):1900038. doi:10.1183/13993003.00038-2019

Hoeper MM, Kramer T, Pan Z, et al. Mortality in pulmonary arterial hypertension: prediction by the 2015 European pulmonary hypertension guidelines risk stratification model. *Eur Respir J.* 2017;50(2):1700740. doi:10.1183/13993003.00740-2017

Kim NH, Delcroix M, Jais X, et al. Chronic thromboembolic pulmonary hypertension. *Eur Respir J.* 2019;53(1):1801915. doi:10.1183/13993003.01915-2018

Kylhammar D, Kjellström B, Hjalmarsson C, et al. A comprehensive risk stratification at early follow-up determines prognosis in pulmonary arterial hypertension. *Eur Heart J.* 2018;39(47):4175-4181. doi:10.1093/EURHEARTJ/EHX257

Lee WTN, Ling Y, Sheares KK, Pepke-Zaba J, Peacock AJ, Johnson MK. Predicting survival in pulmonary arterial hypertension in the UK. *Eur Respir J.* 2012;40(3):604-611. doi:10.1183/09031936.00196611

Price LC, Wort SJ, Finney SJ, Marino PS, Brett SJ. Pulmonary vascular and right ventricular dysfunction in adult critical care: current and emerging options for management: a systematic literature review. *Crit Care.* 2010;14(5):1-22. doi:10.1186/CC9264

Rich JD, Shah SJ, Swamy RS, Kamp A, Rich S. Inaccuracy of Doppler echocardiographic estimates of pulmonary artery pressures in patients with pulmonary hypertension. *Chest.* 2011;139(5):988-993. doi:10.1378/chest.10-1269

Simonneau G, Montani D, Celermajer DS, et al. Haemodynamic definitions and updated clinical classification of pulmonary hypertension. *Eur Respir J.* 2019;53(1):1801913. doi:10.1183/13993003.01913-2018

Sitbon O, Gomberg-Maitland M, Granton J, et al. Clinical trial design and new therapies for pulmonary arterial hypertension. *Eur Respir J.* 2019;53(1):1801908. doi:10.1183/13993003.01908-2018

Vachiéry J-L, Tedford RJ, Rosenkranz S, et al. Pulmonary hypertension due to left heart disease. *Eur Respir J.* 2019;53(1):1801897. doi:10.1183/13993003.01897-2018

Ventetuolo CE, Klinger JR. Management of acute right ventricular failure in the intensive care unit. *Ann Am Thorac Soc.* 2014;11(5):811-822. doi:10.1513/AnnalsATS.201312-446FR

Vonk Noordegraaf A, Chin KM, Haddad F, et al. Pathophysiology of the right ventricle and of the pulmonary circulation in pulmonary hypertension: an update. *Eur Respir J.* 2019;53(1):1801900. doi:10.1183/13993003.01900-2018

Waxman A, Restrepo-Jaramillo R, Thenappan T, et al. Inhaled treprostinil in pulmonary hypertension due to interstitial lung disease. *N Engl J Med.* 2021;384(4):325-334. doi:10.1056/NEJMoa2008470

Weitsman T, Weisz G, Farkash R, et al. Pulmonary hypertension with left heart disease: prevalence, temporal shifts in etiologies and outcome. *Am J Med.* 2017;130(11):1272-1279. doi:10.1016/j.amjmed.2017.05.003

Zamanian RT, Haddad F, Doyle RL, Weinacker AB. Management strategies for patients with pulmonary hypertension in the intensive care unit. *Crit Care Med.* 2007;35(9):2037-2050. doi:10.1097/01.CCM.0000280433.74246.9E

24

Discontinuation of Mechanical Ventilation

Dean R. Hess

I. INTRODUCTION

The safe discontinuation of mechanical ventilation is the goal for most patients on mechanical ventilation. An exception is patients with progressive neuromuscular disease or those with end-stage terminal disease. Advancements in the management of sedation, delirium, and volume status over the past 20 years, as well as improvements to ventilator strategies, have led to shorter time on mechanical ventilation and better hospital outcomes. An understanding of approaches to successful ventilator discontinuation is paramount to the care of the patient who is intubated.

II. DEFINITIONS

A. **Spontaneous Awakening Trial:** the cessation of all sedatives or decreasing doses of sedative infusions to allow a patient to interact and follow commands

B. **Spontaneous Breathing Trial:** a decrease in the amount of support provided by a mechanical ventilator to test the patient's ability to breathe without support

C. **Weaning:** decreasing ventilator settings in a stepwise approach to determine the patient's minimal ventilator needs

D. **Liberation/Discontinuation:** Liberation or discontinuation refers to complete transition from mechanical ventilation to spontaneous breathing (ie, ventilator free).

E. **Ventilator Dependence:** the inability to liberate a patient from mechanical ventilation despite repeated attempts

F. **Extubation:** removal of the endotracheal tube (ETT)

G. **Decannulation:** removal of the tracheostomy tube

III. VENTILATOR DEPENDENCE

This can be due to a variety of reasons and a thorough investigation into each of these is central to the care of patients on ventilation.

A. Nervous System

1. **Primary brain injury:** can lead to damage to respiratory control centers in the brain. Examples include stroke, hemorrhage, mass effect, cerebral edema, seizures, and central apnea.
2. **Sedating medications:** can decrease respiratory drive
3. **Spinal cord and peripheral nerves:** Damage can impair the function of the diaphragm and intercostal muscles.
4. **Critical illness myopathy/critical illness polyneuropathy:** Each is multifactorial, related to length of immobility, degree of critical illness, use of systemic steroids, and paralytic agents. The presence of critical illness myopathy (CIM) or critical illness polyneuropathy (CIP) can lead to impaired function of the diaphragm and accessory muscles of inhalation, resulting in respiratory failure.
5. **Psychological:** Untreated/undertreated anxiety or other psychiatric diseases may lead to unnecessary anxiety surrounding the removal of ventilator support. Reassurance or low-dose anxiolytics may be necessary, depending on the clinical scenario.

6. **Respiratory drive ($P_{0.1}$):** This is a measure of respiratory drive; it is the pressure generated against an occluded airway 0.1 second (100 ms) after the onset of inspiration. Normal $P_{0.1}$ is -0.5 to -1.5 cm H_2O. In patients on mechanical ventilation, it is typically -3 to -6 cm H_2O. Although $P_{0.1}$ is poorly predictive of readiness for spontaneous breathing, a high respiratory drive ($P_{0.1}$ more negative than -6 cm H_2O) is associated with a failed spontaneous breathing trial (SBT).

B. Respiratory Muscles

1. **Electrolyte imbalances:** Phosphate and magnesium are central to muscular function. Severe depletions are associated with muscle weakness and may lead to difficulty with ventilator liberation.
2. **Nutritional factors:** Inadequate nutrition can lead to muscle catabolism, which may result in respiratory muscle weakness and prolonged reliance on mechanical ventilation. Conversely, overfeeding can result in excess CO_2 production and resultant increases in minute ventilation.
3. **Endocrine imbalances:** Cortisol, insulin, and glucagon have been implicated in normal respiratory muscle function, and deficiencies in each have been hypothesized to lead to compromised function. Hypothyroidism may result in diaphragmatic weakness.
4. **Muscle pressures**
   a. **Maximum inspiratory pressure:** This is a measure of inspiratory muscle strength. It is the maximum inspiratory pressure (MIP, P_{Imax}) that can be generated against an occluded airway. Normal individuals can generate a P_{Imax} more negative than -80 cm H_2O. Inability to generate at least -25 cm H_2O suggests respiratory muscle weakness as a contributor to a failed SBT. However, P_{Imax} is a poor predictor of liberation potential.
   b. **Maximum expiratory pressure:** This is a measure of expiratory muscle strength. It is the maximum expiratory pressure (MEP, P_{Emax}) that can be generated against an occluded airway. Normal individuals can generate a P_{Emax} of at least 80 cm H_2O. A low P_{Emax} results in a weak cough and potential benefit for cough assist therapy after extubation.

C. Pulmonary Mechanics: Both increased resistance and decreased compliance increase the amount of inspiratory work. The degree to which resistance and compliance are abnormal determines the degree to which a patient will be reliant on the ventilator.

1. **Resistance:** the opposition to airflow in the respiratory system
   a. Increased airways resistance can be due to bronchospasm, increased respiratory secretions, airway inflammation, ETT or tracheostomy tube obstruction, or small diameter of ETT.
2. **Compliance:** the ability of the thorax and lungs to expand their volume as transmural pressure increases. Measured at end inhalation during a breath hold; the reciprocal of elastic recoil
   a. **Chest wall** compliance may be impaired because of morbid obesity, chest wall bony abnormalities, or intra-abdominal processes that interfere with diaphragm function.
   b. **Lung** compliance can be decreased because of consolidation, fibrosis, or pulmonary edema.
3. **Auto–positive end-expiratory pressure:** increased end-expiratory intra-alveolar pressure caused by incomplete exhalation. Can be caused by increased resistance or tachypnea. Of specific concern in patients with severe obstructive lung disease, which may complicate ventilator liberation
4. **Minute ventilation:** required to maintain normal acid-base status. Increased minute ventilation requirement may indicate increased CO_2 production or increased dead space. High minute ventilation requirements (particularly >10 L/min) may not be tolerated by the patient who is newly extubated

and should suggest to the clinician that a search for undiagnosed underlying causes be undertaken.

a. Rapid-shallow breathing index: The minute ventilation can be divided by respiratory rate to produce tidal volume, and then the tidal volume (in liters) can be divided by the respiratory rate to produce the rapid-shallow breathing index (RSBI). An RSBI greater than 105 has been proposed as predictive of extubation failure conversely, a RSBI < 105 is predictive of success. The RSBI was proposed more than a decade before SBTs became fashionable. Given the safety of SBTs, and that a 30-minute SBT is predictive of extubation success, the RSBI has fallen out of common use.

D. Inadequate Gas Exchange: High levels of fraction of inspired oxygen (FIO_2) and PEEP may be required because of shunt (ie, pneumonia, acute respiratory distress syndrome [ARDS], pulmonary edema, fibrosis).

E. Cardiovascular Disease: Patients with cardiac dysfunction may not tolerate the additional stress to the cardiovascular system that the removal of mechanical ventilation can cause. Underlying coronary artery disease may manifest as chest pressure or pain during an SBT or following extubation that is related to stress-induced cardiac ischemia. Patients with congestive heart failure (CHF) may develop acute pulmonary edema because of the removal of positive pressure and the subsequent increase in venous return.

IV. STANDARDIZED CARE OF THE PATIENT WHO IS INTUBATED

A. The **ABCDEF** bundle. Applied daily to all patients who are intubated:

A: *A*ssess, prevent, and manage pain.
B: *B*oth SAT and SBT
C: *C*hoice of analgesia and sedation
D: *D*elirium—assessment, prevention, and management
E: *E*arly mobility and *E*xercise
F: *F*amily engagement and empowerment

B. Addition of the Spontaneous Awakening Trial to the usual care of patients who are intubated (as opposed to sedation management at the discretion of the clinician) leads to fewer days on mechanical ventilation and in the intensive care unit (ICU), without complications such as self-extubation.

C. Early Mobilization: Physical therapy that begins while intubated, during periods of lightened sedation, is safe and leads to more functional independence after hospital discharge, less delirium, and more ventilator-free days.

V. SEDATION MANAGEMENT

A. Consider an **analgesia-first strategy** to treat pain symptoms, adding a sedative only if the patient remains uncomfortable after pain control is achieved.

B. Short-Acting Agents are preferred to long-acting agents because of both quicker onset of action and shorter duration of effect once discontinued. Renal and liver dysfunction affects timely clearance of medications.

C. Use the **lowest necessary continuous infusion rates**. When possible, use intermittent intravenous (IV) bolus dosing rather than continuous infusion.

D. Use a validated scale to set sedation targets, such as the **RASS** (Richmond Agitation Sedation Scale).

1. −5 (unarousable) to +4 (combative)
2. Target: 0 (alert and calm) to −1 (drowsy)

E. Sedative Choices

1. **Propofol:** γ-aminobutyric acid (GABA) potentiation
   - **a.** Side effects: Hypotension, propofol infusion syndrome (rare), hypertriglyceridemia
2. **Dexmedetomidine** (Precedex): α_2-agonist
   - **a.** Side effects: hypotension, bradycardia
   - **b.** High cost

3. **Midazolam** (Versed): GABA potentiation
    a. Hepatic metabolites are also active GABA potentiators.
    b. Side effects: Prolonged sedation once discontinued, delirium

F. **Analgesia:** Intermittent boluses or continuous infusions of opiates are utilized for pain control in patients who are intubated. Common opiates in the ICU include the following:
1. **Fentanyl:** short acting, fast onset. Most used opiate infusion for intubated patients
2. **Morphine:** short acting, fast onset. Avoid in renal dysfunction because of accumulation of toxic metabolites.
3. **Hydromorphone** (Dilaudid): short acting, fast onset. Seven times stronger than morphine

VI. DELIRIUM IN THE INTENSIVE CARE UNIT

A. Increases risk of longer hospital stays, death, higher hospital costs, and prolonged cognitive impairment at 1 year

B. **Confusion Assessment Method-Intensive Care Unit (CAM-ICU):**
1. Positive (delirium present) or negative (delirium absent)

C. **Treating Delirium**
1. Frequent reorientation, sleep-wake cycle protection (light during the day, dark at night), familiar surroundings
2. Medications
    a. Haloperidol (IV, intramuscular [IM]): short acting, fast onset
    b. Quetiapine (po), olanzapine (po, sublingually [SL]): longer acting, more sedating
    c. **Side effects:** QTc prolongation, rarely neuroleptic malignant syndrome (NMS), torticollis, extrapyramidal symptoms

VII. ASSESSING FOR VENTILATOR DISCONTINUATION POTENTIAL

Patients need to be assessed daily for whether they meet the criteria for the discontinuation of mechanical ventilation. To be considered for ventilator liberation, the following parameters must be considered:

A. **Underlying Pathophysiology:** The initial cause of respiratory failure should be either resolved or significantly improving.

B. **Hemodynamics:** The patient's blood pressure and heart rate should be stable, with either stable or decreasing vasopressor needs and without serious cardiac instability.

C. **Oxygenation:** Generally, an FIO_2 of 0.5 or less and PEEP of 8 cm H_2O or less indicate that any remaining hypoxemia will be able to adequately corrected with supplemental oxygen after extubation.

D. **Ventilation:** The patient must be able to maintain a pH of 7.3 or higher, with a minute ventilation that they can maintain without ventilator assistance.

E. **Weaning Parameters:** In the past, several weaning parameters have been proposed, but none is more predictive than a 30-minute SBT.

VIII. VENTILATOR MODES AND WEANING

A. High-level evidence does not support a gradual, stepwise decrease in ventilatory support.
1. Gradual weaning of **pressure support ventilation (PSV)**, until the patient is tolerating PSV 5/5 cm H_2O
2. Gradually decreasing the ventilator rate for **synchronized intermittent mandatory ventilation (SIMV)** so that the patient takes more spontaneous breaths

B. An SBT with direct transition to PSV 0/0 or 5/0 cm H_2O

1. A **daily SBT** of at least 30 minutes is superior to gradual weaning of either SIMV or PSV.
2. Most patients who tolerate an SBT for 30 minutes tolerate subsequent extubation.

C. Modes that automatically wean

1. **Smartcare** adjusts PSV depending on the patient's tidal volume, respiratory rate, and end-tidal P_{CO_2}. When the patient is weaned to low pressure, an SBT is performed and, if successful, the ventilator prompts to consider extubation.
2. **Adaptive support ventilation** adjusts rate and tidal volume to minimize work of breathing. If the patient is triggering, the number of mandatory breaths decreases and the ventilator chooses a pressure support that maintains a tidal volume sufficient to ensure alveolar ventilation, thus weaning the patient from the ventilator.
3. **Volume support ventilation** adjusts PSV to maintain a constant tidal volume. In this way, the ventilator reduces the pressure as the patient generates a greater inspiratory effort.
4. Despite that these modes have some evidence supporting their use, they are not clearly superior to SBTs. Moreover, their use is limited because they are not available on all ventilator brands.

IX. TECHNICAL APPROACHES TO THE SPONTANEOUS BREATHING TRIAL

A. All sedation should be discontinued. In select patients with agitation, low levels of sedatives may need to be continued, but the patient should typically be alert, interactive, and able to follow commands.

B. Ventilator Settings

1. **Pressure support ventilation 5/5:** Pressure support of 5 cm H_2O and PEEP of 5 cm H_2O are commonly used for SBTs. However, this level of support might result in false positives for extubation readiness because of the level of support provided.
2. **Pressure support ventilation 5/0:** Pressure support of 5 cm H_2O and PEEP of 0 cm H_2O. Although this is recommended in clinical practice guidelines, it does not realistically estimate the patient effort required post extubation.
3. **Tube compensation:** This is a ventilator mode in which pressure support is applied as determined by ETT size and inspiratory flow. If this approach is used, PEEP should be set to zero.
4. **Pressure support ventilation 0/0:** No ventilator support is provided for the SBT. This approach most closely simulates the conditions following extubation. It is most important in patients with CHF or those with auto-PEEP. With CHF, removal of all positive pressure may lead to acute pulmonary edema, which ideally should be identified before extubation. With auto-PEEP, removal of all positive pressure might result in excessive inspiratory effort requirement, which again should ideally be identified before extubation.
5. **Continuous positive airway pressure:** In patients with morbid obesity, continuous positive airway pressure (CPAP) of 10 cm H_2O (or higher in some cases) should be used during the SBT. The same level of CPAP by face mask should be applied post extubation.

C. Duration of Spontaneous Breathing Trial

1. Most SBTs last 30 minutes or shorter if the patient is not tolerating. Longer trials may be used for patients who are more tenuous. However, the SBT should not extend 2 hours.

D. Recognizing a Failed Spontaneous Breathing Trial: There is no single marker of a failed SBT. Many clinical details are monitored simultaneously, and it is the constellation of clinical characteristics that leads to the overall assessment. If SBT failure is determined, the ventilator is set to an appropriate level of support and a search for the etiology of the failure is initiated.

1. **Uncontrolled agitation/anxiety:** Anxiety is a natural part of the extubation process, but the patient should be easily calmed and redirectable. If the patient cannot be refocused, consider whether this is the result of an underlying process that warrants prior correction.
2. **Vital sign instability:** The development of tachycardia, hypertension, diaphoresis, dyspnea, and/or tachypnea during an SBT suggests that the patient is not tolerating the additional work of breathing.
3. A failed SBT often occurs within **the first few minutes.** Therefore, close attention needs to be paid to the patient during this time.

X. FACTORS CONTRIBUTING TO A FAILED SPONTANEOUS BREATHING TRIAL

When patients do not tolerate spontaneous breathing on minimal ventilator support, a search for the contributing factors is initiated. In some instances, the reason for SBT failure may be closely related to the reason for intubation.

A. Resolution of the Disease Process: The most common cause of a failed SBT is insufficient resolution of the underlying disease process. After returning the patient to an appropriate level of support, the underlying disease process is treated aggressively (eg, diuresis, bronchodilators, airway clearance).

B. Mental Status: Depressed mental status, anxiety, agitation

1. If anxiety or agitation is the only barrier to extubation, dexmedetomidine may be considered as a sedative to facilitate SBT because it does not suppress the respiratory drive.

C. Ventilator-Induced Diaphragm Dysfunction: The additional load on the diaphragm during an SBT may overwhelm a patient weakened by ventilator-induced diaphragm dysfunction (VIDD). Either too little support or too much support can lead to VIDD. Thus, it is important to appropriately adjust the level of pressure support to avoid this complication.

D. Volume Status: Pulmonary edema can cause hypoxemia and respiratory distress when positive pressure is removed.

E. Tracheostomy Tube Malposition: In patients for whom a tracheostomy has been placed, the immediate failure of an SBT raises concern for malposition. Obstruction by granulation tissue or the posterior membrane of the trachea may lead to respiratory failure when positive pressure is removed.

F. Daily SBTs are as efficacious as SBTs done multiple times daily. Unless the cause of the failed SBT is rapidly resolved, available evidence does not support that multiple SBTs daily lead to more rapid liberation.

XI. EXTUBATION

Extubation is considered once the patient tolerates an SBT.

A. To be considered **appropriate for extubation**, the patient should:

1. Be awake and calm, able to follow simple commands
   a. **Caveat:** In patients who are intubated for respiratory failure related to neurologic conditions, poor mental status has not been shown to predict extubation failure. If mental status is the only concern, the patient may still be considered for extubation.
2. Require no continuous sedation infusions (or minimal sedation in select cases)
3. Show evidence of cough during suctioning or ETT manipulation
4. Have minimal secretions that are easily managed by infrequent suctioning

B. Cuff Leak Test: The ETT cuff is deflated, and the patient is evaluated for air leaking out of the mouth during application of positive pressure. The presence of a cuff leak suggests that there is space between the ETT and the tracheal wall, implying that there is no airway edema.
   1. The cuff leak test should be reserved for those at risk for postextubation stridor—traumatic intubation, intubation >6 days, large endotracheal tube, female sex, and reintubation after unplanned extubation.
   2. For a failed cuff leak test, administer systemic steroids at least 4 hours before extubation. A repeat cuff leak test is not required.

C. A reasonable reintubation rate is 10% to 20%. If the reintubation rate is less than 10%, it is likely that many patients are subjected to risks associated with excess intubation time. If the reintubation rate is greater than 20%, patients are subjected to risks associated with reintubation.

D. Complications associated with reintubation include developing ventilator-associated pneumonia, longer hospital stay, difficulty with the reintubation procedure and upper airway injury, and excess hospital mortality.

E. The Logistics: The respiratory therapist and nurse should be at the bedside. The patient is positioned upright and the oropharynx and trachea are suctioned. The ETT balloon is deflated, and the ETT is quickly removed. The suction catheter can be passed through the ETT and suction applied during extubation to remove sections from the upper airway as part of the procedure (trailing catheter method). The patient is placed on oxygen by nasal cannula and the flow is titrated per Spo_2. The patient is encouraged to cough and asked to speak to assess vocal cord function.
   1. **A raspy voice** is to be expected for the first day, but if it persists, the patient needs to be evaluated for vocal cord dysfunction, a known complication of intubation.

F. Specific Considerations
   1. **Upper airway edema:** a situation in which a cuff leak may be part of the assessment for extubation readiness
      a. If airway edema is of concern, administer IV steroids at least 4 hours before extubation.
      b. Consider arranging for an anesthesiologist to be present at the bedside at the time of extubation, especially if there is report of a difficult intubation.
      c. If postextubation stridor develops, consider the administration of epinephrine aerosol, heliox, and/or an additional dose of IV steroids. CPAP or noninvasive ventilation (NIV) may stent the airway, allowing time for the abovementioned therapies to work, but it is not a permanent solution.

XII. EXTUBATION TO NONINVASIVE VENTILATION OR HIGH-FLOW NASAL CANNULA

In patients at risk for extubation failure, extubation to NIV or high-flow nasal cannula (HFNC) decreases reintubation risk.

A. Consider immediate postextubation NIV in patients with COPD, CHF, previous reintubation, or respiratory muscle weakness.

B. In those at risk for extubation failure, consider NIV in patients with hypercapnic respiratory failure and consider HFNC in patients with hypoxemic respiratory failure. Some patients benefit from alternating use of NIV and HFNC.

C. NIV should not be used as a rescue technique for patients who develop respiratory distress after extubation because it delays reintubation and has been associated with increased mortality.

D. NIV and/or HFNC should not be used routinely post extubation but be reserved for those deemed at risk for extubation failure.

E. CPAP should be used when asleep post extubation in patients with a history of obstructive sleep apnea. Morbidly obese patients should also be extubated to CPAP or NIV.

XIII. CLINICAL PRACTICE GUIDELINES

A. Guidelines for liberation from mechanical ventilation in adults who are critically ill from the American College of Chest Physicians and the American Thoracic Society:

1. For hospitalized patients ventilated for more than 24 hours, suggest that the initial SBT be conducted with inspiratory pressure support (5-8 cm H_2O) rather than without (T-piece or CPAP).
2. For hospitalized patients ventilated for more than 24 hours, suggest protocols attempting to minimize sedation. There is insufficient evidence to recommend any protocol over another.
3. For patients at high risk for extubation failure who have been receiving mechanical ventilation for more than 24 hours and who have passed an SBT, recommend extubation to NIV.
4. For hospitalized adults who have been mechanically ventilated for more than 24 hours, suggest protocolized rehabilitation directed toward early mobilization.
5. Suggest managing hospitalized adults who have been mechanically ventilated for more than 24 hours with a ventilator liberation protocol.
6. Suggest performing a cuff leak test in adults on mechanical ventilation who meet extubation criteria and are deemed high risk for post extubation stridor. For adults who have failed a cuff leak test but are otherwise ready for extubation, suggest administering systemic steroids at least 4 hours before extubation; a repeated cuff leak test is not required.

XIV. PROLONGED MECHANICAL VENTILATION

A. Definition: at least 6 hours per day of mechanical ventilation for more than 21 consecutive days. The etiology of chronic respiratory failure is often multifactorial.

B. Special Considerations

1. **Ventilator liberation:** Unless an obviously irreversible disease process is responsible for ventilator dependence (ie, spinal cord injury, amyotrophic lateral sclerosis [ALS]), it can take several months to liberate these patients from mechanical ventilation.
   a. Trials of unassisted breathing with a tracheostomy collar, as compared to weaning with PSV, result in a shorter time to ventilator liberation.
2. **Multidisciplinary team approach:** These patients require close attention to adequate nutritional support, intensive physical therapy to strengthen and prevent contractures, speech therapy to combat swallowing dysfunction, and palliative care for longer term goals and discussions.
3. **Long-term weaning units:** Once patients are otherwise hemodynamically stable, specialized care in these units can accomplish all the abovementioned goals. Regular care by physicians, nurses, therapists (respiratory, physical, occupational), and speech-language pathologists is provided in a less intensive manner than in the hospital, which leads to decreased health care costs.
4. Lifelong mechanical ventilation may be necessary in some patients, for whom in-home ventilators can be arranged if ventilator settings are stable and they are not otherwise requiring inpatient monitoring.

C. Tracheostomy: When a patient fails ventilator liberation or requires reintubation, tracheostomy is considered for longer term ventilation.

1. **Benefits:** patient comfort, facilitates talking, less sedation required, possibly more rapid liberation from mechanical ventilation
2. **Timing:** The optimal timing of tracheostomy placement is debated. Traditionally, patients underwent tracheostomy after 14 days because of concerns over tracheomalacia related to ETT cuff pressures and tracheal wall venous insufficiency. This is no longer a concern because of monitoring of cuff pressures by respiratory therapists. Early (usually <1 week) versus late (usually >2 weeks) timing has not been shown to change ICU mortality, ventilator-free days, or length of stay.

XV. DECANNULATION

The removal of the tracheostomy tube once the patient no longer requires mechanical ventilation

A. Readiness for Decannulation: A patient should be considered for decannulation when:

1. No longer requiring mechanical ventilation
2. No respiratory distress with a capped tracheostomy tube and deflated cuff
   a. If respiratory distress prevents capping, the patient should be considered for downsizing of the tracheostomy to a smaller outer diameter. Generally, 6 or 7 mm inside diameter tracheostomy tubes are well tolerated.
   b. If respiratory distress occurs, visual inspection of regions above and below the tracheostomy via bronchoscopy should be conducted to evaluate for granulation tissue, strictures, vocal cord dysfunction, or other anatomic abnormalities that may be preventing independent breathing.
   c. The use of a fenestrated tracheostomy tube offers little additional benefit and can contribute to granulation tissue formation.
3. Effective cough, able to clear secretions
4. No evidence of significant aspiration with a deflated cuff

B. Approaches to Decannulation: The stoma will epithelialize 48 to 72 hours after tracheostomy removal, impairing replacement should respiratory distress develop.

1. **Removal of tracheostomy:** can be accomplished for patients in whom chronic respiratory or other medical conditions are not present
2. **Sequential downsizing of tracheostomy:** performed in patients for whom chronic respiratory or other medical conditions raise concern for possible decannulation failure (ie, COPD, neuromuscular diseases)
3. **Replacement of tracheostomy with a stomal button:** when access to the trachea for continued suctioning is desired

XVI. SUMMARY

The care of intubated patients in intensive care units has drastically changed over the past 20 years, with improvements leading to decreased days on mechanical ventilation and increased success following extubation. Reducing the duration of mechanical ventilation improves ICU outcomes, which is the goal of all care providers in the ICU.

Selected Readings

Barr J, Fraser GL, Puntillo K, et al. Clinical practice guidelines for the management of pain, agitation, and delirium in adult patients in the intensive care unit. *Crit Care Med.* 2013;41(1):263-306.

Blackwood B, Alderdice F, Burns K, Cardwell C, Lavery G, O'Halloran P. Use of weaning protocols for reducing duration of mechanical ventilation in critically ill adult patients: Cochrane systematic review and meta-analysis. *BMJ.* 2011;342:c7237.

Branson RD. Modes to facilitate ventilator weaning. *Respir Care.* 2012;57(10):1635-1648.

Burns KE, Lellouche F, Lessard MR. Automating the weaning process with advanced closed-loop systems. *Intensive Care Med.* 2008;34(10):1757-1765.

Burns KEA, Soliman I, Adhikari NKJ, et al. Trials directly comparing alternative spontaneous breathing trial techniques: a systematic review and meta-analysis. *Crit Care.* 2017;21(1):127.

Fan T, Wang G, Mao B, et al. Prophylactic administration of parenteral steroids for preventing airway complications after extubation in adults: meta-analysis of randomised placebo controlled trials. *BMJ.* 2008;337:a1841.

Girard TD, Kress JP, Fuchs BD, et al. Efficacy and safety of a paired sedation and ventilator weaning protocol for mechanically ventilated patients in intensive care (Awakening and Breathing Controlled trial): a randomised controlled trial. *Lancet.* 2008;371(9607):126-134.

Goligher EC, Dres M, Patel BK, et al. Lung- and diaphragm-protective ventilation. *Am J Respir Crit Care Med.* 2020;202(7):950-961.

Hess DR, MacIntyre NR. Ventilator discontinuation: why are we still weaning? *Am J Respir Crit Care Med.* 2011;184(4):392-394.

Jubran A, Grant BJB, Duffner LA, et al. Effect of pressure support vs unassisted breathing through a tracheostomy collar on weaning duration in patients requiring prolonged mechanical ventilation: a randomized trial. *JAMA.* 2013;309(7):671-677.

Mekontso Dessap A, Roche-Campo F, Kouatchet A, et al. Natriuretic peptide-driven fluid management during ventilator weaning: a randomized controlled trial. *Am J Respir Crit Care Med.* 2012;186(12):1256-1263.

Pun BT, Balas MC, Barnes-Daly MA, et al. Caring for critically ill patients with the ABCDEF bundle: results of the ICU Liberation Collaborative in over 15,000 adults. *Crit Care Med.* 2019;47(1):3-14.

Qaseem A, Etxeandia-Ikobaltzeta I, Fitterman N, Williams JW Jr, Kansagara D. Appropriate use of high-flow nasal oxygen in hospitalized patients for initial or postextubation management of acute respiratory failure: a clinical guideline from the American College of Physicians. *Ann Intern Med.* 2021;174(7):977-984.

Schmidt GA, Girard TD, Kress JP, et al. Liberation from mechanical ventilation in critically ill adults: executive summary of an official American College of Chest Physicians/American Thoracic Society clinical practice guideline. *Chest.* 2017;151(1):160-165.

Schmidt U, Hess D, Kwo J, et al. Tracheostomy tube malposition in patients admitted to a respiratory acute care unit following prolonged ventilation. *Chest.* 2008;134(2):288-294.

Sklar MC, Burns K, Rittayamai N, et al. Effort to breathe with various spontaneous breathing trial techniques. a physiologic meta-analysis. *Am J Respir Crit Care Med.* 2017;195(11):1477-1485.

Stelfox HT, Crimi C, Berra L, et al. Determinants of tracheostomy decannulation: an international survey. *Crit Care.* 2008;12(1):R26.

Thille AW, Gacouin A, Coudroy R, et al. Spontaneous-breathing trials with pressure-support ventilation or a T-piece. *N Engl J Med.* 2022;387(20):1843-1854.

Tobin MJ. Extubation and the myth of "minimal ventilator settings." *Am J Respir Crit Care Med.* 2012;185(4):349-350.

Trivedi V, Chaudhuri D, Jinah R, et al. The usefulness of the rapid shallow breathing index in predicting successful extubation: a systematic review and meta-analysis. *Chest.* 2022;161(1):97-111.

25 Acute Kidney Injury

William J. Benedetto

I. DEFINITION

A. The RIFLE criteria (**R**isk, **I**njury, **F**ailure, **L**oss, and **E**SRD [end-stage renal disease]) were developed in 2004 to standardize the definition of acute kidney injury (AKI), formerly called acute renal failure (ARF). Before this, no consensus was available on the diagnosis or degree of severity.

1. Several modifications were introduced by the Acute Kidney Injury Network (AKIN) soon after, although the main addition with AKIN was a more inclusive Stage 1 (≥0.3 mg/dL increase in creatinine [Cr]).
2. In 2012, the Kidney Disease Improving Global Outcomes Organization (KDIGO) published clinical practice guidelines to create a unified definition with the goal of improving outcome staging and future clinical research (because RIFLE and AKIN did not completely coincide).
3. Although these (see Table 25.1) were created to help standardize clinical outcomes research, they are helpful when assessing the severity of injury and level of management (Figure 25.1).
4. **Serum Cr criteria:** Although well validated, discrepancies exist between various definitions (eg, misclassification of AKI using AKIN in patients in

TABLE 25.1 Classification of Acute Kidney Injury

	Serum creatinine criteria			
	RIFLE	***AKIN***	***KDIGO***	**Urine output criteria**
1—R	>1.5 × baseline or GFR decrease >25%	≥0.3 mg/dL increase or ≥1.5-2 × baseline	1.5-1.9 × baseline or >0.3 mg/dL increase (within 48 h)	<0.5 mL/kg/h for 6-12 h
2—I	>2 × baseline or GFR decrease >50%	>2-3 × baseline	2-2.9 × baseline	<0.5 mL/kg/h for 12 h
3—F	>3 × baseline or Cr >4 mg/dL with an acute rise >0.5 mg/dL	>3 × baseline or ≥4.0 mg/dL with acute increase of ≥0.5 mg/dL or initiation of RRT	3 × baseline or increase in serum Cr ≥4 mg/dL or initiation of RRT	<0.3 mL/kg/h for 24 h or anuria for 12 h
L	*Loss of renal function >4 wk*			
E	*End-stage renal disease*	*←Outcome classes for RIFLE criteria*		

AKIN, Acute Kidney Injury Network; Cr, creatinine; GFR, glomerular filtration rate; KDIGO, Kidney Disease Improving Global Outcomes Organization; RIFLE, Risk, Injury, Failure, Loss, ESRD (end-stage renal disease); RRT, renal replacement therapy.

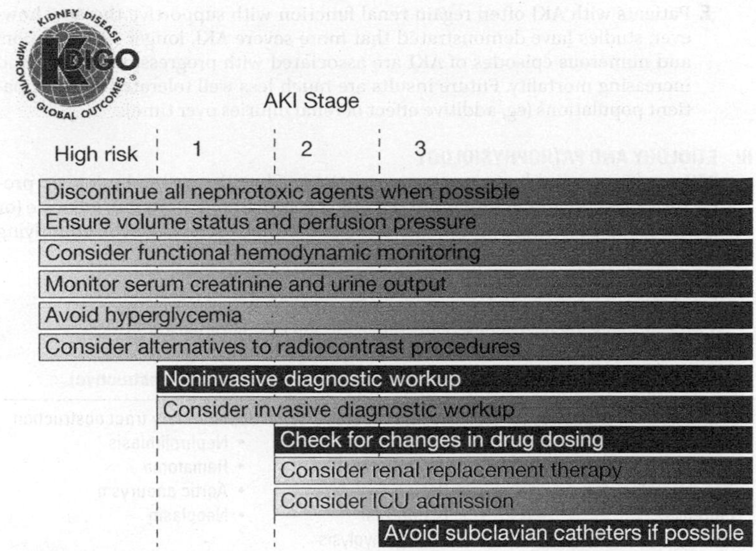

FIGURE 25.1 Stage-based management of AKI. Shading of boxes indicates priority of action—solid shading indicates actions that are equally appropriate at all stages, whereas graded shading indicates increasing priority as intensity increases. AKI, acute kidney injury; ICU, intensive care unit. (Reprinted from Kidney Disease: Improving Global Outcomes [KDIGO] Acute Kidney Injury Work Group. KDIGO clinical practice guideline for acute kidney injury. *Kidney Int Suppl.* 2012;1(2):1-138, with permission from Elsevier.)

postsurgical intensive care unit [ICU] after cardiopulmonary bypass with significant positive fluid balance resulting in hemodilution).

5. Urine volume criteria are the same for all three (RIFLE/AKIN/KDIGO) but oftentimes they are less accurate (eg, morbid obesity).
6. Validation studies are currently underway to establish the utility of these guidelines, particularly with regard to diagnosis and outcome.

II. EPIDEMIOLOGY

A. The historical lack of a standardized definition results in variable epidemiologic data for AKI. Information bias and residual confounding (eg, variability in baseline measures, the use of diagnostic code results), as well as ascertainment bias (AKI vs chronic kidney disease [CKD], which have different pathophysiologic processes, and outcome data), result in differences in reported incidence and outcome measurements.

B. Even with the abovementioned definitions, studies demonstrate significant differences in the incidence of AKI in the ICU when comparing the same populations.

C. Nonetheless, AKI is common in both patient populations—hospitalized (5%-20%) and critically ill (30%-40%).

D. Higher level of severity in AKI classification (by any of the abovementioned definitions) is associated with adverse outcomes, including increased length of stay, progressive kidney disease, and mortality.

E. AKI is an independent risk factor for cardiovascular complications and mortality; AKI requiring renal replacement therapy (RRT) reveals an in-hospital mortality of 50% to 75%. Studies have revealed that up to 28% of surviving patients with AKI died after discharge from the hospital (ie, in-hospital mortality likely underestimates the significance of disease).

F. Patients with AKI often regain renal function with supportive therapy; however, studies have demonstrated that more severe AKI, longer AKI duration, and numerous episodes of AKI are associated with progression to CKD and increasing mortality. Future insults are much less well tolerated in these patient populations (eg, additive effect of renal injuries over time).

III. ETIOLOGY AND PATHOPHYSIOLOGY

AKI is often caused by more than one etiology, but the pathophysiologic processes can be separated into three separate classifications: prerenal, intrinsic (or "renal"), and postrenal injuries. This is helpful both to determine the underlying etiology and for management (Table 25.2).

TABLE 25.2 Etiologies of Acute Kidney Injury in the Intensive Care Unit

Prerenal	**Intrinsic renal**	**Postrenal (obstructive)**

Intravascular volume depletion
• GI fluid loss (eg, vomiting, diarrhea, EC fistula)
• Renal fluid loss (eg, diuretics)
• Burns
• Blood loss
• Redistribution of fluid (eg, "third spacing," pancreatitis, cirrhosis)
	Acute tubular necrosis
	• Ischemic
	• Toxin-induced
	  • Drugs
	  • IV contrast
	• Rhabdomyolysis
	• Massive hemolysis
	• Tumor lysis syndrome
		Upper urinary tract obstruction
		• Nephrolithiasis
		• Hematoma
		• Aortic aneurysm
		• Neoplasm

Decreased renal perfusion pressure • Shock (eg, sepsis) • Vasodilatory drugs • Preglomerular (afferent) arteriolar vasoconstriction • Postglomerular (efferent) arteriolar vasodilation	Acute interstitial nephritis • Drug induced • Infection related • Systemic diseases (eg, SLE) • Malignancy	Lower urinary tract obstruction • Urethral stricture • Hematoma • Benign prostatic hypertrophy • Neurogenic bladder • Malpositioned urethral catheter • Neoplasm
Decreased cardiac output • Congestive heart failure • Myocardial ischemia	Acute glomerulonephritis • Postinfectious • Systemic vasculitis • TTP/HUS • Rapidly progressive GN Vascular • Atheroembolic disease • Renal artery or vein thrombosis • Renal artery dissection • Malignant hypertension Hepatorenal syndrome Increased intra-abdominal pressure	

EC, enterocutaneous; GI, gastrointestinal; GN, glomerulonephritis; HUS, hemolytic uremic syndrome; IV, intravenous; SLE, systemic lupus erythematosus; TTP, thrombotic thrombocytopenic purpura.

Adapted with permission from Barozzi L, Valentino M, Santoro A, Mancini E, Pavlica P. Renal ultrasonography in critically ill patients. *Crit Care Med.* 2007;35(5 suppl):S198-S205; Palevsky PM. Acute renal failure. In: Glassock RJ, ed. *Nephrology Self-assessment Program (NephSAP), Vol. 2.* Lippincott Williams & Wilkins; 2003:42-43.

A. Prerenal (Kidney Hypoperfusion)

1. Decreased intravascular volume

a. Systemic vasodilation (eg, sepsis): Sepsis is the most common cause of AKI in the ICU (~50% can be attributed) and is associated with a very high mortality.

b. Hypovolemia (eg, hemorrhage, gastrointestinal [GI] losses, burns)

c. Hypotension, decreased cardiac output (congestive heart failure [CHF], arrhythmias)

d. Small vessel (renal) vasoconstriction

1. Nonsteroidal anti-inflammatory drugs (NSAIDs): Prostaglandins have important vasodilatory effects on the afferent arteriolar vessels. Cyclooxygenase inhibitors inhibit the production of prostaglandins, resulting in decreased renal blood flow.

2. Angiotensin-converting enzyme inhibitors/angiotensin receptor blockers (ACEis/ARBs): Angiotensin-II is a potent efferent arteriolar vasoconstrictor and the inhibition of its production (ACEis) or the blockage of ARBs results in decreased glomerular perfusion pressure. This is of particular concern when the patient has other risk factors (CKD, renal artery stenosis [RAS], older age) or exposures (diuretics, hypotension, NSAIDs, nephrotoxins).

3. Contrast: Intravenous (IV) contrast is both cytotoxic to renal tubular cells and causes intrarenal vasoconstriction.

4. Hypercalcemia: directly causes vasoconstriction

5. Calcineurin inhibitors (CNIs): Both cyclosporine and tacrolimus, which lead to afferent and efferent arteriolar vasoconstriction, are used as immunosuppressants for patients after renal transplant.

6. Hepatorenal syndrome (HRS): Splanchnic and systemic vasodilation causes an increased neuroendocrine (angiotensin, vasopressin) tone, resulting in renal vasoconstriction. Prognosis is very poor.

7. Intra-abdominal hypertension (IAH; intra-abdominal pressure [IAP] >12 mm Hg) and abdominal compartment syndrome (ACS; IAP >20 mm Hg with new organ failure): The pathophysiology is likely a combination of (initially) intrarenal venous congestion/hypertension (HTN; normally a low-pressure system), followed by decreased cardiac output and elevated catecholamines, neurohormones, and cytokines (inflammation).

8. Cardiorenal syndrome: In addition to decreased cardiac output (acute CHF) resulting in decreased intravascular volume, other pathophysiologic processes are likely involved. Mechanisms likely include a combination of venous congestion (elevated central venous pressure [CVP]) and visceral edema resulting in decreased abdominal perfusion pressure (APP) and elevated neuroendocrine (angiotensin, vasopressin) hormones, resulting in decreased renal perfusion.

e. Large-vessel etiologies

1. Renal artery stenosis (RAS): This usually is in combination with other etiologies (eg, ACEis, hypotension).

2. Aortic or renal artery dissection (or compression)

3. Thrombosis or embolism of the renal vessels

B. Intrinsic Renal Injury

1. Acute tubular necrosis (ATN)

a. Ischemia (prerenal azotemia naturally progresses into ATN): This is the most significant cause of ATN in the ICU.

b. Pigments (hemoglobin, myoglobin): Of note, rhabdomyolysis should be considered with CPK (creatinine phosphokinase) levels greater than 5000 units/L. Injury is secondary to direct tubular toxicity from cast formation, in addition to intrarenal vasoconstriction and hypovolemia (muscle inflammation and third spacing). It is important to remember that CPK levels are a marker for muscle injury and that direct injury is caused by myoglobin.

c. **Drugs**
   1. **Aminoglycosides**, particularly at high doses, are toxic to proximal tubular cells. Once-daily dosing and vigilant dosing of medications can prevent some, but not all, cases.
   2. **Amphotericin B** can cause AKI because of nephrotoxicity and vasoconstriction. It is also associated with the development of distal renal tubular acidosis (RTA). Liposomal and colloid dispersion may decrease the incidence of severe AKI.
   3. **Vancomycin** has been shown to be associated with ATN; however, the incidence has decreased since the preparation has changed. Higher doses/levels may lead to increased incidence.
   4. **Hydroxyethyl starches (HES)** are associated with significant AKI and increased mortality when used as a volume expander in patients with sepsis who are critically ill. Osmotic nephrosis is seen in the proximal tubules.
   5. **Contrast-induced AKI (CIAKI) or contrast-induced nephropathy (CIN):** Contrast is both directly cytotoxic and decreases renal blood flow by vasoconstriction. This usually is in combination with hypovolemia/hypotension.

d. **Proteins (immunoglobulin light chains—multiple myeloma):** Notably, intravenous immunoglobulin (IVIG) therapy has been associated with proximal tubular osmotic nephrosis and, possibly, arterial vasoconstriction.

e. **Crystals** (uric acid, acyclovir, methotrexate)

2. **Acute interstitial nephritis**
   a. **Allergic (drug induced):** The most common drugs include β-lactam antibiotics and sulfonamides. Others include NSAIDs, proton pump inhibitors (PPIs), fluoroquinolones, vancomycin, and phenytoin.
   b. **Infection:** Bacterial and viral infections can lead to AIN by direct (pyelonephritis) and indirect (legionella) renal involvement.
   c. **Infiltrative/autoimmune:** Sarcoidosis, lupus, lymphoma/leukemia, and other systemic diseases can lead to interstitial inflammation.

3. **Glomerulonephritis**
   a. **Intraglomerular inflammation with various timelines of progression and acuity of disease:** Progression can be acute or rapidly progressive and severe, requiring early diagnosis. Pulmonary hemorrhage is a rare but feared complication (can be seen with antineutrophil cytoplasmic antibody [ANCA] or anti-glomerular basement membrane [GBM] disease). Typically classified on the basis of pathology, that is, pauci-immune (ANCA vasculitis), anti-GBM, and immune complex (postinfectious, immunoglobulin A [IgA], lupus nephritis, membranoproliferative, cryoglobulinemia, etc)

4. **Small vessel disease**
   a. **Thrombosis:** various pathophysiologic processes including hemolytic uremic syndrome (HUS), thrombotic thrombocytopenic purpura (TTP), preeclampsia, antiphospholipid antibody syndrome (APLAS), polyarthritis nodosa (PAN), scleroderma, and disseminated intravascular coagulopathy (DIC)
   b. Cholesterol embolism

C. **Postrenal (Obstruction and Hydronephrosis)**

1. **Bilateral ureteral obstruction**
   a. Malignancy (including lymphadenopathy), aneurysmal compression, nephrolithiasis, or retroperitoneal fibrosis or hematoma

2. **Bladder/urethral pathology**

a. Prostate enlargement (from benign prostatic hyperplasia or malignancy), Foley catheter or urethral obstruction, anticholinergic medications, and neurogenic bladder can all contribute to urinary obstruction and postrenal kidney dysfunction.

IV. EVALUATION

A. History should focus on baseline kidney function, risk factors (see **Sections V.A** and **V.B**), including medications, comorbidities, and recent procedures or events.

B. Physical Examination to include vital signs and volume status (intravascular volume), bedside focused ultrasonography (eg, inferior vena cava diameter), and signs/symptoms of vascular disease

C. Renal Function Evaluation

1. Blood urea nitrogen (BUN; nonspecific; increased with GI bleeding, steroids, high-protein tube feeds, hypermetabolism—especially with proteins)
2. Serum Cr (affected by muscle mass, amputation, drugs, and volume status)
3. 24-hour Cr clearance (can also check if more rapid results are desired)
4. Urine output (not sensitive)
5. **Urine evaluation** (Table 25.3)
   a. **Urinalysis and sediment**
      1. **Prerenal:** bland urinalysis and (transparent) hyaline casts
      2. **Intrinsic** etiologies demonstrate the following:
         a. Granular (muddy brown) casts (ATN secondary to ischemia or nephrotoxic injuries) can also be seen in the setting of glomerular disease.
         b. Pigmented casts (ATN secondary to hemoglobin or myoglobin or with hyperbilirubinemia)
         c. Red blood cell (RBC) casts (glomerulonephritis)
         d. White blood cell (WBC) casts (pyelonephritis, AIN, or glomerulonephritis)
         e. Urine eosinophils (AIN and cholesterol emboli, although not very sensitive or specific)
      3. **Postrenal:** bland urinalysis. RBCs with nephrolithiasis

TABLE 25.3 Diagnostic Studies and Indices of Urine

	Prerenal	Renal	Postrenal
Dipstick	0 or trace protein	Mild to moderate protein, hemoglobin, leukocytes	0 or trace protein, red and white cells
Sediment	Few hyaline casts	Granular and cellular casts[a]	Crystals and cellular casts possible
Serum BUN/Cr	20	10	10
Urine osmolality	>500	<350	<350
Urine sodium	<20	>30	
Urine/serum Cr	>40	<20	<20
Urine/serum urea	>8	<3	<3
FeNa	<1%	>1%	>1%
FEUr	<35%	>50%	

Cr, creatinine; FeNa, fractional excretion of sodium = (urine Na/urine Cr) / (serum Na/serum Cr) %; FEUr, fractional excretion of urea.

[a]Composition of casts depends on the cause of renal failure.

b. **Indices** (electrolytes, osmolalities)
 1. Prerenal injuries preserve renal salt and water balance mechanisms (initially), revealing FeNa less than 1% and FeUrea less than 35%; BUN/Cr greater than 20, and Uosm greater than 500.
 2. Intrinsic (eg, ATN) renal injury disrupts such mechanisms, resulting in FeNa greater than 2% and FeUrea greater than 50%. Note that diuretic use will prevent FeNa from maintaining utility [FeNa = (UNa / PNa) / (UCr / PCr)]; [FeUrea = (UUr / PUr) / (UCr / PCr)]. Note: FeNa may not be accurate in the setting of sepsis, CHF, cirrhosis, or pigment-induced injury.

6. **Serologic testing** (primarily for glomerular etiologies): antinuclear antibody (ANA), complement (C3, C4), ANCA, anti-GBM, cryocrit, hepatitis C virus (HCV), hepatitis B virus (HBV), serum protein electrophoresis (SPEP), serum-free light chains, urine Bence Jones proteins, phospholipase A2 receptor antibody (PLA2R Ab; membranous nephropathy; involve nephrology to assist with workup and to assess the need for RRT)
7. **Imaging studies**
 a. **Renal ultrasound:** can assess for hydronephrosis and estimate chronicity of kidney disease (small kidneys <10 cm suggest dysplasia or chronic disease). Color Doppler flow can evaluate perfusion and assess for thrombosis or RAS.
 b. **Computed tomography (CT)** scan, pyelography, and angiography have select roles in specific, select circumstances.
 c. **Magnetic resonance imaging (MRI):** Patients with moderate to severe CKD **should not** receive gadolinium because of concern for **nephrogenic systemic fibrosis (NSF)**, which results in skin and internal organ fibrosis with significant mortality.
8. **Renal biopsy:** If the abovementioned workup does not reveal the underlying etiology, biopsy may help evaluate intrinsic AKI.

V. RISK FACTORS

Risk factors can be divided into susceptibilities and exposures; this can be helpful when assessing who is most at risk for developing AKI (susceptible) and what can be minimized or avoided (exposures) to either prevent or minimize injury.

A. Susceptibilities

1. Advanced age (estimated glomerular filtration rate [eGFR] declines by ~1 mL/min/yr/1.73 m^2 after age 30)
2. Body mass index (BMI) greater than 30
3. Chronic kidney disease
4. Diabetes mellitus
5. Sepsis/septic shock (very high risk)
6. Liver disease
7. Congestive heart failure
8. Lymphoma/leukemia
9. Low baseline Cr (less muscle mass—suggested to be a surrogate marker of overall health and age)

B. Exposures

1. Nephrotoxic medications (see drugs listed in **Section III**)
2. Angiotensin-converting enzyme inhibitors, angiotensin receptor blockers
3. Nonsteroidal anti-inflammatory drugs
4. Chronic HTN plus shock (see SEPSISPAM study in **Section VI.B.1.c**)
5. Prolonged arterial cross-clamp (aorta, renal artery)
6. Cardiopulmonary bypass
7. Emergent surgery
8. Blood product transfusion
9. IV contrast (CIN): Risk from contrast exposure may be dose dependent. Patients with hypovolemia are more susceptible to CIN.

VI. MANAGEMENT OF ACUTE KIDNEY INJURY (FIGURE 25.1)

A. The management of AKI Stage I focuses primarily on (i) assessing and treating the etiology (see **Sections IV** and **V**), (ii) removing and avoiding insults (see **Section V.B**), (iii) optimizing hemodynamics, and (iv) managing complications. If AKI Stages 2 to 3 develop, (v) check for renal dosing of medications and (vi) assess for RRT.

B. Assessing and Treating Specific Etiologies

1. Prerenal

a. Optimize hemodynamics and establish appropriate monitoring, including invasive monitors when appropriate.

b. Fluid resuscitation: In general, crystalloid-based resuscitation with balanced salt solutions is preferred initially. In patients with septic shock and hypoalbuminemia, albumin supplementation may have an improved effect on mortality (the albumin replacement in patients with severe sepsis or septic shock [ALBIOS] trial). Increasing evidence suggests that large volumes of chloride-containing fluids (such as normal saline) may be associated with worse renal outcomes and, perhaps, even worse mortality. Although these data need confirmation, it seems prudent to avoid the exclusive use of normal saline in most patients. Patients with traumatic brain injuries and other central nervous system (CNS) lesions that need hyperosmolar therapy are an exception and will need saline-based resuscitation.

c. Managing blood pressure: Clinicians often raise the mean arterial pressure (MAP) target from the conventional 65 mm Hg to 75 to 80 mm Hg in patients who have a history of chronic HTN. The high versus low blood-pressure target in patients with septic shock (SEPSISPAM) trial compared the use of elevated MAP goals with conventional goals in patients with septic shock and found that in a predefined cohort of patients with chronic HTN, there was a decreased incidence of AKI and a decreased need for RRTs (but no mortality benefit) with higher MAPs. However, targeting a higher MAP was also associated with an increased incidence of atrial fibrillation. The primary methods for increasing MAP (fluids vs vasoactive drugs) probably affect outcomes and need to be further investigated.

d. Diuretics, mannitol, and renal-dose dopamine have not demonstrated any outcome benefits (but diuretics may be used to manage volume in the setting of hypervolemia).

e. Hepatorenal syndrome: possible role for midodrine and octreotide as temporizing measures. Liver transplantation is the definitive therapy.

f. Intra-abdominal hypertension/abdominal compartment syndrome: Medical therapy includes deep anesthesia, neuromuscular blockade, paracentesis, nasogastric and rectal decompression, minimizing/correction of positive fluid balance (including ultrafiltration/hemodialysis), and vasopressors (for APP >60 mm Hg) but surgical decompressive laparotomy may be required.

g. Cardiorenal syndrome: Focus should be on (i) optimizing cardiac output/perfusion and (ii) decreasing venous congestion (judicious diuresis).

h. Renal artery stenosis: angiography and stent placement in selected circumstances (bilateral RAS with progressive AKI/CKD, refractory HTN, or recurrent pulmonary edema)

2. Intrinsic renal injury

a. Acute tubular necrosis: Remove and avoid possible inciting agent(s).

b. Acute interstitial nephropathy: Consider steroids if no improvement with removal of the offending agent.

c. Contrast-induced nephropathy

1. Prevention

a. Minimize the number of contrast exposures. Use iso-osmolar and nonionic contrast.

b. **Hydration:** Hydration with isotonic crystalloids is likely as efficacious as the use of bicarbonate drips.
c. **N-acetylcysteine (NAC):** Some studies suggest the addition of NAC (600 or 1200 mg po bid for 2 days) plus hydration was superior to hydration alone for the prevention of CIN, whereas others have not shown a benefit. Given the low-risk profile of NAC, its use may be considered for CIN prophylaxis.

d. **Glomerulonephritis:** Steroids and immunosuppressive therapies may have a role. Specialty consultation should be requested for the management of these patients.

3. **Postrenal**
   a. Relieve obstruction (eg, ureteral stent placement, nephrostomy, and Foley manipulation or placement) with close monitoring because complications can occur with rapid decompression (hemorrhagic cystitis) and hypotonic diuresis.

VII. MANAGING COMPLICATIONS OF ACUTE KIDNEY INJURY

RRT may be required for the management of the complications of AKI (see **Section VIII**). RRT is usually initiated when more conservative measures have proved ineffective.

A. Volume Overload

1. Minimize fluid administration.
2. Diurese (when possible or responsive). Favor IV over oral loop diuretics. Use high-dose loop diuretics in the setting of oliguric AKI (general rule: starting IV Lasix dose = 30 × Cr, ie, if Cr: 4, use 120 mg IV Lasix). The combination of a thiazide diuretic (such as chlorothiazide or metolazone) and a loop diuretic may be used if a loop diuretic alone is ineffective. Diuretics have not been shown to have an outcome benefit in the setting of AKI but their use may make management of volume status easier.

B. Metabolic Acidosis

B. Metabolic Acidosis: Kidney injury can cause a mixed gap and nongap metabolic acidosis (see **Chapter 8**). Acidemia is generally not treated symptomatically unless it is severe (pH <7.15). Sodium bicarbonate infusions may be used for severe metabolic acidemia provided the resulting increase in CO_2 production can be offset by increased minute ventilation. See **Chapter 8** for details of symptomatic management of academia. The use of bicarbonate may be considered therapeutic if the primary reason for acidosis is renal bicarbonate wasting.

C. Electrolyte Abnormalities

1. **Hyperkalemia** (assess for electrocardiogram [ECG] changes, although this is not a sensitive measure to predict subsequent arrhythmias—do not delay treatment of marked hyperkalemia because ECG changes have not yet appeared)
   a. **Antagonism of the effects of potassium (membrane stabilization)**
      1. **Calcium:** Calcium gluconate (or calcium chloride) acts as a physiologic antagonist of potassium at the cell membrane. Initially, 10 mL of a 10% calcium gluconate solution should be used. If calcium chloride is used instead, remember that it provides about three times the amount of calcium per volume compared with calcium gluconate.
   b. **Promoting an intracellular shift of potassium**
      1. **Insulin:** A typical initial dose is 10 units of **regular insulin IV** with an ampule of **50% dextrose** (in patients who are **normoglycemic**). This therapy takes 15 to 20 minutes to begin to take effect.
      2. **α-Adrenergic agonists:** High-dose albuterol (10-20 mg, nebulized) has been shown to be effective in the treatment of hyperkalemia. The onset of effect is evident by 30 minutes and lasts for up to 6 hours. Tachycardia may be dose limiting, although initial studies that used high-dose albuterol did not report significant tachycardia.

3. **Increasing blood pH**: If pH is less than 7.3, an ampule (50 mEq) of $NaHCO_3$ can be given IV. If possible (within limits of lung-protective ventilation), minute ventilation should be increased.

c. **Removal of potassium from the body**

1. **Renal replacement therapy:** See **Section VIII.**
2. **Ion-exchange resins:** Lokelma (sodium zirconium cyclosilicate) can effectively remove potassium from the gut and has a more rapid onset (~1 hour) than do older therapies (eg, Kayexalate). If Lokelma is not available, Kayexalate (sodium polystyrene sulfate) may be used but its onset of action may require 12 to 24 hours and it may cause intestinal necrosis. Sodium polystyrene sulfate should be used with extreme caution in the setting of GI illness, particularly ileus or bowel obstruction.
3. **Loop diuretics** will decrease total body potassium and may be used as adjunctive therapy.

2. **Hyponatremia, hyperphosphatemia, and hypermagnesemia:** See **Chapter 8.**

D. **Uremic Encephalopathy:** The critically ill may have multiple competing reasons for becoming encephalopathic and the presence of encephalopathy should prompt a detailed evaluation for other metabolic derangements, infection, or drug toxicity. Uremic encephalopathy usually improves with RRT.

E. **Coagulation Abnormalities:** usually due to uremic platelet dysfunction. Management is discussed in **Chapter 27.**

F. **Anemia:** Multifactorial etiology is common. In the absence of active bleeding or ongoing coronary ischemia, it is recommended that hemoglobin values as low as 7 g/dL not be treated in the critically ill (blood transfusion, erythropoietin supplementation, and iron supplementation are all associated with risks in the critically ill).

G. **Infectious Complications** are a major cause of death in patients with AKI. Both uremia and RRT (particularly continuous RRT) blunt the ability of patients to mount an effective response to infections and typical signs (such as fever) may be masked.

H. **Uremic Pericarditis** occurs for unknown reasons and can lead to cardiac tamponade. It is an indication of RRT.

I. **Decreased Drug Elimination:** Assess medications for renal clearance and adjust doses accordingly. It should be kept in mind that in evolving AKI, the calculated Cr clearance may be inaccurate and typically an overestimate.

J. **Nutritional Support** is an important component of the management of patients who are critically ill with AKI—see **Chapter 11** for details.

VIII. RENAL REPLACEMENT THERAPY

Can be classified into intermittent or continuous methods. Prototypical examples are intermittent hemodialysis (IHD) or continuous venovenous hemofiltration (CVVH), although other modalities are occasionally used. IHD is used for patients who are hemodynamically stable, whereas CVVH may be more appropriate for patients who are hemodynamically unstable, have intracranial HTN, or are encephalopathic secondary to cirrhosis. The choice between intermittent versus continuous RRT is often based on institutional experience and culture. Although continuous RRT intuitively seems to be preferable when dealing with patients who are hemodynamically unstable and critically ill, the data do not support a robust benefit for continuous RRT over intermittent modes.

A. **Indications:** The classic indications for RRT initiation are listed here. Early initiation of RRT in the critically ill has been recommended by some authorities—however, the data do not show improved outcomes for early CVVH compared with conventional use.

1. **A**cidemia
2. **E**lectrolyte abnormalities (hyperkalemia, tumor lysis)
3. **I**ntoxication (lithium, methanol, salicylates, nephrotoxic medications)
4. **O**verload (volume)
5. **U**remia (if pericarditis, bleeding, or encephalopathy present)

B. Intermittent Hemodialysis (Figure 25.2A)

1. Semipermeable membrane with countercurrent flow between blood and a dialysate
2. Fluid removal driven by pressure gradient, solute removal by concentration gradient
3. **Complications:** hypotension, infection, arrhythmias

C. Continuous Venovenous Hemofiltration (Figure 25.2B)

1. Pressurized blood flows next to a highly permeable membrane
2. Fluid and solute removal via pressure gradient (convection)
3. Replacement fluid buffer required, either HCO_3 or citrate (provides local anticoagulation by binding calcium in the circuit). Citrate is subsequently metabolized by the liver to HCO_3. Use of citrate in patients with significant liver dysfunction can lead to life-threatening acidosis.

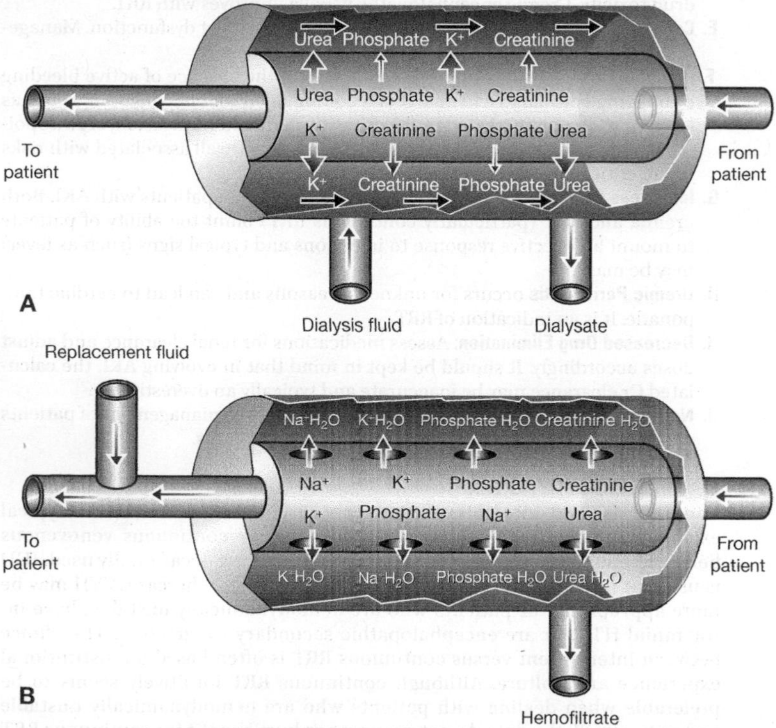

FIGURE 25.2 A: Hemodialysis achieves solute clearance by diffusion across a semipermeable membrane from a higher concentration (in the patient's blood) to a lower concentration (in the dialysis fluid). **B:** Hemofiltration (which is the mechanism used in continuous venovenous hemofiltration [CVVH]) achieves solute clearance by convection across a semipermeable membrane from a higher hydrostatic pressure (in a patient's blood) to a lower hydrostatic pressure (in the hemofiltrate). (Modified from Forni LG, Hilton PJ. Continuous hemofiltration in the treatment of acute renal failure. *N Engl J Med.* 1997;336:1303-1309.)

4. Complications: hypotension (much less common than with IHD), infection, citrate toxicity (in the setting of poor hepatic function), complications associated with anticoagulation (may be required with HCO_3)

D. **Access for Renal Replacement Therapy:** In the acute setting, double-lumen temporary hemodialysis catheters (14 Fr) are commonly used. The catheters are typically inserted percutaneously using the Seldinger technique and ultrasound guidance. The right internal jugular vein is the most frequent site of cannulation, often preferred for optimal catheter function. However, a large, randomized study comparing internal jugular with femoral site insertions found that the rate of catheter colonization and bloodstream infection was equivalent between the jugular and femoral sites in patients who are **non-obese, bed-bound**, and critically ill. The subclavian site is often avoided because of concerns for subclavian vein stenosis, which can limit the future success of arteriovenous fistulas and grafts.

Selected Readings

Allegretti AS, Steele DJ, David-Kasdan JA, et al. Continuous renal replacement therapy outcomes in acute kidney injury and end-stage renal disease: a cohort study. *Crit Care.* 2013;17:R109.

Asfar P, Meziani F, Hamel JF, et al. High versus low blood-pressure target in patients with septic shock. *N Engl J Med.* 2014;370:1583-1593.

Barrett BJ, Parfrey PS. Clinical practice. Preventing nephropathy induced by contrast medium. *N Engl J Med.* 2006;354:379-386.

Bellomo R, Ronco C, Kellum JA, et al. Acute renal failure—definition, outcome measures, animal models, fluid therapy and information technology needs: the Second International Consensus Conference of the Acute Dialysis Quality Initiative (ADQI) Group. *Crit Care.* 8:R204-R212.

Bosch X, Poch E, Grau JM. Rhabdomyolysis and acute kidney injury. *N Engl J Med.* 2009;361:62-72.

Friedrich JO, Adhikari N, Herridge MS, et al. Meta-analysis: low-dose dopamine increases urine output but does not prevent renal dysfunction or death. *Ann Intern Med.* 2005;142:510-524.

John S, Eckardt KU. Renal replacement strategies in the ICU. *Chest.* 2007;132:1379-1388.

Kidney Disease: Improving Global Outcomes (KDIGO) Acute Kidney Injury Work Group. KDIGO clinical practice guideline for acute kidney injury. *Kidney Int Suppl.* 2012;1:1-138.

Lameire N, Van Biesen W, Vanholder R. Acute renal failure. *Lancet.* 2005;365(9457):417-430.

Mohmand H, Goldfarb S. Renal dysfunction associated with intra-abdominal hypertension and the abdominal compartment syndrome. *J Am Soc Nephrol.* 2011;22:615-621.

Okusa MD, Davenport A. Reading between the (guide)lines—the KDIGO practice guideline on acute kidney injury in the individual patient. *Kidney Int.* 2014;85:39-48.

Parienti JJ, Thirion M, Megarbane B, et al. Femoral vs jugular venous catheterization and risk of nosocomial events in adults requiring acute renal replacement therapy: a randomized controlled trial. *JAMA.* 2008;299(20):2413-2422.

Pickkers P, Darmon M, Hoste E, et al. Acute kidney injury in the critically ill: an updated review on pathophysiology and management. *Intensive Care Med.* 2021;47:835-850.

Prowle JR, Forni LG, Bell M, et al. Postoperative acute kidney injury in adult non-cardiac surgery: joint consensus report of the Acute Disease Quality Initiative and Perioperative Quality Initiative. *Nat Rev Nephrol.* 2021;17:605-618.

26 Critical Care of Patients With Liver Disease

Paige McLean Diaz, Hovig V. Chitilian, Parsia Vagefi, and Esperance A. K. Schaefer

I. CIRRHOSIS

A. Pathophysiology: Through various mechanisms—inflammatory, apoptotic, or necrotic injury to the liver—epithelial cells, endothelium, and hepatocytes converge to recruit and activate stellate cells. These activated stellate cells then become myofibroblasts that deposit collagen matrix and begin an unequal remodeling involving fibrogenesis and fibro-resorption among hepatic sinusoids. Understood as an end pathway, cirrhosis is characterized as a process that replaces healthy liver architecture with diffuse sinusoidal fibrosis and regenerative nodules predominantly within portal tracts. The liver receives two-thirds of its blood supply from the portal system and the derangement of its architecture directly impacts the venous portal pressures. Clinically significant portal hypertension is diagnosed when the hepatic venous gradient is greater than 10 mm Hg (normal <6 mm Hg). The complications of portal hypertension and synthetic dysfunction are intimately associated with critical illness in patients affected with cirrhosis.

B. Epidemiology: Nearly 2% to 3% (~26 000 individuals) are admitted annually for cirrhosis-related complications, acute-on-chronic liver failure (ACLF), or acute liver failure (ALF). In cirrhosis, acute decompensations (ascites, variceal bleeding, spontaneous bacterial peritonitis [SBP], hepatic encephalopathy [HE], hepatorenal syndrome [HRS], hepatic hydrothorax) are common reasons for ICU admission. ACLF, which additionally manifests with extrahepatic organ failure, is a highly morbid pathway in the natural history of chronic liver disease with high short-term mortality approaching 60%. Studies suggest that 5% of intensive care unit (ICU) admissions belong to this subset of illness, and it may be the first acute decompensation in up to 20% of patients with cirrhosis. Globally, the triggering etiologies differ because alcohol-associated hepatitis (AH) and bacterial infection are more frequently recognized in the Western hemisphere, in contrast to the East, where reactivation of viral hepatitis from hepatitis B and superinfection with hepatitis E are more likely to be seen.

Acute AH is an important and rapidly increasing cause of liver-related hospitalizations in the United States. It is a clinical diagnosis, with diagnostic criteria including onset of jaundice and active alcohol use within 8 weeks, alcohol intake of greater than 40 g in women and greater than 60 g in men, aspartate aminotransferase (AST) greater than 50 and AST:ALT (alanine aminotransferase) ratio of greater than 1.5 (and both AST/ALT <400 IU/L), and T bilirubin greater than 3 mg/dL, with absence of other etiologies. Severe AH is generally defined when the Model for End-Stage Liver Disease (MELD) score is greater than 20. Approximately 70% of patients with severe AH have underlying cirrhosis, but even in the absence of cirrhosis there is a significant risk of mortality (30% at 90 days). Although therapeutic options are limited, early identification and management of this disease entity is imperative and more than 50% of transplant centers in the United States offer liver transplantation (LT) for carefully selected patients.

C. Prognostication: The MELD score was created in 2001 to risk stratify patients before transjugular intrahepatic portosystemic shunt (TIPS) placement. It has replaced the Child-Pugh score as the preferred mechanism to stratify the risk of short-term (within 90 days) mortality in patients with cirrhosis. In 2008, sodium was added to the measure, improving its predictive accuracy of mortality. Patients who have an acute decompensating event may have a transiently increased MELD score; however, in a subset of patients, the MELD score remains persistently elevated. LT candidacy evaluation typically begins when a patient has a persistent MELD score of 15 or higher. Owing to the limited availability of organs and relatively poor uptake of liver donation, most patients with cirrhosis do not begin to receive offers until their MELD score is much higher, and often when it is greater than 30 (short-term mortality risk ~50%).

D. Fundamentals: A few concepts are essential when caring for a patient with advanced liver disease complications.

1. **Infection:** Patients with cirrhosis are at an exceptionally high risk for infection, which carries great morbidity and mortality (2-fold) compared to the general population. The incidence of infections in patients with decompensated cirrhosis ranges between 25% and 40%. Portal hypertension leads to enhanced intestinal permeability, enhanced activation of inflammatory cytokines, and compromised immune system function. Reduced bacterial clearance facilitates overgrowth and translocation via a more permeable intestinal tract. Activated proinflammatory cytokines such as tumor necrosis factor (TNF)-α and interleukin (IL)-6 promote the development of sepsis. Infections are often the etiology of acute decompensations, especially spontaneous bacterial peritonitis (SBP) and variceal hemorrhages (VHs). The most common infections identified include SBP (25%-30%), bacteremia, urinary tract infections, community-acquired pneumonia, and soft tissue infections.
2. **Volume status:** Decompensated cirrhosis is characterized by intravascular volume depletion, renal hypoperfusion, and extravascular volume overload. The extravascular volume overload is addressed with diuretics, and 20% to 40% of patients on diuretic therapy for ascites develop an adverse effect (typically, prerenal acute kidney injury [AKI], electrolyte abnormalities [hyponatremia, hypomagnesemia, hypo- or hyperkalemia], and, less commonly, HRS II). Best practices dictate the cessation of diuretic therapy in the presence of comorbid gastrointestinal (GI) bleeding, active uncontrolled infection, AKI, or severe hyponatremia (Na <125).
3. **Bleeding/coagulopathy:** Among patients with cirrhosis, gastroesophageal varices (GEVs) are present in 30% to 40% of patients with compensated cirrhosis and greater than 60% of patients with decompensated cirrhosis, and VH occurs at a rate of 5% to 15% per year. There remains a 15% to 20% risk of mortality from VH but uncontrolled bleeding is not the most common cause: ACLF, HRS, and infection all are important contributors to mortality. The coagulopathy related to cirrhosis also represents a complex physiology and manifestations include both bleeding issues and abnormal clotting.
4. **Metabolic alterations:** Another consideration is that medications may be metabolized differently in patients with cirrhosis. This can be secondary to multifactorial changes, including bowel edema and portal gastropathy, which can impair absorption, impaired renal excretion, the presence of portosystemic shunts that remove first-pass metabolism and subsequently increase bioavailability, and hypoalbuminemia that can reduce protein binding, potentially decreasing the therapeutic efficacy because the free drug is more rapidly cleared from sera. It is worth noting, however, that more than 90% of the liver's metabolic capacity must be lost before dose adjustments for hepatic impairment are generally required.

II. EVALUATION

A. Infectious Evaluation/Paracentesis: Prompt recognition of infection includes a thorough diagnostic approach, which is not complete without a diagnostic paracentesis. This is particularly important in patients with clinically known or evident decompensated cirrhosis. Delayed (>12 hours from presentation) paracentesis is associated with an average of 3.3% higher in-hospital mortality even when the MELD score and renal dysfunction are accounted for. A large cohort study showed a 24% decrease in mortality in patients who received a diagnostic paracentesis on admission compared with those who did not.

B. Hemodynamics/Renal Function: The physiology of decompensated liver disease generally involves a decrement in systemic perfusion pressures and high risk of renal impairment due to hypoperfusion. Initial evaluation should include careful monitoring of hemodynamics, urine output, and renal function. Some data suggest that cystatin C may be more reliable than creatinine in estimating glomerular filtration rate (GFR) in this patient population that is often sarcopenic. Hypotension is common: Despite evidence of a hyperdynamic state, patients may be hypotensive and unresponsive to volume challenges, which is rarely due to cardiac dysfunction. Generally, targeting a mean arterial pressure (MAP) of 65 to 75 mm Hg is standard practice. However, recent data suggest that a higher MAP (75 mm Hg) may be associated with decreased mortality and, thus, higher MAPS should be considered, particularly in patients with AKI. It should be noted that increased intra-abdominal pressure from tense ascites is associated with reduced ventricular preload and can lead to renal, cardiovascular, and respiratory dysfunction. Therefore, a therapeutic paracentesis (5 L) should be considered when this condition is present, with 6 to 8 g albumin replacement per liter removed. Norepinephrine is the vasoactive agent of choice for volume-insensitive hypotension. When a patient is suspected of having HRS, octreotide and terlipressin (or vasopressin when unavailable or if respiratory concerns preclude the use of terlipressin) should be considered as first-line therapy.

C. Mental Status/Airway Protection: Patients are at increased risk for respiratory distress secondary to aspiration in the setting of hepatic or another metabolic encephalopathy. A standard measurement for mentation is the Glasgow Coma Scale. Endotracheal intubation is indicated when scores are persistently less than 8 or in the presence of active upper GI bleeding. Lung-protective ventilation strategies include low tidal volumes (4-8 mL/kg of predicted body weight) with permissive hypercapnia, use of positive end-expiratory pressure (PEEP) to maintain oxygenation, and minimized plateau pressures in patients with respiratory failure or acute lung injury. Prolonged endotracheal intubation is optimally avoided but percutaneous tracheostomy can be performed even in coagulopathy.

D. Bleeding/Coagulopathy: Bleeding is a common complication of end-stage liver disease, and may manifest with GI losses (hematemesis, melena, bright red blood per rectum), and, less commonly, hematuria or spontaneous hematoma. It is essential to avoid reacting to laboratory abnormalities with the absence of active bleeding. Elevations in the international normalized ratio (INR) are commonly seen and do not reflect a patient's actual ability for clots secondary to secondary mechanisms that are robustly activated, promoting thromboembolism. Other common derangements include thrombocytopenia (related to splenic sequestration) and low fibrinogen. Vitamin K deficiency is prevalent in decompensated cirrhosis and it is reasonable to offer intravenous (IV) vitamin K repletion for 3 to 5 days to replete nutritional stores.

III. MANAGEMENT OF ACUTE DECOMPENSATION

A. Variceal Hemorrhage: Patients with cirrhosis need a portal pressure of at least 12 mm Hg to develop clinically significant GEVs. Without assessment of portal pressures by means of a hepatic venous pressure gradient (HVPG, obtained invasively via venous access), a low platelet count is the most common sign of portal hypertension in patients. It correlates slightly with elevated HVPG and GEV presence. VH is associated with a greater than 10% in-hospital mortality rate, and, in combination with other complications of cirrhosis (ascites or HE), has an up to 80% 5-year mortality rate. Endoscopic and interventional radiologic techniques have dramatically decreased the mortality associated with VH, but non-bleeding complications (ACLF, infection, hepatorenal failure) remain important contributors to mortality. As such, ICU medical management remains critical.

1. **Resuscitation:** Return of hemodynamic stability is the goal of resuscitation. A restrictive packed red cell strategy with a transfusion threshold of 7 g/dL to maintain hemoglobin (Hgb) 7 to 9 g/dL has been studied and is associated with a significant decrease in mortality and early rebleeding rates compared with a liberal strategy (transfusion threshold ≥9 g/dL). Massive bleeding with hemodynamic changes, age, and cardiovascular status are considerations for individualized treatment. Endoscopic therapy is recommended within 12 hours of admission and once the patient is hemodynamically stable.
2. **Addressing coagulopathy:** Randomized clinical trials of recombinant factor VIIa administration have not shown a clear benefit for acute VH, so it is not recommended to attempt to correct the INR with cryoprecipitate or fresh frozen plasma (FFP) routinely because this is not a reliable marker of coagulation status in cirrhosis. Platelet administration is reasonable with massive transfusion protocols per hospital. Patients with a history of prior bleeding with disseminated intravascular coagulation or uremia with thrombocytopenia may benefit from desmopressin (DDAVP) administration to address bleeding on an individualized basis.
3. **Vasoactive agents:** A meta-analysis of 30 randomized trials showed that using vasoactive agents such as IV octreotide is associated with lower short-term all-cause mortality and lower transfusion requirements. Options include IV somatostatin (SMT), octreotide, and terlipressin where available. If TIPS is not performed, vasoactive agents should be continued for 2 to 5 days, and then nonselective β-blockers for secondary VH prophylaxis should be started if hemodynamics permit. Rescue TIPS may be required if bleeding recurs despite vasoactive drugs and endoscopic variceal ligation (EVL).
4. **Antibiotic prophylaxis:** Antibiotic prophylaxis has been consistently shown to decrease mortality in patients hospitalized with VH. IV ceftriaxone is preferred for treatment (1 g every 24 hours for 5-7 days); it was superior to norfloxacin in a head-to-head comparison, and fluoroquinolone resistance has risen recently. However, in some patients with low-protein ascites, continued prophylaxis may be considered indefinitely.
5. **Rescue therapy:** Early recurrence of VH is considered new variceal bleeding within 5 days of the inciting event. Repeat upper endoscopy is the first line; however, if this demonstrates a failure to control bleeding via endoscopic technique (repeat EVL), then interventional radiology should be involved to consider TIPS to control bleeding, typically within 72 hours of admission. For gastric VH, balloon occluded retrograde transvenous obliteration (BRTO) with or without TIPS placement should be considered. Relative contraindications for TIPS include age older than 75, MELD scores greater than 18, infiltrating malignancy, and significant right heart dysfunction.

B. **Ascites-Hepatic Hydrothorax:** Refractory ascites develops in 5% to 10% of patients, and this complication has high morbidity because up to 50% will die within 6 months of its onset. The diagnostic evaluation for ascites includes assessment of liver and renal function, urine electrolytes, abdominal ultrasound with Doppler to rule out new thrombosis as a source of rapidly accumulating ascites, and a diagnostic paracentesis. A diagnostic paracentesis should be performed in all patients who present with clinically significant ascites, and if their presentation is suspected to be the first, obtaining serum albumin and ascitic albumin for the calculation of the serum albumin ascites gradient (SAAG) can help rule out secondary causes for ascites accumulation (infectious, malignant, pancreatic). A SAAG greater than 1.1 is expected in ascites accumulation secondary to portal hypertension with an accuracy of around 97%. A SAAG greater than 1.1 with high ascitic protein (>2.5 g/dL) is more often related to right heart failure; thus, echocardiography to rule out ventricular dysfunction may be indicated. When the SAAG is low (<1.1), peritoneal disease, which may have infectious or malignant etiologies, should be ruled out with cytology, culture, and cross-sectional imaging. Owing to the relatively high incidence of comorbid renal dysfunction, the standard practice is discontinuing diuretic therapy in patients with suspected refractory ascites and managing volume with serial large-volume paracentesis (LVP). LVPs are safe in patients with coagulopathy related to cirrhosis, with studies showing that even with INR greater than 1.5 and severe thrombocytopenia ($<50 \times 10^9$/L), the risk of minimal cutaneous bleeding was only 1%. Elevated INR is never a contraindication in a patient with cirrhosis for paracentesis, nor do patients need routine transfusions of clotting factors or platelets.

Four percent to 12% of patients with cirrhosis will have clinically significant pleural effusions. These are typically unilateral and often recur upon thoracentesis; right-sided effusions have a prevalence of 77%, according to one study. Spontaneous infectious can also occur in patients with hepatic hydrothorax, albeit with lower incidence when compared to ascites. Both grade 2 to 3 ascites and hepatic hydrothorax can be considerations for orthotopic liver transplantation (OLT) and TIPS placement. Patients with specific characteristics (young age, low MELD score, complete resolution of ascites) may substantially improve with TIPS placement because this offers a survival advantage compared to serial LVP.

1. **Hyponatremia:** Mild hyponatremia between 126 and 135 mEq/L does not require aggressive treatment, but management should focus on improving renal perfusion: holding diuretics and β-blockers, monitoring, and initiating free water restriction less than 2 L. Data are limited, but there may be benefit with initiating midodrine in subjects not on vasopressor support. Further management (1 L fluid restriction) should be considered when Na is persistently less than 120 to 125. Symptomatic hyponatremia, rapid onset, and proximity to OLT may dictate the consideration of advanced therapies, including hypertonic saline administration and vasopressin receptor antagonists, in consultation with nephrologists. Osmotic demyelinating syndromes are more frequently seen in patients with a history of alcoholism, malnutrition, prior encephalopathy, and comorbid severe metabolic derangements. They often have a delayed onset compared with the episode of overcorrection, so care should be taken to use the lower range correction of 4 to 6 mEq/L per 24-hour period and not exceed an increase of 8 mEq/L per 24-hour period.
2. **Volume shifts:** There is a high rate of post-paracentesis circulatory dysfunction with serial LVPs greater than 8 L, even with albumin repletion of 6 to 8 g/L. High-volume paracentesis should be avoided in these patients. If patients are young with relatively low MELD (10-18), consider TIPS—the gradual transition of blood volume back to the systemic circulation is associated with significant diuresis within 4 to 6 months of placement.
3. **Spontaneous bacterial peritonitis:** Spontaneous infections arise in approximately 36% of patients with cirrhosis and half are health care associated or nosocomial in origin. Patients with decompensated alcohol-related

liver disease may be at particular risk because of the higher prevalence of intestinal bacterial overgrowth. The organisms tend to be monobacterial, especially enteric gram-negative species such as *Escherichia coli*. Some of the less common ones are infections from organisms such as *Klebsiella pneumoniae, Staphylococcus aureus, Enterococcus faecalis, or Enterococcus faecium*. However, ascitic fluid cultures commonly return a negative result and a positive culture result is *not* required for the diagnosis of SBP. Diagnostic paracentesis with a culture of ascitic fluid at the bedside before initiating empiric antibiotic therapy is ideal for treating SBP. When ascitic fluid total neutrophil counts are greater than 250/mm^3, the patient should be treated empirically. Although third-generation cephalosporins are first-line therapy with IV albumin (1 mg/kg on the first day, 40-50 g/kg on the second day) for the treatment of SBP, rising rates of multidrug-resistant organisms may require the use of carbapenems or other broad-spectrum antibiotics.

4. **Hepatorenal syndrome:** Patients with cirrhosis are vulnerable to impaired renal perfusion related to the splanchnic vasodilation and recurrent prerenal insults associated with the development of clinically significant ascites. An AKI is diagnosed when a patient's serum creatinine increases 0.3 mg/dL or higher in 48 hours, or there is a 50% or higher increase in the serum creatinine that is known or presumed to have occurred within the preceding 7 days. HRS-AKI is the newest terminology for the spectrum of severe prerenal injury without parenchymal disease or another reversible process that affects patients with cirrhosis. Urinalysis with sediment microscopy and updated imaging to rule out secondary processes (bile cast nephropathy, immunoglobulin [Ig]A glomerulonephritis in alcohol-associated cirrhosis, and renal obstruction) are typically sought. The risk of HRS is exceptionally high when patients have a comorbid infection (SBP). Vasoconstrictive agents are considered first-line therapy (terlipressin, norepinephrine, vasopressin) along with albumin infusions. Improvement in the serum creatinine toward baseline or duration of 14 days is used to determine the length of treatment. Renal replacement therapy is generally reserved for selected patients with reversible causes of comorbid organ failure if not already listed for an LT, given the exceptionally high rates of short-term mortality in patients with advanced liver disease who initiate renal replacement while not listed.

C. **Hepatic Encephalopathy:** HE encompasses a spectrum of reversible neuropsychiatric impairments. In the minimal stage, the changes may be as subtle as mild inattention or executive function difficulties. In more severe cases, patients may demonstrate neuromuscular abnormalities (asterixis), become lethargic, develop disorientation, or become comatose, culminating in death secondary to cytotoxic brain edema if not reversed with therapy. Overt HE (OHE) develops in most patients with cirrhosis, and it is a marker of poor prognosis because its onset is associated with a projected 1-year survival of 41% without LT. Among complications of cirrhosis, OHE is the greatest determinant of short-term readmission. Common HE triggers include dehydration, sarcopenia, medications, GI bleeding, and infection. Although arterial hyperammonemia is present in up to 90% of patients with HE, the presence of elevated ammonia is neither sensitive nor specific for this condition; thus, HE remains a clinical diagnosis. The standard therapy is oral lactulose, and rifaximin added to lactulose has been shown to decrease recurrent episodes of HE. Nonabsorbable disaccharides such as oral lactulose pass mostly unabsorbed from the small bowel to the colon, where colon bacteria ferment it, trapping ammonia in the process. Rifaximin is a minimally absorbed antibiotic that depletes ammoniagenic bacteria from the gut lumen.

For patients without enteral access, rectal lactulose may be substituted. When given with oral lactulose, it can accelerate recovery for patients with evidence of severe OHE (>grade II). More frequent administration (every 2 hours) may be necessary for patients without enteral access to see clinical improvement.

D. Nutrition: Critical illness and cirrhosis are both metabolically demanding conditions. Patients without access to an enteral source, or with diminished oral intake (such as can occur with large-volume ascites, encephalopathy, or active alcohol use), are at high risk for worsened malnutrition, and advanced liver disease increases the risk of hypoglycemia because glycogen storage can become impaired. Prealbumin can be checked as one element of nutritional evaluation. Nutritional support via enteral access should be secured within 7 days of ICU admission. Sarcopenia is associated with poor outcomes in patients with end-stage liver disease, and thus there should be a particular focus on protein intake. Guidelines suggest that patients with cirrhosis with muscle depletion should receive 30 to 45 kcal/kg/d and 1.5 g protein/kg/d.

A common question is the relative safety of nasogastric tube (NGT) placement in the presence of esophageal varices. Little data exist in the literature on this topic. Still, four clinical trials have shown a low risk of hemodynamically significant upper GI bleeding with the blind placement of NGTs. Although this procedure appears safe overall, a slightly higher risk of GI bleeding has been shown in patients with high MELD and known lower esophageal varices. In the short term, post an intervention for variceal bleeding, endoscopically placed enteral access with direct visualization is likely the safest approach.

IV. EVALUATION AND MANAGEMENT OF ACUTE LIVER FAILURE

A. Definition: ALF is defined as liver injury accompanied by the development of impaired coagulation (INR >1.5) and HE in a patient without preexisting liver disease and an illness duration of less than 26 weeks. In large studies, symptom duration and time to jaundice is widely variable, with a range between 2 and 75 days between onset and clinical presentation to a referral center. Exceptions to the criterion of absence of preexisting cirrhosis may be made for patients with an acute exacerbation of Wilson disease, vertically transmitted hepatitis B virus (HBV) infection and autoimmune hepatitis because these can be marked by a fulminant course. ALF remains uncommon, with an incidence of six cases per million population in Western countries. Although the epidemiology has changed with the advent of therapy for acetaminophen toxicity, viral hepatitis A virus (HAV)/HBV vaccination efforts, and the cure for the hepatitis C virus, the etiology of a considerable proportion of episodes of ALF is unknown.

B. Common Etiologies: On the basis of data from 17 referral centers in the United States of 308 consecutively enrolled patients with ALF, drug-induced liver injury via acetaminophen ingestion was the most common cause in the early 2000s with 39% representation. It is important to mention that 57% of acetaminophen ALF cases were related to therapeutic misadventure (repeated ingestion for treatment of pain or other illness) and 37% of cases were secondary to overt suicidal intent. The median dose associated with ALF was 13.2 g/d and the vast majority (83%) ingested more than 4.2 g/d. Idiosyncratic drug-induced liver injuries were the next most common cause of ALF in 13% of patients. More recently, studies have suggested that non–acetaminophen drug-induced injury has emerged as the leading cause and antibiotics and supplements are among the leading culprits. The Adverse Drug Reaction Probability Scale (Naranjo Scale) is a method to assess whether there is a causal relationship between an identified untoward clinical event and a drug using a simple questionnaire to assign probability scores (from 0 to 9) with different values (−1, 0, +1, or +2) granted on the basis of certainty of answer.

ALF related to viral hepatitis was most frequently attributed to HBV (7%), then HAV with 4% of cases. Hepatitis C virus (HCV) and hepatitis E virus (HEV) made up less than 1% of viral hepatitis–related ALF.

C. Uncommon Etiologies: These causes of ALF are seen in less than 10% of cases. They include ischemic hepatitis (6%), autoimmune hepatitis (4%), Wilson disease (3%), and Budd-Chiari syndrome (2%). Pregnancy-related liver disease is seen in less than 2% of cases, most often from acute fatty liver of pregnancy, HELLP (*h*emolysis, *el*evated *l*iver enzymes, *l*ow *p*latelet count), or eclampsia; it is important to note that the typical causes of ALF are more common in pregnant women. Overwhelming metastatic burden, heat stroke, vascular shunt procedures, peri-transplant hepatic artery thrombosis (HAT), or hepatectomy are historically the remaining rare (<2%) etiologies.

D. Diagnosis: It is paramount in ALF to confirm the acuity of the insult and then stratify the severity of their HE with arterial ammonia given the risk of intracranial hypertension (ICH; levels >100 are high risk and >200 are predictive). The evaluation for common and uncommon etiologies entails a careful historical review of recent medication or toxin use, including over-the-counter medicines, dietary supplements, alcohol, and illicit substances given the overwhelming likelihood of a drug-induced injury. A pregnancy test is warranted in women of childbearing age. Collaborative information from the patient's family and chart review are especially important toward this goal. Patients with ischemic and drug-induced hepatitis tend to have a marked (>10 times the upper reference limit) compared with patients with autoimmune hepatitis (>5 but <10 times the upper reference limit).

Understanding serologic patterns with strong predictive value can be very helpful in guiding diagnosis, particularly for Wilson disease. More than half of the patients with ALF have low ceruloplasmin levels; thus, if there is suspicion for Wilson disease, the rapid diagnostic criteria should be employed (alkaline phosphatase:bilirubin ratio <4, AST:ALT ratio >2.2) because these criteria are 100% sensitive and specific for fulminant Wilson disease. Conversely, markedly elevated AST levels with low bilirubin (anicteric hepatitis) can be seen in ischemic hepatitis, acetaminophen overdose, and acute herpes simplex virus (HSV). Acetaminophen has a readily available but time-sensitive assay that should be done as soon as ALF is suspected, along with toxicology urine and serum assays. The Rumack-Matthew nomogram is a valuable tool to assess likelihood of severe toxicity based on serum levels and time of ingestion.

Time is of the essence to assess for viral and autoimmune etiologies. Viral testing should be part of the initial evaluation (and should include HAV IgM, HBV surface Ab, core IgM, HCV RNA, HDV IgM, HEV IgM, and Epstein-Barr virus/herpes zoster virus/varicella zoster virus [EBV/HZV/VZV] serologies when risk factors are present) because antiviral therapy may be beneficial. Autoimmune markers should also be assessed (including antinuclear antibody [ANA], ferritin, serum protein electrophoresis [SPEP], and anti-smooth muscle antibodies) to readily identify autoimmune hepatitis and less frequently seen myeloproliferative disorders. Ultrasound vascular imaging is expedient and can rapidly identify structural changes (large hepatic tumor burden, thrombosis) as well as Budd-Chiari syndrome. Finally, in a significant proportion of cases of ALF (~17%), a clear etiology is not readily identified and there should be a low threshold for liver biopsy in such patients. It is believed that autoimmune hepatitis and unrecognized acetaminophen poisoning make up the largest proportion of etiologies in this category.

E. Management Basics

1. **Supportive care:** Multisystem organ failure and cerebral edema are typically the outcome most feared in ALF; their risk is directly tied to severity of HE at presentation. Frequent monitoring of acid-base status given the

common renal dysfunction, mental status assessments with low threshold for airway protection, arterial ammonia monitoring, and a broad-spectrum infectious evaluation make up the cornerstones of supportive care.

a. **Infection:** Nearly half of the patients in a large multicenter epidemiology study had a culture-positive infection finding while hospitalized for ALF and infection is a leading cause of death in ALF. Further, control of active infections is vital if a patient develops an indication for LT. Although prophylactic antibiotics have not shown benefit, patients with ALF merit heightened vigilance and surveillance for infection, with a low threshold for antibiotic initiation.

b. **Encephalopathy/risk of cerebral edema:** Previous studies showed that in patients with ALF, a serum ammonia concentration of 75 uM/L was identified as an important threshold below which patients rarely develop ICH. Conversely, arterial ammonia levels greater than 100 uM/L on admission represent an independent risk factor for the development of high-grade HE and baseline levels of ammonia greater than 200 uM/L are predictive of clinically significant ICH. Thus, although routine serum ammonia monitoring is not recommended in chronic liver disease, it is a cornerstone of management in ALF. Arterial ammonia should be checked every 6 to 8 hours. Given the risk of ICH, it is recommended to maintain MAP greater than 75 mm Hg to preserve cerebral perfusion pressure. In the setting of rising ammonia levels, it is also suggested to ensure head of bed elevation and to increase serum sodium to a goal of 145 to 155 mEq/L. Neurology and neurosurgery consultations are warranted if cerebral edema develops.

c. **Bleeding:** Bleeding complications can occur related to the severe coagulopathy associated with ALF. However, prophylactic FFP is not recommended. Careful clinical monitoring for signs of bleeding (including intracranial and intramuscular) is warranted, and if bleeding should occur, FFP, cryoprecipitate, and platelets may confer benefit.

2. **Indications for OLT evaluation:** Owing to the fulminant nature of ALF, most patients with a nonrecoverable etiology risk death within 4 weeks of presentation. Causes of death are typically related to cerebral edema, cardiac arrhythmias, respiratory failure, multi-organ dysfunction, or sepsis. Certain etiologies (liver disease of pregnancy, autoimmune hepatitis, HBV, HSV, acetaminophen poisoning, Budd-Chiari syndrome) are readily treatable when diagnosed in a timely manner. The most important features that dictate recovery are rapid stabilization of synthetic dysfunction (INR <2), and a lower severity of HE at presentation. Several scoring systems exist for predicting risk of death or transplantation (such as the King's College criteria) but these should not be used in isolation to assess trajectory. A transplant hepatology consultation is necessary for any candidacy evaluation and if the patient is not showing signs of recovery, develops ICH, or the etiology is known to be nonrecoverable, they may be listed as status 1A (highest priority) for transplant, in the absence of a clear contraindication for surgery (active uncontrolled malignancy, overwhelming uncontrolled sepsis, brain death). In general, a transplant hepatology consultation is recommended early for any patient with ALF.

3. **Specific therapies:** Acetaminophen poisoning is readily treated with *N*-acetyl-cysteine (NAC) but this is most beneficial when administered within 8 hours of ingestion. However, all patients with confirmed acetaminophen overdose should receive NAC. Additional data suggest potential mortality benefit for NAC for non–acetaminophen-related liver failure and it should be considered when etiology is uncertain. Ischemic hepatitis is generally self-limited when the primary underlying causes are

addressed and corrected (hypotension with vasopressor support, cardiac intervention as indicated). IV acyclovir is the standard therapy for acute disseminated HSV. Pulse-dose steroids may be indicated for autoimmune liver disease. For thrombotic causes, vascular interventions such as catheter-guided thrombolysis, systemic anticoagulation, and/or TIPS may be employed. Prompt delivery of the fetus is definitive management of liver disease of pregnancy.

V. POSTOPERATIVE MANAGEMENT OF THE PATIENT UNDERGOING ORTHOTOPIC LIVER TRANSPLANTATION

A. Overview: The success of an LT is dependent on a true multidisciplinary effort between all involved in the patient's care. Because there can be significant variation between transplant programs in terms of types of donors utilized and the severity of illness within the waitlist candidate population, there are often center-specific practices for postoperative management of these recipients. Thus, overall, it is of paramount importance that there be always an open line of communication, with a primary point of contact established between the critical care team and the transplant service in advance to expedite decision-making and care of this patient population.

B. Survival Rates: Current estimates of the 1-year unadjusted survival rate for a recipient are nearly 90%.

C. Donor Factors: Consideration must be given to donor factors that influence graft function in the immediate postoperative period. Given the disparity in organ supply and demand, there has been an increased application of expanded criteria donors (ECDs). Indeed, the use of certain ECD liver grafts may result in slower initial graft function and/or portend a higher risk of primary nonfunction (PNF) or vascular/biliary complications. Although the definition of these more marginal grafts may vary depending on institution, they are generally thought to encompass donors of advanced age (older than 60 years), higher degree of steatosis (>30% macrosteatosis), donation after cardiac death (vs donation after brain death), and split LTs. Additional donor factors to consider because they relate to immediate graft function are donor instability before procurement, cold ischemia time, and warm ischemia time.

D. Intraoperative Factors: Sign-out from the anesthesia and surgical team should include occurrence of hypotension, vasopressor use, degree of acidosis, urine output, intraoperative bile production, and technical concerns that may affect outcome.

E. Systems-Based Considerations for Postoperative Management: The majority of patients are admitted to the ICU in the initial postoperative period for a typical 24- to 48-hour stay.

1. Neurologic

a. Analgesia: Poor pain control can lead to prolonged recovery and increased pulmonary complications.

1. Delivery route: Patient-controlled analgesia or IV drips/boluses are reasonable alternatives until an enteral route can be used. Epidural catheter placement is avoided given the risk of post-LT bleeding from resolving the coagulopathy.

2. Analgesics: Because the majority of analgesics are metabolized and excreted by the liver or the kidney, poor liver graft function or concomitant renal failure may impact clearance of these medications.

a. Paracetamol (acetaminophen) can be used safely at reduced dosing or in combination therapy for mild to moderate postoperative pain.

b. Nonsteroidal anti-inflammatories are typically avoided because of potential effects on coagulation and renal function.

c. Morphine use has been shown to lead to increased sedation in patients undergoing liver surgery.
d. Hydromorphone and fentanyl are alternative opioids that are less affected by renal impairment and are reasonable alternatives to morphine use. Tramadol has also been used safely to provide post-LT analgesia.

b. **Mental status:** It should be noted that although hepatic synthetic function often recovers quickly following implantation of the liver, encephalopathy can linger in the postoperative period necessitating standard precautions for patients with alterations in mental status. With any change in mental status, in addition to routine workup, attention should be paid to reevaluation of graft function as well as electrolyte and glucose levels, which may be directly affected by hepatic function. Antipsychotics should be avoided if possible because they are often hepatotoxic; however, if needed, low-dose Haldol or quetiapine may be used.

2. **Cardiovascular**

a. **Preoperative baseline:** Preoperative cardiovascular testing is uniformly used for the waitlisted population but may vary in type depending on institutional preference. Cardiovascular testing should be reviewed in all patients in whom it was performed. Special consideration should be given to those with known coronary artery disease, a history of nonalcoholic steatohepatitis and diabetes, valvular stenosis or insufficiency, and known portopulmonary hypertension.

b. **Perioperative hypotension** may result postoperatively given the risk of bleeding, as well as the fact that the vasodilatory and hyperdynamic state of liver failure often takes times to resolve after an LT. Unremitting acidosis or vasopressor requirement should warrant further investigation.

c. **Venous pressures:** Increased venous pressures may lead to hepatic congestion and graft dysfunction due to outflow obstruction. Invasive monitoring can help distinguish cardiac from vasodilatory hypotension and guide appropriate use of inotropic agents, vasopressors, and fluid administration.

d. **Perioperative hypertension** may be seen following an LT in the patient with adequate graft function who may have inadequate analgesia.

e. **Atrial fibrillation:** Post-LT atrial fibrillation may result because of significant perioperative fluid shifts and electrolyte fluxes. If possible, it should be managed without the use of amiodarone because of this medication's potential for hepatotoxicity.

3. **Respiratory**

a. **Weaning and extubation:** Early weaning and extubation from the ventilator is recommended in patients after LT to decrease risk of infection, deconditioning, and prolonged recovery. Care should be taken for those patients with hepatopulmonary syndrome (HPS) because the hypoxemic state can persist in the postoperative period.

b. **Ventilator management:** In optimizing ventilator settings, given the theoretical risks of decreased venous return and hepatic outflow, PEEP should be limited up to 15 cm of H_2O, which has been shown to not impair overall hemodynamics in the patient following LT.

c. **Hepatopulmonary syndrome:** The postoperative management of the patient with HPS is difficult because the timing of the resolution of hypoxemia is variable and can take up to 12 months to return to baseline. A lowered expectation of a resting O_2 saturation is needed in the postoperative period. Extubation postoperatively should be undertaken after careful assessment of the patient. The clinical decompensation of these patients post the extubation can be rapid and unexpected. Thus, preparedness for reintubation or noninvasive positive pressure ventilation (NIPPV) is paramount in the management of these complex cases.

d. **Hypoxemia:** Other etiologies for post-LT hypoxemia include the presence of ascites, atelectasis, and pleural effusion, causing restrictive lung disease. All patients should be optimized with adequate analgesia, rigorous chest physiotherapy, and incentive spirometry. Thoracentesis may be considered for a hydrothorax-limiting extubation but should be approached with caution given the coagulopathy and thrombocytopenia in the immediate postoperative period. Placement of an indwelling chest tube is avoided given the infectious risk.

4. **Gastrointestinal**
   a. **Liver function tests:** There is a typical rise in transaminase levels due to hepatocellular ischemia/reperfusion injury often peaking within 24 hours. Persistent rise, however, may indicate ongoing ischemia. Laboratory abnormalities should be communicated with the surgeon because they may prompt further investigation with Doppler ultrasound. Alkaline phosphatase and bilirubin rise may indicate biliary obstruction.
   b. **Synthetic function laboratory tests:** Platelet count, prothrombin INR, fibrinogen level, and activated partial thromboplastin times (aPTTs) are markers of coagulation, and abnormalities may reflect insufficient liver synthetic function.
   c. **Graft ultrasound with Doppler:** A hepatic graft ultrasound with Doppler can evaluate the patency of the vasculature and biliary system.
5. **Genitourinary**
   a. **Fluids:** Excessive fluid administration to decrease the pressor requirement, generate urine output, or decrease an elevated creatinine should not be attempted in the setting of a normal central venous pressure (CVP) and normal cardiac output because this may lead to venous congestion and graft dysfunction. Non–lactate-containing solutions may be beneficial in those patients with rising lactate levels secondary to decreased consumption of lactate because of decreased liver gluconeogenesis in the transplanted graft. Thus, generally, 5% dextrose with 0.45% normal saline is used unless the recipient has a serum sodium of less than 130 mEq/L, at which point 5% dextrose with 0.9% normal saline may be more appropriate. If volume expansion is needed, colloid solutions, or if indicated, packed red blood cells should be considered.
   b. **Pretransplant renal dysfunction:** present in up to 25% of recipients. If renal replacement therapy is needed in the immediate postoperative period, continuous venovenous hemodialysis (CVVH) is the preferred route. Reinstitution of standard hemodialysis posttransplant should not be attempted until the patient has been stabilized. Transplant nephrology is often consulted to aid in the management of dialysis, as well as any electrolyte abnormalities related to renal dysfunction. Because fresh patients undergoing LT will not metabolize citrate in the setting of liver dysfunction, dialysis replacement fluid should be bicarbonate based in most cases. Even in patients without renal dysfunction before LT, some degree of AKI can be observed postoperatively depending on the duration of vena caval clamping, degree of ischemia/reperfusion injury, and presence of hemodynamic instability during the operation. Given the varying degrees of AKI observed with concomitant oliguria or anuria,

assessment of intravascular status by CVP measurement will allow avoidance of over- or underresuscitation.

c. Electrolytes: Abnormalities should be appropriately addressed promptly.

1. Hyponatremia: Sodium should be corrected carefully keeping in consideration that the patient should be kept euvolemic or marginally hypovolemic in the early postoperative period following LT.

2. Hypocalcemia: Calcium should be optimized because it is an important element in the coagulation cascade, which may already be challenged in the early post-LT period.

3. Hypophosphatemia: Phosphate is important in cellular energy metabolism, and a deficiency can have respiratory, cardiac, neurologic, and endocrine system consequences.

4. Hypomagnesemia: Patients with cirrhosis often have decreased magnesium, which is often further depleted through operative blood loss as well as certain immunosuppressants (ie, tacrolimus).

6. Endocrine

a. Glucose levels: Hyperglycemia may be present because of postsurgical stress and use of steroid therapy for immunosuppression. This should be managed using ICU protocols and may require insulin drips with minimization of dextrose-containing fluids. If hypoglycemia is noted, graft ultrasound with Doppler should be performed because this may be indicative of graft dysfunction.

7. Hematologic

a. Monitoring: In the early post-LT period (first 24-48 hours), patients should receive serial complete blood count tests and coagulation labs to assess for bleeding and hepatic synthetic function. Any significant changes should prompt notification of the transplant team and triggers for transfusion should be clarified for each patient.

1. General considerations

a. A gradual decline of the INR should be expected with a functioning liver and should not require further FFP; thus, a rising INR should prompt concern for early graft dysfunction and consideration for repeat Doppler ultrasound and notification of the transplant team.

b. More aggressive correction of an INR with FFP should be undertaken in the setting of continued drops in the hematocrit.

c. Patients with cirrhosis can often demonstrate a significant degree of thrombocytopenia due to splenomegaly and sequestration, which is only exacerbated by the immunosuppressive and antiviral/antibiotic medications administered. Consideration for administration of platelets should be given for platelet counts less than 50 for the first 12 hours postoperatively and should be continued beyond 12 hours only if clinical signs of bleeding exist. The latter must be balanced with the understanding that a numerical increase in peripheral platelet counts with continued platelet transfusions will be small and unlikely to be sustained in the setting of splenomegaly.

d. Consideration for desmopressin acetate (DDAVP) should be given if there is preexisting renal disease.

e. Cryoprecipitate can be considered for fibrinogen levels less than 100.

f. If bleeding persists, use of ε-aminocaproic acid (Amicar) can be considered after discussion with the transplant team because the management of bleeding must be balanced with the risk of graft thrombosis.

8. **Infectious disease**
   a. **Bacterial prophylaxis:** Standard perioperative antibacterial prophylaxis is utilized, with consideration for organism-specific antibiotics of longer duration if the recipient has an infectious history or if the donor carries an infectious history.
   b. **Viral prophylaxis:** HSV reactivation is the most common opportunistic viral infection in the immediate posttransplant period (first month) and can be reduced by prophylactic antiviral administration. Additional considerations include mismatch of cytomegalovirus (CMV)-seronegative recipients with grafts from CMV-seropositive donors because these patients benefit from antiviral therapy. For those with lower risk of CMV, antiviral administration can be pursued, or, alternatively, monitoring by CMV polymerase chain reaction can be done and therapy instituted if the virus is detected.
   c. **Fungal prophylaxis:** *Pneumocystis jirovecii* infection can be prevented by routine use of prophylactic trimethoprim-sulfamethoxazole after an LT. Additional widespread use of antifungal prophylaxis is not standard practice; however, special consideration should be given to patients requiring retransplantation, reoperation, renal replacement therapy pre- or posttransplant, and those receiving transplant for fulminant hepatic failure.
9. **Nutrition:** Enteral nutrition is preferred to the parenteral route because it is associated with a lower incidence of wound infections and complications and should be started as soon as possible postoperatively. Early enteric feeding aids in nourishing enterocytes and thus decreasing bacterial translocation in addition to stimulating enterohepatic circulation. Validated data on the use of probiotics in this patient population is lacking. Special consideration for NGT or nasal jejunal tube feeds should be given for those patients with prolonged intubation or with encephalopathy and at risk for aspiration.
10. **Immunosuppression:** Immunosuppressive medications are managed by the transplant team, and typical regimens include triple therapy with a calcineurin inhibitor such as tacrolimus or cyclosporine, an antiproliferative agent such as mycophenolate mofetil, and a steroid such as prednisone.
    a. **Calcineurin inhibitors (tacrolimus or cyclosporine):** weight based, usually started at a low-dose and increased, trough levels needed every morning. Common side effects include nephrotoxicity and mental status changes.
    b. **Antiproliferative agent (mycophenolate mofetil):** no levels needed. Common side effects include thrombocytopenia and GI upset.
    c. **Steroid (prednisone):** varying regimens depending on cause of liver disease. Steroids are tapered and no levels checked. Common side effects include altered mental status and hyperglycemia.
11. **Tube/lines/drains**
    a. **Surgical intra-abdominal drains:** Decisions on management of surgical drains are made by the surgical team and are dependent on the volume and type of fluid draining. Any significant change in drainage (such as increasing bilious drainage or bloody drainage) should be immediately communicated to the surgical team. Patients with long-standing portal hypertension and ascites before transplant will often have high serous output from the surgical drains until the portal hypertension begins to resolve.
    b. **Nasogastric tube (NGT):** The standard patient undergoing LT should have NGT removal once they are alert, awake, and able to take their medications orally. Patients with Roux-en-Y creation for biliary drainage will often have an NGT in the postoperative period.

c. **Foley catheter:** Although patients who are stable can have their Foley removed on postoperative day 2 to decrease the risk of catheter-associated urinary tract infection, complex cases or those who are debilitated or with renal dysfunction may require bladder drainage for longer periods.
d. **Endotracheal tube (ETT) and invasive vascular lines:** ETT and invasive vascular lines should be removed as soon as clinically indicated to decrease the risk of ventilator-associated pneumonia and central line–associated blood stream infection.

12. **Prophylaxis**
    a. **Thromboprophylaxis:** Definitive data on the use of routine prophylactic chemoprophylaxis for deep venous thrombosis or pulmonary embolism are currently lacking; however, mechanical thromboprophylaxis is often employed. Patients in the post-LT period are often thought to be in a hypocoagulable state because coagulation may take time to normalize and it takes the new liver time to make sufficient coagulation factors and for thrombocytopenia to resolve.
    b. **Stress ulcer prophylaxis:** Stress ulcer prophylaxis should be utilized, especially in the setting of high-dose steroid use and should be instituted per ICU protocol.

F. Postoperative Complications After Liver Transplantation

1. **Primary nonfunction (PNF):** PNF is the most devastating post-LT complication and is defined as an AST greater than or equal to 3000 U/mL and either an INR greater than or equal to 2.5 and/or evidence of acidosis (arterial pH $\leq$7.3 or a venous pH of 7.25 and/or a lactate level $\geq$4 mmol/L) within 7 days of transplantation. The etiology of PNF is often multifactorial and the only therapy for PNF is retransplantation, with the majority of patients not surviving past 5 days after initial LT.
2. **Vascular complications**
   a. **HAT or stenosis:** HAT occurs in approximately 3% of patients after an LT and is the most common technical complication. Early HAT (within 1 week of LT) may clinically result in rapid-onset hepatic failure, sepsis, fever, altered mental status, and coagulopathy, with laboratory studies suggestive of transaminitis. Delayed diagnosis can result in peritonitis due to biliary necrosis because the bile duct receives its blood supply from the hepatic artery. Hepatic artery stenosis, on the other hand, is often detected incidentally when a graft ultrasound is obtained for another indication or upon workup for transaminitis or biliary complications. Diagnostic studies include graft ultrasound with Doppler or either computed tomography angiography (CTA) or magnetic resonance angiography (MRA) if they can be done expeditiously and tolerated from a renal function standpoint. Treatment for both HAT and stenosis in the early post-LT period is often through operative arterial reconstruction in the immediate postoperative period or, alternatively, through an interventional approach in select patients. If extensive hepatic necrosis is present at the time of exploration, the patient may need emergent retransplantation.
   b. **Portal vein thrombosis (PVT) or stenosis:** PVT occurs in 1% to 3% post-LT cases and may clinically result in ascites, sepsis secondary to bacterial translocation due to intestinal congestion, GI bleeding, and rapid-onset hepatic failure, with laboratory studies suggestive of transaminitis. Graft ultrasound with Doppler is preferable to CTA or MRA, which has decreased sensitivity. If portal vein stenosis is of concern, percutaneous transhepatic portography may be used to measure pressures across the area of concern (generally considered to be significant if the gradient is >5 mm Hg). Treatment of early PVT in the early post-LT period

may necessitate operative exploration and vascular reconstruction. Often, portal vein stenosis can initially be managed with angioplasty and stenting.

c. **Hepatic vein and inferior vena cava (IVC) anastomosis complications:** These complications are relatively uncommon, resulting from kinking, thrombosis, or stenosis and often clinically present with dependent edema and/or ascites because of impeded hepatic outflow. Similar to other vascular complications, diagnostic studies include graft ultrasound with Doppler. Depending on the degree of outflow obstruction, hepatic outflow anastomosis complications can often be managed through interventional methods including angioplasty and/or stenting.

3. **Biliary complications**
   a. **Etiology:** typically multifactorial; however, often related to decreased arterial flow (from the hepatic artery)
      1. **Biliary leak:** Defined by the International Study Group of Liver Surgery to be based on drain fluid bilirubin concentration greater than 3 times the serum concentration on or after postoperative day 3 of surgery or the need for either radiologic or operative intervention because of bile collection or biliary peritonitis. Clinically, it often presents as increased abdominal pain, nausea, increased ascites, and fever. In addition to checking drain bilirubin levels, graft ultrasound with Doppler should be performed to assess for concomitant HAT or stenosis. Endoscopic retrograde cholangiopancreatography (ERCP) can be both diagnostic and therapeutic. CT scan may help localize biloma or other intra-abdominal collections. Treatment options included biliary drainage, biliary stents, possible reconstructive surgery, use of intra-abdominal drains, and, possibly, antibiotics.
      2. **Biliary stricture:** Biliary stricture clinically may present with jaundice, pruritus, or as cholangitis, with laboratory studies suggestive of increased serum bilirubin with persistently elevated alkaline phosphatase. In addition to checking drain bilirubin levels, graft ultrasound with Doppler should be performed to assess for concomitant HAT or stenosis. ERCP can be both diagnostic and therapeutic. Treatment is similar to that of biliary leak. Surgical conversion from a biliary duct-to-duct anastomosis to Roux-en-Y drainage can also be considered.
4. **Infectious complications:** These are the most common cause of postoperative morbidity and mortality and include bacteremia, fungemia, pneumonia, wound infection, urinary infection, and *Clostridium difficile* colitis given the immunosuppressed state of the recipient. Prevention and source control/treatment form the main principles in management and can be complemented with reductions in immunosuppression when indicated.
   a. **Line- and tube-related infections:** Catheter-associated urinary tract infections, central line–associated blood stream infection, and ventilator-associated pneumonias can be minimized by removal of invasive lines and tubes as expeditiously as possible.
   b. **Pneumonia:** Early-onset hospital-acquired pneumonia within 7 days of LT occurs in approximately 15% of patients and is associated with prolonged ventilation (>48 hours). Early diagnostic bronchoscopy is favored over empiric treatment whenever possible.
   c. ***C. difficile* colitis:** *C. difficile* colitis occurs in approximately 19% of liver recipients, compared with 1% of patients without transplants, and is likely due to empiric antibiotic use, immunosuppression, and increased nosocomial exposure. These patients should be managed with close attention given to consequences on allograft function induced by

diarrhea and associated hypovolemia and hypotension, as well as electrolyte abnormalities.

5. **Renal complications**
   a. **Definition:** AKI can be stratified on the basis of the *R*isk, *I*njury, *F*ailure, *L*oss, and *E*nd-stage kidney disease (RIFLE) criteria or the Acute Kidney Injury Network (AKIN) staging system, both of which use creatinine and urine output as criteria.
      1. In the post-LT period, AKI has been associated with reduced patient and graft survival in the perioperative and long-term periods.
      2. Baseline creatinine levels in patients with cirrhosis can lead to overestimation of renal function because of lower creatinine production rates secondary to malnutrition and decreased muscle mass in these patients.
   b. **Etiology and risk factors:** Post-LT AKI is often multifactorial and includes intraoperative factors such as hypotension, bleeding, vena cava clamping, increased transfusion requirement, and ischemia/reperfusion injury.
   c. **Management:** Hemodynamic optimization and initiation of renal support may be necessary in the management of post-LT AKI. Consideration for modification of immunosuppression regimen to decrease calcineurin inhibitors as well as decreasing potentially nephrotoxic prophylactic medications should also be performed in patients with post-LT AKI.
6. **Early immunologic complications**
   a. **Hyperacute rejection:** Hyperacute rejection, also known as antibody-mediated rejection, is a rare complication that usually occurs within minutes to hours of LT. In this case, rejection is secondary to preformed recipient antibodies that are present at the time of LT depositing in the newly transplanted graft, resulting in activation of the complement and coagulation cascade causing subsequent graft thrombosis and necrosis. This is typically secondary to ABO incompatibility and attempts at plasma exchange, IV γ-globulin, B-cell depletion therapy, and splenectomy can be performed. However, if acute hepatic failure ensues, emergent retransplantation may be necessary.
   b. **Acute cellular rejection (ACR):** ACR typically occurs within 6 weeks of LT and is secondary to cytotoxic and helper T-cell activation. The clinical manifestation of ACR is usually nonspecific but laboratory studies typically manifest with increasing ALT followed by elevations in AST and bilirubin. After other etiologies of laboratory abnormalities are ruled out, diagnosis is typically made through biopsy. Management typically involves optimization of immunosuppressive therapy for mild ACR, steroid pulse therapy for moderate ACR, and adjunctive therapy utilizing T-cell depletion therapy for severe ACR.
7. **Bleeding:** Post-LT bleeding may be secondary to insufficient surgical hemostasis or more commonly due to coagulopathy and thrombocytopenia.
   a. Coagulopathy may occur secondary to dilution associated with massive transfusion, inadequate replacement of components, hypothermia, hyperfibrinolysis, or inadequate hepatic synthetic function.
   b. Ongoing bleeding may require surgical reintervention to assess for surgical hemostasis or may be indicative of graft dysfunction in the patient following the LT.

Selected Readings

Aldenkortt F, Aldenkortt M, Caviezel L, Waeber JL, Weber A, Schiffer E. Portopulmonary hypertension and hepatopulmonary syndrome. *World J Gastroenterol.* 2014;20(25):8072-8081.

Bajaj JS, Kamath PS, Reddy KR. The evolving challenge of infections in cirrhosis. *N Engl J Med.* 2021;384:2317-2330.

Biggins SW, Angeli P, Garcia-Tsao G, et al. Diagnosis, evaluation, and management of ascites, spontaneous bacterial peritonitis and hepatorenal syndrome: 2021 practice guidance by the American Association for the Study of Liver Diseases. *Hepatology*. 2021;74:1014-1048.

Bischoff SC, Bernal W, Dasarathy S, et al. ESPEN practical guideline: clinical nutrition in liver disease. *Clin Nutr*. 2020;39:3533-3562.

European Association for the Study of the Liver. EASL Clinical Practice Guidelines for the management of patients with decompensated cirrhosis. *J Hepatol*. 2018;69:406-460.

Farid SG, Prasad KR, Morris-Stiff G. Operative terminology and post-operative management approaches applied to hepatic surgery: trainee perspectives. *World J Gastrointest Surg*. 2013;5:146-155.

Fernandez TMA, Gardiner PJ. Critical care of the liver transplant recipient. *Curr Anesthesiol Rep*. 2015;5:419-428.

Garcia-Tsao G. Current management of the complications of cirrhosis and portal hypertension: variceal hemorrhage, ascites, and spontaneous bacterial peritonitis. *Dig Dis*. 2016;34:382-386.

Ginès P, Krag A, Abraldes JG, Solà E, Fabrellas N, Kamath PS. Liver cirrhosis. *Lancet*. 2021; 398(10308):1359-1376.

Martens K, McMurry HS, Koprowski S, et al. Anticoagulation in cirrhosis: evidence for the treatment of portal vein thrombosis and applications for prophylactic therapy. *J Clin Gastroenterol*. 2022;56:536-545.

O'Leary JG, Greenberg CS, Patton HM, Caldwell SH. AGA clinical practice update: coagulation in cirrhosis. *Gastroenterology*. 2019;157:34-43.e1.

Olson JC. Intensive care management of patients with cirrhosis. *Curr Treat Options Gastroenterol*. 2018;16:241-252.

Olson JC, Karvellas CJ. Critical care management of the patient with cirrhosis awaiting liver transplant in the intensive care unit. *Liver Transpl*. 2017;23:1465-1476.

Passi NN, McPhail MJ. The patient with cirrhosis in the intensive care unit and the management of acute-on-chronic liver failure. *J Intensive Care Soc*. 2022;23(1):78-86.

Patidar KR, Peng JL, Pike F, et al. Associations between mean arterial pressure and poor ICU outcomes in critically ill patients with cirrhosis: is 65 the sweet spot? *Crit Care Med*. 2020;48:e753-e760.

Paugam-Burtz C, Levesque E, Louvet A, et al. Management of liver failure in general intensive care unit. *Anaesth Crit Care Pain Med*. 2020;39:143-161.

Rifaie N, Saner FH. Critical care management in patients with acute liver failure. *Best Pract Res Clin Anaesthesiol*. 2020;34:89-99.

Ruf A, Dirchwolf M, Freeman RB. From Child-Pugh to MELD score and beyond: taking a walk down memory lane. *Ann Hepatol*. 2022;27:100535.

Tocia C, Dumitru A, Alexandrescu L, Popescu R, Dumitru E. Timing of paracentesis and outcomes in hospitalized patients with decompensated cirrhosis. *World J Hepatol*. 2020; 12:1267-1275.

27

Coagulopathy and Hypercoagulability

Robert D. Sinyard, III, Noelle N. Saillant, and
Katherine H. Albutt

I. OVERVIEW OF COAGULATION

A. Classical Versus Cell-Based Model of Coagulation

1. Classically, coagulation has been taught as a series of separate processes involving a primary plug of platelet aggregation and a secondary activation via a cascading series of factors resulting in the activation of fibrin to strengthen this primary plug through vigorous cross-linking.
2. Newer cell-based models of coagulation replace the traditional "cascade" hypothesis and propose that coagulation takes place on different cell surfaces in three overlapping steps. In highlighting the importance of cellular control during coagulation, the cell-based model allows a more thorough understanding of how hemostasis works in vivo and sheds light on the pathophysiologic mechanisms behind certain coagulation disorders.
3. In the cell-based model, coagulation occurs in three overlapping stages: (i) initiation, which occurs on a tissue factor–bearing cell; (ii) amplification, in which platelets and cofactors are activated to set the stage for large-scale thrombin generation; and (iii) propagation, in which large amounts of thrombin are generated on the platelet surface.
4. Coagulopathy in the critically ill covers a range of abnormal states of coagulation. Simply, coagulopathy can be defined as the blood's inability to clot normally, which may be a deficiency of clot formation, hypocoagulability, or an overactivation of the coagulation process, hypercoagulability.

B. Monitoring of Coagulation

1. History and physical exam
   a. Early investigation should include a family history as well as a review of therapeutic agents contributing to the coagulopathy, considering medications received both in and out of the hospital before critical illness. Current nutritional status, history of bleeding in the past, and nonmedication causes of coagulopathy should also be assessed. In patients who are critically ill, concurrent illnesses such as sepsis, multiple organ failure, recent heparin exposure, and mechanical circulatory device requirements are just a few of the many contributors to coagulation pathology.
   b. Exam findings may help differentiate between diagnoses that present with similar laboratory findings. For example, major vascular sources of bleeding as opposed to petechiae and oozing from vascular catheter sites and mucosal surfaces point to markedly different causes and treatments.
2. Laboratory studies
   a. **Activated partial thromboplastin time** is performed by adding an activator of the intrinsic pathway, phospholipids, and calcium to a citrated plasma sample. Normal values of activated partial thromboplastin time (aPTT) vary widely depending on the reagent and analyzer used, making it a poor comparison across institutions. The test is sensitive to decreased amounts of coagulation factors of the intrinsic pathway (prekallikrein); factors XII,

XI (hemophilia C), IX (hemophilia B), and VIII (hemophilia A); and common pathway factors (X, V, II, and fibrinogen). In addition, unfractionated heparin (UFH), direct thrombin inhibitors (DTIs), antibodies to factor VIII or IX (acquired hemophilia), and antiphospholipid antibodies such as lupus anticoagulant (LA) also affect the aPTT. Antiphospholipid antibodies prolong aPTT by reducing the availability of phospholipids—required for coagulation—in plasmatic coagulation tests (in vitro). Notably, aPTT prolongation due to an antiphospholipid syndrome (APS) is not associated with bleeding but with thrombosis. aPTT can be used to guide UFH therapy but is not sensitive enough to measure the effects of low-molecular-weight heparin (LMWH), which should be monitored via anti–factor Xa assays. The clinician should be aware that the positive and negative predictive value for bleeding is low for aPTT, which means that neither a prolonged aPTT has to be associated with bleeding (eg, in APS) nor does a normal aPTT exclude bleeding. Correction of an abnormal aPTT in patients undergoing surgery is not always indicated unless the patient is bleeding.

b. **Anti–factor Xa assays** are chromogenic assays that facilitate the measurement of inhibition of factor Xa by UFH, LMWH, fondaparinux, and direct factor Xa inhibitors (DXaIs). Because LMWH, fondaparinux, and DXaIs minimally prolong aPTT, anti–factor Xa assays should be used for monitoring therapeutic levels of these drugs. Furthermore, the aPTT cannot be used to monitor UFH in some instances, for example, in the presence of antiphospholipid antibodies or in the case of factor XII deficiency. In these cases, monitoring of UFH with anti–factor Xa assays is more appropriate.

c. **Prothrombin time** is performed by adding thromboplastin (tissue factor = factor III), as the activator of the extrinsic pathway, phospholipids, and calcium to a citrated plasma sample. The test is sensitive to decreased amounts of coagulation factors of the extrinsic (factor VII) and common pathway (factors X, V, II, and fibrinogen). Because most vitamin K–dependent coagulation factors (II, VII, IX, and X) are involved in the extrinsic and common pathway (except factor IX), prothrombin time (PT) has been designed for monitoring of vitamin K antagonists (VKAs) such as warfarin. However, reagents used for PT measurement vary widely regarding their tissue factor activity, and therefore, the **international normalized ratio (INR)** was instituted in 1983 to permit comparability of results in patients treated with warfarin between different laboratories. Warfarin therapy can be guided by a targeted INR value independent of the performing laboratory. Although the INR is frequently used to assess coagulation impairment in patients with trauma and liver disease (eg, to verify trauma-induced coagulopathy [TIC] or to calculate the Model for End-Stage Liver Disease [MELD] score), it may not truly represent their coagulation profile.

d. **Fibrinogen** is the first factor to drop to a critical level in case of hemorrhage. The normal range for fibrinogen is 150 to 400 mg/dL and in the third trimester of pregnancy 450 to 600 mg/dL. In acute-phase reaction, it can rise to about 1000 mg/dL. In severe bleeding, it is crucial to maintain the plasma fibrinogen level above 150 to 200 mg/dL. Fresh frozen plasma (FFP) is often not effective in reaching this target; thus, transfusion of cryoprecipitate or fibrinogen concentrate is required. Fibrinogen levels can be measured by several methods. The more classical optical methods are influenced by infused colloids, resulting in wrong high fibrinogen values by 15% to 90% depending on the reagent used. In contrast, viscoelastic testing using the **fibrinogen thromboelastometry (FIBTEM; rotational thromboelastometry [ROTEM])** or **functional**

fibrinogen (FF) assay (thromboelastography [TEG]) demonstrates impaired fibrin polymerization after colloid infusion, associated with increased blood loss and transfusion requirements.

e. **Fibrin(ogen) degradation products** are peptides produced from the action of plasmin on fibrinogen or on fibrin monomers. They are measurable by serum assays and may aid in the diagnosis of primary fibrinolysis or disseminated intravascular coagulation (DIC). Furthermore, fibrin(ogen) degradation products (FDPs) modulate clotting assays by interfering with fibrin monomer polymerization and by impairing platelet function. FDPs are often elevated in cirrhosis because of impaired clearance from circulation.

f. **D-Dimer** is a specific fragment produced when plasmin cleaves cross-linked fibrin and can be measured by a serum assay. Almost all patients with acute venous thromboembolism (VTE) present with an elevated D-dimer level. However, elevated D-dimer is not specific to VTE because it can be associated with several other conditions, including DIC, patients who are postsurgical or posttraumatic, pregnancy, and malignancy. However, a normal D-dimer test usually excludes the diagnosis of VTE.

g. **Single-factor assays** are specialized tests quantifying the activity of individual coagulation factors. They can be used to clarify prolonged global plasmatic coagulation tests, such as aPTT, PT, and thrombin time (TT). On the one hand, isolated prolongation of aPTT is suspicious for hemophilia A (factor VIII), B (factor IX), or C (factor XI), but can be prolonged significantly in factor XII deficiency, too, which is not associated with bleeding. On the other hand, isolated prolongation of PT can be a sign of factor VII deficiency. Notably, factor XIII deficiency is not associated with a prolongation of aPTT, PT, or TT but can be the cause of unexpected postoperative bleeding. Single-factor analyses are usually performed in concert with a clinical pathology or hematology consultation.

h. **Activated clotting time** is a clotting test in which kaolin, celite, or glass beads are added to a noncitrated whole-blood sample to activate the intrinsic pathway. Activated clotting time (ACT) usually is performed as a point-of-care test in the acute setting, for example, during cardiopulmonary bypass or extracorporeal membranous oxygenation (ECMO), to monitor high heparin concentrations where aPTT cannot be measured any more (>180 seconds). Because ACT is a nonspecific whole-blood test, it can not only be influenced by heparin and protamine but also by a lot of other variables, such as hemodilution, fibrinogen, platelets, aprotinin, and glycoprotein IIb/IIIa receptor antagonists. This is important for a meaningful interpretation of ACT test results. Because normal ACT depends on the test system used, it should be standardized by an institution.

i. **Rotational thromboelastometry and thromboelastography** are viscoelastic test devices used most often at the point of care in the emergency room (ER), the operating room (OR), or in the intensive care unit (ICU). Both devices are assessing the change in viscoelasticity of a small amount of whole blood activated by different agents in a system where a heated cup and a pin are oscillating against each other. Viscoelastic testing provides real-time, dynamic information about the whole coagulation process, including clot initiation (thrombin generation), clot kinetics, clot strength, and clot stability (lysis). ROTEM and TEG differ in some technical points, definition of parameters, and reagents used; therefore, results are not completely interchangeable between tests. The definition of ROTEM/TEG parameters and their clinical relevance are displayed in Figure 27.1. Specific patterns of the trace are characteristic

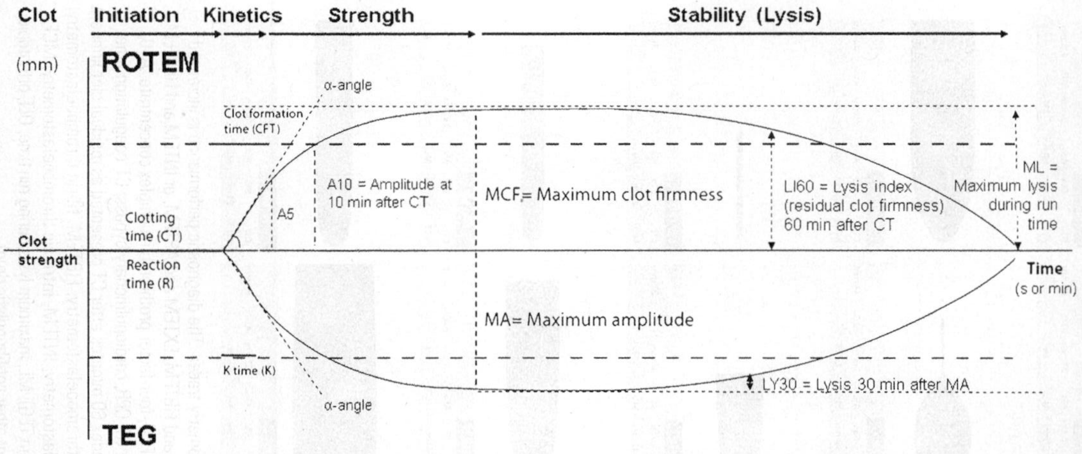

	ROTEM	TEG	Hemostatic factors
Clot initiation	CT (clotting time) in s	R (reaction time) in min	Enzymatic coagulation factors, anticoagulants, FDPs, tissue factor expression on monocytes
Clot kinetics	CFT (clot formation time) in s α (angle) in degrees	K (kinetic time) in min α (angle) in degrees	Enzymatic coagulation factor, anticoagulants, fibrinogen, platelets
Clot strength	(A5) A10 (amplitude (5) 10 min after CT) in mm MCF (maximum clot firmness) in mm	MA (maximum amplitude) in mm	Platelets, fibrinogen, FXIII, colloids
Clot stability (lysis)	LI60 (lysis index (residual clot firmness) 60 min after CT) in % of MCF ML (maximum lysis during run time) in % of MCF	LY30 (lysis 30 min after MA) in % of MA	Fibrinolytic enzymes, fibrinolysis inhibitors, FXIII

FIGURE 27.1 Rotational thromboelastometry/thromboelastography (ROTEM/TEG) parameters. FDPs, fibrin(ogen) degradation products; FXIII, factor XIII.

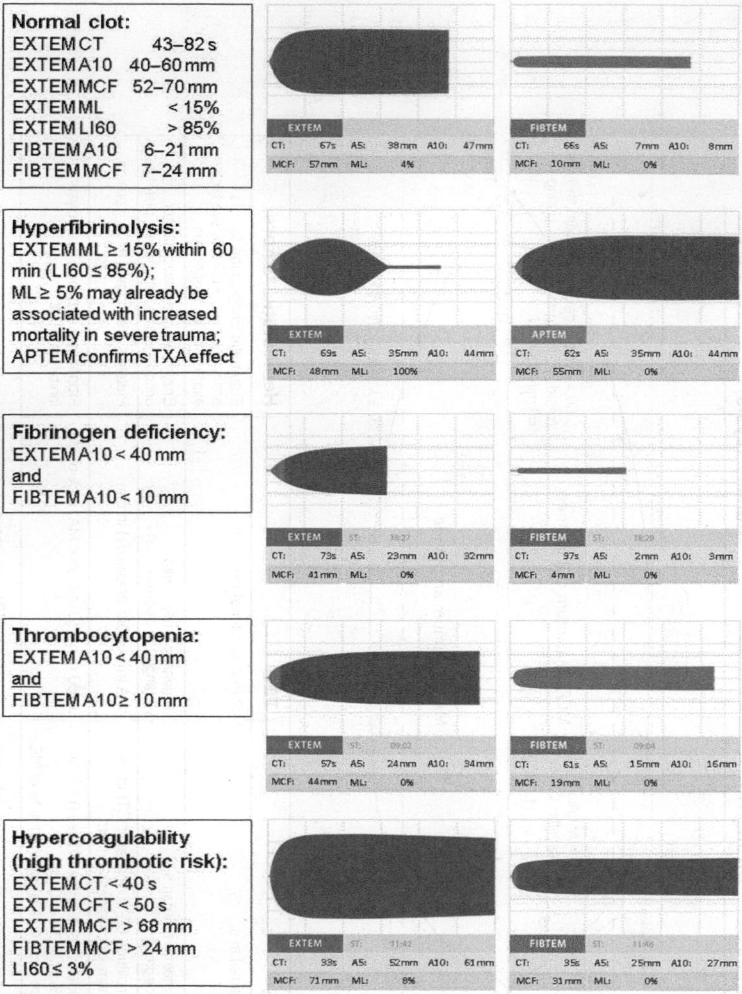

FIGURE 27.2 Characteristic thromboelastometry traces. The diagnostic performance is increased by test combinations, for example, EXTEM and FIBTEM, EXTEM and APTEM, or INTEM and HEPTEM (for assay description, see Figure 27.1). 4F-PCC, four-factor prothrombin complex concentrate; A10, amplitude of clot firmness 10 minutes after CT; CPB, cardiopulmonary bypass; CT, coagulation time (corresponds to r-time in TEG); LI60, lysis index 60 minutes after CT presented as residual clot firmness in percentage of MCF; EXTEM, extrinsic thromboelastometry; FIBTEM, fibrin thromboelastometry; HEPTEM, heparinase modified thromboelastometry; INTEM, intrinsic thromboelastometry; MCF, maximum clot firmness (corresponds to MA in TEG); ML, maximum lysis during run time; OLT, orthotopic liver transplantation; TXA, tranexamic acid (or other antifibrinolytic drug).

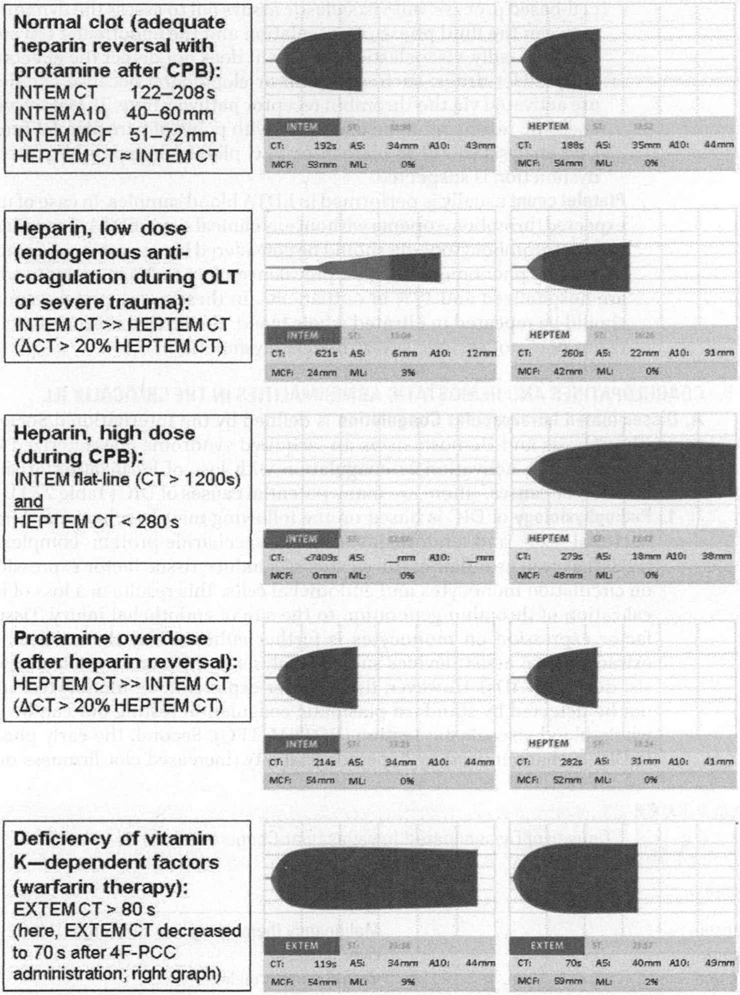

FIGURE 27.2 *(continued)*

of several coagulation abnormalities (eg, hyperfibrinolysis, fibrinogen deficiency, thrombocytopenia, factor deficiencies of the extrinsic and intrinsic pathways, heparin effects; see Figure 27.2), assisting the clinician with the diagnosis and appropriate treatment. Here, the use of ROTEM/TEG-guided bleeding management algorithms is highly recommended, and their clinical- and cost-effectiveness has been proven in several studies and health technology assessments. More on use of viscoelastic measures for guiding therapeutic interventions is detailed later in this chapter.

1. Two major **limitations** of viscoelastic assays are (i) the in vitro nature of the assay and (ii) the lack of assessment of antiplatelet drugs. As mentioned in the opening part of this chapter, coagulation is a

cell-based process, but viscoelastic assays fail to assess the dynamics between the fluid phase of coagulation and the endothelial cell surface. Secondly, viscoelastic assessment does not detect the effects of antiplatelet drugs, such as aspirin or clopidogrel because platelets are activated via the thrombin receptor pathway here. Therefore, viscoelastic testing must be combined with point-of-care platelet function analysis (ROTEM platelet or TEG platelet mapping) if platelet dysfunction is suspected.

j. **Platelet count** usually is performed in EDTA blood samples. In case of unexpected thrombocytopenia without any clinical signs, EDTA-dependent pseudothrombocytopenia should be considered because it is a common laboratory phenomenon with a prevalence of up to 2% in patients who are hospitalized and 17% in outpatients. In these cases, platelet count should be repeated in citrated whole blood. However, a normal platelet count does not exclude severe platelet dysfunction.

II. COAGULOPATHIES AND HEMOSTATIC ABNORMALITIES IN THE CRITICALLY ILL

A. **Disseminated Intravascular Coagulation** is defined by the International Society on Thrombosis and Hemostasis as an "acquired syndrome characterized by the intravascular activation of coagulation with loss of localization arising from different causes." There are many potential causes of DIC (Table 27.1).

1. **Pathophysiology** of DIC is based on the following main mechanisms. First, bacterial exo- and endotoxins (lipopolysaccharide-protein complexes [LPSs]) as well as inflammatory cytokines induce tissue factor expression on circulation monocytes and endothelial cells. This results in a loss of localization of thrombin generation to the site of endothelial injury. Tissue factor expression on monocytes is further enhanced by the surfaces of extracorporeal assist devices such as dialysis, ECMO, and ventricular assist devices (VADs). However, tissue factor expression on monocytes cannot be detected by standard plasmatic coagulation testing but can be by whole-blood viscoelastic testing (ROTEM/TEG). Second, the early phase of DIC is characterized by hypercoagulability (increased clot firmness due

TABLE 27.1 Causes of Disseminated Intravascular Coagulation

Acute	Chronic
Sepsis	Malignancy (hematologic or solid organ)
Shock	Liver disease
Trauma	Vascular abnormalities
Head injury	Aortic aneurysm
Crush injury	Aortic dissection
Burns (extensive)	Peritoneovenous shunt
Extracorporeal circulation (eg, ECMO)	Intra-aortic balloon pump
Pregnancy catastrophes	
Placental abruption	
Amniotic fluid embolus	
Septic abortion	
Embolism of fat or cholesterol	
Hepatic failure (severe)	
Toxic/immune reactions (severe)	
Snake bites	
Hemolytic transfusion reactions	

ECMO, extracorporeal membranous oxygenation.

to acute-phase reaction with high fibrinogen levels), consumption of physiologic coagulation inhibitors (antithrombin [AT] and protein C), platelet dysfunction, and inhibition of fibrinolysis (upregulation of plasmin activator inhibitor-1 [PAI-1]). This results in thrombosis of the microcirculation and multiple organ failure. Finally, when coagulation factors and fibrinolytic inhibitors are consumed, hypocoagulation and secondary fibrinolysis can result in severe bleeding. Early detection of pathologic thromboelastometric results and platelet dysfunction detected by whole-blood impedance aggregometry on admission at the ICU are associated with worse outcomes.

2. **Clinical features** of DIC include hemorrhage from operative or traumatic wounds, oozing from venipuncture sites, petechiae, and ecchymosis. Micro- and macrovascular thrombosis can lead to organ failure.
3. **Diagnosis** includes clinical and laboratory data. Recommendations include the use of a DIC scoring system, of which three use different criteria for different types of DIC.
4. **Laboratory tests** such as prolonged PT and INR, reduction of platelet counts, and reduced fibrinogen and AT levels may overlap with other coagulopathies. Elevation of fibrin-related markers such as D-dimer, FDPs, and soluble fibrin are common findings not specific to DIC. Peripheral blood smears can reveal schistocytes (fragmented red blood cells [RBCs]), which are formed as RBCs that flow through fibrin strands in the microvasculature are severed. Point-of-care testing includes ROTEM/TEG and aPTT waveforms to support the diagnosis.
5. **Treatment** of DIC is aimed at correcting the underlying cause, blood product transfusion when indicated, and pharmacologic treatment. Blood products should be transfused to correct for active bleeding or in preparation for life-saving procedures. Fibrinogen levels should then be corrected to 150 to 200 mg/dL. Platelet transfusion should be considered in patients who are actively bleeding and who have a platelet count of less than 50 000/mm^3. However, platelet transfusion should be considered carefully because it may aggravate multiple organ failure and result in secondary bacterial infections. In patients who are not bleeding, the threshold for platelet transfusion should be 10 000 to 20 000/mm^3. Other blood components such as FFP and packed red blood cells (pRBCs) should be transfused only in patients with active bleeding or who are at high risk for bleeding. Pharmacologic treatment depends on the type of DIC and includes anticoagulation or antifibrinolytics. The balance of coagulation and fibrinolysis can be further characterized with point-of-care testing (ROTEM/TEG and whole-blood impedance aggregometry) to guide treatment, but hematologic consult should be considered in complicated cases of DIC.

B. Trauma-Induced Coagulopathy is accepted to be a discrete clinical entity different from DIC (Figure 27.3). In contrast to DIC, hypoperfusion-induced activation of protein C with subsequent cleavage of activated factors V and VIII and downregulation of PAI-1 result in endogenous anticoagulation and primary hyperfibrinolysis. Furthermore, shedding of the endothelial glycocalyx leads to liberation of heparinoids, which intensifies endogenous anticoagulation. In addition, TIC is modulated by hemodilution, hypothermia, and acidosis. TIC is functionally characterized by a reduction in clot strength. With a threshold of clot amplitude at 5 minutes of less than or equal to 35 mm, ROTEM can identify acute traumatic coagulopathy at 5 minutes and predict the need for massive transfusion. Concepts to treat TIC vary widely between the United States and Europe, with some using a fixed transfusion ratio of pRBCs, FFP, and platelets; and others an individualized goal-directed bleeding management using coagulation factor concentrates (fibrinogen and four-factor prothrombin complex concentrate [4F-PCC]) guided by viscoelastic testing (ROTEM/TEG). Randomized clinical trials (RCTs) are missing to show which

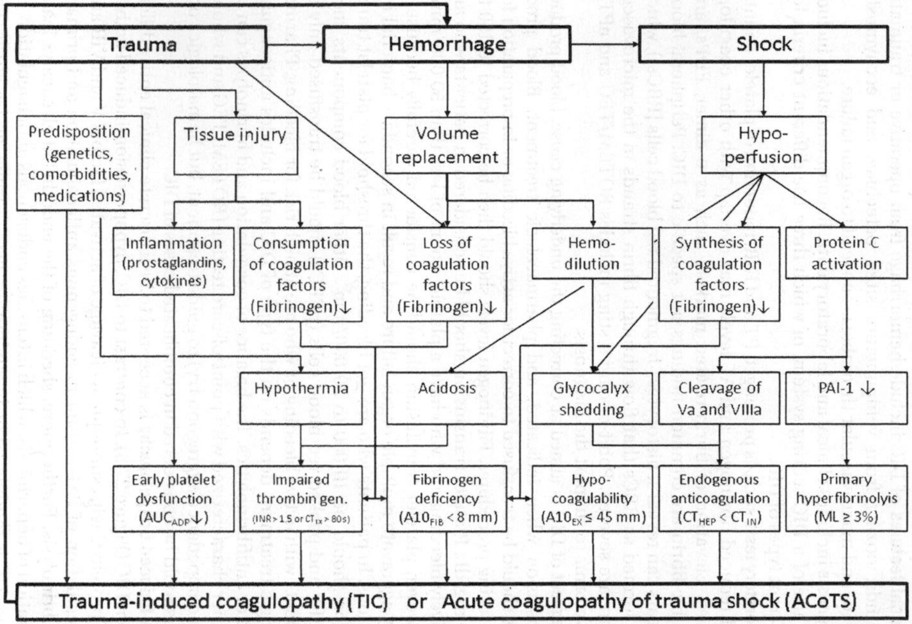

FIGURE 27.3 Pathophysiology of trauma-induced coagulopathy (TIC) and corresponding triggers of thromboelastometry and whole-blood impedance aggregometry. A10, amplitude of clot firmness 10 minutes after CT; AUC, area under the curve; CT, coagulation time; EX, extrinsic thromboelastometry (EXTEM); FIB, fibrin thromboelastometry (FIBTEM); HEP, heparinase modified thromboelastometry (HEPTEM); IN, intrinsic thromboelastometry (INTEM); INR, international normalized ratio; ML, maximum lysis.

approach is superior in severe trauma. In traumatic brain injury (TBI), the risk of bleeding and thrombosis is high.

1. Increasing evidence supports viscoelastic testing for guidance of transfusion in the trauma bay, OR, and ICU setting. Early evidence suggests at least two to three distinct phenotypes of TIC that may be linked to patient characteristics, injury patterns, and comorbidities. TEG allows for distinct characterization of these phenotypes and individualization of therapy. For patients undergoing massive transfusion protocols, RCT evidence has demonstrated that viscoelastic guidance of transfusion improves survival and increases ventilator-free and ICU-free days.
2. Increased viscoelastic testing has also resulted in the identification of a spectrum of disorders related to fibrinolysis associated with TIC. On the one end of the spectrum, hyperfibrinolysis is common in patients who are severely injured and may warrant the use of antifibrinolytics. Conversely, inhibition of fibrinolysis, or "**fibrinolysis shutdown**," has also been observed in patients after an operation and in those with TIC, often resulting in deep vein thrombosis (DVT) and multiorgan failure. Given this complexity, many have argued against blanket administration of antifibrinolytic therapy in exchange for goal-directed therapy for hyperfibrinolysis based on viscoelastic testing. Suggested algorithms can be found in **Section III** of this chapter.

C. Mechanical Cardiac Support is increasingly common in patients in critical care and associated with significant complexities in terms of management of coagulopathy both due to devices and critical illness. Beyond the mechanical forces on RBCs, tissue factor expression on monocytes is enhanced by the surfaces of devices such as VADs or ECMO.

a. Ventricular assist devices may function either as pulsatile or nonpulsatile with anticoagulation varying between differing devices but typically focused on targeting either aPTT 1.5 to 2.5 times normal, an INR 1.5 to 3.5, and/or the use of a low-dose acetylsalicylic acid. Event rates for bleeding and thromboembolic complications in patients with VAD approach 45% and are frequently associated with poor outcomes and high costs. Regarding bleeding, patients with nonpulsatile VADs may develop a similar acquired von Willebrand factor (vWF) syndrome (type 2A), most commonly presenting as gastrointestinal (GI) bleeding, due to the high shear stress induced by the device resulting in cleavage of vWF multimers. This should be managed with antifibrinolytics, desmopressin, factor VIII concentrates, or transfusion. Acquired factor XIII deficiency may also occur because of continuous device-related thrombin generation resulting in factor XIII consumption. Viscoelastic testing is helpful for identification of coagulopathy due to factor XIII deficiency and management. Factor XIII appears to be helpful only when plasma levels are 70% of the normal value. Regarding thromboembolic complications, patients with VADs may experience these events even with aPTT or INR in the therapeutic range given the limitations of these tests. This further emphasizes the need for repeated viscoelastic-guided therapy, including platelet function testing. The detection of heparin-induced thrombocytopenia (HIT) is also complex in patients with VAD given the thrombocytopenia experienced by virtually all patients requiring mechanical support. Although less common in this population, HIT can and should be evaluated as a cause of thrombosis by the use of the 4T score and laboratory workup. Finally, the risk of complications due to allogeneic transfusion (transfusion-related acute lung injury [TRALI], transfusion-associated circulatory overload [TACO], and transfusion-related immunomodulation [TRIM]) is higher in patients with VAD, resulting in many coagulation management algorithms to prioritize fibrinogen and PCCs combined with point-of-care testing. Although this currently exists in the trauma bay and OR, it is likely to make its way to ICUs in the near future.

b. Extracorporeal membranous oxygenation may also in significant circuit-related thrombosis as well as in vivo bleeding. Etiologies for such coagulopathy are usually attributed to deficiency of factor XIII, thrombocytopenia, acquired vWF syndrome, platelet function defects, hyperfibrinolysis, and intravascular hemolysis. Patients on ECMO are typically anticoagulated with UFH and followed by either aPTT or anti-Xa levels, although DTIs may be used for those with heparin resistance. An ECMO circuit primed only with crystalloid and/or RBCs (without plasma), an initial dilutional thrombocytopenia and coagulopathy often result. Similar to VADs, ECMO circuits result in continuous thrombin formation, thus resulting in fibrinogen consumption, and levels should be monitored and maintained greater than 150, potentially greater than 200 if concerns for bleeding exist. Unexplained bleeding may be attributable to factor XIII deficiency, which should be kept above 70%, and acquired vWF should be managed similarly to the VAD management mentioned earlier. Lastly, intravascular hemolysis often results in renal damage for patients on ECMO. Given that intravascular hemolysis may be an early sign of thrombus formation within the circuit or at the cannula position, free plasma hemoglobin (Hb) should be regularly monitored. Elevated levels are associated with higher mortality, and, when greater than 150 mg/dL, should be managed with therapeutic plasma exchange with FFP as a replacement fluid.

D. Organ Dysfunction

1. Liver disease affects coagulation because the majority of factors, except factor VIII and vWF, are produced in the liver. In chronic liver disease, coagulation factors (I, II, V, VII, IX, X, and plasminogen) and inhibitors (AT, protein C and S, α_2-antiplasmin, as well as the vWF-cleaving enzyme ADAMTS13) synthesized by the liver, are decreased, whereas the vascular endothelium-derived factor VIII, vWF, tPA, and PAI-1 are elevated. Clinically, this results in a rebalanced hemostasis, although standard plasmatic coagulation tests such as PT and aPTT may be elevated. In fact, thrombin generation assays containing thrombomodulin and viscoelastic tests demonstrate that patients with long-standing liver disease tend to be hypercoagulable. They should be considered for thromboprophylaxis unless contraindicated. Similarly, in acute liver failure, overt bleeding is less common than would be expected because of a "rebalanced" coagulation dysfunction. Thrombocytopenia frequently occurs as the result of splenic sequestration but may be compensated by high vWF levels.

a. Prophylactic transfusion of FFP and platelets should be avoided, and hemostatic interventions should only be performed in case of clinically relevant bleeding. There is usually response to vitamin K supplementation. Antifibrinolytic drugs or coagulation factor concentrates such as fibrinogen, PCC, or activated recombinant factor VII (rFVIIa) may be appropriate in certain patients. However, the potential benefit of improving hemostasis at the expense of increasing the thrombotic risk should be carefully evaluated in individual patients. Here, viscoelastic testing seems to be helpful to guide therapy in patients with bleeding. Notably, procoagulant agents such as rFVIIa have been shown to improve laboratory values such as PT, without improving control of bleeding during liver transplant or upper GI hemorrhage.

2. GI dysfunction may result in **vitamin K deficiency**. Vitamin K, a fat-soluble vitamin, depends on the normal flow of bile and pancreatic exocrine function that is absorbed in the jejunum and ileum and transported via chylomicrons in the lymphatic system. Vitamin K is important in the synthesis of coagulation factors in the liver, including the clotting factors II, VII, IX, and X, as well as the anticoagulant factors protein C and protein S. Vitamin K deficiency is common in prolonged illness and can be repleted 2.5 to 25 mg subcutaneously once or 10 mg subcutaneously daily for 3 days. Vitamin K can be given via an intravenous (IV) line, although both anaphylaxis and subsequent resistance to VKAs thereafter are well documented (eg, a patient who will need to be therapeutically anticoagulated again after temporary reversal). In severe and life-threatening bleeding due to VKAs, for example, in intracerebral hemorrhage or GI bleeding, the effect can be reversed rapidly by the administration of 4F-PCCs. 4F-PCC has been approved by the U.S. Food and Drug Administration (FDA) for this indication since 2013.

3. Kidney disease may result in **uremia** and associated platelet dysfunction. The primary therapy is hemodialysis and should be strongly considered before invasive procedures in the event of uremia-related coagulopathy. IV desmopressin as a slow infusion increases multimers of factor VIII: vWF. Cryoprecipitate and treatment of anemia with transfusion of pRBCs in the acute setting can be considered as well. Therapy with less immediate response time includes conjugated estrogens (over the course of 4-7 days) and erythropoietin (over the course of weeks to months).

E. Postoperative Bleeding, for example, after cardiac surgery or liver transplant, usually is multifactorial. Here, hyperfibrinolysis, fibrinogen deficiency, fibrin polymerization disorders, thrombocytopenia, thrombocytopathy, and impaired thrombin generation can play a major role. Standard plasmatic coagulation tests are limited because of their long turnaround time and their inability to predict bleeding and guide hemostatic therapy in the perioperative setting. Here, ROTEM/TEG as well as point-of-care platelet function analysis have been shown to be superior in reducing transfusion requirements, transfusion-associated adverse events, thromboembolic events, and improving patient outcomes. The use of perioperative bleeding management algorithms guided by ROTEM/TEG is highly recommended here (Figure 27.4). Their clinical- and cost-effectiveness has been proven in several studies and health technology assessments.

F. Clotting

1. **Hypercoagulability abnormalities** include congenital conditions such as factor V Leiden (activated protein C resistance), prothrombin mutation, protein C and S deficiencies, AT deficiency, antiphospholipid antibodies (LAs), and hyperhomocysteinemia. Evaluation includes thorough history and labs, supported by genetic testing for the patient and family members. However, in the setting of acute illness and elevation of acute-phase reactants, these tests may not be specific. Expert hematologic consultation is recommended in patients who are critically ill.
   - **a.** Medications such as oral contraceptives and smoking or obesity and diabetes should be taken into consideration when patients who are critically ill with hypercoagulability are evaluated. Pregnancy, trauma, and surgery predispose and contribute to the multifactorial process of hypercoagulability.
   - **b.** Treatment is individually tailored. Compression stockings, sequential compression devices, and prophylactic and therapeutic anticoagulation are determined on the basis of history and clinical setting.
2. **Heparin-induced thrombocytopenia** is classified as nonimmune mediated (HIT type 1) or immune mediated (HIT type 2).

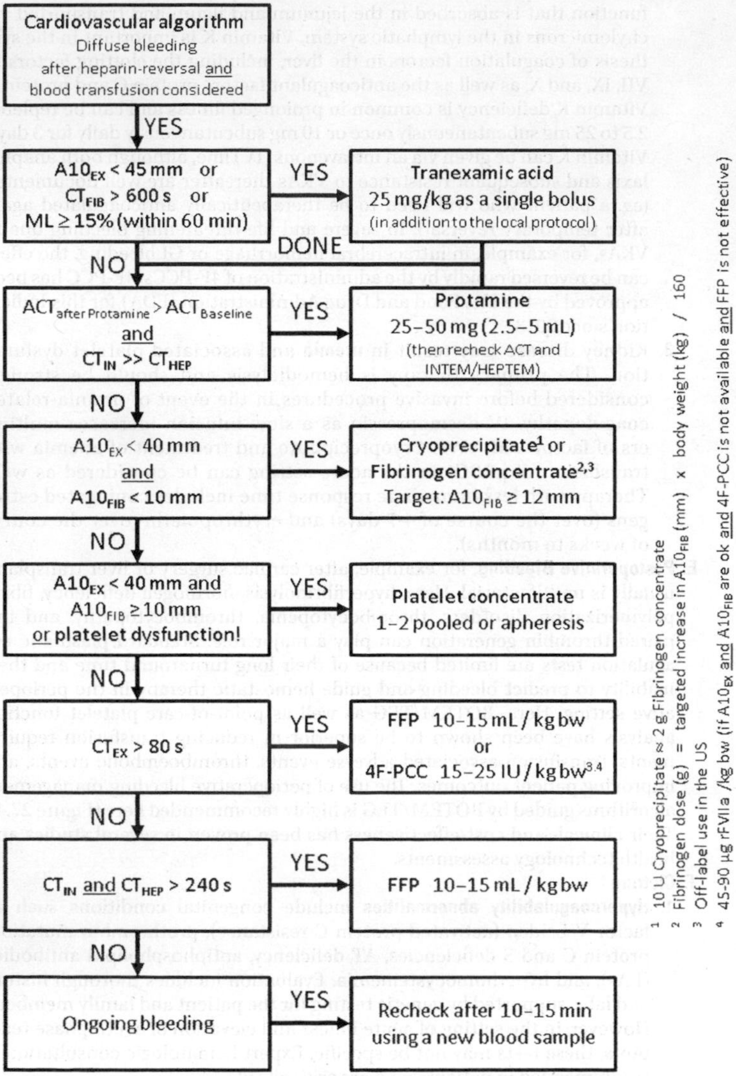

FIGURE 27.4 Point-of-care algorithm for bleeding management in cardiovascular surgery guided by thromboelastometry and whole-blood impedance aggregometry. 4F-PCC, four-factor prothrombin complex concentrate; A10, amplitude of clot firmness 10 minutes after CT; ACT, activated clotting time; bw, body weight; CT, coagulation time; EX, extrinsic thromboelastometry (EXTEM); FIB, fibrin thromboelastometry (FIBTEM); HEP, heparinase modified thromboelastometry (HEPTEM); IN, intrinsic thromboelastometry (INTEM); ML, maximum lysis; rFVIIa, activated recombinant factor VII.

a. HIT type 1 is a benign fall in platelet count, usually within 5 days of initiating heparin. The platelet count usually does not fall below 100 000 mm^3 and heparin does not have to be discontinued or avoided in the future.

b. HIT type 2 is immune mediated. IgG antibodies are formed against heparin-platelet factor 4 (PF-4) complexes. This results in platelet activation and aggregation, leading to pathologic platelet aggregation, thrombocytopenia, and vascular thrombosis. HIT antibodies binding to endothelial cell surfaces may result in tissue factor expression and a prothrombotic state.

c. Up to half of patients undergoing cardiac surgery and 15% of those undergoing orthopedic surgery develop HIT type 2 by immunologic assays (enzyme-linked immunosorbent assay [ELISA]). However, only 1% to 3% of these patients develop clinically significant HIT type 2. This can be significantly reduced using LMWH and eliminated with fondaparinux or DTIs such as argatroban (Figure 27.5). Argatroban is approved for prophylaxis and treatment of thrombosis in patients with or at risk for HIT. In patients with hepatic impairment or multiple organ failure, the argatroban dosage should be decreased to 0.1 to 0.2 μg/kg/min to avoid bleeding complications. Argatroban therapy can be monitored by aPTT. Because aPTT reaches a plateau at higher argatroban plasma concentrations, an overdose may not be recognized. Therefore, ecarin-based assays are more reliable for monitoring DTIs.

d. Diagnosis is made by history and physical, as well as a decrease in platelet count by 50% from baseline (but usually not <50 000 mm^3) within 5

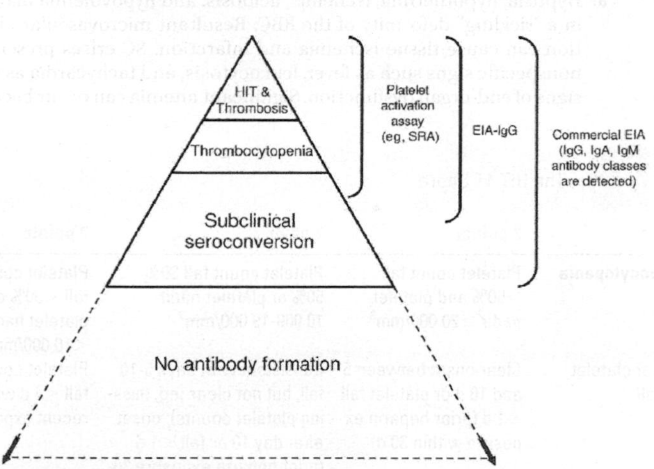

Patient population	ELISA antibody detected	Positive platelet activation / Functional assay (SRA)	Thrombocytopenia	HIT and thrombosis
Post Open Heart Surgery	50%	20%	2%	1%
Post Orthopedic Surgery—unfractionated heparin (UFH)	15%	10%	5%	3%
Post Orthopedic Surgery—low-molecular-weight heparin (LMWH)	8%	3%	1%	0.5%
Patients in ICU	< 1%	< 1%	41%–54%	—

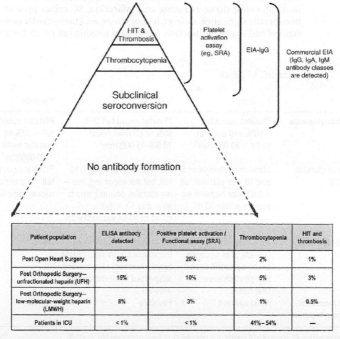

FIGURE 27.5 Iceberg model of HIT. EIA, enzyme immunoassay; ELISA, enzyme-linked immunosorbent assay; HIT, heparin-induced thrombocytopenia; ICU, intensive care unit; Ig, immunoglobulin; SRA, serotonin release assay.

to 14 days of heparin exposure. Previous heparin exposure can lead to a quicker decrease in platelets. Platelet recovery after ceasing exposure to heparin and tachyphylaxis or resistance to heparinization is also suggestive. The clinical 4T score can be used to estimate the probability of HIT type 2 (Table 27.2). For patients with a 4T score of less than 4 points, the probability of having immune HIT is less than 5%. Platelet serotonin release assays (SRAs) are more specific than are ELISA assays, but take longer to obtain. Whole-blood impedance aggregometry can be used as a functional assay for platelet-activating HIT antibodies with a sensitivity and specificity similar to that of SRAs but with a shorter turnaround time. A high index of suspicion in the correct clinical setting (4T score ≥4 points) should be treated as positive for HIT type 2.

e. **Treatment** involves discontinuing all exposure to heparin, including heparin-coated catheters, flushes, hemodialysis, or extracorporeal circuitry. Appropriate anticoagulation is essential because 50% to 75% of patients with HIT type 2 develop thrombotic complications. Appropriate anticoagulation is patient specific and would include DTIs such as argatroban. Platelet transfusion should be restrictive because of thrombotic concerns. Longer term anticoagulation (at least 6-8 weeks) will generally be required.

3. **Sickle cell** disease is caused by substitution of the amino acid valine for glutamic acid on the β-chain of Hb and is most common in African Americans. Clinical presentation occurs with homozygotes. Similar presentations can occur for homozygotes of sickle cell (SC) or β-thalassemia. Heterozygote carriers usually do not present clinically.

a. Hypoxia, hypothermia, ischemia, acidosis, and hypovolemia may result in a "sickling" deformity of the RBC. Resultant microvascular obstruction can cause tissue ischemia and infarction. SC crises present with nonspecific signs such as fever, leukocytosis, and tachycardia as well as signs of end-organ dysfunction. Significant anemia can occur because of

TABLE 27.2 The HIT 4T Score

4T score	2 points	1 point	0 points
Thrombocytopenia	Platelet count fall >50% and platelet nadir ≥20 000/mm^3	Platelet count fall 30%-50% or platelet nadir 10 000-19 000/mm^3	Platelet count fall <30% or platelet nadir <10 000/mm^3
Timing of platelet count fall	Clear onset between 5 and 10 d or platelet fall ≤1 d (prior heparin exposure within 30 d)	Consistent with days 5-10 fall, but not clear (eg, missing platelet counts); onset after day 10 or fall ≤1 d (prior heparin exposure 30-100 d ago)	Platelet count fall <4 d without recent exposure
Thrombosis or other sequela	New thrombosis (confirmed); skin necrosis; acute systemic reaction postintravenous UFH bolus	Progressive or recurrent thrombosis; non-necrotizing (erythematous) skin lesions; suspected thrombosis (not proven)	None
Other causes for thrombocytopenia	Nonapparent	Possible	Definite

For patients with a 4T score of <4 points, the probability of having immune HIT is <5%.
HIT, heparin-induced thrombocytopenia; UFH, unfractionated heparin.

the shortened lifespan and destruction of the RBCs. Treatment involves addressing the precipitating causes, providing adequate pain relief, and transfusion only when indicated.

G. Frequent Hematologic Diseases

1. **Hemophilia A** is a hereditary disorder of factor VIII and hemophilia B is a hereditary disorder of factor IX. History and physical findings are supported by laboratory findings of an elevated intrinsic pathway clotting time, with a normal PT/INR. Platelet function is normal but the blood clot is unable to be stabilized, so bleeding will recur. Treatment includes factor VIII, factor IX, cryoprecipitate, and desmopressin (DDAVP). rFVIIa and activated PCC (FEIBA [factor eight inhibitor bypassing activity]) are indicated in patients with acquired hemophilia due to inhibitors. Expert hematology consultation is recommended in patients who are critically ill.
2. **Von Willebrand disease** is a primarily autosomal-dominant genetic disorder resulting from defects in vWF. vWF normally anchors platelets to collagen while strengthening clotted platelets and stabilizing factor VIII. Treatment includes DDAVP, human factor VIII-vWF complex concentrates, and cryoprecipitate preferably over FFP. In certain patients with acquired von Willebrand disease, high-dose IV gamma globulin has been used successfully. Again, expert hematology consultation is recommended in patients who are critically ill.

III. TREATMENT

A. Transfusion

Traditionally, transfusion of blood products has been based on conventional laboratory tests such as Hb, platelet count, aPTT, and PT/INR. Most evidence of current transfusion practice is derived from chronic anemia, minor surgical bleeding, or preparation for surgery. However, in massive trauma and hemorrhage, a massive transfusion strategy of transfusing pRBCs and FFP in a ratio of 1:1 or 2:1 is widely practiced because conventional plasmatic coagulation tests are typically not timely available to guide decision-making during major hemorrhage. The pragmatic, randomized, optimal platelet and plasma ratios (PROPPR) trial, an RCT published in 2015, demonstrated no differences in mortality for patients receiving 1:1:1 as compared to 2:1:1 (RBCs, platelets, FFP), with better hemostasis and fewer deaths due to exsanguination in 24 hours in the 1:1:1 cohort. Some data suggest even increased incidence of acute respiratory distress syndrome (ARDS), sepsis, and multiple organ dysfunction in patients receiving FFP in nonmassive transfusion, and there is no evidence supporting FFP transfusion in patients who are nonmassively transfused. Furthermore, ABO-compatible but nonidentical plasma transfusion seems to be associated with a high complication rate of ARDS and sepsis up to 70% and even an increased mortality by 15% compared with transfusion of ABO-identical plasma only. Of note, administration of specific coagulation factor concentrates (fibrinogen and 4F-PCC) guided by ROTEM is increasingly used rather than FFP in Europe. However, despite promising results in several clinical studies, efficacy, safety, and cost-effectiveness of this new approach have to be proved in large observational studies and RCTs.

B. Anticoagulation is indicated for underlying medical conditions such as atrial fibrillation with high CHADS2 scores, pulmonary embolism, DVT, DIC, and underlying hypercoagulable states. Mechanical support devices from intra-aortic balloon pumps to extracorporeal life support and renal replacement circuits may be indications for anticoagulation.

1. **Heparin** is administered subcutaneously or via IV and acts by binding and accelerating the action of AT. This resultant complex inactivates thrombin and factor X in the coagulation cascade. Therapeutic anticoagulation for

DVT or PE requires aPTT of 1.5 to 2 times baseline and should be reached within 24 hours of initiation. Usual dosing includes an IV bolus followed by titration of a continuous infusion. With a half-life of 90 minutes, the therapeutic effects of heparin will be gone by 4 to 6 hours after cessation. Protamine (1 mg/100 units of remaining heparin in circulation) can be slowly administered to reverse heparin sooner if needed.

   a. Resistance to heparin occurs in patients who are critically ill because of acute-phase reactants that bind heparin, depleted levels of AT, or because of HIT. Increasing the dose of heparin and transfusing AT concentrate or FFP would be appropriate in the first two causes for resistance. Development of HIT requires immediate cessation of heparin and treatment for HIT (see **Section II.F.2**).

2. Factor Xa inhibitors include subcutaneous LMWH such as enoxaparin and dalteparin, which inhibit factor Xa. They do not prolong the aPTT and if therapeutic monitoring is needed, anti-Xa levels must be measured. LMWHs have improved efficacy for prophylaxis of DVT and PE in certain patients with high-risk orthopedic, trauma, and spinal cord injuries. The therapeutic predictability of LMWH is improved with less binding of acute-phase reactants compared with heparin. In addition, the incidence of HIT is dramatically reduced with LMWH when compared with UFH. However, LMWH is more expensive, and if reversal is needed, it has a longer half-life of 4 hours, is incompletely reversed by protamine, and depends on renal clearance.

   a. Fondaparinux selectively inhibits factor Xa and shares many of the advantages and disadvantages of the other LMWHs. It is unique in its long half-life of 14 hours and lack of interaction with platelets or PF-4. The combination of renal elimination and long half-life makes fondaparinux less suitable for patients who are critically ill.

   b. Rivaroxaban and apixaban are oral DXaIs that do not require AT. In the outpatient setting, they are generally considered safe with less drug-drug interactions and do not require monitoring of therapeutic levels, but have less usefulness in patients who are critically ill. Reversal is more challenging than is reversing VKAs. 4F-PCC, activated PCC (FEIBA), and rFVIIa have been suggested in emergent situations.

   c. Andexanet alfa for reversal of anti-Xa drugs has demonstrated promise for emergent situations, especially intracranial hemorrhage. Data on whether andexanet alfa is superior to 4F-PCC are still under investigation, especially given the significant cost difference between the two therapeutics.

3. Warfarin (vitamin K antagonist) is administered orally and inhibits vitamin K epoxide reductases effectively. By blocking the epoxide reductases, factors II, VII, IX, X, and proteins C and S cannot be carboxylated to their active forms. The long half-life of warfarin (35 hours) makes it difficult to titrate therapeutic goals rapidly. Since 2013, 4F-PCC is FDA approved for urgent reversal of VKAs, for example, in intracerebral hemorrhage or GI bleeding. To avoid a warfarin rebound, PCC should be combined with vitamin K. In contrast to FFP, 4F-PCC reverses the effect of VKAs quicker, more effectively, and in a smaller volume. If 4F-PCC is not available, FFP can be used for warfarin reversal; however, it is associated with a higher complication rate, for example, volume overload, and a significantly longer time to correct the INR. Vitamin K can be administered, but it takes 6 hours or more for reversing the anticoagulation effects of warfarin. Therapeutic goals are monitored with PT and INR levels. Exaggerated effects of warfarin are seen in patients who are nutritionally deficient in vitamin K or are also on amiodarone. In an acute setting with patients who are critically ill, warfarin is not a first-line agent of anticoagulation.

4. **Platelet inhibitors** such as aspirin and other nonsteroidal anti-inflammatory drugs (NSAIDs) affect the cyclooxygenase (COX) pathway and inhibit platelet aggregation. Owing to the irreversible COX inhibition, the effect of aspirin lasts 7 to 10 days, whereas the reversible COX inhibition of other NSAIDs lasts about 3 days.
   a. In recent multicenter, randomized control trials (PeriOperative ISchemic Evaluation-2 trail, POISE-2), aspirin was not shown to decrease perioperative cardiac events in patients undergoing noncardiac surgery compared with placebo. The FDA removed primary prevention as an indication for daily aspirin use. It is important to note that patients with cardiac or vascular comorbidities such as recent coronary stents or carotid artery stenosis are still recommended to take aspirin for secondary prevention.
   b. Other platelet inhibitors include clopidogrel and ticlopidine, which are potent antiplatelet drugs that inhibit adenosine diphosphate (ADP)-mediated platelet aggregation. Abciximab and eptifibatide are IV glycoprotein IIb/IIIa receptor antagonists. Fibrinogen and vWF are prevented from binding to the platelet and prevent aggregation.
   c. Point-of-care platelet function analysis such as whole-blood impedance aggregometry can help guide the need for platelet transfusion if emergent reversal of antiplatelet therapy is required.
   d. For patients requiring dual antiplatelet therapy (DAPT) and nondeferrable noncardiac surgery, current American College of Cardiology guidelines recommend stratifying patients into low-, intermediate-, and high-risk categories for both hemorrhagic and thrombotic risks. Risk of surgical hemorrhage is attributed based on complexity and the organ system involved in the operation. Thrombotic risk is derived from time from PCI and type of stent placed. The 12- and 6-month cutoffs stratify patients with recently placed drug-eluting stents into low, intermediate, and high thrombotic risk categories. For patients with low and intermediate thrombotic risk, guidelines are conserved across the spectrum of hemorrhagic risk: continue aspirin, discontinue $P2Y_{12}$ receptor inhibitor with resumption within 24 to 72 hours postoperatively via a loading dose. For patients with high thrombotic and low hemorrhagic risks, guidelines recommend continuation of both aspirin and $P2Y_{12}$ inhibitor throughout the perioperative period. Finally, for patients with high thrombotic risk and undergoing operations with intermediate or high hemorrhagic risk, guidelines recommend continuation of aspirin, cessation of $P2Y_{12}$ inhibitor until 24 to 72 hours postoperatively, and consideration of short-acting IV antiplatelet therapy as a bridge.
5. **Direct thrombin inhibitors** do not require cofactors to inhibit circulating and clot-bound thrombin. Laboratory tests include ACT, dilute thrombin time (dTT), ecarin clotting time (ECT), and aPTT to guide therapeutic range. ECT and dTT show the highest sensitivity and a strong linear correlation to drug levels. Because aPTT reaches a plateau at higher DTI plasma concentrations, an overdose may not be recognized. There is no active reversal medication for these potent anticoagulants, but most have short half-lives.
   a. Argatroban has a half-life of 40 minutes and is approved by the FDA for treatment and prophylaxis of HIT. Patients with hepatic dysfunction or multiple organ failure require dose reduction to 0.1 to 0.2 μg/kg/min to avoid bleeding complications. Argatroban falsely interferes with the PT/INR values; thus, consideration must be taken when bridging to warfarin anticoagulation. It also crosses the blood-brain barrier and may play a role in the treatment of ischemic or thrombotic stroke.
   b. Bivalirudin has a half-life of 25 minutes and is used for percutaneous coronary interventions. Off-label, it has been used successfully in the treatment of HIT and for cardiopulmonary bypass in patients with HIT.

c. Lepirudin has a half-life of 80 minutes, but undergoes renal excretion, and thus should be dose adjusted or avoided in patients with renal failure.

d. Oral DTIs include dabigatran etexilate, which requires conversion to dabigatran. It was shown to be as effective as enoxaparin in preventing DVT after total hip replacement, but as with most oral agents its usefulness in the critical care setting is limited. Furthermore, dabigatran plasma levels cumulate significantly in patients with renal impairment (creatinine clearance <50 mL/min), which is associated with an increased risk of bleeding. Dabigatran is contraindicated in patients with severe renal impairment (creatinine clearance <30 mL/min). Dabigatran can be eliminated by hemodialysis. 4F-PCC and activated PCC, but not rFVIIa, seem to be effective in reducing the anticoagulant effect of dabigatran.

e. Idarucizumab was recently developed as a monoclonal antibody fragment for reversal of dabigatran. Several studies have demonstrated laboratory measures of dabigatran-associated coagulopathy, but scarcity of data exists regarding clinical effectiveness.

6. Thrombolytics convert plasminogen to plasmin to lyse fibrin clots. These include tissue plasminogen activator (tPA), streptokinase, and urokinase. There is a high risk of bleeding in a perioperative setting because of the hypofibrinogenemic state. In the setting of acute coronary, pulmonary, cerebral, or other major vascular artery occlusion, they can be life or limb saving. Emergent reversal may require administration of aminocaproic acid, tranexamic acid (TXA), or transfusion of fresh frozen plasma (FPP) or cryoprecipitate.

C. Hemostatic Agents

1. Desmopressin: DDAVP increases release of multimer factor VIII: vWF and plasminogen activator from endothelial cells. It is useful in certain coagulopathic states, such as uremia, von Willebrand deficiency, or hemophilia A, that involve factor VIII deficiency.

2. Lysine analogs (aminocaproic acid, tranexamic acid): TXA was demonstrated in the CRASH-2 (Clinical Randomisation of an Antifibrinolytic in Significant Haemorrhage 2) trial to reduce mortality from bleeding if given within 3 hours of injury, but, notably, mortality was increased if TXA was administered more than 3 hours after the injury. This likely speaks of the spectrum of fibrinolysis disorders and thus suggests goal-directed therapy with viscoelastic testing. One common parameter used by institutions is LY30 greater than or equal to 3%, indicating hyperfibrinolysis and thus a potential benefit from TXA administration. Aminocaproic acid (Amicar) also inhibits fibrinolysis through decreasing plasmin conversion upstream. Its effects have been variable, but it has been used in cardiac surgery (10 g IV load over 1 hour followed by 1-2 g/h), prophylaxis for dental procedures in patients with hemophilia, and during liver transplantation surgeries.

3. Coagulation factor concentrates are available as plasma-derived or recombinant products. In the United States, most of the factor concentrates are FDA approved for congenital deficiencies only, for example, fibrinogen concentrate for congenital fibrinogen deficiency, factor VIII for hemophilia A, vWF/factor VIII complex concentrates for von Willebrand disease, factor IX and 3F-PCCs for hemophilia B, and factor XIII for congenital factor XIII deficiency. Some other coagulation factor concentrates are FDA approved for acquired coagulation factor deficiencies: 4F-PCCs for urgent reversal of VKAs, such as warfarin, in case of major bleeding, rFVIIa and FEIBA (activated PCC) for acquired hemophilia due to inhibitors, and a solvent detergent–treated pooled plasma (SD plasma) product for replacement of multiple coagulation factors in patients with acquired deficiencies, for example, due to liver disease, liver transplant, cardiac surgery, or for plasma exchange in thrombotic thrombocytopenic purpura (TTP). In general, expert hematology consultation is recommended if coagulation factor concentrates are considered to be used in patients who are critically ill.

Selected Readings

Adamzik M, Görlinger K, Peters J, et al. Whole blood impedance aggregometry as a biomarker for the diagnosis and prognosis of severe sepsis. *Crit Care.* 2012;16:R204.

Adamzik M, Langemeier T, Frey UH, et al. Comparison of thrombelastometry with simplified acute physiology score II and sequential organ failure assessment scores for the prediction of 30-day survival: a cohort study. *Shock.* 2011;35:339-342.

Ageno W, Gallus AS, Wittkowsky A, et al. Oral anticoagulant therapy: antithrombotic therapy and prevention of thrombosis, 9th ed: American College of Chest Physicians evidence-based clinical practice guidelines. *Chest.* 2012;141(2 suppl):e44S-e88S.

Ahn Y, Görlinger K. Coagulopathy and hypercoagulability. In: Bigatello L, Allain RM, Haspel KL, et al, eds. *Critical Care Handbook of the Massachusetts General Hospital.* 5th ed. Lippincott Williams & Wilkins; 2015.

Beiderlinden M, Treschan TA, Görlinger K, et al. Argatroban anticoagulation in critically ill patients. *Ann Pharmacother.* 2007;41(5):749-754.

Benson G. Rotational thromboelastometry and its use in directing the management of coagulopathy in the battle injured trauma patient. *J Perioper Pract.* 2014;24:25-28.

Bernal W, Wendon J. Acute liver failure. *N Engl J Med.* 2013;369:2525-2534.

Breuer G, Weiss DR, Ringwald J. "New" direct oral anticoagulants in the perioperative setting. *Curr Opin Anaesthesiol.* 2014;27:409-419.

Brohi K, Cohen MJ, Davenport RA. Acute coagulopathy of trauma: mechanism, identification and effect. *Curr Opin Crit Care.* 2007;13:680-685.

Collins PW, Solomon C, Sutor K, et al. Theoretical modelling of fibrinogen supplementation with therapeutic plasma, cryoprecipitate, or fibrinogen concentrate. *Br J Anaesth.* 2014;113(4):585-595. doi:10.1093/bja/aeu086

CRASH-2 Collaborators; Roberts I, Shakur H, et al. The importance of early treatment with tranexamic acid in bleeding trauma patients: an exploratory analysis of the CRASH-2 randomised controlled trial. *Lancet.* 2011;377:1096-1101.

Davenport R, Manson J, De'Ath H, et al. Functional definition and characterization of acute traumatic coagulopathy. *Crit Care Med.* 2011;39:2652-2658.

Devereaux PJ, Mrkobrada M, Sessler DI, et al. Aspirin in patients undergoing noncardiac surgery. *N Engl J Med.* 2014;370:1494-1503.

Fawole A, Daw HA, Crowther MA. Practical management of bleeding due to the anticoagulants dabigatran, rivaroxaban, and apixaban. *Cleve Clin J Med.* 2013;80:443-451.

Gerlach R, Krause M, Seifert V, et al. Hemostatic and hemorrhagic problems in neurosurgical patients. *Acta Neurochir.* 2009;151:873-900.

Gonzalez E, Moore EE, Moore HB, et al. Goal-directed hemostatic resuscitation of trauma-induced coagulopathy: a pragmatic randomized clinical trial comparing a viscoelastic assay to conventional coagulation assays. *Ann Surg.* 2016;263(6):1051-1059.

Gonzalez E, Moore EE, Moore HB, Chapman MP, Silliman CC, Banerjee A. Trauma-induced coagulopathy: an institution's 35 year perspective on practice and research. *Scand J Surg.* 2014;103(2):89-103.

Görlinger K, Bergmann L, Dirkmann D. Coagulation management in patients undergoing mechanical circulatory support. *Best Pract Res Clin Anaesthesiol.* 2012;26:179-198.

Görlinger K, Dirkmann D, Solomon C, et al. Fast interpretation of thromboelastometry in non-cardiac surgery: reliability in patients with hypo-, normo-, and hypercoagulability. *Br J Anaesth.* 2013;110:222-230.

Görlinger K, Jambor C, Hanke AA, et al. Perioperative coagulation management and control of platelet transfusion by point-of-care platelet function analysis. *Transfus Med Hemother.* 2007;34:396-411.

Görlinger K, Schaden E, Saner F. Perioperative hemostasis in hepatic surgery. In: Marcucci CE, Schoettker P, eds. *Perioperative Hemostasis: Coagulation for Anesthesiologists.* Springer; 2015.

Görlinger K, Shore-Lesserson L, Dirkmann D, et al. Management of hemorrhage in cardiothoracic surgery. *J Cardiothorac Vasc Anesth.* 2013;27(4 suppl):S20-S34.

Greinacher A, Althaus K, Krauel K, et al. Heparin-induced thrombocytopenia. *Hämostaseologie.* 2010;30(1):1-50.

Haas T, Görlinger K, Grassetto A, et al. Thromboelastometry for guiding bleeding management of the critically ill patient: a systematic review of the literature. *Minerva Anestesiol.* 2014;80:1320-1335.

Hagemo JS, Stanworth S, Juffermans NP, et al. Prevalence, predictors and outcome of hypofibrinogenaemia in trauma: a multicentre observational study. *Crit Care.* 2014;18:R52.

Holbrook A, Schulman S, Witt DM, et al. Evidence-based management of anticoagulant therapy: antithrombotic therapy and prevention of thrombosis, 9th ed: American College of Chest Physicians evidence-based clinical practice guidelines. *Chest.* 2012;141(2 suppl):e152S-e184S.

Holcomb JB, del Junco DJ, Fox EE, et al. The prospective, observational, multicenter, major trauma transfusion (PROMMTT) study: comparative effectiveness of a time-varying treatment with competing risks. *JAMA Surg.* 2013;148:127-136.

Holcomb JB, Pati S. Optimal trauma resuscitation with plasma as the primary resuscitative fluid: the surgeon's perspective. *Hematology Am Soc Hematol Educ Program.* 2013;2013:656-659.

Hunt BJ. Bleeding and coagulopathies in critical care. *N Engl J Med.* 2014;370:847-859.

Innerhofer P, Westermann I, Tauber H, et al. The exclusive use of coagulation factor concentrates enables reversal of coagulopathy and decreases transfusion rates in patients with major blunt trauma. *Injury.* 2013;44:209-216.

Khan S, Brohi K, Chana M, et al. Hemostatic resuscitation is neither hemostatic nor resuscitative in trauma hemorrhage. *J Trauma Acute Care Surg.* 2014;76:561-568.

Kinard TN, Sarode R. Four factor prothrombin complex concentrate (human): review of the pharmacology and clinical application for vitamin K antagonist reversal. *Expert Rev Cardiovasc Ther.* 2014;12:417-427.

Konkle BA. Acquired disorders of platelet function. *Hematology Am Soc Hematol Educ Program.* 2011:391-396.

Korte W. F XIII in perioperative coagulation management. *Best Pract Res Clin Anaesthesiol.* 2010;24:85-93.

Kozek-Langenecker SA, Afshari A, Albaladejo P, et al. Management of severe perioperative bleeding: guidelines from the European Society of Anaesthesiology. *Eur J Anaesthesiol.* 2013;30:270-382.

Kutcher ME, Redick BJ, McCreery RC, et al. Characterization of platelet dysfunction after trauma. *J Trauma Acute Care Surg.* 2012;73:13-19.

Levi M. Coagulation in sepsis. *Int J Intensive Care.* 2013;20:77-81.

Maegele M, Schöchl H, Cohen MJ. An update on the coagulopathy of trauma. *Shock.* 2014;41(suppl 1):21-25.

Mallett SV, Chowdary P, Burroughs AK. Clinical utility of viscoelastic tests of coagulation in patients with liver disease. *Liver Int.* 2013;33:961-974.

Moore HB, Moore EE, Gonzalez E, et al. Hyperfibrinolysis, physiologic fibrinolysis, and fibrinolysis shutdown: the spectrum of postinjury fibrinolysis and relevance to antifibrinolytic therapy. *J Trauma Acute Care Surg.* 2014;77(6):811-817.

Müller MC, Meijers JC, Vroom MB, et al. Utility of thromboelastography and/or thromboelastometry in adults with sepsis: a systematic review. *Crit Care.* 2014;18:R30.

Sarode R, Milling TJ Jr, Refaai MA, et al. Efficacy and safety of a 4-factor prothrombin complex concentrate in patients on vitamin K antagonists presenting with major bleeding: a randomized, plasma-controlled, phase IIIb study. *Circulation.* 2013;128:1234-1243.

Schaden E, Saner FH, Goerlinger K. Coagulation pattern in critical liver dysfunction. *Curr Opin Crit Care.* 2013;19:142-148.

Schöchl H, Maegele M, Solomon C, et al. Early and individualized goal-directed therapy for trauma-induced coagulopathy. *Scand J Trauma Resusc Emerg Med.* 2012;20:15.

Spahn DR, Bouillon B, Cerny V, et al. Management of bleeding and coagulopathy following major trauma: an updated European guideline. *Crit Care.* 2013;17:R76.

Stensballe J, Ostrowski SR, Johansson PI. Viscoelastic guidance of resuscitation. *Curr Opin Anaesthesiol.* 2014;27:212-218.

Thomas J, Kostousov V, Teruya J. Bleeding and thrombotic complications in the use of extracorporeal membrane oxygenation. *Semin Thromb Hemost.* 2018;44(1):20-29.

Tripodi A, Mannucci PM. The coagulopathy of chronic liver disease. *N Engl J Med.* 2011;365:147-156.

Wada H, Thachil J, Di Nisio M, et al. The Scientific Standardization Committee on DIC of the International Society on Thrombosis Haemostasis. Guidance for diagnosis and treatment of DIC from harmonization of the recommendations from three guidelines. *J Thromb Haemost.* 2013;11:761-767.

Yanamadala V, Walcott BP, Fecci PE, et al. Reversal of warfarin associated coagulopathy with 4-factor prothrombin complex concentrate in traumatic brain injury and intracranial hemorrhage. *J Clin Neurosci.* 2014;21:1881-1884.

28 Acute Gastrointestinal Diseases

Katherine H. Albutt and Kristin Kennedy

I. INTRODUCTION

Gastrointestinal (GI) diseases are common in the intensive care unit (ICU) and include both surgical and nonsurgical problems. There are several GI diseases that present in an acute manner and require critical care, including, but not limited to, hemorrhage, obstruction, perforation, ischemia, or following a major surgical procedure involving the GI tract. In addition, those critically ill may also develop acute GI complications as a result of their critical illness. This chapter focuses on the most common GI diseases that may lead to ICU admission and those GI diseases that may arise from being critically ill.

II. EVALUATION OF SUSPECTED GASTROINTESTINAL PATHOLOGY

The diagnosis of a GI disorder in the critically ill can be challenging because these patients may not be able to articulate their symptoms and often do not present with classic clinical findings. A nonspecific finding such as a change in mental status, fever, leukocytosis, hypotension, or decreased urine output may be the only sign of intra-abdominal pathology. Thus, clinicians must maintain a high index of suspicion for an undiagnosed GI problem as a cause of hemodynamic instability.

A. Signs and Symptoms that suggest GI pathology are numerous and can include abdominal pain, chest pain, bleeding (hematemesis, melena, rectal bleeding), emesis, distension, change in bowel habits, and tube feed intolerance.

B. Initial Evaluation includes assessing for abdominal tenderness and distension, fever, tachycardia, hypotension, and/or change in vasopressor requirement. Correct positioning and functioning of existing nasogastric (NG) tubes and abdominal drains must be confirmed. Laboratory tests such as a complete blood count (CBC), serum chemistries, liver function tests (LFTs), and amylase may be helpful adjuncts.

C. Increased vigilance is required when caring for recipients of solid **organ transplants** or patients with chronic inflammatory or autoimmune disorders treated with immunosuppressive medications. These patients who are chronically **immunosuppressed** may not demonstrate typical signs and symptoms of ongoing GI pathology.

D. Diagnostic Studies and Procedures are often necessary to establish a diagnosis and are guided by the initial assessment. Portable plain radiographs can reveal the presence of pneumoperitoneum or intestinal obstruction or confirm the correct placement of an enteral tube (Figure 28.1). Ultrasound is a useful adjunct that can be performed at the bedside, particularly to assess the biliary tree. However, more sophisticated studies are often required to establish a diagnosis. The risks associated with a diagnostic study must be weighed against the expected benefits. Commonly performed tests such as an abdominal computed tomography (CT) scan pose a higher risk to the patient who is critically ill and at increased risk for contrast-induced nephropathy, ventilator-associated pneumonia, as well as airway and hemodynamic complications while traveling to the radiology department. Commonly available diagnostic modalities and their advantages and disadvantages in an ICU setting are summarized in Table 28.1.

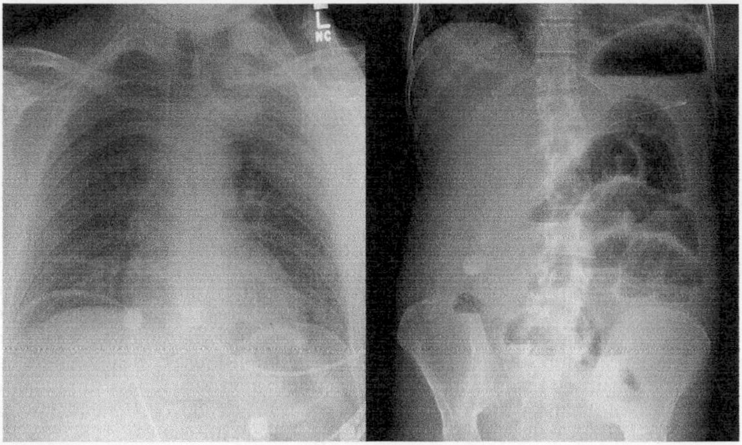

FIGURE 28.1 A plain chest radiograph demonstrating pneumoperitoneum (left) and an abdominal film demonstrating small bowel obstruction and nasogastric tube placement (right). (Courtesy of Hasan Alam, MD.)

III. GASTROINTESTINAL BLEEDING

GI hemorrhage is commonly seen in an ICU setting (Table 28.2). GI bleeding may originate from the upper (proximal to the ligament of Treitz) or lower GI tract. Risk factors include liver disease, alcoholism, uremia, diverticulosis, peptic ulcer disease (PUD), critical illness, and the intake of a variety of medications, including nonsteroidal anti-inflammatory drugs (NSAIDs), antiplatelet agents, and anticoagulants.

A. Signs and Symptoms include shock, hematemesis, coffee ground emesis, melena, hematochezia, or hematocrit drop with occult blood present in the stool.

B. Initial Evaluation may need to proceed expeditiously depending on the rate of blood loss and hemodynamic stability of the patient.

1. A **history** focusing on risk factors for GI bleeding, prior abdominal operations, significant medical comorbidities, and thorough medication review should be obtained.
2. **Physical examination** should focus on assessing end-organ perfusion. Certain physical findings such as stigmata of liver disease may suggest an underlying etiology.
3. **Laboratory studies** including CBC, coagulation studies, and chemistries should be obtained. Initial hemoglobin values do not reflect the degree of acute blood loss and thus should not be used as a marker for the presence or absence of GI hemorrhage.

C. Stabilization is accomplished by ensuring an adequate airway, hemodynamic stability, and adequate monitoring. A patient with an altered level of consciousness and copious hematemesis will likely require endotracheal intubation. Adequate large-bore peripheral intravenous (IV) access should be secured. Central venous access, an arterial catheter, and a urinary catheter placement may be appropriate for patients in shock. Initial resuscitation with isotonic crystalloid solution is appropriate while preparations for blood transfusions are made. Blood resuscitation should be balanced and titrated to effect depending on the patient's clinical status and not necessarily their hemoglobin and hematocrit. Laboratory adjuncts such as thromboelastography (TEG) can be used to monitor the clotting process and further guide resuscitation. Severe coagulopathy should be corrected (see **Chapter 27**).

TABLE 28.1 Diagnostic Modalities for Acute Gastrointestinal Diseases in the Intensive Care Unit

Modality	Advantages and usefulness	Disadvantages
Plain radiographs	• Portable and fast • Assess for free air. • Confirm tube placement (nasogastric, postpyloric).	• Findings are usually nonspecific. • Overlying tubes, monitors, cables, and other ICU equipment obscure images.
Ultrasound	• Portable • Assess gall bladder/biliary tree. • Can guide procedures (paracentesis, biliary drains)	• Image quality is operator dependent. • Air-filled intestines can obscure images.
CT	• Characterizes many forms of intra-abdominal pathology • CT angiography can assess mesenteric vessels.	• Patient transport out of the ICU • Optimum study requires IV contrast, which can cause nephropathy and allergic reactions.
MRI	• Noninvasive method to assess for choledocholithiasis	• Patient transport out of the ICU • Time consuming • Requires patient cooperation
Angiography	• Diagnostic and therapeutic in mesenteric ischemia • Useful to localize and intervene on GI bleeding and intra-abdominal/pelvic bleeding following trauma	• Patient transport out of the ICU • Requires IV contrast • Risk of vascular injury (arterial injury at the access site, pseudoaneurysms, hematoma, bleeding, arterial dissection, and embolization of vessel plaque)
Radionuclide imaging	• HIDA scan may help characterize suspected biliary pathology such as cholecystitis. • Technetium scan can confirm ongoing GI bleeding.	• Never an initial diagnostic test • Patient transport out of the ICU
Endoscopy	• Diagnostic and therapeutic • EGD and colonoscopy can be performed at the bedside. • ERCP can be lifesaving in cholangitis.	• Requires sedation • Colonoscopy requires colonic purge for optimum study. • Small risk of intestinal perforation • ERCP can cause pancreatitis.
Bedside laparoscopy	• Direct visualization facilitates diagnosis of acalculous cholecystitis and mesenteric ischemia, according to several reports (small case series). • Can potentially avoid nontherapeutic laparotomy	• Invasive • Inability to evaluate some areas (retroperitoneum) • Patient must be mechanically ventilated and sedated. • Utility as a diagnostic modality in the ICU has not been rigorously studied.

CT, computed tomography; EGD, esophagogastroduodenoscopy; ERCP, endoscopic retrograde cholangiopancreatography; GI, gastrointestinal; HIDA, hepatobiliary iminodiacetic acid; ICU, intensive care unit; IV, intravenous; MRI, magnetic resonance imaging.

TABLE 28.2 Causes of Gastrointestinal (GI) Bleeding

Upper GI source	Lower GI source
Variceal bleeding • Esophageal, gastric, duodenal Mallory-Weiss tears Peptic ulcers • Gastric, duodenal Gastritis and erosions Malignancy Dieulafoy lesions Arterial-enteric fistula • Rupture of aneurysm or ulcer • Postaortic surgery Diverticulum (duodenal) Angiodysplasia (duodenal) Hemobilia	Diverticulum • Small bowel, colonic Inflammatory bowel disease Mesenteric ischemia, including ischemic colitis Infectious colitis Malignancy Angiodysplasia • Small bowel, colonic Hemorrhoids

D. Localization of Bleeding

1. **Nasogastric tube lavage** of the stomach is easy to perform and is the first maneuver performed to assess for an upper GI source. A clear lavage of the stomach with some bile staining reassures the clinician that the source is not the upper GI tract.
2. **Endoscopy**
   a. **Esophagogastroduodenoscopy** is the diagnostic test of choice for suspected upper GI bleeding and is diagnostic in 90% to 95% of cases. Often, the precise source of bleeding is identified, allowing for immediate endoscopic therapy; however, this can be challenging if a copious amount of blood and clot is present.
   b. **Colonoscopy** for lower GI bleeding is diagnostic in 53% to 97% of cases. Colonoscopy is usually undertaken after a colonic purge to increase diagnostic accuracy and visualization. Colonoscopy allows for examination of the rectum, colon, and, potentially, the distal small bowel; however, the mid small bowel remains difficult to access endoscopically. Without a prep, it is often challenging to definitively localize and intervene on a bleed. Even when prepped, localization is challenging and less successful than in the upper GI tract. It is possible to perform therapeutic maneuvers as well, but these are less successful than in upper GI bleeds. Inking of the affected segments may facilitate subsequent identification of the bleeding segment by surgeons intraoperatively. Complications, including perforation, are rare, but the index of suspicion for their occurrence must be high in the critically ill, older adults, and patients who are immunosuppressed.
3. **Angiography** may be required if endoscopy cannot localize bleeding. Angiography may be performed via computed tomographic angiography (CTA) or on-table angiography in the interventional suite.
   a. Ongoing bleeding is required for successful angiographic detection (0.5-1 mL/min, ~3 U of blood per day).
   b. Angiography may direct further endoscopic or surgical treatment or may be therapeutic via embolization or selective intra-arterial

vasopressin infusion. The risk of significant bowel ischemia as a result of embolization, even in the small or large bowel, is less than 5% but the patient must be monitored for ischemia with serial abdominal exams.

c. Other complications associated with angiography include contrast-induced nephropathy, distal embolization of vessel wall plaque, and access site complications.

d. Provocative angiography may be performed if no bleeding is able to be detected by conventional angiography. This technique involves the use of pressors to drive the systolic pressure high (160-180 mm Hg), vasodilators to dilate the mesenteric vessels, and heparin. If heparin fails, a low dose of tissue plasminogen activator (tPA) may be considered. By provoking the bleeding, the angiographer may then perform the embolization of the affected segment. A provocative angiogram demonstrates the bleeding in approximately 50% of the cases. If the angiographer cannot control the bleeding, the patient must go to the operating room for a resection immediately. Performance of provocative angiography in a hybrid operating room allows for the angiographic procedure and surgical intervention in the same location, although hybrid rooms may not be accessible at all institutions. A multidisciplinary approach with radiology, gastroenterology, and surgery is key.

4. Radionuclide imaging involves the use of one or two available tracers: technetium-^{99m}–labeled sulfur colloid (^{99m}Tc-SC), and technetium-99m–labeled red blood cells (^{99m}Tc-RBC). ^{99m}Tc-SC can be used immediately but is taken up by the liver and spleen, which can obscure interpretation of the images when bleeding is located adjacent to these structures. ^{99m}Tc-RBC is not taken up by the liver and spleen but requires preparation before use.

a. ^{99m}Tc-labeled scans are sensitive and can confirm ongoing bleeding. Their specificity in determining a precise anatomic site of bleeding is debatable.

b. Their utility in an ICU setting is limited, but radionuclide imaging may be helpful in patients who are hemodynamically stable with slow lower GI bleeding not localized by colonoscopy.

5. A **capsule study** can occasionally help identify a bleeding source in the small bowel of patients who are hemodynamically stable.

E. Specific Causes of Gastrointestinal Bleeding

1. Upper gastrointestinal bleeding

a. Variceal bleeding may originate in the esophagus, stomach, or duodenum and is usually the result of cirrhosis and portal hypertension. Splenic vein thrombosis can also result in the development of gastric varices.

1. Prognosis is related mainly to the severity of the patient's underlying liver disease. Mortality following an episode of variceal bleeding ranges from 10% to 70%. The risk of rebleeding is 70% within 6 months.

2. Early endoscopy is crucial for diagnosis and management. Between 30% and 50% of patients with known varices bleed from other upper GI sources. Endoscopic variceal band ligation and sclerotherapy can control bleeding in 80% to 90% of cases.

3. Balloon tamponade is indicated when endoscopic interventions cannot control esophageal or gastric variceal bleeding. Available balloon tamponade devices include the Sengstaken-Blakemore tube and Minnesota tube. Because of the risk of pressure necrosis, balloon deflation must occur within 24 to 48 hours and should be followed by another attempt at endoscopy with band ligation or sclerotherapy. *It is important to protect the airway with endotracheal intubation before placement of the balloon tube.*

4. Medical management should occur concurrently with endoscopy or balloon tamponade. **Somatostatin** and its synthetic analog **octreotide**, as well as **vasopressin** and **high-dose proton-pump inhibitor (PPI) therapy**, are important procedural adjuncts.
5. After the bleeding has stopped and the patient is stabilized, treatment with **nonselective α-blockers** (propranolol or nadolol) should be initiated. These agents decrease the risk of rebleeding and have a proven survival benefit.
6. In patients with cirrhosis, **antibiotic administration** is associated with reduced mortality, bacterial infections, rebleeding events, and hospitalization length of stay. The data here are strong, with a number need to treat of 1 in 22 to prevent death and 1 in 4 to prevent infectious complications.
7. **Transjugular intrahepatic portosystemic shunting** controls refractory variceal bleeding in up to 90% of cases by reducing the portal pressure gradient to less than 15 mm Hg. Using a transjugular approach, a stent is placed in the liver to connect a branch of the portal vein with a hepatic vein. Complications include occlusion, accelerated liver failure, and hepatic encephalopathy.
8. **Surgical therapy** for refractory bleeding includes splenorenal shunt and portacaval shunt and should generally be undertaken after the patient is determined to not be a candidate for liver transplant. These shunting methods are rarely used in the present day. **Splenectomy** is indicated in patients who are bleeding from gastric varices due to splenic vein thrombosis.

b. **Mallory-Weiss tears** are mucosal lacerations within 2 cm of the gastroesophageal (GE) junction that are likely due to increases in pressure occurring during vomiting. Most of these lesions stop bleeding spontaneously and have less than a 10% chance of rebleeding. However, actively bleeding Mallory-Weiss tears are best addressed endoscopically.

c. **Peptic ulcer disease** is a disruption of the inner lining of the GI tract that occurs in either the stomach or duodenum. PUD has various causes; however, *Helicobacter pylori*–associated PUD and NSAID-associated PUD account for most cases. It can present with intractable symptoms related to oral intake, hemorrhage, obstruction, or perforation.

1. **Esophagogastroduodenoscopy** is the initial diagnostic and therapeutic choice. The **endoscopic appearance** of an ulcer has prognostic significance. Ulcers with a spurting artery or a visible vessel have a high rebleeding risk (50%-100%). Ulcers with an adherent clot or a red or black spot are at moderate risk, whereas ulcers with a clean base are at low risk (<5%) for rebleeding. Repeat esophagogastroduodenoscopy (EGD) may be necessary to control bleeding in some circumstances. In refractory cases, angiographic embolization has been reported to stop bleeding in 80% to 88% of cases. Uncontrolled bleeding in a patient who is hemodynamically unstable may necessitate surgical intervention.
2. **Acid suppression** with PPIs has evolved as a crucial component in the management of ulcer disease. In the acute setting, PPIs are administered via an IV line as a continuous infusion or as twice-daily boluses. Patients are then transitioned to an oral regimen. PPIs produce more consistent acid suppression than do histamine receptor (H2) blockers. Patients with large ulcerations greater than 2 cm have a high risk of failing medical therapy and surgical resection/acid reduction should be considered.
3. ***H. pylori* infection** (see **Section IV.B.2**), if present, should be eradicated to decrease the rate of future rebleeding.

4. Mucosal ulcerations may be due to a **neoplasm** rather than to PUD. The endoscopic appearance in conjunction with a biopsy will help establish the correct diagnosis. If ulceration fails to resolve, it should be biopsied to ensure there is no concurrent malignancy

d. Stress gastritis, also called stress ulceration, stress-related erosive syndrome, erosive gastritis, or hemorrhagic gastritis, leads to upper GI bleeding in 1% to 7% of patients in the ICU. Mucosal hypoperfusion and increased gastric acidity occurring in patients who are critically ill are postulated to play a role in pathogenesis. In the case of head injury, these ulcerations are also known as a Cushing ulcer and in burn injury as a Curling ulcer.

1. Endoscopic findings include mucosal erosions.

2. Management is with PPIs, as discussed earlier. *H. pylori* infection should be excluded. Rarely, angiography with selective embolization (often of the left gastric artery) is necessary. Operative management is reserved for severe refractory hemorrhage.

e. Aortoenteric fistulae are communications between the GI tract, most commonly the distal duodenum, and either the native aorta (primary) or an aortic vascular graft (secondary). Secondary fistulas are more common, occurring in 0.6% to 1.5% of patients after an open aortic reconstructive surgery. An initial "herald" bleed followed by massive hemorrhage has been described. Patients may also present with graft infection. Accurate and timely diagnosis is facilitated by a high index of suspicion.

1. Endoscopy demonstrating an eroding aortic graft is uncommon. CT scan is the diagnostic study of choice and may demonstrate hematoma or air at the aortic graft. Once the diagnosis is established, **emergency surgery** is indicated.

f. Dieulafoy lesion is an abnormally large artery protruding through the mucosa, most often into the gastric lumen (fundus or body). There is no mucosal ulceration. Bleeding can be massive and can recur in 5% to 15% despite endoscopic therapy. When rebleeding occurs despite endoscopic intervention, surgical ligation or excision of the vessel is indicated.

g. Duodenal diverticulum is a rare cause of upper GI bleeding. The diagnosis can be made endoscopically. Bleeding duodenal diverticula are treated with surgical excision.

h. Angiodysplasia can be located throughout the entire GI tract and can cause brisk bleeding. Endoscopy can detect and treat these lesions. Surgical excision is indicated when lesions continue to bleed despite medical management.

i. Pseudoaneurysms arising in the celiac vasculature may manifest as hematemesis, bleeding from the NG tube, melena, by bleeding from drains, or an abdominal wound or intra-abdominal bleeding. Such bleeding may be intraluminal, extraluminal, or a combination of both. It is usually associated with a sentinel bleeding event. Postpancreatectomy hemorrhage, seen in less than 10% of patients, is an example of bleeding often attributable to a pseudoaneurysm or disruption of the gastroduodenal artery (GDA) stump.

j. Hemobilia can result from trauma, procedures such as liver biopsy, biliary stent placement, malignancy, gallstones, or erosion of blood vessels into the biliary tree. The treatment of choice is angioembolization.

2. Lower gastrointestinal bleeding accounts for approximately 25% of GI bleeding and has a mortality rate of 2% to 4%.

a. Intestinal ischemia can involve either the small bowel or the colon and can present with lower GI bleeding. Intestinal ischemia is discussed later in greater detail (**Section IV.F.1**).

b. **Small bowel bleeding** can be a challenging diagnosis and should be suspected after two negative EGDs and a negative colonoscopy.
   1. **Angiodysplasia** is the most common cause of GI hemorrhage between the ligament of Treitz and the ileocecal valve. Other causes include tumors, inflammatory bowel disease, Meckel diverticulum, NSAID-induced ulcers, and Dieulafoy lesions.
   2. **Diagnosis** is difficult but may be made in approximately 50% to 70% of cases by push enteroscopy (which examines the jejunum) or capsule study. If the bleeding is brisk, radionuclide scans or angiography may be useful. Again, a provocative angiogram (see earlier text) is an option followed by embolization or operative resection. The angiographer may leave the catheter in place and the surgeon may inject the catheter during the laparotomy with methylene blue to visualize the segment of bowel with the bleeding site.
   3. **Treatment** of small intestinal sources of bleeding is directed at the underlying disease.

c. **Diverticular bleeding** accounts for 20% of colonic bleeding and is the most common cause of massive lower GI bleeding. Hemorrhage occurs when the *vasa recta* ruptures into an adjacent diverticular lumen. Bleeding is self-limited in 85% of cases but can recur in 14% to 53% of patients. Colonoscopy can locate the site of bleeding, but therapeutic maneuvers are difficult. Angiography can also localize the bleeding and is potentially therapeutic. Urgent operative resection is indicated when bleeding and hemodynamic instability persists. Elective colectomy can be considered after multiple episodes of diverticular bleeding.

d. **Colonic angiodysplasias** are more frequent in patients older than age 60. Most lesions are found in the ascending colon and most patients have multiple lesions. Colonoscopy and angiography are very successful for diagnosis and treatment, and colon resection is reserved for failures of these modalities.

e. **Neoplasm** (adenocarcinoma as well as polyps) can present with acute lower GI bleeding, although chronic or occult blood loss and microcytic anemia is a more common presentation. Treatment is multidisciplinary, including surgical resection. Postpolypectomy bleeding can be treated with colonoscopy and coagulation.

f. **Hemorrhoids and other benign anorectal diseases** make up nearly 10% of acute hematochezia. In patients with portal hypertension, hemorrhoidal bleeding can be life-threatening, and treatment must be aggressive and may involve a portosystemic shunting procedure.

g. **Colitis** may be ischemic, infectious, or a result of inflammatory bowel disease (**Crohn disease** or **ulcerative colitis**) and can present with bloody diarrhea, hematochezia, or melena. Colonoscopy usually reveals diffuse mucosal inflammation. Management of inflammatory bowel disease is best directed by a gastroenterologist and consists of hydration, bowel rest, and steroids. Ischemic and infectious colitis are discussed in **Sections IV.F.1** and **IV.F.4.**

IV. SPECIFIC GASTROINTESTINAL PROBLEMS BY ORGAN

A. Esophagus

1. **Esophageal perforation** may arise from increased intraluminal pressure at the anatomic sites of narrowing, as well as sites narrowed by a malignancy, foreign body, or physiologic dysfunction. More than half of esophageal perforations are iatrogenic and may follow upper endoscopy procedures, NG tube placement, balloon tamponade of bleeding varices, dilation of strictures, endotracheal tube placement, or transesophageal echocardiography.

Abnormal anatomy such as a Zenker diverticulum may predispose the patient to this complication. Perforation can occur in the cervical, thoracic, or abdominal esophagus, leading to cervical abscess, mediastinitis, empyema, or peritonitis.

a. **Diagnosis:** Patients may have pain, fever, subcutaneous crepitus, leukocytosis, pneumomediastinum, or a pleural effusion. A contrast swallow study, CT scan, or an esophagoscopy can confirm and localize esophageal perforations.

b. **Treatment** is urgent and includes broad-spectrum antibiotics, drainage, and gastric acid suppression. Some patients may be candidates for primary repair at the time of drainage. Most patients will remain npo for a prolonged period and will require nutritional support via a feeding tube.

2. **Boerhaave syndrome** refers to spontaneous esophageal perforation, which may have no obvious precipitant or may be related to retching/vomiting, blunt trauma, weightlifting, or childbirth. Predisposing factors include reflux esophagitis, esophageal infections, PUD, and alcoholism.

3. **Ingestion** of foreign bodies and caustic substances can cause significant esophageal injury.

a. Ingested **foreign bodies**, most commonly food boluses, can present with dysphagia, odynophagia, chest pain, or airway obstruction. Blunt objects less than 2 cm in size may traverse the GI tract uneventfully, whereas objects larger than 6 cm can obstruct within the duodenum if not in the esophagus. Most objects that do not pass spontaneously may be removed endoscopically—this should be done early to minimize the risk of perforation from pressure-induced necrosis of the esophageal wall.

b. **Acids** (pH <2) and **alkalis** (pH >12) cause severe burns when ingested. Vomiting after the ingestion exposes the esophagus to the caustic substance a second time.

1. **Initial management** includes a careful assessment of the airway. Intraoral burns, edema of the uvula, and inability to swallow saliva may suggest impending airway compromise. Assessment of the airway should be ongoing as the injury evolves. Patients may also require significant **resuscitation** because of the inflammation of the mediastinal tissues. Radiographs of the chest and abdomen are helpful to evaluate for perforation. There is no role for gastric lavage, induced emesis, or activated charcoal.

2. **Endoscopy** early in the patient's course is controversial but can be helpful to assess the degree of injury. Endoscopy is helpful in evaluating and managing esophageal strictures that develop later on as a complication of caustic ingestions.

B. Stomach

1. **Stress ulceration** is discussed in **Section III.E.1**.

2. Risk factors for PUD include *H. pylori* infection, NSAIDs, and aspirin use. Patients can present with pain, upper GI bleeding, obstruction, or peritonitis from perforation.

a. The **diagnosis** of active *H. pylori* infection can be made during endoscopy utilizing the biopsy specimen and include histology, culture, urease testing, and polymerase chain reaction (PCR).

b. **Treatment** of *H. pylori* is indicated in most patients on the basis of its association with peptic ulcers, gastric carcinoma, and gastric lymphoma. First-line regimens consist of a PPI plus two antibiotics such as amoxicillin + clarithromycin (first-line therapy), amoxicillin + metronidazole (for macrolide allergy), or metronidazole + clarithromycin (for penicillin allergy).

c. Complications of PUD include upper GI bleeding (**Section III.E.1**), perforation, and obstruction. Perforation requires an operation with either a laparoscopic or an open approach.

C. Pancreas

1. Acute pancreatitis

a. Most common etiologies are alcohol and gallstones (70%-80% of cases). Other causes include biliary reflux, contrast reflux, hypercalcemia, hyperlipidemia, trauma, and others.

b. The **pathogenesis** of acute pancreatitis is related to the release of activated pancreatic enzymes that autodigest the pancreatic parenchyma and cause inflammation, microvascular injury, and necrosis. Activated enzymes may also circulate to distant organs, causing activation of the complement and coagulation cascades, vasodilatation, and endothelial injury. Systemic consequences may include shock, acute lung injury and acute respiratory distress syndrome (ALI/ARDS), and acute renal failure.

c. Symptoms of acute pancreatitis include severe epigastric pain radiating to the back, nausea and vomiting, and fever.

d. The **diagnosis** is established with a consistent history and physical examination and increased serum amylase or lipase levels. An abdominal CT scan demonstrating pancreatic inflammation, edema, or necrosis may be a useful adjunct (Figure 28.2).

e. The **prognosis** for the majority of patients is good and they experience mild, self-limiting disease. Severe acute pancreatitis, defined as acute pancreatitis with organ dysfunction, develops in 10% to 20% of patients, necessitating admission to the ICU. Various tools have been developed to assess the severity of acute pancreatitis—the most commonly used is the Ranson criteria (Table 28.3).

f. Clinical course

1. The early phase is characterized by local inflammation, significant retroperitoneal fluid sequestration, and a systemic inflammatory response that can be robust and may lead to **multiple organ system failure.**

a. Initial treatment is largely supportive. Aggressive fluid resuscitation and electrolyte repletion should be undertaken. NG tube decompression can be helpful to alleviate nausea but does not shorten the clinical course. Pain relief, supplemental oxygen, invasive monitoring, mechanical ventilation, and inotropic support may be necessary.

b. Prophylactic antibiotics are not indicated in severe pancreatitis without overt signs of sepsis or positive culture or aspiration. Even in patients with a large amount of necrosis (≥30%), routine use of antibiotics has been associated with no improvement in outcomes.

c. Nutrition should be provided. Several trials support the use of early enteral feeding via an NG or a nasojejunal tube within the first 48 hours. Total parenteral nutrition (TPN) should only be considered for patients who cannot tolerate adequate enteral nutrition.

d. Patients with mild gallstone pancreatitis should undergo **cholecystectomy during the index hospitalization** to prevent recurrence. The type of intervention and timing for patients with severe gallstone pancreatitis must be individualized. Patients who are too sick to undergo cholecystectomy may be treated with endoscopic retrograde cholangiopancreatography (ERCP) and sphincterotomy.

2. The later phase of severe acute pancreatitis is characterized by local complications and can carry on for weeks or months.

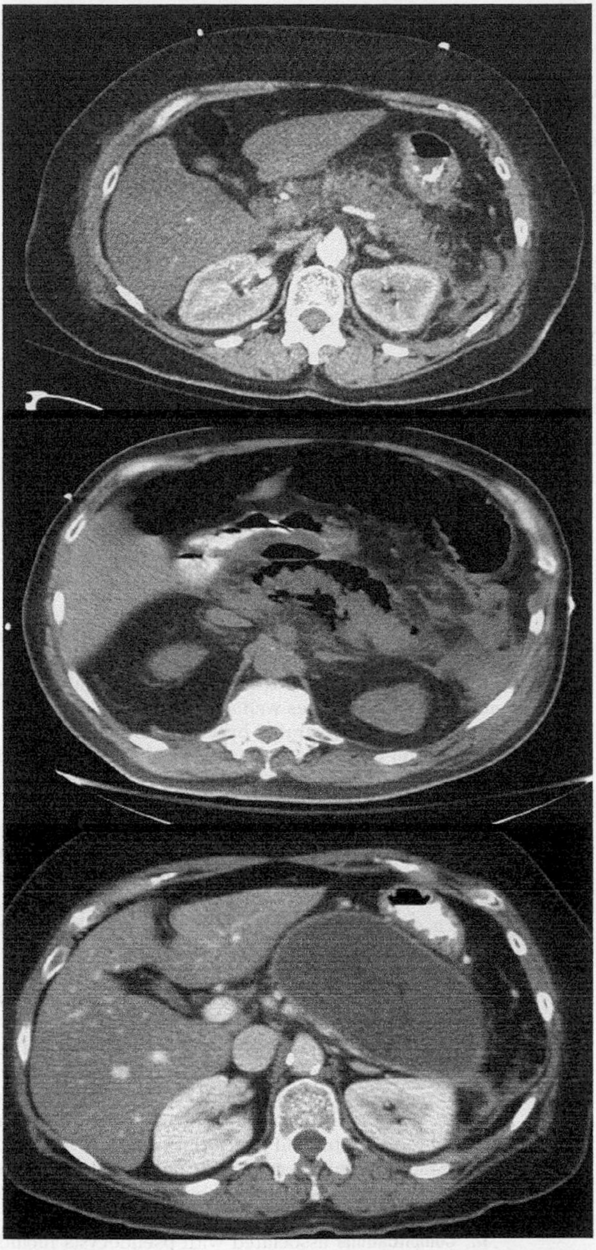

FIGURE 28.2 Acute pancreatitis. Axial computed tomography (CT) images demonstrating acute pancreatitis with prominent pancreatic inflammation (top), pancreatic necrosis with air around the pancreas (middle), and a giant pancreatic pseudocyst that developed several weeks after the acute episode (bottom). (Courtesy of Hasan Alam, MD.)

TABLE 28.3 Ranson Criteria for Prognosis of Acute Pancreatitis

At admission
- Age >55 yr
- WBC count >16 000/μL
- Blood glucose >200 mg/dL
- Serum lactate dehydrogenase (LDH) >350 IU/L
- Serum glutamic oxaloacetic transaminase (SGOT, aspartate aminotransferase [AST]) >250 IU/L

During initial 48 h
- Hematocrit decrease of >10%
- Blood urea nitrogen (BUN) increase of >5 mg/dL
- Serum calcium <8 mg/dL
- Arterial Pa_{O_2} <60 mm Hg
- Base deficit >4 mEq/L
- Estimated fluid sequestration >6 L

Number of criteria met	Expected mortality (%)
<3	<1
3 or 4	15
5 or 6	40
7 or 8	90

a. **Pancreatic necrosis** (Figure 28.2) should be suspected in patients who fail to improve or suffer clinical deterioration. Necrosis is not present in the first 2 to 3 days of symptoms. The extent of pancreatic necrosis correlates well with the amount of devascularized pancreas, as demonstrated by a contrast-enhanced CT scan. Superinfection of the necrosis may occur. New organ failure, new fever, or an increasing leukocytosis should prompt CT-guided aspiration of necrotic tissue. Gram stain and culture aid in establishing the diagnosis of infected pancreatic necrosis. Patients with infected pancreatic necrosis should be treated with antibiotics and drainage. There has been evidence to suggest that percutaneous treatment as a bridge to definitive drainage is an option, using a step-up approach. The use of transgastric endoscopic debridement, video-assisted retroperitoneal debridement, and sinus tract endoscopy are newer modalities that may be considered if debridement is needed. The morbidity is significantly less than that with a laparotomy.

b. **Pancreatic pseudocysts** (Figure 28.2) are encapsulated fluid collections, rich in pancreatic enzymes, which form 4 to 6 weeks after an episode of acute pancreatitis. Typically, they communicate with the pancreatic duct. Collections that are observed earlier are referred to as acute fluid collections and may spontaneously regress. Small, asymptomatic pseudocysts can be observed safely.
   i. Large (>6 cm) or symptomatic pseudocysts can be drained either endoscopically or surgically.
   ii. **Complications** associated with pseudocysts include rupture into the peritoneal cavity (resulting in pancreatic ascites), rupture into the pleural space (resulting in pancreaticopleural fistula), erosion into an adjacent vessel (resulting in upper

GI bleeding), compression of intra-abdominal structures, and infection (resulting in abscess formation).

c. **Pseudoaneurysms** occur most commonly in the **splenic artery** because of the proximity of this structure to the inflamed pancreas. Splenic artery pseudoaneurysms have a 75% bleeding rate and may rupture into a pseudocyst or intraperitoneally. Hemorrhage requires immediate intervention, either angiographically or surgically.

d. **Splenic vein thrombosis** may occur and lead to the later development of portal hypertension. Patients may require splenectomy if variceal bleeding develops. Thrombosis of the mesenteric vessels leading to gut ischemia is rare.

D. Biliary Tree

1. **Acute acalculous cholecystitis** is an inflammatory disease of the gallbladder occurring in the absence of gallstones. Predisposing factors include critical illness, trauma, sepsis, burns, hypotension, TPN, atherosclerosis, and diabetes.

a. The **pathogenesis** of acute acalculous cholecystitis (AAC) is multifactorial and appears to be related to chemical and ischemic injury of the gallbladder. Pathology specimens reveal an occluded or impaired gallbladder microcirculation, possibly due to inflammation or inappropriate activation of the coagulation cascade.

b. **Diagnosis** requires a high index of suspicion because fever may be the only symptom. Other signs and symptoms can include right upper quadrant or epigastric pain, nausea/vomiting, and new intolerance of enteral feeding. Laboratory findings may be limited to leukocytosis and LFT abnormalities, which may already be present in the patient who is critically ill and in the ICU. Ultrasound and CT scans are used to confirm the diagnosis.

1. **Ultrasound** can be performed at the bedside. Diagnostic findings include gallbladder wall thickness greater than 3.5 mm, gallbladder distension greater than 5 cm, sludge or gas in the gallbladder, pericholecystic fluid, mucosal sloughing, and intramural gas or edema. However, the sensitivity of ultrasound in diagnosing AAC may be as low as 30%.
2. **Computed tomography** scan (Figure 28.3) may be helpful when the diagnosis is uncertain and other intra-abdominal pathology needs to be excluded.
3. **Hepatobiliary iminodiacetic acid** scan is another option to establish the diagnosis. A nonfilling gallbladder confirms the diagnosis.

c. **Treatment** involves antibiotics and cholecystectomy if the patient can tolerate an operation, or more commonly in the critically ill the placement of a percutaneous cholecystostomy tube for drainage. There are now also endoscopic options for the treatment of cholecystitis.

2. **Cholangitis** is an infection of the biliary tract, often associated with septic shock and is described in **Chapter 30.**

E. Spleen: Patients may be admitted to the ICU for management of a splenic laceration or rupture following blunt abdominal trauma. Other splenic pathology encountered in the ICU includes splenomegaly, infarction, or abscess. Splenic infarcts usually occur in patients with preexisting splenomegaly due to portal hypertension or hematologic disorders such as leukemia, sickle cell disease, polycythemia, or hypercoagulable states. **Splenic abscess** usually requires splenectomy or percutaneous drainage and can be due to direct extension of infection or hematogenous seeding. Thus, the possibility of endocarditis should be entertained in the setting of splenic abscess. Patients who undergo

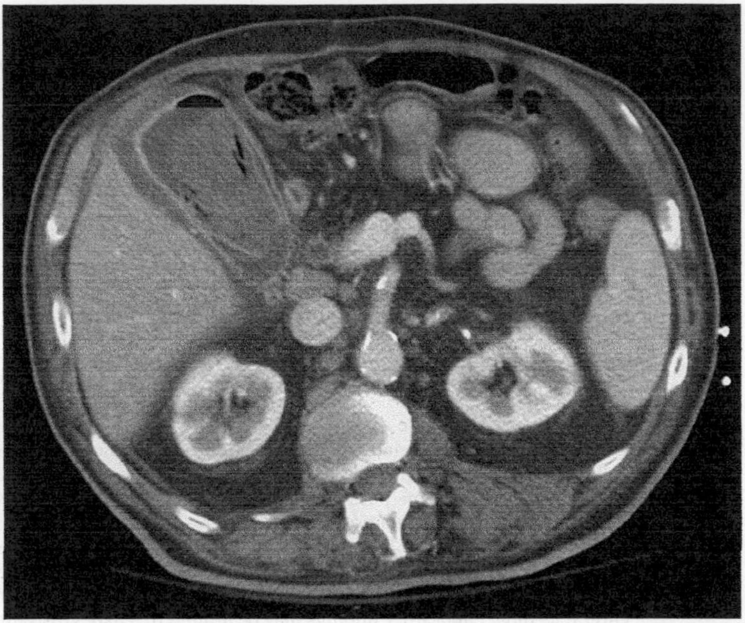

FIGURE 28.3 Acute acalculous cholecystitis (AAC). Axial computed tomography (CT) image demonstrating several common findings of AAC, including an enhancing gallbladder wall, distended gallbladder, pericholecystic fluid, and air within the gallbladder. (Courtesy of Hasan Alam, MD.)

splenectomy should receive vaccination against *Streptococcus pneumoniae*, *Haemophilus influenzae*, and *Neisseria meningitides* and should be counseled about their immunocompromised state and the need for revaccination.

F. **Intestines**

1. **Enteritis and colitis** are common causes of abdominal pain and may affect variable portions of the small or large intestine. Their differential diagnosis is broad, including ischemic, infectious, and inflammatory pathologies.
2. **Ischemic enterocolitis** refers to a spectrum of pathology wherein inflammation of and injury to the intestine result from inadequate blood supply.
   a. **Acute mesenteric ischemia** occurs as a result of arterial obstruction (embolic, thrombotic, or due to aortic dissection) or venous obstruction. Acute mesenteric ischemia (AMI) can also be nonocclusive and result from hypoperfusion, vasoconstriction, or vasospasm.
      1. AMI typically presents with severe abdominal pain out of proportion to physical examination findings. Other signs include sudden intolerance of enteral feeding, nausea, vomiting, fever, intestinal bleeding, abdominal distension, and altered mental status.
      2. **Leukocytosis** and **metabolic acidosis** are common early laboratory abnormalities, whereas elevated serum lactate and amylase are late findings.
      3. **Abdominal radiograph** may show an ileus. **CT scan** may show a thickened bowel. Portal venous gas and *pneumatosis intestinalis* are late findings of intestinal ischemia and suggest infarction. **CTA** may reveal the site of arterial occlusion. **Conventional angiography** can also be used to establish the diagnosis and may be therapeutic. **Duplex**

ultrasound can be used to assess proximal celiac and superior mesenteric artery (SMA) flow. However, overlying edematous bowel can make ultrasonography nondiagnostic.

4. **Treatment** of AMI should be prompt and is aimed at restoring intestinal blood flow to avoid intestinal infarction. Patients should be given volume resuscitation, correction of hypotension, broad-spectrum antibiotics, and NG drainage. Systemic anticoagulation is appropriate after aortic dissection and is ruled out as a cause of mesenteric ischemia. Depending on the cause of ischemia, patients may require surgical or endovascular revascularization or observation. A second-look laparotomy may be necessary in 12 to 24 hours to reassess bowel viability.
   a. **SMA emboli** cause 50% of AMI. Emboli typically originate from the left atrium, left ventricle, and cardiac valves. The SMA is susceptible because of its anatomy (large caliber, nonacute angle off the aorta). Most emboli lodge in the SMA, just distal to the origin of the middle colic artery. Vasoconstriction of surrounding nonobstructed arteries further exacerbates intestinal hypoperfusion. Treatment involves aggressive resuscitation and anticoagulation. Laparotomy and embolectomy are performed before evaluating bowel viability.
   b. **SMA thrombosis** generally occurs acutely in patients with chronic mesenteric ischemia from atherosclerosis. Blunt trauma to the abdomen is also a risk factor, presumably from endothelial disruption. Surgical revascularization usually requires thrombectomy, a bypass graft, or an endovascular stent.
   c. **Nonocclusive mesenteric ischemia** results from mesenteric arterial vasospasm and accounts for 20% to 30% of AMI. Vasopressors, diuretics, cocaine, arrhythmia, and shock predispose patients to this condition. Therapy involves resuscitation, anticoagulation, administration of vasodilator agents, and discontinuation of the offending agent.
   d. **Mesenteric venous thrombosis** is a less common cause of intestinal ischemia. Risk factors include inherited or acquired hypercoagulable states, abdominal trauma, portal hypertension, pancreatitis, and splenectomy. Diagnosis is by CT scan. Treatment is with systemic **anticoagulation** (heparin followed by warfarin). Laparotomy is indicated only in cases of suspected bowel infarction.

b. **Ischemic colitis** is a common form of mesenteric ischemia typically affecting the "watershed" areas (splenic flexure and rectosigmoid junction) of the colon. It is usually caused by underlying atherosclerotic disease in the setting of hypotension, although embolism, vasculitis, hypercoagulable states, vasospasm, and inferior mesenteric artery (IMA) ligation during aortic surgery are other causes.
   1. The **diagnosis** of ischemic colitis is suspected in patients with left-sided crampy abdominal pain, often associated with mild lower GI bleeding, diarrhea, abdominal distension, nausea, and vomiting. Other signs and symptoms include fever, leukocytosis, and abdominal tenderness to palpation. The diagnosis is confirmed by CT scan or by endoscopy.
   2. Most cases resolve within days to weeks with **supportive care** including bowel rest, fluid resuscitation, and broad-spectrum antibiotics. Fifteen percent of patients will develop transmural necrosis. Indications for colon resection include peritonitis, colonic perforation, and clinical deterioration despite adequate medical therapy. Long-term complications include chronic colitis and colonic strictures.

c. **Infectious enterocolitis** is due to bowel inflammation caused by bacteria, viruses, or parasites. Common pathologies include diverticulitis,

Clostridium difficile colitis (see subsequent text), cytomegalovirus enterocolitis (particularly in the immunosuppressed), and other infectious entities.

d. **Diverticulitis** is a condition affecting one or more colonic or small bowel diverticula (outpouchings). It most commonly affects the sigmoid colon, although it may affect the entire colon and, rarely, the small bowel. Secondary infectious pathology is common and antibiotic therapy is warranted.
   1. The diagnosis of diverticulitis is suspected in patients with left lower quadrant abdominal pain, nausea, vomiting, fevers, and leukocytosis. CT scan is typically used to confirm diagnosis.
   2. Uncomplicated disease can be managed conservatively with bowel rest and antibiotics. Complicated disease may include perforation, abscess formation, or frank peritonitis. Antibiotics and percutaneous drainage of abscesses are the mainstays of treatment in the absence of peritonitis.

e. **Inflammatory enterocolitis** can be primary (inflammatory bowel disease, vasculitis) or secondary (chemotherapy, radiation therapy, graft-versus-host disease, and others). Two common forms of inflammatory bowel disease are **ulcerative colitis** and **Crohn disease.** Ulcerative colitis always involves the rectum and a variable amount of colon, whereas Crohn disease typically involves the distal ileum.

3. **Adynamic or paralytic ileus** refers to an alteration in GI motility that leads to failure of intestinal contents to pass. Ileus can affect the entire GI tract or a localized segment. **Ogilvie syndrome** refers to isolated colonic ileus (pseudo-obstruction). This most often affects the more proximal colon up to the level of the splenic flexure.
   a. Ileus may be related to a number of predisposing factors. After an uncomplicated abdominal operation, small bowel motility generally returns within 24 hours. Gastric motility follows within 48 hours and colonic motility returns in 3 to 5 days. Early feeding decreases the incidence of ileus.
   b. **Diagnosis** is clinical and radiologic. Patients may present with nausea/vomiting, abdominal distension, intolerance of enteral feeding, and diffuse abdominal discomfort. Abdominal radiographs show distension of the affected part of the GI tract with intraluminal air throughout. Contrast studies are sometimes needed to exclude mechanical obstruction.
   c. **Complications** of ileus depend on the portion of the GI tract involved. A severe ileus can lead to increased intra-abdominal pressure and even abdominal compartment syndrome. Ileus can also lead to bacterial overgrowth and reflux of bowel contents into the stomach can predispose to aspiration. **Fluid sequestration** due to intestinal wall edema can compromise the gut's microcirculation. **Colonic dilation** can lead to ischemia, necrosis, and perforation. Patients with a cecal diameter more than 12 cm or duration more than 6 days are at higher risk for perforation, although perforations have been reported with smaller cecal diameters. Patients with chronic colonic dilation may tolerate much larger diameters.
   d. **Treatment** begins with **supportive care**, which consists of fluid and electrolyte repletion and NG tube drainage. Potential causes of ileus should be reviewed and corrected (Table 28.4). If tolerated, fiber-containing enteral diets or minimal enteral nutrition can promote GI motility. Patients should be encouraged to ambulate. Medications such as metoclopramide, erythromycin, and neostigmine have been used with mixed results. Osmotic laxatives are contraindicated.
      1. **Neostigmine** (2-2.5 mg IV given over 3 minutes) can successfully treat Ogilvie syndrome (colonic pseudo-obstruction) in approximately 80% of cases. Close monitoring for bradycardia is required. Atropine should be readily available at the bedside, if needed, during the administration.
      2. If conservative measures fail or if perforation appears imminent, **colonoscopic** or **operative decompression** is indicated.

TABLE 28.4 Causes of Ileus

Postoperative
Intraperitoneal or retroperitoneal pathology:
- Inflammation, infection
- Hemorrhage
- Intestinal ischemia
- Bowel wall edema (may be due to massive fluid resuscitation)
- Ascites

Systemic sepsis
Trauma
Uremia
Sympathetic hyperactivity
Electrolyte derangements
Drugs:
- Catecholamines
- Calcium channel blockers
- Narcotics
- Anticholinergics
- Phenothiazines
- β-blockers

4. **Bowel obstruction** presents with signs and symptoms similar to that of ileus. As with ileus, plain x-rays (Figure 28.1) and CT scan (Figure 28.4) can confirm the diagnosis. Unlike ileus, the diagnosis of bowel obstruction requires a mechanical blockage and there are usually decompressed loops of intestine more distal to the obstruction.

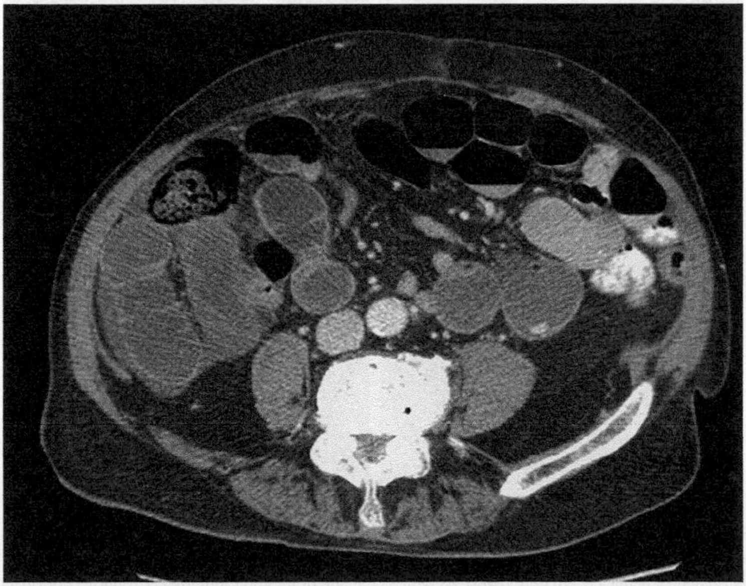

FIGURE 28.4 Small bowel obstruction. Axial computed tomography (CT) image demonstrating several dilated loops of small bowel, consistent with small bowel obstruction.

a. **Small bowel obstruction** is most often due to adhesions. Other causes include abdominal wall and internal hernias, tumors, foreign bodies, and gallstones. Patients with partial small bowel obstruction (SBO) often respond to nonoperative management, which consists of fluid and electrolyte repletion and NG tube drainage. Fevers, leukocytosis, persistent pain, and tenderness on examination are indications to proceed with exploratory laparotomy. Complete SBO should be managed surgically because of the high risk of bowel ischemia, necrosis, and perforation.

b. **Large bowel obstruction** is commonly due to malignancy and develops insidiously over time. Other causes include sigmoid or cecal volvulus (Figure 28.5), diverticular strictures, and fecal impaction. **Treatment** of large bowel obstruction (LBO) is usually operative. Complete LBO represents a surgical emergency in patients with a competent ileocecal valve because ischemia and perforation are imminent.

   1. **Sigmoid volvulus** commonly presents in older males with diabetes and/or neuropsychiatric disorders. Primary management in the absence of peritonitis includes colonoscopic decompression and rectal tube placement, followed by elective sigmoidectomy.
   2. **Cecal volvulus** presents more commonly in younger females and is only corrected by surgical management.

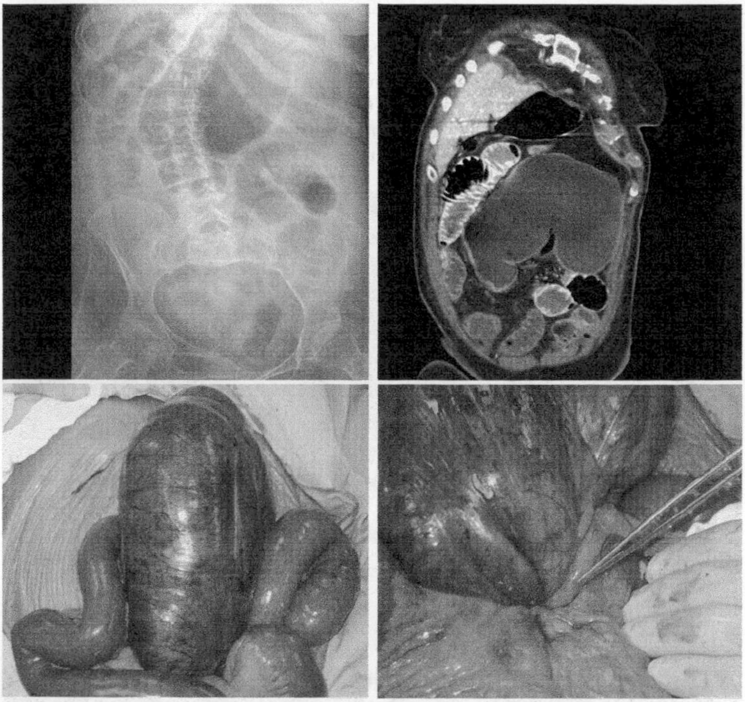

FIGURE 28.5 Cecal volvulus. A plain abdominal radiograph (left upper) and a coronal computed tomography (CT) image (right upper) demonstrating cecal volvulus. Intraoperative photographs reveal a dilated and ischemic cecum (left lower), as well as the site of torsion (right lower). (Courtesy of Hasan Alam, MD.)

5. **Diarrhea** occurs when fluid intake into the gut lumen does not match fluid absorption from the GI tract.
   a. Under normal conditions, 9 to 10 L of fluid enters the bowel lumen each day from oral intake and intestinal secretions. The majority is absorbed in the small bowel, leaving the remaining 1 to 1.5 L to be absorbed in the proximal half of the colon, with approximately 100 mL lost daily in stool.
   b. Water is absorbed secondary to osmotic flow as well as active and passive transport of sodium. Changes in GI motility and epithelial mucosal integrity can drastically affect fluid absorption.
   c. Common **etiologies** of diarrhea in the patient who is critically ill include infections, enteral nutrition, medications, ischemic colitis, fecal impaction, intestinal fistula, pancreatic insufficiency, and hypoalbuminemia.
      1. **Infectious diarrhea** in the ICU setting is usually due to *C. difficile* infection in patients treated with antibiotics.
         a. **Clinical presentation** varies from asymptomatic leukocytosis to severe colitis and toxic megacolon.
         b. Because the sensitivity of the toxin assay for *C. difficile* is no greater than 90%, testing three separate stool samples is the standard for diagnosis if the clinical suspicion is there, unless PCR is available. PCR has a sensitivity nearing 100%. First-line treatment is with oral vancomycin, as described in **Chapter 12**.
         c. Indications for operative management, subtotal colectomy, are failure of medical therapy in the face of escalating cardiopulmonary support. The mortality approaches 80% for those who need a subtotal colectomy; however, earlier intervention seems to be associated with a mortality closer to 30%.
      2. **Enteral nutrition** causing diarrhea is a diagnosis of exclusion. Osmotic diarrhea is secondary to malabsorption of nutrients and usually stops with fasting. Malnutrition and hypoalbuminemia can also cause malabsorption.
         a. An **osmolar gap** in the stool of greater than 70 mOsm suggests an osmotic diarrhea. The osmolar gap is the difference between the measured stool osmolarity and the predicted osmolarity, which is $2 \times ([Na^+] + [K^+])$, based on serum electrolyte measurements.
         b. **Treatment** of enteral nutrition–related diarrhea involves slowing the rate of feeding, diluting the tube feeds, changing the formula, or temporarily stopping enteral nutrition. Enteral nutrition should be lactose free. In some patients, peptide-based, fiber-rich, or elemental diets with reduced fat and residue may be helpful.
      3. **Fecal impaction** can paradoxically lead to diarrhea as a result of decreased fecal tone, mucus secretion, and impaired anorectal sensation.
      4. An **altered enterohepatic circulation**, leading to increased bile acid in the colon, can induce net fluid secretion. This is seen in diseases of the ileum, fatty acid malabsorption, and altered bowel flora.
   d. **Management** of diarrhea consists of replacement of lost fluids and electrolytes and treatment of the underlying cause. After excluding infectious etiologies, diarrhea can be treated symptomatically with agents such as **diphenoxylate with atropine** (Lomotil 5 mg/dose, 4 doses/d, reduce dose once controlled), **loperamide** (Imodium 4-16 mg/d), **bismuth subsalicylate** (Pepto-Bismol 262 mg/dose up to 8 doses/d), and **deodorized or camphorated opium tincture** (0.3-1 mL/dose every 2-6 hours up to 6 mL/d).
6. **Constipation** may affect up to 83% of patients in the ICU and has been associated with prolonged ICU length of stay, infectious complications, pulmonary complications, and increased mortality in some studies.

a. The **etiology** of constipation in the ICU is incompletely understood. Proinflammatory mediators, poor perfusion, dehydration, immobilization, and medications (vasopressors and opiates) likely contribute to the problem.

b. A **bowel regimen** should be initiated and titrated to avoid constipation and can include **stool softeners** (Colace), **bulking agents** (methylcellulose, psyllium), **stimulants** (castor oil, senna), **lubricants** (mineral oil), or **osmotic agents** (lactulose, magnesium).

Selected Readings

Batke M, Cappell MS. Adynamic ileus and acute colonic pseudo-obstruction. *Med Clin North Am.* 2008;92:649-670.

Cheatham ML, Malbrain ML, Kirkpatrick A, et al. Results from the International Conference of Experts on intra-abdominal hypertension and abdominal compartment syndrome. II. Recommendations. *Intensive Care Med.* 2007;33:951-962.

Chey WD, Wong BC; Practice Parameters Committee of the American College of Gastroenterology. American College of Gastroenterology guideline on the management of *Helicobacter pylori* infection. *Am J Gastroenterol.* 2007;102:1808-1825.

Crandall M, West MA. Evaluation of the abdomen in the critically ill patient: opening the black box. *Curr Opin Crit Care.* 2006;12:333-339.

Dellinger EP, Tellado JM, Soto NE, et al. Early antibiotic treatment for severe acute necrotizing pancreatitis. A randomized, double blind, placebo-controlled study. *Ann Surg.* 2007;245:674-683.

Haney JC, Pappas TN. Necrotizing pancreatitis: diagnosis and management. *Surg Clin North Am.* 2007;87:1431-1446.

Heinrich S, Schafer M, Rousson V, et al. Evidence-based treatment of acute pancreatitis. *Ann Surg.* 2006;243:154-168.

Jaramillo EJ, Treviño JM, Berghoff KR, et al. Bedside diagnostic laparoscopy in the intensive care unit: a 13-year experience. *JSLS.* 2006;10:155-159.

Maerz L, Kaplan LJ. Abdominal compartment syndrome. *Crit Care Med.* 2008;36:S212-S215.

Proctor DD. Critical issues in digestive diseases. *Clin Chest Med.* 2003;24:623-632.

Raju GS, Gerson L, Das A, et al. American Gastroenterological Association (AGA) Institute technical review on obscure gastrointestinal bleeding. *Gastroenterology.* 2007;133:1697-1717.

Ramasamy K, Gumaste VV. Corrosive ingestion in adults. *J Clin Gastroenterol.* 2003;37:119-124.

Stewart D, Waxman K. Management of postoperative ileus. *Am J Ther.* 2007;14:561-566.

Villanueva C, Colomo A, Bosch A, et al. Transfusion strategies for acute upper gastrointestinal bleeding. *N Engl J Med.* 2013;368:11-21.

Villatoro E, Bassi C, Larvin M. Antibiotic therapy for prophylaxis against infection of pancreatic necrosis in acute pancreatitis. *Cochrane Database Syst Rev.* 2006;(4):CD002941.

29 Endocrine Disorders and Glucose Management

Devan Cote and Katarina J. Ruscic

I. GLUCOSE HOMEOSTASIS, INSULIN RESISTANCE, AND INSULIN DEFICIENCY

A. Normal Blood Glucose Dynamics: In the normal fasting state, blood glucose (BG) is regulated between **70 and 110 mg/dL**. Despite significant prandial glucose loading, serum levels do not increase to more than 200 mg/dL in normal individuals. A 70-kg patient with a blood volume of 5 L and mean BG of 100 mg/dL has a BG content of 5 g. Absorption of a typical meal may lead to 150 g of glucose (a 30-fold excess of the steady-state amount in the blood) moving through the circulation and into storage within a few hours. A 2-fold rise in BG (>200 mg/dL) during this process is abnormal and sufficient to diagnose **diabetes mellitus (DM)** in the outpatient setting. Glycated hemoglobin (**HbA_{1c}**) can be used to evaluate average plasma glucose concentration over the preceding 3 months, with a level of 6.5% or greater being diagnostic of DM (corresponding to an average serum BG of around 140 mg/dL).

B. Endocrine Control of Blood Glucose: In the fed state, pancreatic β-cells secrete **insulin** directly into the portal circulation in response to BG elevations. In the liver and muscle, glucose is converted to glycogen for storage. In the liver and adipose, excess glucose is converted to triglycerides through a series of metabolic pathways including glycolysis (glucose to pyruvate), pyruvate decarboxylation (pyruvate to acetyl-CoA [acetyl coenzyme A]), fatty acid synthesis (acetyl-CoA to fatty acids), and triglyceride synthesis (fatty acids to triglycerides). In the fasting state, pancreatic α-cells secrete **glucagon** to promote breakdown of glycogen stores and release of glucose into the blood. Elevated glucagon and decreased insulin levels are the body's primary defense against hypoglycemia.

C. Insulin Resistance and Deficiency: Insulin stimulates glucose uptake and promotes cell growth and survival. In states of insulin resistance, such as type 2 DM and critical illness, higher levels of insulin are required to achieve adequate glucose uptake. Insulin resistance is mediated by **counterregulatory hormones** such as glucagon, epinephrine, norepinephrine, cortisol, and growth hormone, as well as inflammatory cytokines and intracellular free fatty acids altering postreceptor insulin signaling. Counterregulatory hormones stimulate glycogen breakdown, gluconeogenesis, and release of fatty acids from lipids. If pancreatic β-cells cannot sufficiently increase insulin production in response to insulin resistance, relative insulin deficiency leads to hyperglycemia. In long-standing type 2 DM, toxicity of cytokines and hyperglycemia itself can lead to β-cell failure and absolute insulin deficiency superimposed on insulin resistance.

D. Hypoglycemia: Hypoglycemia that is not secondary to therapeutic use of insulin or other hypoglycemic agents is rare. Because insulin is largely renally cleared, patients with acute or chronic kidney disease are at increased risk for hypoglycemia due to insulin therapy. Critical illness hypoglycemia not secondary to hypoglycemic drugs may arise from ethanol intoxication (inhibition of gluconeogenesis), sepsis (increased glucose utilization outpacing gluconeogenesis), severe liver failure (impaired gluconeogenesis), and adrenal insufficiency (inadequate glucocorticoids). Hypoglycemia in the intensive care unit (ICU) is exacerbated by withholding nutrition and is frequently observed following abrupt cessation of parenteral nutrition. Critical hypoglycemia may be corrected with boluses of dextrose-containing solutions (eg, 50 mL [1 amp] of D50 containing 25 g dextrose), infusions of dextrose-containing solutions (eg, D10 infusion at 30-100 mL/h), or glucagon (1 mg intravenous [IV] or intramuscular [IM]).

II. HYPERGLYCEMIA OF CRITICAL ILLNESS

A. Pathophysiology: Patients who are critically ill but without preexisting DM frequently become insulin resistant and hyperglycemic because of elevated levels of stress hormones, such as cortisol, glucagon, and catecholamines, as well as cytokines, such as interleukin (IL)-1, IL-6, and tumor necrosis factor (TNF). Treatment with glucocorticoids and sympathomimetic drugs, increased nutrition to compensate for a catabolic state, and administration of IV dextrose all contribute to hyperglycemia. Patients with preexisting DM have insulin resistance and almost always need higher levels of insulin to maintain normal glucose levels while critically ill.

B. Hyperglycemia and Outcomes: Hyperglycemia appears to be a **marker for severity of illness** and is **associated with poor outcomes** including increased infarct volume after stroke, decreased cardiac function after myocardial infarction, increased wound complications after heart surgery, and increased mortality.

1. Although hyperglycemia attributed to critical illness is associated with worse outcomes, hyperglycemia attributed to preexisting diabetes is also associated with increased mortality. In one study, preoperative hyperglycemia (>200 mg/dL) was associated with a 2-fold increase in 30-day mortality and a 4-fold increase in 30-day cardiovascular mortality. Studies also suggest that patients with diabetes in particular have an increased risk of wound infections, renal failure, and rehospitalization following heart surgery.

C. Treatment of Hyperglycemia

1. Moderately permissive insulin therapy: Several studies have tested the efficacy of **intensive insulin therapy (IIT)**, or using insulin to tightly regulate BG to normal or near normal, a much narrower range than had been historically customary in the ICU. In 2001, Van den Berghe (Leuven Surgical Trial) found that targeting a BG of 80 to 110 mg/dL led to a reduction of in-hospital mortality of patients post surgery in the ICU by as much as 34%, in addition to reducing acute renal failure, bloodstream infections, critical illness polyneuropathy, duration of mechanical ventilation, and duration of ICU stay. However, follow-up studies (one of which was in the same Leuven center) failed to show a mortality benefit to IIT and found high rates of severe hypoglycemia, prompting the premature termination of some investigations. A multicenter randomized controlled trial on tight glucose control (Glucontrol) and volume substitution and insulin therapy in severe sepsis (VISEP) trial both noted no difference in mortality between IIT and conventional glucose control. In 2009, the largest multicenter trial to date on this topic, NICE-SUGAR, randomized 6104 patients in the medical and surgical ICU to a goal BG of 80 to 110 versus conventional glucose control of less than or equal to 180 mg/dL. In the conventional group, insulin infusion was discontinued when BG was below 144 mg/dL (8 mmol/L). The study found a small increase in 90-day mortality with intensive glucose control with a number needed to harm of 38. Furthermore, there was no difference in median number of ICU days, duration of mechanical ventilation, or need for renal replacement therapy. Retrospective analysis suggests that this mortality difference may be due to whether a patient has preexisting diabetes. Those without diabetes who develop hyperglycemia in the acute setting seem to be at greater mortality risk; however, it is unclear whether intensive glucose control benefits this subpopulation.

a. The reason for such wide discrepancy among large, controlled clinical trials is not entirely clear. Confounding factors may include methodology, different ranges of BG goals tested, preexisting diabetes, proportions of medical versus surgical cases, and the different provision of total calories as well as their source (enteral vs parenteral). Although not proved, it may also be that the benefits of IIT derive not only from glucose control but also from the anabolic effects of insulin. Insulin has been shown to improve protein synthesis, stimulate anti-inflammatory effects, and modulate energy usage.

2. **Risks of intensive insulin therapy:** The primary risk of IIT is **hypoglycemia.** Throughout various IIT trials, severe hypoglycemia (BG <40 mg/dL) occurred in 5% to 19% of study patients and was in some cases identified as an independent risk factor for death. Because the brain depends on glucose as its primary fuel source, severe hypoglycemia may exacerbate neurologic damage in the brain injured. The risk of hypoglycemia to other organ systems is not as well defined, but hypoglycemia due to excess insulin is also associated with low blood levels of free fatty acids, the preferred fuel for the heart. This suggests that IIT may contribute to cardiac stress. In patients with poorly controlled diabetes, IIT may also stimulate a maladaptive hypoglycemic stress response.
   a. The consequences of hypoglycemia may counteract some or all of the benefits of IIT. In the ICU, the most common cause of hypoglycemia is **interruption of nutrition** in the setting of ongoing insulin therapy. This can occur because of unintended occlusion of feeding tubes, depletion of total parenteral nutrition (TPN) or IV dextrose bags, or accidental removal of tubes or lines. The BG level can fall very rapidly when feeding is interrupted, requiring a **high degree of vigilance** from staff. If enteral feeding or TPN is interrupted, a dextrose infusion (eg, D10) should be started immediately and the rate of insulin infusion decreased to prevent a precipitous fall in BG.
3. **Implementation of insulin therapy:** Intensive glucose control to normoglycemic levels is no longer advised. Given the lack of uniformity of the results of the IIT trials, a wider target range for BG control may confer most of the potential benefit with less risk of hypoglycemia. From the **Surviving Sepsis Campaign's** 2016 guidelines on implementing insulin therapy:
   a. Insulin should be used to treat hyperglycemia targeting an upper BG level of less than or equal to 180 mg/dL rather than less than or equal to 110 mg/dL.
   b. All patients receiving IV insulin should have BG monitored as frequently as every 1 to 2 hours until BG values are stable, then every 4 hours.
   c. Low BG levels obtained from capillary blood by point-of-care testing should be confirmed with a full blood or plasma sample because the former may not be accurate.
4. **Dosing algorithms for insulin:** In our surgical ICU, we use a BG of 140 to 180 mg/dL as our standard goal. No consensus has emerged on the best algorithms to use for control of BG with IV insulin. There has been interest in developing automated "closed-loop" systems for glucose regulation in the ICU to improve the quality of BG control and safety. Very high doses of insulin may be required to control BG in the critically ill. Insulin infusion rates of greater than 10 U/h are not uncommon and some patients require rates in excess of 50 U/h. Tables 29.1 and 29.2 provide sample insulin infusion protocols.
   a. **Appropriate use of insulin dosing algorithms:** Exercise caution when implementing generalized insulin protocols because they may not address individualized insulin needs. For example, those with type 1 diabetes require a basal rate of insulin administration to prevent lipolysis and ketone body formation; thus, protocols calling for holding the insulin infusion when BG declines below a threshold value may inadvertently lead to ketoacidosis. In addition, generalized insulin infusion protocols are not appropriate for diabetic ketoacidosis (DKA) and hyperglycemic hyperosmolar state (HHS) because rapid correction of hyperglycemia can result in severe hypokalemia and osmotic shifts, risking cerebral edema.
   b. **Transition from intravenous to subcutaneous insulin:** The transition from IV to subcutaneous (SC) insulin injections requires careful attention. The first dose of a long-acting analog of insulin (usually **NPH [neutral protamine hagedorn] insulin, twice daily**) should be given at least **2 hours before**

TABLE 29.1 Insulin Infusion Initial Dosing[a]

Current glucose (mg/dL)	Bolus (units)	Infusion rate (units/h)
<150	0	0.5
150-179	2	1
180-240	4	2
241-300	6	3
301-360	8	4
>360	10	5

[a]Blood glucose to be checked hourly until steady state is reached.

TABLE 29.2 Insulin Infusion Adjustment[a]

	Change in glucose since prior reading				
Current glucose (mg/dL)	↓31+	↓11-30	±10	↑11-30	↑31+
70-110	×0.25	×0.50	×0.75	Continue	×1.5
111-150	×0.50	×0.75	Continue	×1.25	×1.5
151-180	×0.75	Continue	×1.25	×1.5	×2.0
181-210	Continue	Continue	×1.5	×1.5	×2.0
>210	Continue	×1.5	×1.5	×2.0	×2.0

[a]Current insulin infusion rate to be multiplied by factor specified by current blood glucose level and change in blood glucose since previous reading.

discontinuation of the infusion. The total daily dose of long-acting insulin (divided into two daily doses if using NPH insulin) should be at least half of the total daily insulin dose. The remainder of the insulin requirement may be provided with a sliding scale of **regular** or **rapid-acting** formulation (insulin aspart, lispro, or glulisine). Correctional or "sliding scale" insulin alone, without any scheduled basal or prandial insulin, is not recommended because of the high likelihood of recurrent hyperglycemia. Insulin regimens should be reevaluated daily in the ICU. A useful rule of thumb is to add at least half of the sliding scale given on the previous day to the basal insulin dosing for the upcoming day and repeat the process until all or most of the BG values are in the desired range. Conversely, hypoglycemia should usually prompt reduction in the basal insulin dose unless it occurred after a large sliding scale bolus to treat hyperglycemia. **All patients with type 1 diabetes require basal insulin**, whether or not they are eating, to prevent development of DKA. A modest reduction from the home basal insulin dose may be appropriate upon hospital admission depending on the form of basal insulin and tightness of control.

III. DIABETIC KETOACIDOSIS

A. Pathophysiology: DKA occurs because of severe insulin deficiency, often accompanied by excessive counterregulatory hormones or inflammatory cytokines. Clinical triggers involve extreme stress and include infection, myocardial infarction, and postoperative inflammation. The pathophysiology of DKA involves lipolysis and ketogenesis due to insulin deficiency resulting in anion gap (AG) acidemia. In addition, hyperglycemia and hyperosmolarity lead to osmotic diuresis, hypovolemia, and electrolyte losses. On presentation, hyperkalemia is common despite whole-body potassium depletion because insulin is an important mediator of potassium uptake into cells. Osmotic diuresis causes loss of water in excess of sodium, resulting in dehydration and volume depletion in addition to prominent potassium and phosphate wasting. Elevated levels of prostaglandins are thought to play a role in the decreased peripheral vascular resistance, nausea, vomiting, and abdominal pain that are frequently observed clinically.

B. Symptoms of Diabetic Ketoacidosis: Symptoms may include polyuria, polydipsia, polyphagia, weight loss, vomiting, abdominal pain, dehydration, weakness, and confusion. Physical examination may reveal poor skin turgor, ileus, Kussmaul respirations (very deep breaths without tachypnea), tachycardia, hypotension, the fruity aroma of ketones on the breath, coffee-ground emesis (hemorrhagic gastritis), and altered mental status. The patient may have a warm and well-perfused periphery despite severe volume depletion.

C. Causes of Diabetic Ketoacidosis: DKA can evolve rapidly, in less than 24 hours. DKA occurs when **insulin is mistakenly withheld or reduced**, or when an **acute illness** increases insulin requirements. Patients with type 1 DM are most at risk but patients with type 2 DM can also develop DKA in the setting of critical illness, not infrequently as the initial presentation of their diabetes. Thus, DKA should be considered in any patient with diabetes who is critically ill. Drugs can uncommonly precipitate DKA. A partial list of causes for DKA is shown in Table 29.3.

TABLE 29.3 Causes of Diabetic Ketoacidosis

- Omission of insulin, inappropriate reduction in dose, inadvertent use of denatured insulin (insulin exposed to heat)
- Infection/sepsis
- Infarction
  - MI, bowel ischemia, stroke
- Endocrine abnormalities:
  - Pheochromocytoma
  - Acromegaly
  - Thyrotoxicosis
  - Glucagonoma
  - Pancreatectomy
- Medications/drugs:
  - Ethanol abuse (DKA can be confused with alcoholic ketosis)
  - Atypical antipsychotics—olanzapine, clozapine, risperidone
  - SGLT2 inhibitors—empagliflozin, canagliflozin, dapagliflozin, ertugliflozin
  - Anticalcineurin drugs—FK506
  - HIV protease inhibitors
  - a-Interferon/ribavirin therapy
  - Corticosteroids
  - Sympathomimetics (cocaine, terbutaline, dobutamine)
  - Pentamidine
  - Thiazides
- Other conditions that may predispose to DKA:
  - Pancreatitis (reduced insulin secretion and insulin resistance)
  - Surgery
  - Trauma
  - Pregnancy
- Eating disorder

DKA, diabetic ketoacidosis; MI, myocardial infarction.

D. **Diagnosis of Diabetic Ketoacidosis:** Diagnosis requires the presence of serum ketones and is supported by AG greater than 12 mEq/L (AG = Na − [Cl + HCO_3]), plasma glucose greater than 250 mg/dL, pH less than 7.3, serum bicarbonate less than 18 mEq/L, and moderate to large ketones in the urine. Patients compensating for volume losses by increasing their fluid intake may excrete enough ketones as sodium salts with retention of chloride so that they present with a hyperchloremic non-AG metabolic acidosis. Treatment of DKA with extra insulin, either by patient or provider, may decrease BG to less than 200 mg/dL without clearing ketones to produce a euglycemic DKA. A euglycemic DKA is also more likely to occur during pregnancy and in patients taking SGLT2 inhibitors. See Table 29.4 for the differential diagnosis of AG acidosis. See Figure 29.1 for a summary of the diagnosis and management of hyperglycemic emergencies.

E. **Measurement of Serum Ketones:** The three ketone bodies are β-hydroxybutyrate, acetoacetate, and acetone. β-hydroxybutyrate is the dominant ketone produced in DKA. Quantitative serum β-hydroxybutyrate assays are now widely available. Traditional assays such as the nitroprusside test detected only acetoacetate and acetone and were therefore less reliable. Most urinalysis ketone assays detect acetoacetate; thus, serum β-hydroxybutyrate is the best test to rule in or rule out DKA. Ketone levels are best used for diagnostic purposes and should not be monitored serially.

F. **Goals of Therapy and Search for the Cause of Diabetic Ketoacidosis:** Glucose normalization is not the first priority in managing DKA. The **primary goals of therapy are to treat hypovolemia, to replete potassium stores, to suppress further ketone formation, and to address the underlying cause of DKA.** Initial evaluation for triggers should include a comprehensive history, physical exam, and diagnostics with consideration of cultures to look for source of infection, chest radiograph, electrocardiogram, and other imaging. Some laboratory anomalies that are common in DKA may obscure the underlying cause, including nonspecific elevations of amylase and lipase, liver enzymes, and the white blood cell count.

G. **Volume Repletion:** Typical volume deficits in DKA are 10% of body mass (eg, for a 70-kg adult, 7 L). Fluid repletion should **begin with 2 L of isotonic crystalloid,** with the remaining fluid deficit to be corrected over 24 hours as an infusion. More rapid administration of fluid may delay resolution of acidemia by diluting bicarbonate. Particularly in children, rapid repletion of volume may be associated with cerebral edema. In all patients, excess normal saline (NS) administration contributes to the non-AG **hyperchloremic metabolic acidosis** that often follows the resolution of ketoacidosis. Patients with end-stage renal

TABLE 29.4 Differential Diagnosis of Anion Gap Acidosis

- Starvation ketosis—bicarbonate rarely <18, no hyperglycemia
- Alcoholic ketoacidosis—glucose usually <250, may be hypoglycemic
- Lactic acidosis—serum lactate
- Renal failure—BUN, Cr (Note that the measured Cr can be artifactually elevated by acetoacetate depending on the assay used.)
- Salicylate intoxication—salicylate level
- Methanol—methanol level
- Ethylene glycol—calcium oxalate and hippurate crystals in urine
- Paraldehyde ingestion—usually hyperchloremic, strong odor on breath

BUN, blood urea nitrogen; Cr, creatinine.

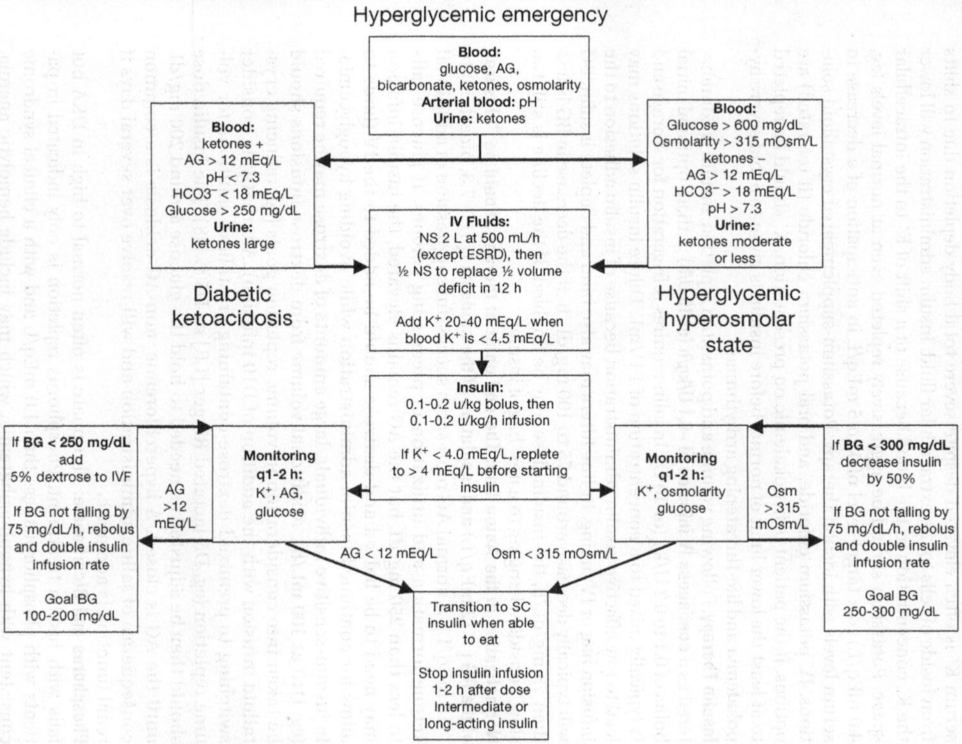

FIGURE 29.1 Diagnosis and management of hyperglycemic emergencies. Not all elements are required for diagnosis—key elements for diabetic ketoacidosis (DKA) are blood ketones and anion gap (AG) greater than 12; for hyperglycemic hyperosmolar state (HHS), blood glucose (BG) greater than 600 mg/dL and Osm greater than 315 mOsm/L. ESRD, end-stage renal disease; IVF, intravenous fluids; NS, normal saline; SC, subcutaneous.

failure who are anuric are a special case and are likely to need little IV fluid because they are not capable of osmotic diuresis in response to hyperglycemia.

H. **Potassium Repletion:** Potassium (K^+) depletion is almost universal in DKA (with the exception of patients who are oliguric or anuric) with a typical deficit of 3 to 5 mEq K^+ per kilogram body weight that requires aggressive repletion. Glucosuria can result in the loss of 70 mEq of potassium for each liter of volume lost. Some patients also have gastrointestinal (GI) losses. The initial serum K^+ is often elevated despite severe total body depletion due to shifts from inside of cells to the extracellular fluid. Insulin administration will lower the K^+ concentration in the blood because of a shift of K^+ to the intracellular space. Potassium should be aggressively repleted even at normal levels (eg, 4.0 mEq/L) to a target level of 4 to 5 mEq/L in anticipation of a decrease in serum levels with insulin therapy. Potassium-supplemented crystalloid solutions, IV potassium chloride, and oral potassium chloride (if tolerated) are options. If the patient is hypokalemic on presentation, K^+ should be repleted to at least the lower limit of normal before insulin is given to avoid severe hypokalemia and life-threatening arrhythmias.

I. **Insulin Therapy:** Following volume and potassium repletion, insulin is administered as a **continuous IV infusion of ~0.1 U/kg/h (or 10 U/h)** with an optional initial bolus of 0.1 to 0.2 U/kg (or 10 U). Insulin requires refrigeration for storage and is typically mixed to a concentration of 1 U/mL. Dilute insulin solutions may lead to low effective insulin administration because of insulin adhesion to the infusion bag or IV tubing. In-line filters may also bind and deplete insulin. BG will typically decrease around 75 to 100 mg/dL/h. If the decrease in BG is less than 75 mg/dL/h, the insulin dose may be doubled. If the decline is still too slow, consider changing to a new bag of insulin.

J. **Normalization of the Anion Gap: The end point of therapy should be "closure" of the AG** ($<$12 mEq/L) **and resolution of the acidosis** (pH $>$7.3, bicarbonate $>$18 mEq/L). A normal AG represents successful suppression of additional ketone formation and utilization of preexisting ketones. If glucose falls to less than 250 mg/dL but the AG remains elevated, the insulin infusion may need to be halved and dextrose should be added to the IV fluids to allow for continued insulin administration while avoiding hypoglycemia. In insulin-sensitive individuals, large amounts of dextrose may be required (eg, D10 at 100 mL/h). Additional volume from dextrose infusions should be taken into consideration in volume repletion goals (eg, reducing crystalloid infusion with the addition of D10 infusion). Alternatively, consider switching to premixed dextrose-containing crystalloid solutions for volume repletion (eg, D5 lactated Ringer [LR] or D5 ½ NS). The insulin dose should then be adjusted as needed to hold the glucose around 200 mg/dL until the AG is closed. A hyperchloremic, non-AG acidosis is a common consequence of saline administration and will resolve over several days if renal function is adequate.

K. **Phosphorus and Bicarbonate:** Phosphate is often normal to high in DKA but falls with insulin treatment. Phosphorus repletion is only indicated in patients with phosphorous less than 1.0 mEq/L and with a clinical syndrome consistent with hypophosphatemia, which may include hemolytic anemia, platelet dysfunction with petechial hemorrhage, rhabdomyolysis, encephalopathy, seizure, heart failure, and weakness of respiratory or skeletal muscles. There is **no benefit of bicarbonate treatment in patients with pH greater than 6.9**. Administration of insulin will result in utilization of ketones in the tricyclic antidepressant (TCA) cycle and regeneration of bicarbonate. Extra bicarbonate can increase potassium requirements, may increase hepatic production of ketones, and may delay resolution of cerebral acidosis.

L. **Complications of Diabetic Ketoacidosis:** The most feared complication of DKA is **cerebral edema**, which occurs in up to 1% of children with DKA, but rarely in adults. However, the mortality in cerebral edema can be as high as 24%.

Cerebral edema as a complication of DKA is a diagnosis of exclusion in adults, and other causes of depressed mental status should be carefully investigated. **Noncardiogenic pulmonary edema** can occur from the high fluid load given during treatment.

M. Transition from IV to SC insulin should begin when the patient is able to eat. A dose of the long-acting insulin (eg, NPH, glargine, or detemir) should be administered 2 to 3 hours before the insulin infusion is stopped. In cases of uncomplicated DKA, the patient's home regimen can be restarted if glucose control on that regimen was adequate (as judged by HbA_{1c}). Making the transition to SC insulin in the morning or evening is preferred so that there is a smooth transition to the patient's usual insulin schedule.

IV. HYPEROSMOLAR HYPERGLYCEMIC STATE

A. Pathophysiology: Insulin is able to suppress lipolysis and ketogenesis at much lower concentrations than is required to stimulate glucose uptake. In contrast to patients with type 1 DM, patients with type 2 DM usually have sufficient insulin production to prevent the excessive production of ketones. When **severe hyperglycemia occurs in the absence of ketosis**, the syndrome is called hyperosmolar hyperglycemic state (**HHS**) or previously hyperosmolar nonketotic coma (**HONKC**). BG may rise to levels that are unusual in DKA, often greater than 1000 mg/dL. The blood pH and bicarbonate levels are typically normal and test results for ketones are negative. Both HHS and DKA are associated with hyperosmolarity, polyuria, polydipsia, volume depletion, and whole-body potassium depletion, although the serum potassium is usually normal or elevated before treatment. The two syndromes are part of a spectrum and approximately one-third of patients have some aspects of both syndromes. **Altered mental status**, including obtundation and coma, are more common in HHS because the degree of hyperglycemia and hyperosmolarity are higher. Patients with HHS may also develop seizures or focal neurologic signs, and up to 50% of patients present with coma. Although DKA is more common than is HHS, HHS has 10 times greater mortality. As in DKA, patients with oliguric renal failure have a different presentation. Although glucose levels are high, the serum sodium is reduced to compensate so that there is minimal hyperosmolarity and few neurologic symptoms.

B. Diagnosis: The diagnosis of HHS requires **severe hyperglycemia** (>600 mg/dL, often >1000 mg/dL) and **hyperosmolarity without an AG acidosis.** A serum osmolality greater than 320 mOsm/kg and a pH greater than 7.3 support a diagnosis of HHS. HHS exists on a spectrum with DKA and some patients with HHS may have modest ketonemia, whereas some patients with DKA may have more severe hyperosmolarity than is typical of DKA. See Figure 29.1 for a summary of diagnosis and management of hyperglycemic emergencies.

C. Treatment: IV fluid replacement and insulin therapy are the mainstays of treatment for HHS, just as they are for DKA, but the goals of insulin therapy differ. Fluid replacement in HHS is similar to that in DKA, although the fluid requirement may be greater because of more extreme hyperosmolarity. By lowering plasma tonicity, IV fluid also improves insulin responsiveness and stress hormone levels. In cases of extreme hyperglycemia, sodium levels corrected according to glucose level may be more informative of prognosis. There is an expected decrease in sodium of about 2 mEq/L for every 100 mg/dL increase in serum glucose above normal (about 100 mg/dL). Thus, a patient with a sodium of 126 mEq/L and a BG of 800 mg/dL has a corrected sodium of 140 mEq/L. **Insulin therapy starts with an initial bolus of 0.1 to 0.2 U/kg and an infusion rate of approximately 0.1 to 0.2 U/kg/h.** Instead of normalizing the AG, **the goal is to bring the glucose into a reasonable range and then to normalize the osmolarity.** Although most patients with DKA are insulin sensitive, **many patients with HHS are very insulin resistant.** Much higher doses of insulin may be required. Once the BG falls to less than 300 mg/dL, the insulin infusion rate should be reduced by 50%. The serum glucose should be maintained between 250 and 300 mg/dL by adjusting the insulin infusion rate until the plasma osmolality is less than 315 mOsm/L. If the corrected serum sodium is less than 135 mEq/L, continue isotonic saline. For normal or elevated sodium, use ½ NS. **Potassium repletion** is similar to that in DKA with 20 to 40 mEq/L of supplemental K^+ added to IV fluids immediately. Just as in DKA, there is typically a substantial total body potassium deficit. It is appropriate to check serial electrolytes during treatment and adjust supplementation accordingly to keep serum K^+ within 4 to 5 mEq/L.

V. NORMAL ADRENAL PHYSIOLOGY AND PATHOPHYSIOLOGY OF ADRENAL INSUFFICIENCY

A. Adrenal Functional Anatomy: Each adrenal gland is made up of a **cortex**, which produces sex steroids (androgens, estrogens), mineralocorticoids (aldosterone), and glucocorticoids (cortisol), and a **medulla**, which produces adrenergic hormones (such as epinephrine). The term "adrenal insufficiency" is commonly used to describe deficiency of both **cortisol** (which may be isolated) and **aldosterone** (which is almost always associated with cortisol deficiency).

B. Regulation of Adrenal Hormone Production (Figure 29.2): Cortisol production by the adrenal glands is dependent on **adrenocorticotrophic hormone (ACTH)**, which is produced by the pituitary gland. ACTH is regulated by corticotropin-releasing hormone (CRH), which is produced in the hypothalamus. Cortisol feeds back to inhibit CRH and ACTH release, closing the control loop. Cortisol deficiency

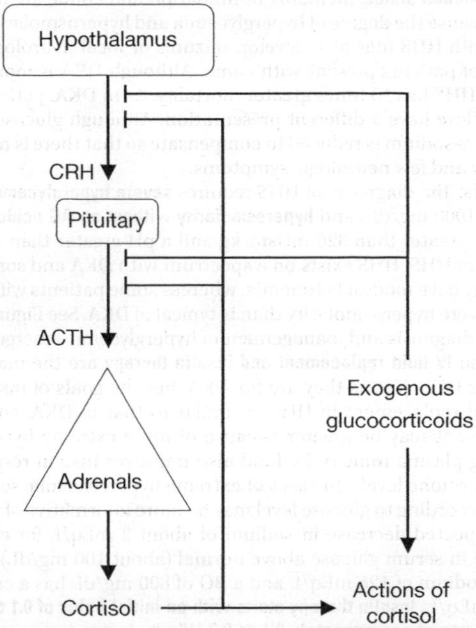

FIGURE 29.2 Regulation of adrenal hormone secretion. Arrows indicate positive action, production, or conversion. Lines ending in crossbars indicate inhibition. ACTH, adrenocorticotrophic hormone; CRH, corticotropin-releasing hormone.

may be caused by injury either to the adrenal cortex (primary adrenal insufficiency with elevated ACTH) or to the pituitary or hypothalamus (secondary or central adrenal insufficiency with low or "inappropriately normal" ACTH). Primary adrenal insufficiency is often associated with aldosterone deficiency, but central forms of adrenal insufficiency are limited to a deficit in cortisol production because aldosterone production is not dependent on ACTH.

C. **Classification of Adrenal Insufficiency:** Adrenal insufficiency can be defined on the basis of the origin of the disease.
   1. **Primary:** The adrenal gland is unable to produce steroid hormones despite adequate corticotropin from the pituitary gland (eg, Addison disease, autoimmune diseases).
   2. **Secondary:** a lack of ACTH from the pituitary or CRH from the hypothalamus to stimulate the adrenal gland (eg, brain tumors, infarction, granulomatous disease)
   3. **Tertiary:** adrenal deficiency due to the withdrawal of exogenous glucocorticoids (eg, chronic steroid use)

D. **Signs of Adrenal Insufficiency: The adrenal gland is activated in states of stress, activating the release of catecholamines, glucocorticoids, mineralocorticoids, and factors of the renin-angiotensin-aldosterone axis.** Cortisol deficiency is acutely dangerous and causes **circulatory collapse** with **refractory hypotension** that may be fatal within hours to days without glucocorticoid replacement. Symptoms and signs of glucocorticoid deficiency include nausea, vomiting, anorexia, weight loss and wasting, weakness, hyponatremia, and eosinophilia. Suspicion of glucocorticoid deficiency is sufficient cause to begin treatment immediately; treatment can be discontinued if adequate adrenal function is demonstrated.

E. **Causes of Adrenal Insufficiency:** A "functional" or "relative" deficiency in cortisol secretion **may occur in critical illness**, but this is controversial and there are no universally accepted criteria for diagnosis of this condition. Adrenal insufficiency may be caused by drugs that inhibit cortisol production, notably ketoconazole and etomidate. Drugs that accelerate the metabolism of cortisol, such as phenytoin, barbiturates, and rifampin, can contribute to the development of adrenal insufficiency in patients with limited physiologic reserve. The **most common cause of adrenal insufficiency is exogenous glucocorticoids** (or drugs with glucocorticoid activity such as megestrol acetate) that cause feedback inhibition of ACTH production, which in turn causes atrophy of the cortisol-producing cells in the adrenal gland. Iatrogenic adrenal insufficiency should be considered in all patients taking glucocorticoids, including patients chronically on as little as 5 mg of prednisone daily. **Complete recovery** from iatrogenic adrenal insufficiency **may take months or even years.** Causes of adrenal insufficiency are listed in Table 29.5.

F. **Aldosterone Deficiency:** Aldosterone production is regulated by the **renin-angiotensin system.** The most important action of aldosterone is to promote sodium retention by the kidney. Deficiency of aldosterone causes sodium wasting, hypovolemia, and hypotension. Aldosterone deficiency can be managed in the short term with sufficient sodium and fluid intake, but long-term deficiency is managed with medications having aldosterone receptor agonist activity, such as fludrocortisone. The most common cause of aldosterone deficiency is injury to the adrenal gland itself, which is typically also associated with glucocorticoid deficiency. Isolated mineralocorticoid deficiency is rare.

VI. DIAGNOSTIC TESTING AND TREATMENT FOR ADRENAL INSUFFICIENCY

A. **Diagnosis of Adrenal Insufficiency in Critical Illness:** The diagnosis of cortisol deficiency in the setting of critical illness is challenging. Under normal conditions, cortisol is secreted diurnally; however, during critical illness, this

TABLE 29.5 Differential Diagnosis of Adrenal Insufficiency

Primary adrenal insufficiency	Central adrenal insufficiency

• Hemorrhagic infarction
  • Sepsis
  • Adrenal vein thrombosis
  • Anticoagulation
  • Coagulopathy
  • Thrombocytopenia
  • Hypercoagulable state
  • Trauma
  • Postoperative
  • Severe stress
• Cancer metastasis/lymphoma
• Autoimmune
  • Addison disease
  • Polyglandular autoimmune syndromes I and II
• Infectious process
  • Disseminated fungal infections (histoplasmosis)
  • Tuberculosis
  • HIV (CMV, MAC, cryptococcus)
• Infiltrative process
• Iatrogenic
  • Ketoconazole
  • Etomidate
  • Metyrapone
  • Suramin
	• Iatrogenic
	  • Glucocorticoids
	  • Megestrol acetate (glucocorticoid activity)
	• Tumor or other mass lesion
	  • Pituitary adenoma
	  • Metastasis
	  • Lymphoma
	  • Primary tumor of brain or meninges
	  • Rathke cleft cyst
	  • Empty sella
	• Pituitary apoplexy
	  • Sheehan syndrome (postpartum hemorrhage)
	• Infiltrative process
	  • Hemochromatosis
	  • Histiocytosis
	  • Tuberculosis

CMV, cytomegalovirus; MAC, mycobacterium avium complex.

diurnal variation is lost. Cortisol secretion is naturally increased during times of physiologic stress, which can result in unmasking of preexisting subclinical adrenal insufficiency. Critical illness may also cause a functional deficiency in cortisol production or responsiveness. Improvement of critical illness in response to glucocorticoids does not necessarily imply diminished adrenal function. It is important to make a conceptual distinction between treatment of adrenal insufficiency and pharmacologic treatment with glucocorticoids, which may improve clinical outcomes independent of adrenal functional status.

B. Total Versus Free Cortisol: Cortisol binds to cortisol-binding globulin (CBG) in the blood. Widely available cortisol assays measure total cortisol, although unbound "free" cortisol is physiologically active. Critical illness is often associated with reductions in the level of CBG, as is cirrhosis; thus, total cortisol may be reduced without reduction of free cortisol, leading to overdiagnosis of adrenal insufficiency. As a result of the wide variation in total cortisol levels in septic shock, total cortisol is not a useful test for adrenal insufficiency. Free cortisol assays are not widely available.

C. Adrenocorticotrophic Hormone Stimulation Test: The main test for cortisol deficiency is the ACTH stimulation test. A blood sample for cortisol and ACTH is obtained, and synthetic ACTH (cosyntropin) is administered IV or IM. A blood sample for a second cortisol measurement is obtained 30 to 60 minutes after cosyntropin administration. The dose of cosyntropin administered in the stimulation test is a matter of debate.

1. **High-dose adrenocorticotrophic hormone stimulation test:** This test uses an IV dose of 250 μg cosyntropin. One prospective study suggested that a high baseline serum cortisol (>34 μg/dL) level coupled with a diminished cortisol increase (<9 μg/dL) to a high-dose stimulation test is predictive of increased mortality.
2. **Low-dose adrenocorticotrophic hormone stimulation test:** This test uses 1 μg of cosyntropin for stimulation. Advocates of the low-dose stimulation test have argued that the 250 μg cosyntropin stimulation test stimulates cortisol release even in patients who are adrenally insufficient. The low-dose ACTH stimulation test identifies more patients with adrenal insufficiency. In a study comparing the low-dose versus high-dose cosyntropin test, it was found that a cortisol response to the high-dose, but not low-dose, cosyntropin test was predictive of increased mortality.
3. **Diagnostic criteria for adrenal insufficiency:** Because glucocorticoid levels are normally elevated in response to stress, a very low baseline plasma cortisol (**<3 μg/dL**) in the setting of critical illness is diagnostic of adrenal insufficiency. Moderate levels of baseline cortisol (**<10 μg/dL**) suggest adrenal insufficiency but may be misleading in the setting of a low CBG where free cortisol may be appropriately elevated. A **baseline (nonstimulated) cortisol of more than 18 μg/dL** effectively rules out adrenal insufficiency in most patients. For intermediate cortisol levels, **a stimulated rise of less than 9 μg/dL has been proposed to identify patients who would benefit from glucocorticoid therapy. A peak level of more than 18 μg/dL effectively excludes primary adrenal insufficiency**, although CBG may be elevated in response to oral estrogen and liver inflammation limiting the clinical significance of total cortisol levels.
4. **Limitations:** The utility of the ACTH stimulation test and the appropriate stimulation dose remains unresolved. The ACTH stimulation test does not determine whether sufficient cortisol is being produced by the hypothalamic-pituitary-adrenal axis; it measures only the ability of the adrenal cortex to respond to exogenous ACTH. As a result, it should not be used to diagnose secondary adrenal insufficiency. It may also be altered in the case of etomidate administration due to pharmacologic suppression. In the case of recent-onset central adrenal insufficiency, the adrenal cortex may not yet have atrophied and the stimulated cortisol response may be normal.

D. **Therapy: Therapy should be directed at addressing the cause of the adrenal insufficiency and steroid replacement.** Ideally, cortisol and ACTH levels should be drawn before any empiric therapy is begun. Empiric therapy with dexamethasone (1 mg q6h) does not interfere with the ACTH stimulation test. Once the post-cosyntropin cortisol sample has been drawn, **hydrocortisone**, which provides complete glucocorticoid and mineralocorticoid replacement, should be used at a total daily dose of **300 mg in divided doses every 6 or 8 hours, or given via continuous infusion at 10 mg/h.** Although dexamethasone lacks mineralocorticoid activity, it can nevertheless be used in an adrenal crisis because glucocorticoid deficiency is the primary driver of hemodynamic instability. It should be noted that the appropriate "stress" dose of glucocorticoids is a matter of controversy. Commonly used dosages may provide glucocorticoid activity in excess of that produced by the normal adrenal gland during critical illness. There is no reliable test to determine the appropriateness of the replacement dose, so the dosing must be adjusted empirically. Doses of hydrocortisone should not be reduced below a replacement dose for a patient who is hospitalized with known adrenal insufficiency, 50 to 60 mg orally (PO) divided in two doses, until follow-up testing demonstrates adequate adrenal function.

The equivalent dose of prednisone is 10 to 15 mg daily, whereas the equivalent for dexamethasone is 1.5 to 2.5 mg daily. Doses of hydrocortisone less than 50 mg daily do not provide sufficient mineralocorticoid activity for patients with primary adrenal insufficiency. Note that prednisone and dexamethasone have minimal mineralocorticoid activity. Patients requiring mineralocorticoid replacement should be treated with fludrocortisone at doses of 0.1 to 0.2 mg po daily. Long-term risks of glucocorticoids include hyperglycemia, weight gain, and hypertension. See Table 29.6 for the relative glucocorticoid and mineralocorticoid activities of various steroids.

E. **Identifying the Cause of Adrenal Insufficiency:** An adrenocorticotropin (ACTH) level drawn before initiation of empiric glucocorticoid therapy can help localize the cause of adrenal insufficiency. An elevated ACTH suggests primary adrenal insufficiency and a low (or inappropriately normal) ACTH is consistent with central adrenal insufficiency. If the test suggests primary cortisol insufficiency (elevated ACTH levels), the evaluation should include imaging of the adrenal glands to evaluate for neoplastic, inflammatory, or infiltrative processes. Adrenal protocol computed tomography (CT) scans include a noncontrast series, portal venous phase contrast-enhanced series, and delayed contrast-enhanced series. In the setting of central cortisol deficiency, imaging of the pituitary and hypothalamus is indicated. Pituitary protocol magnetic resonance imaging (MRI) is the most appropriate test, although CT can rule out large tumors or gross hemorrhage. See Table 29.5 for the differential diagnosis of adrenal insufficiency.

F. **Pituitary Apoplexy:** Pituitary apoplexy, also known as Sheehan syndrome, is a clinical syndrome caused by hemorrhage or infarct within a preexisting pituitary mass lesion. It is a rare cause of adrenal insufficiency but it deserves special mention in the ICU because it is one of the true **endocrine emergencies.** Pituitary apoplexy can lead to abrupt and severe adrenal insufficiency in the setting of severe physiologic stress, a combination that may prove fatal if not treated promptly. In addition, mass effect on surrounding structures, including the optic nerve and cranial nerves III and VI, can lead to permanent visual deficits or blindness. Therefore, pituitary apoplexy should always be considered in the differential diagnosis of adrenal insufficiency. Unfortunately, the signs and symptoms of apoplexy (headache, visual disturbance)

TABLE 29.6 Glucocorticoid and Mineralocorticoid Activity

Steroid	Glucocorticoid potency	Glucocorticoid equivalent dose	Mineralocorticoid potency	Mineralocorticoid equivalent dose
Cortisol/ hydrocortisone	1	10 mg[a]	0.0125	10 mg
Prednisone/ prednisolone	4	2.5 mg	0.01	12.5 mg
Methylprednisolone	5	2 mg	0.003	40 mg[b]
Dexamethasone	25	0.4 mg	0	NA[b]
Fludrocortisone	10	1 mg[c]	1.6	0.08 mg
Aldosterone	0	NA	1	0.125 mg[a]

NA, not applicable.
[a]Average daily production in healthy adult subjects.
[b]Not used for mineralocorticoid replacement therapy.
[c]Not used for glucocorticoid replacement therapy.

may be masked in the critically ill. Imaging is key to making the diagnosis. Noncontrast head CT is not reliable for detection of pituitary hemorrhage or infarction but is sensitive for detecting pituitary masses greater than 1 cm, the substrate for most cases of apoplexy. MRI can be used to identify hemorrhage or infarction if a mass is found. Management of pituitary apoplexy involves high-dose glucocorticoids and rapid surgical decompression.

VII. ADRENAL INSUFFICIENCY IN SEPTIC SHOCK

A. Sepsis and the Hypothalamic-Pituitary Axis: The hypothalamic-pituitary axis (HPA) is activated in states of physiologic stress. The normal physiologic response includes reduced cortisol metabolism, decreased cortisol protein binding, and increased free cortisol levels. Critical illness can impair the ability of the HPA to generate an adequate stress response. Studies have demonstrated increased mortality in patients with sepsis who do not respond to a cosyntropin stimulation test. Unfortunately, there is no clear consensus for what constitutes adrenal insufficiency in sepsis.

B. Steroid Supplementation: Steroids have been used in septic shock because of their known anti-inflammatory properties and inhibition of endothelial cell activation, capillary leak, complement activation, and free radical formation.

1. In clinical trials, glucocorticoid use has decreased vasopressor requirements and improved systemic vascular resistance in septic shock. Multiple studies have demonstrated quicker withdrawal of pressors following supplemental steroid initiation. A randomized control trial in 2002 by Annane et al showed a 10% reduction in all-cause mortality among nonresponders to a high-dose cosyntropin stimulation test who received supplemental steroids. No mortality benefit was observed in cosyntropin responders. However, the 2008 Corticosteroid Therapy of Septic Shock (CORTICUS) trial, a multicenter, randomized, controlled trial of 499 patients, found no benefit to stress-dose hydrocortisone in both responders and nonresponders to a high-dose stimulation test. The two trials are notable for several methodological differences, including that Annane et al used both hydrocortisone and fludrocortisone, whereas the CORTICUS trial used only hydrocortisone. Annane et al also initiated steroids closer to the time of onset of shock.
2. In the 2021 Surviving Sepsis Guidelines, steroids (hydrocortisone 200 mg total daily) are recommended for patients with septic shock and an ongoing pressor requirement. An ACTH stimulation test is not advised to determine steroid eligibility. There is no clear consensus on when to discontinue steroids in sepsis, although a rapid taper over 3 to 5 days has been recommended when patients clinically improve and have substantially reduced vasopressor requirements.

VIII. CUSHING SYNDROME

A. Diagnosis: Cushing syndrome is caused by chronic exposure to excess endogenous or exogenous glucocorticoid. Signs and symptoms include central obesity, hypertension, and insulin resistance. Cushing syndrome may be caused by glucocorticoid medications, cortisol-secreting adrenal adenoma, or ACTH-secreting pituitary adenoma (Cushing disease). In states of excessive cortisol production, there is loss of the normal diurnal circadian rhythm of cortisol in the serum. Because the normal response to critical illness is to dramatically increase cortisol production, the usual screening tests for Cushing syndrome cannot be used in the ICU. Suspicion of Cushing syndrome should be prompted by examination of body habitus, enlarged supraclavicular and dorsal cervical fat pads, wide (>1 cm) violaceous (not pink) striae, and proximal weakness.

B. Treatment: For disease caused by exogenous therapy, the treatment is to stop the glucocorticoid via gradual withdrawal. Definitive treatment of tumor-related Cushing syndrome is surgical. Medical treatment options include adrenal enzyme inhibitors (eg, ketoconazole), agents reducing ACTH levels (cabergoline, pasireotide), antineoplastic agents for adrenocortical carcinoma (eg, mitotane), and glucocorticoid antagonists for the treatment of hyperglycemia (eg, mifepristone).

IX. THYROID FUNCTION AND DISEASE

A. Physiology (Figure 29.3): There are two forms of thyroid hormone, **T4 (levothyroxine)**, which contains four iodine atoms, and **T3 (triiodothyronine)**, which contains three iodine atoms. Both T4 and T3 are produced in the thyroid gland and are stored in the form of thyroglobulin. The production and release of thyroid hormone is controlled by **thyroid-stimulating hormone (TSH)** secreted by the pituitary gland. TSH stimulates the cleavage of thyroglobulin to release thyroid hormone and promotes the conversion of T4 to T3 before release into the bloodstream. TSH secretion is regulated by thyrotropin-releasing hormone (TRH), which is secreted by the hypothalamus. TRH and TSH secretion are under negative regulation by the thyroid hormone, thereby completing a feedback regulatory loop.

1. Thyroid hormone signaling mostly acts through receptors for T3, whereas T4 is essentially a prohormone. Approximately 10% of T3 is directly released by the thyroid, whereas 80% of T3 is produced in other tissues by

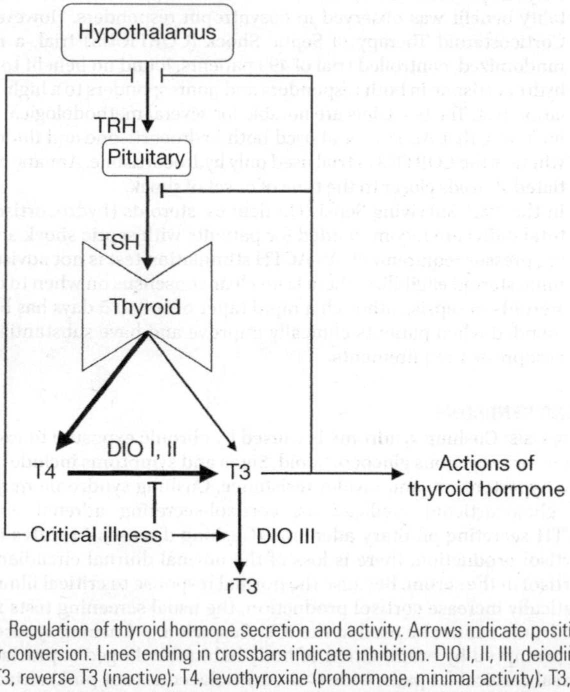

FIGURE 29.3 Regulation of thyroid hormone secretion and activity. Arrows indicate positive action, production, or conversion. Lines ending in crossbars indicate inhibition. DIO I, II, III, deiodinase types I, II, and III; rT3, reverse T3 (inactive); T4, levothyroxine (prohormone, minimal activity); T3, triiodothyronine (active thyroid hormone); TRH, thyrotropin-releasing hormone; TSH, thyroid-stimulating hormone.

conversion of T4 to T3 by deiodinase enzymes. Deiodinase activity is suppressed by conditions common to the ICU, including malnutrition, diabetes (insulin resistance or relative insulin deficiency), high levels of free fatty acids, inflammatory cytokines, illness in general, and drugs including β-blockers and amiodarone (see **Section X.A**). The production of active T3 is increased by high caloric intake and insulin.

B. Functions of Thyroid Hormone and Symptoms and Signs of Thyroid Dysfunction: Thyroid hormone is an important modulator of metabolic rate and protein synthesis and turnover. Thyroid hormone increases inotropy and chronotropy, whereas it reduces systemic vascular resistance. **Hyperthyroidism** is associated with tachycardia, systolic hypertension, widened pulse pressure, high-output heart failure, atrial fibrillation, and myocardial ischemia. **Hypothyroidism** is associated with bradycardia and hypertension and can precipitate congestive heart failure in those with underlying cardiac disease. Myopathy associated with thyroid dysfunction can cause inadequate ventilation. Poor ventilation can be especially problematic in hyperthyroidism, where oxygen consumption and CO_2 production are increased. Thyroid hormone promotes gut motility, leading to constipation in hypothyroidism and diarrhea and malabsorption in hyperthyroidism. Free water clearance is dependent on thyroid hormone, leading to hyponatremia in hypothyroidism. The metabolism of many medications and endogenous substances is regulated by thyroid hormone; thus, certain drugs (eg, propranolol, digoxin, warfarin) may need dosing adjustments in thyroid dysfunction. It is important to note that cortisol clearance is also promoted by thyroid hormone. Thus, treatment of hypothyroidism with thyroid hormone has been known to unmask coexisting adrenal insufficiency. Hypothyroidism is associated with accumulation of matrix glycosaminoglycans in many tissues, which can lead to coarse skin and hair, enlargement of the tongue, hoarseness, and nonpitting edema. Graves disease, the most common cause of hyperthyroidism, can also cause autoimmune infiltration of the fatty tissue of the orbit and autoimmune attack on the eyes, which can cause ocular inflammation and proptosis.

X. THYROID FUNCTION IN CRITICAL ILLNESS

A. Nonthyroidal Illness Syndrome (formerly sick euthyroid syndrome): TSH levels in patients who are hospitalized can be misleading, especially in patients with critical illness. In nonthyroidal illness syndrome, patients have **low T3** levels from the **inhibition of type 1 deiodinase** that converts T4 to T3. Low T3 is often accompanied by elevated reverse T3, normal T4, and normal TSH. However, in chronic critical illness, T4 and TSH levels often become low. The weight of evidence suggests that **treatment of the critically ill with nonthyroidal illness syndrome is not beneficial** and may in fact be harmful. It is theorized that relative hypothyroidism reduces catabolism and may be protective.

B. Lab Testing

1. **Thyroid testing in the intensive care unit:** Because nonthyroidal illness syndrome is so common in critical illness, **thyroid studies should not be sent unless there is a strong suspicion of preexisting hypothyroidism or hyperthyroidism requiring treatment**. If such suspicion exists, a reasonable starting point is to check TSH and free T4 level.
2. **Interpretation of a low thyroid-stimulating hormone:** A normal or low TSH is an expected component of critical illness. If the TSH is low and hyperthyroidism is suspected on clinical grounds, the **serum T3** may be helpful. Patients with nonthyroidal illness syndrome should have low or low-normal T3 values, whereas those with hyperthyroidism should have high or high-normal T3 values. A patient with an **undetectable TSH** using a modern

high-sensitivity assay is likely to have hyperthyroidism, and this diagnosis can be supported by an elevated or high-normal T3.

3. **Interpretation of an elevated thyroid-stimulating hormone:** An elevated TSH can be seen in patients recovering from nonthyroidal illness syndrome, although the TSH rarely rises to more than 20 mU/L. In a patient who is still critically ill, an elevated TSH is suggestive of primary hypothyroidism due to a defect in thyroid hormone synthesis or release by the thyroid gland. A diagnosis of hypothyroidism is supported by a TSH greater than 20 mU/L accompanied by low free T4. In this scenario, treatment with levothyroxine is appropriate.
4. **Interpretation of free T4 levels:** T4 is highly bound by serum proteins, primarily by thyroid-binding globulin, but also transthyretin, albumin, and lipoproteins. A very small fraction of T4 is unbound. Reduction of binding proteins, which is common in critical illness, will reduce T4 binding and total T4 levels. In critical illness, an elevated free T4 supports a diagnosis of hyperthyroidism. A low free T4 level associated with TSH elevation greater than 10 mU/L can support a diagnosis of hypothyroidism.

C. Treatment of Thyroid Dysfunction in Patients in the Intensive Care Unit

1. **Treatment of hypothyroidism:** Although nonthyroidal illness syndrome is probably a state of relative hypothyroidism, **treatment with thyroid hormone does not improve outcomes in patients with critical illness** or in patients post surgery. Patients with preexisting hypothyroidism should not have their usual dose of thyroid hormone adjusted. Treatment of newly diagnosed hypothyroidism should be with synthetic T4 (levothyroxine), and initial dosing should be weight based. A replacement dose of T4 by the enteral route is approximately 1.6 μg/kg daily, although individual patients may require substantially more or less. A somewhat lower initial dose is appropriate for patients who are older and frail or if there is a concern for precipitating cardiac ischemia or atrial fibrillation. Before levothyroxine administration, enteral feeds should be paused until there is minimal gastric residue and should not be started for 30 minutes afterward. Levothyroxine should also be given separately from all other medications. In cases where this is not practical, IV administration is preferred. IV levothyroxine should be dose reduced by 20% to account for improved bioavailability. Because it takes at least 6 weeks after a change in dose for the T4 and TSH to reach a new equilibrium, dosage changes must be made with caution. Treatment of hypothyroidism with synthetic T3 (liothyronine) is generally not indicated except in cases of myxedema coma.
2. **Treatment of hyperthyroidism:** Patients who are critically ill undergoing treatment for hyperthyroidism should be monitored by an endocrinologist because antithyroid medications can have significant toxicities and large iodine loads from medications (such as amiodarone and iodinated contrast) can alter thyroid homeostasis. If a new diagnosis of hyperthyroidism is suspected, endocrine consultation should be obtained to confirm the diagnosis and to monitor treatment. Thyroid hormone action **increases the number of cardiac and peripheral adrenergic receptors**, explaining many of the symptoms of hyperthyroidism. Therapy for hyperthyroidism typically includes β-blockade. **Propranolol** (nonselective β-blocker, IV/po), **esmolol** (β-1 selective, IV infusion), and **metoprolol** (β-1 selective, IV/po) are commonly prescribed to inhibit T4 to T3 conversion by deiodinase. A typical course of therapy also includes treatment with thionamide antithyroid drugs such as **methimazole** (more potent) and **propylthiouracil** (less potent). These drugs **block new production of thyroid hormone but do not prevent release of thyroid hormone** that has already been synthesized, so thionamide drugs have little immediate effect on their own. However, once the thionamide has blocked new thyroid hormone synthesis, large doses of **iodine may be given to block release of T3 and T4** from the thyroid.

XI. SPECIAL CONSIDERATIONS IN THYROID DISORDERS

A. Myxedema Coma

1. **Clinical syndrome:** Myxedema coma is a medical emergency associated with high mortality. Owing to long-standing severe hypothyroidism, patients with myxedema coma present with altered mental status (usually lethargy but occasionally psychosis; actual coma is rare), hypothermia, bradycardia, hypotension, hypoventilation, hyponatremia (usually syndrome of inappropriate antidiuretic hormone [SIADH]), and hypoglycemia. **Myxedema coma can occur acutely** in persons with preexisting untreated or inadequately treated hypothyroidism who are exposed to the stress of an illness, cold ambient temperatures, dehydration, or sedative drugs. Owing to the loss of thermoregulation, patients can be profoundly hypothermic with temperatures less than 86 °F (30 °C). Myxedema coma will not occur quickly after **discontinuation of thyroid hormone** even in a patient with severe hypothyroidism because the **half-life of thyroid hormone is long** (~1 week).
2. **Diagnosis and treatment:** The severity of hypothyroidism required to produce this clinical syndrome is extreme, so high levels of TSH are to be expected. Owing to a mortality rate as high as 60%, myxedema coma should be immediately treated without waiting for laboratory testing if suspicion is high. Treatment of the precipitating illness is essential. Supportive care including rewarming, ventilatory support, hemodynamic support, and electrolyte correction are paramount. Passive warming should be immediately initiated, whereas active rewarming should be avoided because it could precipitate rapid vasodilation and circulatory collapse. Myxedema coma can be associated with adrenal insufficiency. **Administration of thyroid hormone** to a patient with adrenal insufficiency can acutely **precipitate an adrenal crisis.** Therefore, a cosyntropin test should be performed at the time thyroid tests are obtained and **stress-dose glucocorticoid therapy** must be started before initiation of thyroid hormone therapy. Glucocorticoids can be discontinued if the cosyntropin stimulation test demonstrates sufficient adrenal reserve. The appropriate treatment for myxedema coma is controversial, with different authorities preferring T4 alone versus T4 in combination with T3.

B. Thyroid Storm

1. **Clinical syndrome:** Thyroid storm is a life-threatening presentation of severe hyperthyroidism with exaggerated symptoms and signs, usually occurring as an acute exacerbation of preexisting hyperthyroidism. Because thyroid hormone concentrations are similar to those observed in uncomplicated thyrotoxicosis, the diagnosis of thyroid storm is made clinically. TSH is often undetectable. Signs and symptoms include fever, tachycardia, mental status changes, delirium, tremor, congestive heart failure, nausea, diarrhea, sweating, dehydration, and abdominal pain. Although thyroid surgery was previously a more common trigger for thyroid storm, it is now less common because of routine treatment of hyperthyroidism. Triggers include infection, stress, and trauma.
2. **Treatment** consists of supportive therapy and medications targeted specifically at the excessive action, production, and release of thyroid hormone. Initial therapy should include an **IV β-blocker**, such as esmolol or propranolol, titrated to control tachycardia. Stress-dose **glucocorticoids** (eg, 100 mg hydrocortisone IV every 8 hours) are administered to reduce T4 to T3 conversion by deiodinase and to ensure thyroid storm is not complicated by adrenal insufficiency due to rapid glucocorticoid metabolism. Thionamide medications, such as propylthiouracil or methimazole, are used to reduce the production of thyroid hormone. Iodides, although useful, should not be given first because they may increase the synthesis of new

thyroid hormones. Cholestyramine (4 g PO QID) can be considered to reduce thyroid hormone levels by interrupting the enterohepatic circulation. Supportive care includes hyperpyrexia management, fluid resuscitation, rate control of atrial fibrillation, and the diagnosis and treatment of any precipitating conditions.

XII. REGULATION OF CALCIUM HOMEOSTASIS

A. Calcium Uptake From the Gut and Secretion by the Kidney: Calcium is essential for many functions, including neural transmission, intracellular signaling, blood coagulation, skeletal structure, and myocardial contractility. Under ordinary circumstances, the intake and excretion of calcium are balanced. From a typical daily intake of 1000 mg, there may be 200 mg net absorption from the gut and a similar amount excreted in the urine. Calcium is filtered by the glomerulus and must be actively reabsorbed. **Parathyroid hormone (PTH)** promotes the absorption of calcium and phosphate from the gut and promotes the liberation of calcium and phosphate from bone. In addition to direct effects on the gut, PTH promotes the activation of vitamin D to **1,25-dihydroxyvitamin D**, which also promotes calcium and phosphorus absorption from the gut. In the kidney, PTH promotes calcium reabsorption and phosphate excretion. The net effect of PTH is to raise the serum calcium and reduce serum phosphorus. Calcitonin opposes the action of PTH and inhibits bone and renal resorption of calcium. Most **calcium reabsorption** by the kidney occurs paracellularly in the proximal tubule, following shifts of sodium and water. Thus, calcium reabsorption is promoted in sodium-avid states (eg, dehydration) and calcium excretion is promoted by saline infusion.

B. Calcium Equilibrium Between the Blood and Bone: Almost all of the body's calcium is found along with phosphorus in hydroxyapatite crystals within the bone. If bone reabsorption is increased out of proportion of bone mineralization, quite large amounts of calcium can be released into the blood. Equilibrium between the blood and the bone is primarily regulated by PTH. A small fraction (~1%) of the total body calcium is found within cells and in the extracellular fluid. Approximately half of the serum calcium concentration is protein bound (mostly to albumin) while the other half is ionized.

C. Measurement of Serum Calcium: Approximately 50% of serum calcium is found as free, ionized calcium, approximately 40% is bound (mostly to albumin), and 10% is complexed with anions. In patients who are hypoalbuminemic, the total serum calcium can be corrected for the serum albumin level (corrected Ca^{2+} = total $Ca^{2+} + 0.8 \times$ [normal albumin − patient albumin]). The resulting "corrected calcium" can be interpreted against the normal total calcium reference range (8.8-10.3 mg/dL), but this correction is not entirely reliable. In the critically ill, it is often preferable to measure the ionized calcium, although laboratory testing for ionized calcium remains comparatively expensive.

D. Causes of Hypercalcemia

1. **Primary hyperparathyroidism:** This syndrome is typically caused by **benign parathyroid tumors.** It is the most common cause of hypercalcemia in the outpatient setting, typically occurring in the third to fifth decades of life. The sensitivity of parathyroid tumors to ambient calcium levels is reduced so that higher levels of calcium are required to fully suppress PTH production. A new equilibrium is reached in which serum calcium is elevated, yet PTH is not fully suppressed. **PTH levels are not usually elevated, but are not appropriately suppressed to undetectable levels** in the setting of elevated calcium levels.
2. **Secondary hyperparathyroidism** (renal osteodystrophy): Renal insufficiency reduces the ability to excrete phosphorus. **Elevated phosphorus**, similar to low calcium, is a **stimulus for PTH secretion.** The elevation of calcium may be exacerbated by administration of calcium-containing phosphate binders

(eg, calcium citrate). PTH is usually not elevated but is inappropriately high ("normal") in the setting of hypercalcemia.

3. **Tertiary hyperparathyroidism:** Long-standing secondary hyperparathyroidism may lead to a degree of **parathyroid autonomy** from calcium feedback regulation. Once this occurs, PTH production is not appropriately suppressed even if phosphate levels are controlled by dialysis or phosphate binders. The consequence is inappropriately high PTH levels in the setting of hypercalcemia.
4. **Hypercalcemia of malignancy:** This syndrome may develop in the setting of large lytic lesions of bone but is more commonly associated with **PTH-related protein (PTHrP)** from tumors, which circulates systemically and acts similarly to PTH. PTHrP is classically associated with multiple myeloma, breast cancer, lung cancer, and squamous cell carcinoma but may be found with tumors of many types. PTH production from the parathyroid glands is suppressed by the elevated calcium and PTH is typically undetectable.
5. **Paget disease:** Localized patches of increased bone resorption and disorganized reformation are the hallmark of Paget disease. Paget disease does not typically cause hypercalcemia because bone resorption is balanced by bone formation. However, immobilization can lead to the abrupt development of hypercalcemia. Paget disease is present in up to 3% of individuals older than 50 years.
6. **Drugs and ingestions:** Excess ingestion of vitamin D can cause hypercalcemia. Other drugs that may cause hypercalcemia include vitamin A (increased bone turnover), lithium (increasing PTH secretion), theophylline (increased bone turnover), and thiazide diuretics (reduced calcium excretion).
7. **Endocrinopathies:** Non-parathyroid endocrinopathies that may cause hypercalcemia include hyperthyroidism (increased bone turnover), adrenal insufficiency (decreased calcium excretion), and pheochromocytoma (PTHrP secretion).

XIII. DIAGNOSIS AND TREATMENT OF HYPERCALCEMIA

A. Diagnosis

1. **Signs and symptoms of severe hypercalcemia** include polyuria, abdominal pain, nausea, vomiting, constipation, headache, altered mental status, lethargy, weakness, and depression. Hyporeflexia, hypertension, and bradycardia may occur. In the critical care setting, hypercalcemia is primarily diagnosed by laboratory studies.
2. **Parathyroid hormone–dependent hypercalcemia:** Serum PTH is not usually elevated even when PTH is the cause of hypercalcemia. Rather, PTH is "inappropriately normal" in the setting of hypercalcemia. A frankly elevated PTH may also be found, but extreme elevations of PTH are rare and suggest the diagnosis of parathyroid carcinoma. In the setting of hypercalcemia, any detectable PTH suggests hyperparathyroidism as the cause. Primary hyperparathyroidism can be distinguished from secondary and tertiary hyperparathyroidism by renal function studies and history.
3. **Parathyroid hormone–independent hypercalcemia:** If PTH is undetectable, past medical history and medication history will provide important clues. Additional laboratory workup should include PTHrP (for hypercalcemia of malignancy), 25-hydroxyvitamin D (if ingestion is suspected), 1,25-dihydroxyvitamin D (for granulomatous disease), and thyroid studies (TSH, free T4, T3). Alkaline phosphatase is usually strikingly elevated in Paget disease and less so in other causes of increased bone turnover.

B. Treatment

1. **Promotion of renal calcium excretion:** Calcium is freely filtered into the urine and most of it is actively reabsorbed along with sodium. Delivery of sodium

in the form of **saline hydration** (eg, 200 mL/h) can be very effective in lowering serum calcium in patients who are volume depleted. The goal in most cases should be to adequately hydrate the patient, although saline therapy may be limited by development of volume overload and edema. In such cases, a loop diuretic such as furosemide may be required and may further promote calcium excretion. Loop diuretics should not be used without saline treatment because dehydration may worsen hypercalcemia. The combination of saline and furosemide for **forced diuresis has fallen out of favor** as the first-line therapy for hypercalcemia. In the setting of renal failure, renal replacement therapy with dialysis or continuous hemofiltration with a low calcium dialysate is usually necessary to treat hypercalcemia. **Dialysis** may also be used for emergency treatment of severe hypercalcemia in patients with normal or only modestly impaired renal function.

2. **Inhibiting calcium release from bone: Calcitonin** inhibits bone resorption as well as renal calcium resorption. Treatment with calcitonin, at 4 to 8 U/kg SC every 6 hours, can be very effective in **rapidly lowering serum calcium**, often within hours. The combination of calcitonin and saline hydration is probably the most appropriate **first-line therapy** for hypercalcemia. **Tachyphylaxis** to the effects of calcitonin usually occurs after a few days of treatment, so it is usually used in the acute phase of treatment only. Rebound hypercalcemia can occur upon development of tachyphylaxis when calcitonin is the sole therapy. Either the underlying cause should be treated or **bisphosphonates** should be given concurrently with calcitonin and saline hydration. Bisphosphonates are deposited in the mineral matrix of bone and inhibit the release of calcium from bone. Pamidronate and zoledronic acid can be administered IV. **Pamidronate is given at 60 to 90 mg IV over 2 to 4 hours, zoledronic acid at 4 mg IV over 30 minutes.** The peak effect of both drugs occurs after 48 to 72 hours. These drugs are indicated for treatment of **hypercalcemia of malignancy** but should be used cautiously in other settings because their effects may last for years. They inhibit bone loss in high-turnover states but also delay bone formation when conditions would otherwise favor it. Bisphosphonates may cause **hypocalcemia** in certain clinical situations, such as patients with **vitamin D deficiency.** These drugs should be used when the ultimate cause of hypercalcemia cannot be reversed in the short-to-medium term (malignancy) or when they directly address the pathophysiology of hypercalcemia (Paget disease of bone). Bisphosphonates are relatively contraindicated in renal failure. Glucocorticoids may also provide benefit in combination with bisphosphonates for hypercalcemia of malignancy due to osteolytic lesions.
3. **Inhibition of parathyroid hormone and vitamin D production: Cinacalcet** is a drug that increases the sensitivity of the **calcium-sensing receptor**, found on parathyroid cells, to extracellular calcium. It is useful in PTH-dependent hypercalcemia by decreasing PTH secretion and serum calcium levels. Cinacalcet is approved for the treatment of secondary hyperparathyroidism and parathyroid carcinoma. It is also clinically used for the treatment of primary hyperparathyroidism. It has no role in the treatment of PTH-independent hypercalcemia. **Glucocorticoids** are primarily used to treat hypercalcemia due to granulomatous disease but may obscure a pathologic diagnosis if used before a biopsy.

XIV. CARCINOID SYNDROME

A. Carcinoid Tumor Physiology: Carcinoid tumors are slowly growing neoplasms most frequently found in the **GI tract (70%)** and in the **bronchi (20%)**. Because carcinoid tumors originate from neuroendocrine cells, they can secrete a wide variety of products, including serotonin, histamine, tachykinins, kallikrein, and prostaglandins. Less common products include norepinephrine, dopamine, gastrin, glucagon, ACTH, and growth hormone. Because the liver inactivates most of the products of carcinoid tumors, most GI tumors do not cause symptoms until they metastasize to the liver. Primary lung tumors can cause symptoms without metastasis. High levels of serotonin may lead to cardiac valvular abnormalities, typically involving fibrous thickening of the right heart valves and leading most commonly to tricuspid regurgitation and/or pulmonic stenosis or regurgitation. Almost all carcinoid tumors take up and metabolize tryptophan, resulting in hypoproteinemia due to the depletion of this essential amino acid. In most cases, carcinoid tumors convert tryptophan to **serotonin**, which is then metabolized to 5-hydroxyindoleacetic acid (5-HIAA). 5-HIAA can be measured in the blood and urine to diagnose carcinoid syndrome.

B. Symptoms of carcinoid syndrome: Secretory diarrhea, flushing, and itching are the most common manifestations of excess serotonin, histamine, and kinins. The diarrhea can be explosive and result in substantial fluid loss and malabsorption. Peripheral vasodilation may lead to hypotension and tachycardia, although hypertensive episodes have been observed. Episodes are usually spontaneous and last less than 30 minutes. Flushing may be associated with bronchospasm, particularly when associated with bronchial carcinoids. In nonfunctional tumors, patients do not develop the hormonal effects, but rather present with abdominal pain, GI obstruction, or bleeding.

C. Diagnosis: In patients with carcinoid syndrome, typical urinary levels of 5-HIAA are more than 10-fold above the upper limit of normal. Serotonin levels greater than 25 mg/24 h are considered diagnostic for carcinoid, although the sensitivity is only 80%. Many drugs and foods can give falsely elevated levels of 5-HIAA including acetaminophen, phenobarbital, and ephedrine. Bronchial and gastric carcinoids may have normal urinary 5-HIAA levels even in the absence of interfering substances. In such cases, blood measurements of chromogranin A and serotonin may be helpful. In the ICU, the provocation of paradoxical flushing and hypotension by epinephrine should prompt consideration of carcinoid syndrome. Multiple imaging modalities, including endoscopy, ultrasound, CT, MRI, and barium radiography, can be used to locate the tumor. Radiolabeled somatostatin analog scintigraphy is the gold standard for location confirmation. Echocardiography is useful if cardiac lesions are suspected.

D. Treatment: Definitive treatment of carcinoid syndrome involves surgical removal of the tumor. However, most patients who develop the classic syndrome have gut carcinoids with metastasis to the liver, so definitive surgical management is not possible. **Somatostatin** is a GI peptide that can reduce serotonin release. **Octreotide** is a somatostatin analog used to control symptoms such as flushing and diarrhea associated with carcinoid syndrome, prevent progression of carcinoid cardiac valvular disease, and prevent carcinoid crisis during anesthesia. Levels of urinary 5-HIAA can be followed up to monitor response to treatment. Octreotide may be administered in conjunction with **telotristat**, a tryptophan hydroxylase inhibitor reducing serotonin levels effective in reducing the frequency of bowel movements. The treatment of hypotension in carcinoid crisis is unusual because **catecholamines can exacerbate secretion** and further lower blood pressure (BP). Hypotension should be treated with IV octreotide (IV bolus of 300 µg followed by an infusion of up to 150 µg/h) and fluid resuscitation. Bronchospasm can be treated with albuterol.

XV. PHEOCHROMOCYTOMA AND PARAGANGLIOMA

A. Diagnosis: These are tumors of neural crest origin that secrete catecholamines (norepinephrine, epinephrine, and/or dopamine) in an unpredictable manner. They are found arising from the adrenal medulla or from the sympathetic ganglia along the aorta up to the carotid bifurcation. Approximately 5% of all incidentally discovered adrenal masses are pheochromocytomas. The classic presentation is of episodic palpitations, headache, and pallor associated with **hypertension**. However, sustained hypertension is also common. Testing typically includes urinary and plasma-fractionated metanephrines and catecholamines. However, these tests are best performed in the outpatient setting because reference ranges are poorly defined in the population in the ICU. In patients for whom biochemical testing is not appropriate, MRI and specialized tests such as meta-iodobenzylguanidine (MIBG) scintiscanning may be used to support the diagnosis.

B. Treatment: All patients with catecholamine-secreting tumors require **preparation for surgery**. The traditional regimen includes loading with **phenoxybenzamine**, an irreversible α-blocker, followed by β-blockade for arrhythmia management. **Doxazosin** is a shorter acting reversible option for α-blockade that has been increasingly used with favorable results. It is important not to initiate β-blockade before α-blockade to avoid an uncontrolled α-adrenergic response resulting in hypertensive crisis. Pheochromocytomas are often associated with tonic vasoconstriction and volume contraction; thus, despite being hypertensive, patients may be hypovolemic. Optimal blockade occurs when the patient has nasal congestion, orthostatic hypotension (but BP no less than 80/45), an electrocardiogram (ECG) free of ST changes, and no more than one premature ventricular contraction (PVC) every 5 minutes. In the operating room, vigilance is essential because extreme hemodynamic lability is expected with tumor manipulation.

C. Postoperative Management of Pheochromocytoma: Patients can be either hypertensive or hypotensive following resection. If residual tumor exists, catecholamine levels may remain elevated and require antihypertensive treatment. However, patients can also be hypotensive because of the sudden decrease in catecholamines and ongoing adrenergic blockade. In this scenario, vasopressors and IV fluids may be needed to maintain hemodynamics and phenoxybenzamine can be discontinued. Because hypoglycemia is known to complicate the immediate postoperative period, glucose monitoring should occur at regular intervals during the first postoperative day.

Selected Readings

Annane D, Bellissant E, Bollaert PE, et al. Corticosteroids for treating sepsis in children and adults. *Cochrane Database Syst Rev*. 2019;12:CD002243.

Annane D, Sébille V, Charpentier C, et al. Effect of treatment with low doses of hydrocortisone and fludrocortisone on mortality in patients with septic shock. *JAMA*. 2002;288(7):862-871.

Body J-J, Bouillon R. Emergencies of calcium homeostasis. *Rev Endocr Metab Disord*. 2003;4(2):167-175.

Devos P, Preiser J, Melot C. Impact of tight glucose control by intensive insulin therapy on ICU mortality and the rate of hypoglycaemia: final results of the Glucontrol study. *Intensive Care Med*. 2007;33:S189.

Hamrahian AH, Oseni TS, Arafah BM. Measurements of serum free cortisol in critically ill patients. *N Engl J Med*. 2004;350:1629-1638.

Ito T, Lee L, Jensen RT. Carcinoid-syndrome: recent advances, current status and controversies. *Curr Opin Endocrinol Diabetes Obes*. 2018;25(1):22-35.

Karslioglu French E, Donihi AC, Korytkowski MT. Diabetic ketoacidosis and hyperosmolar hyperglycemic syndrome: review of acute decompensated diabetes in adult patients. *BMJ*. 2019;365:l1114.

Krinsley JS, Grover A. Severe hypoglycemia in critically ill patients: risk factors and outcomes. *Crit Care Med*. 2007;35:2262-2267.

Kwaku MP, Burman KD. Myxedema coma. *J Intensive Care Med*. 2007;22:224-231.

Mancuso K, Kaye AD, Boudreaux JP. Carcinoid syndrome and perioperative anesthetic considerations. *J Clin Anesth*. 2011;23:329-341.

Naranjo J, Dodd S, Martin YN. Perioperative management of pheochromocytoma. *J Cardiothorac Vasc Anesth*. 2017;31(4):1427-1439.

NICE-SUGAR Study Investigators. Intensive versus conventional glucose control in critically ill patients. *N Engl J Med.* 2009;360:1283-1297.

Rhodes A, Evans LE, Alhazzani W, et al. Surviving sepsis campaign: international guidelines for management of sepsis and septic shock: 2016. *Intensive Care Med.* 2017;43(3):304-377.

Schimmer BP, Funder JW. ACTH, Adrenal steroids, and pharmacology of the adrenal cortex. In: Brunton LL, Chabner BA, Knollmann BC, eds. *Goodman & Gilman's: The Pharmacological Basis of Therapeutics.* 12th ed. McGraw-Hill Education; 2011.

Siraux V, De Backer D, Yalavatti G, et al. Relative adrenal insufficiency in patients with septic shock: comparison of low-dose and conventional corticotropin tests. *Critical Care Med.* 2005:33:2479-2486.

Van den Berghe G. On the neuroendocrinopathy of critical illness. Perspectives for feeding and novel treatments. *Am J Respir Crit Care Med.* 2016;194(11):1337-1348.

Van den Berghe G, Wilmer A, Hermans G, et al. Intensive insulin therapy in the medical ICU. *N Engl J Med.* 2006;354:449-461.

Ylli D, Klubo-Gwiezdzinska J, Wartofsky L. Thyroid emergencies. *Pol Arch Intern Med.* 2019;129(7-8):526-534.

Young WF Jr. Adrenal causes of hypertension: pheochromocytoma and primary aldosteronism. *Rev Endocr Metab Disord.* 2007;8:309-320.

30 Acute Weakness

Kristin Parlman and Karen Waak

There is a myriad of causes that can lead to acute weakness in a patient in the intensive care unit (ICU). These include diseases affecting the central nervous system (CNS), the peripheral nervous system (PNS), the neuromuscular junction (NMJ), and the muscles (myopathic disorders). Other etiologic causes include the effects of drugs/medication and injuries. A patient may have acute onset weakness that necessitates admission to the ICU or develop weakness over the course of the critical illness. A thorough history and physical exam are critical in identifying the etiology of weakness, accompanied by relevant diagnostic studies such as computed tomography, lumbar puncture, electrophysiologic studies, and complete laboratory assessment. Physical exam should include evaluation for upper and lower motor neuron signs of impairment, which can be helpful in directing the clinician toward a CNS or PNS problem. An exhaustive review of causes for acute weakness is beyond the scope of this chapter, with selected conditions described subsequently.

I. CNS CAUSES

A. Stroke

Patients being treated in an ICU can present with an acute onset of weakness caused by an ischemic or hemorrhagic stroke. An acute focal change in neurologic status, such as facial droop, arm and/or leg weakness, and speech difficulties, ought to be recognized as a potential stroke. A noncontrast head CT should be performed as soon as possible to assess the situation (eg, ischemic stroke vs hemorrhage) and determine the need for additional imaging and specific interventions (eg, intravenous tPA, intra-arterial tPA, mechanical recanalization, and external ventricular drain).

B. Infection

Infections (including meningitis and meningoencephalitis) and abscesses of the CNS are other causes that could lead to acute weakness in patient who is in ICU. Although multiple clinical manifestations frequently accompany such an infection, including confusion, high fever, and/or seizure, weakness may be one of the presenting signs. For example, patients with herpes simplex virus encephalitis can present with focal neurologic deficits including hemiparesis, in addition to altered mental status. A small percentage of patients with West Nile virus develop rapidly progressive weakness, similar to poliomyelitis, in the context of destruction to the anterior horn cells of the spinal cord. Careful evaluation of the serum lab work, cerebrospinal fluid (CSF) studies, and brain imaging is required to reach a diagnosis. Treatment will be goal directed (eg, antibiotics, antiviral meds, surgical treatment for abscesses).

C. Osmotic Demyelination Syndrome (Formally Called Central Pontine Myelinolysis)

Symptoms of progressive tetraparesis along with dysarthria, dysphagia, weakness of respiratory muscles, and decreased level of consciousness, presenting in the setting of a recent rapid serum sodium correction, should prompt the clinician to think of osmotic demyelination syndrome (ODS). Symptoms typically present 2 to 6 days after an overly rapid correction of serum sodium. An overly rapid serum sodium correction is not likely to occur in patients experiencing severe hyponatremia for a few hours but demonstrates an increasingly higher incidence when it has been present for more than 2 to 3 days. Although the exact mechanism of ODS is unclear, the natural process by which the brain adapts to hyponatremia in the early stages to prevent cerebral edema makes the brain much more susceptible to a decrease in brain volume and demyelination in prolonged hyponatremia during an overly rapid serum sodium correction. Demyelination primarily occurs in the pons, but extrapontine demyelination could occur in locations such as the cerebellum, basal ganglia, corpus callosum, and internal capsule. MRI would confirm the diagnosis. Supportive therapy is the primary approach to treatment, with other interventions such as early relowering of sodium still being studied.

II. PNS CAUSES

A variety of conditions impacting the PNS can lead to weakness, with the impact ranging from mild and isolated to broad and severe. Many acquired polyneuropathies such as those resulting from vascular disease, diabetes, or alcohol use occur over time and thus do not typically present as an acute loss of strength. However, it is important to consider such conditions in weak patient who is in ICU who cannot provide a functional history. Infections, toxins, endocrine disorders, and vitamin B_{12} deficiency can also lead to polyneuropathy.

A. Guillain-Barré Syndrome: Guillain-Barré syndrome (GBS) describes a syndrome of acute, immune-mediated, inflammatory polyneuropathies that consist of several different forms. GBS is typically preceded by an infection or illness and is characterized by widespread, patchy areas of peripheral nerve demyelination that translates into weakness and paralysis. Acute inflammatory demyelinating polyneuropathy (AIDP) is interchangeably used with GBS. Variant forms of GBS including Miller Fisher syndrome (MFS), acute motor axonal neuropathy, and acute sensorimotor axonal neuropathy are less frequently seen in the United States. Clinical presentation includes migrating, symmetrical paralysis, typically starting in the legs with absent or diminished deep tendon reflexes. Patients with MFS present with ophthalmoplegia, ataxia, and areflexia. Paresthesias and neuropathic pain are common. Symptoms usually progress over a 2- to 3-week period before reaching a nadir, followed by subsequent improvement. Degree of weakness can vary from mild to severe with complete paralysis. Approximately 25% to 30% of patients will have sufficient involvement of the respiratory muscles to require mechanical ventilation. Autonomic dysfunction including dysrhythmias, hypotension, and hypertension is common and may be fatal; thus, close monitoring is warranted.

1. Diagnosis is based on clinical exam and confirmed with an analysis of CSF and electrophysiology studies. Treatment in the acute phase includes supportive care with particular attention to the respiratory and cardiovascular systems. Daily bedside pulmonary function tests such as measurements of negative inspiratory force (NIF) may be monitored in those patients at risk for respiratory decline. Response to intravenous vasoactive drugs is often exaggerated and thus should be used with caution. Rehabilitation in the acute phase includes a focus on preventing secondary complications and initiating gentle active exercises, titrating to patient response. More intense rehabilitation is often indicated after the acute phase to restore function. Specific therapies to treat GBS include plasma exchange and IV immunoglobulin (IVIG); treatment with either plasma exchange or IVIG is associated with improved recovery and expedited time to independent ambulation. Remyelination and functional recovery occur over a period of weeks to months. Approximately 80% of patients return to independent ambulation by 6 months; 5% to 10% of patients have delayed and/or incomplete recovery. Prediction models such as the Modified Erasmus GBS Outcome Score can be used to predict ambulation using data collected on

admission or at 7 days (including strength scores, age, and ± preceding diarrhea). Relapses occur in approximately 7% of patients and are generally treated with the initial regimen. Deterioration after initial improvement and stabilization, or prolongation of symptoms beyond 8 weeks may indicate the presence of chronic inflammatory demyelinating polyneuropathy (CIDP).

B. Critical Illness Polyneuropathy

Critical illness polyneuropathy (CIP) is a sensorimotor neuropathy characterized by distal axonal degeneration. CIP frequently coexists with critical illness myopathy (CIM; see later in the chapter). Clinically, these two conditions can be difficult to distinguish, although doing so may inform functional prognosis. The alternative term "ICU-acquired weakness" (ICU-AW) is used extensively in the literature to describe more broadly the weakness of extremities and respiratory muscles detected on the clinical exam, which cannot be explained by causes other than the presence of critical illness. ICU-AW may be attributed to CIP, CIM, disuse atrophy, or a combination of all three. ICU-AW is common in critical illness, affecting 25% to 70% of patients requiring mechanical ventilation greater than or equal to 7 days, with increasing incidence in those with sepsis and multi-organ failure. The specific etiology of CIP is multifactorial, with inflammation, impaired perfusion, and altered permeability all potentially contributing. Typically, CIP becomes apparent as the patient regains arousal and is noted to have a profound weakness with an inability to wean from the ventilator. It is characterized by flaccid, usually symmetrical weakness, diminished sensation, and reduced or absent deep tendon reflexes. Lower extremities may be more affected than upper extremities, and distal extremities often more than proximal. Cranial nerves are frequently spared; therefore, it is important to include an assessment of facial movements when determining command-following ability in patients who are not moving their extremities. Muscle atrophy will be present.

1. Formal diagnosis of CIP requires electrophysiology testing: Nerve conduction studies (NCS) will show evidence of sensorimotor *axonal* neuropathy including the decreased amplitude of compound motor and sensory action potentials, with the absence of a conduction block. Needle electromyography (EMG) will demonstrate resting fibrillation potentials. In CIP, electrodiagnostic studies will not show evidence of demyelination.
2. The less formal diagnosis of ICU-AW can be made via bedside manual muscle testing of 12 specific muscle groups in cooperative patients. Patients who demonstrate global weakness with a Medical Research Council strength sum score of less than 48 out of 60 can be identified as having "ICU-AW" (<36/60 indicating more severe impairment), once other causes for weakness are ruled out (see Table 30.1). Furthermore, dominant handgrip strength via dynamometry of less than 11 kg for males and less than 7 kg for females is also suggestive of a diagnosis of ICU-AW. Electrophysiology studies should be considered in cases where a patient cannot be accurately examined at the bedside and/or where weakness does not show improvement with time despite rehabilitation efforts.
3. Strategies to prevent or minimize the development of ICU-acquired weakness should be incorporated into clinical practice as feasible. Although robust, cause-effect evidence is limited, associations have been found among several critical care variables and ICU-AW and CIP. In particular, immobility contributes directly to muscle atrophy, and thus it is key to integrate exercise and mobilization into patient care as early as clinically appropriate. Early mobility pathways or algorithms can be helpful in facilitating safe, targeted, incremental activity in critically ill patients. Regular screening for participation in spontaneous awakening trials is encouraged in order to

TABLE 30.1 Manual Muscle Testing Screen for ICU-Acquired Weakness in Cooperative Patients

	Right	Left
Abduction of the shoulder		
Flexion of the elbow		
Extension of the wrist		
Flexion of the hip		
Extension of the knee		
Dorsal flexion of the foot		

Sum score (max 60): Test the six muscle groups listed above, bilaterally in sufficiently alert and attentive patients. Grade each muscle on a score of 0-5. All grades can be combined for a "sum score" out of 60. Sum scores ≤48 may be associated with ICU-acquired weakness. MRC strength grading scale: 0, no muscular contraction; 1, trace or flicker of contraction; 2, active movement with gravity eliminated; 3, active movement against gravity; 4, active movement against gravity and some resistance; 5, active movement against gravity and full resistance.

minimize oversedation, which in turn perpetuates immobilization. Similarly, when clinically acceptable, it is important to enable spontaneous breathing to facilitate diaphragm activation in order to minimize diaphragmatic atrophy. More well-designed, prospective studies investigating the specific effects of early exercise and mobility on ICU-AW are needed.

a. Prevention efforts may also include aggressive management of sepsis to minimize systemic inflammation and oxidative stress, as these conditions appear linked to ICU-AW and CIP. Consider early nutrition when appropriate to help mediate muscle catabolism, although studies specifically evaluating the impact of nutrition regimen and ICU-AW are needed. There is some evidence to show that intensive insulin therapy reduces the incidence of CIP; however, because other potential risks exist with this practice, it cannot be broadly recommended. The association between the use of neuromuscular blocking agents (NMBAs) and the development of ICU-AW is not clear-cut. Although NMBAs have an apparent role in the management of select conditions (eg, severe ARDS), it is probably wise to avoid prolonged use when possible.

4. Once present, treatment of ICU-AW and CIP ought to include the aforementioned considerations, as well as good supportive care and rehabilitation. Prognosis for recovery with CIP is variable and can be prolonged, given axonal involvement. CIP is associated with increased length of stay, time on the ventilator, mortality, and reduced functional outcomes. Although most patients gradually recover over weeks to months, evidence suggests that a sizable portion of patients with severe involvement are not fully recovered at 1 year.

C. Isolated Peripheral Nerve Injury

Patients who present with isolated, focal, peripheral weakness should be evaluated for a local injury to a peripheral nerve. Nerves can be injured through a variety of mechanisms including ischemia or disruption of fibers through stretch injury or laceration. Patients will demonstrate weakness and sensory impairment (if the impacted nerve is responsible for both) in the regions supplied by the nerve and may have diminished associated deep tendon reflex. Degree of deficit may vary from mild weakness to full paralysis of the muscle(s) innervated by the nerve, depending on the extent of the injury. For long nerves such as the sciatic, a detailed exam can help localize the area of injury along the nerve's path. Certain fractures are more commonly associated with concomitant nerve injuries and should be investigated accordingly. For example, radial nerve injuries are reported in up to 18% of patients with humeral shaft fractures; acetabular fractures have been associated with sciatic nerve injuries. Given the proximity of the femoral nerve to the femoral artery, patients who develop groin hematomas should be monitored for clinical signs of compression to the nerve. Patients experiencing prolonged immobility are at risk for direct compression to the fibular nerve near the fibular head, resulting in foot drop which may be unilateral or bilateral. Similarly, patients may experience nerve compression in the context of operative or procedural positioning (eg, lower extremity nerve injury has been noted to be 0.3%-1.8% in vaginal births). Consider NCS to characterize the injury, in addition to diagnostic studies to evaluate for causation. Interventions include treatment of underlying cause (eg, hematoma evacuation, revascularization, removal of peripheral compression), rehabilitation and compensatory bracing as indicated, and/or direct surgical repair.

III. NEUROMUSCULAR JUNCTION DISORDERS

There are different etiologies for neuromuscular junction disorders (NMJD) discussed in the literature whereby myasthenia gravis (MG), belonging to the autoimmune category, is the most common form. Other causes are congenital or toxic (eg, botulism).

A. Myasthenia Gravis

MG is a disease that interferes with the transmission of acetylcholine at the neuromuscular junction, leading to proximal muscle weakness and fatigue. In the majority of cases, it is caused by the binding of circulating autoantibodies to postsynaptic nicotinic Ach receptors. This in turn prevents acetylcholine, the neurotransmitter that is responsible for muscle contraction at the motor end plate, from connecting to its receptor. There is a generalized, an ocular, and a paraneoplastic variant of MG. The abovementioned autoantibodies can be found in about 80% of those with the generalized form of MG. In about 10% of patients with MG, a thymoma can be detected, which goes along with anti-titin antibodies.

1. The lead symptom of MG is general fatigue associated with progressive proximal muscle weakness, especially upon activity and improving with rest. There is a typical progression during the day, with a peak weakness during the evening hours. Facial, oropharyngeal, ocular, and neck muscles are as susceptible as skeletal muscles. Ocular involvement with diplopia and ptosis is frequently the initial sign. Further symptoms include dysarthria and dysphagia with severe cases affecting the respiratory muscles as well. *Myasthenic* crisis is a life-threatening condition with respiratory failure and aspiration that develops usually over days, rarely acutely. It is caused by infections, errors in the intake of medication, and insufficient immunosuppression. Intensive care support and plasma exchange or IVIG are vital in these cases. Despite these measures, the mortality can be still as high as 5%.
2. A *cholinergic* crisis can present clinically in a similar fashion to the myasthenic crisis with flaccid paralysis; however, the underlying pathophysiology, and thus the therapy, is very different. Treatment with excess doses of cholinesterase inhibitors can lead to a cholinergic crisis by the nonresponsiveness of ACh receptors to abundant acetylcholine. Applying edrophonium (an ACh-esterase inhibitor) can distinguish both forms of crises by worsening the cholinergic crisis and by improving the symptoms of a myasthenic crisis. There is no specific treatment for cholinergic crisis other than discontinuing the responsible agents and applying supportive measures like intubation and mechanical ventilation. Atropine, a blocking

agent at the muscarinergic ACh receptor, has only a limited impact on the muscle weakness component, which is triggered through nicotinic acetylcholine receptors. Several medications can exacerbate symptoms of MG (Table 30.2).

3. A thorough history and a physical examination, especially with a focus on the muscle groups, are essential. If MG is suspected with symptoms that can be objectified (important!), pharmacologic testing with neostigmine, edrophonium, or pyridostigmine with atropine at the bedside should be carried out to look for improvement of muscle strength, which occurs rapidly after the administration of the abovementioned drugs. Careful documentation of the affected muscles is mandatory. A nonpharmacologic but unspecific test is the "ice-on-eyes" test that leads to an improvement of symptoms by decreasing the activity of ACh esterase due to low temperature. Additional neurophysiologic testing with 3-Hz repetitive nerve stimulation (accessory or facial nerve) with evidence of a decrement of more than 10% further underscores the diagnosis. Laboratory testing should include anti-ACh-receptor antibodies (high yield in generalized and paraneoplastic MG forms), anti-MuSK (muscle-specific-kinase) antibodies (in 40%-70% positive in ACh receptor antibody "seronegative" MG), and anti-titin antibodies (frequently associated with thymoma), besides general labs to assess complex comorbidities (eg, diabetes, autoimmune thyroid disease) and for the guidance of immune therapy. The autoantibody status is merely used for classification and has essentially no impact on management. Further studies should include imaging (chest CT or MRI) to rule out a thymoma.
4. Patients with suspected MG in the ICU should be stabilized first from the respiratory and, if necessary, cardiovascular standpoints. This might implicate intubation and mechanical ventilation. Symptomatic treatment is achieved with acetylcholine esterase inhibitors such as pyridostigmine or neostigmine. Frequently intravenous administration is required in severe MG exacerbations, but attention should be paid to their rather high side-effect profile (eg, bronchial secretions). Glucocorticoids have good efficacy on muscle weakness in MG with frequent initial deterioration of symptoms. The average onset of action, however, is 4 to 8 weeks in 70%

TABLE 30.2 Medications That Can Exacerbate Symptoms of Myasthenia Gravis (MG)

Substance group	Examples
Analgesics	Morphine derivatives
Antibiotics	Aminoglycosides, macrolides, quinolones, sulfonamides, tetracyclines, polymyxins, and penicillin in high doses
Antiarrhythmics	Procainamide, ajmaline, chinidine
Anticonvulsants	Benzodiazepines, gabapentin, carbamazepine, phenytoin
β-Blockers	Propranolol, pindolol, timolol
Calcium antagonists	Verapamil, nifedipine, diltiazem
Diuretics	Loop diuretics (furosemide), acetazolamide, hydrochlorothiazide
Statins	Different statins reported
Psychotropic agents	Chlorpromazine, promazine
Muscle-relaxing agents	Curare derivatives, suxamethonium

Note: These are merely examples of drugs that can cause a worsening of MG symptoms, and this list cannot be considered complete.

to 80% of the cases. Thus, they are combined with other immunosuppressants, for example, azathioprine or cyclosporine A; an escalation therapy would include more potent immunomodulators like mycophenolate, cyclophosphamide, or methotrexate. Challenging courses might require off-label applications of agents like tacrolimus or monoclonal antibodies like rituximab or alemtuzumab. In refractory cases or in a myasthenic crisis, IVIG therapy or plasma exchange should be considered. Thymectomy should be considered after clinical stabilization in all patients with evidence of thymoma and also in patients aged 15 to 50 years with generalized MG, without detected thymomas.

B. Lambert-Eaton Myasthenic Syndrome

A more uncommon disorder of neuromuscular junction transmission is Lambert-Eaton myasthenic syndrome (LEMS), which is also an autoimmune disorder. Most often it presents with progressive proximal muscle weakness, especially in the lower extremities, autonomic dysfunction, and areflexia. Different than myasthenia gravis, strength may temporarily improve with exertion due to buildup of acetylcholine. The pathophysiology of LEMS is based on antibodies directed against presynaptic voltage-gated calcium channels (VGCC), and there is a strong association with malignancy, especially with small-cell lung cancer (SCLC). Treatment is focused on the underlying cause (removal of the tumor). Immune-directed therapy with steroids and plasma exchange is applied as well.

C. Botulism

Acute onset of symmetric descending weakness associated with bilateral cranial neuropathies (diplopia, nystagmus, ptosis, dysphagia, facial weakness) should raise red flags to consider botulism. Urinary retention and constipation can occur as well. Botulism is a rare potentially life-threatening disease caused by the toxin of the ubiquitously appearing gram-positive, spore-forming, obligate anaerobic bacterium *Clostridium botulinum.* There are different forms, namely, foodborne, infant, wound, adult enteric, and inhalational botulism. Foodborne botulism, for instance, is caused by the consumption of these pathogens in home-canned foods like vegetables or fruits. When botulism is suspected, the clinician ought to contact the State Health Department instantly to obtain antitoxin as the treatment of choice. Equine serum heptavalent botulism antitoxin is used for adults. Wound botulism requires antibiotics (penicillin G or metronidazole) after the administration of antitoxin.

IV. MYOPATHIC CAUSES

A. Critical Illness Myopathy

CIM is a primary myopathy acquired during critical illness. The incidence of isolated CIM is unknown as there is significant overlap with CIP, although it is thought to be more common than CIP, and tends to have an earlier onset. Similar to CIP, CIM is thought to arise from a complex interaction of inflammatory processes, reduced microperfusion, and metabolic changes as well as muscle protein breakdown. In CIM, generally symmetrical, flaccid weakness is observed; proximal weakness may be more pronounced than distal, and facial muscles are more commonly affected than in CIP. In patients with pure CIM, reflexes are often normal and sensation intact, thus examination of the latter is useful when trying to distinguish between the two entities. Patients with significant weakness from CIM may grimace in response to painful stimulation in the extremities, without producing a motor response in the limb. When both CIM and CIP are present, the term "critical illness polyneuromyopathy" is used.

1. Formal diagnosis of CIM requires confirmation via electrodiagnostic studies. These tests typically show increased duration of compound motor

action potentials, normal sensory action potentials, decreased muscle excitability with direct stimulation, and low amplitude motor unit potentials, with or without fibrillation. Muscle biopsy (when performed) will show loss of myosin, fiber atrophy (more so type 2 fibers), and varying degrees of necrosis. Lab values may demonstrate elevated CK levels. As with CIP, treatment for CIM is largely supportive, including addressing underlying causes of critical illness. There is evidence suggesting increased risk for CIM in patients receiving IV glucocorticoids; thus, treatment includes minimizing glucocorticoids when possible. There is literature to support physical therapy for strengthening in patients with CIM, although no dose-response relationship has been established. Additional preventative and treatment measures appear similar to those described for CIP. Prognosis for functional recovery varies, but evidence suggests it is better and more rapid than in CIP. Recovery frequently takes weeks to months; however, many patients with isolated CIM will be largely recovered within 6 months to 1 year.

B. Rhabdomyolysis

Muscular symptoms including acute weakness and myalgias are present in some patients with rhabdomyolysis, with typical findings including myoglobinuria and elevated creatine kinase. Common causes of rhabdomyolysis are severe muscle injury with ensuing muscle necrosis. Complications that go along with this clinical entity are acute kidney injury, compartment syndrome, and disseminated intravascular coagulation. Treatment includes prompt correction of the abovementioned manifestations and complications and identification of the trigger with appropriate management of the same (eg, discontinuation of drugs causing rhabdomyolysis).

V. OTHER CAUSES

Nutritional deficiencies can result in changes to the central and/or peripheral nervous systems, in addition to other multisystem sequala (hematologic, cardiac, etc). Although clinical presentation is often subacute or chronic, neurologic manifestations may present more acutely in some patients. Nutritional deficiencies may be a function of, but not limited to, inadequate oral intake, excessive losses (eg, diarrhea, diuresis), or malabsorption (eg, individuals post-bariatric surgery). The precise impact on the nervous system depends on the specific vitamin or mineral deficiency and the extent thereof. For example, patients with thiamine deficiency may present with signs of acute, progressive sensorimotor neuropathy, similar to GBS. In addition to central signs such as cerebellar ataxia, patients with vitamin E deficiency may exhibit evidence of peripheral neuropathy including weakness. Full laboratory evaluation and thorough patient history are important in establishing a diagnosis, supplemented by additional studies such as CSF assessment and CT imaging to rule out other causes, as warranted. Treatment is aimed at repleting the deficiency and addressing underlying contributing factors.

Transverse myelitis (TM) is an acute to subacute inflammatory insult to the spinal cord, frequently impacting one or two levels of the cord, although the degree of impact can vary widely. TM may be idiopathic in nature or associated with other conditions such as known infectious diseases, inflammatory disease (eg, sarcoidosis), or CNS disorders (eg, multiple sclerosis). In many patients with idiopathic TM, this is preceded by an infection without a clearly defined link. Clinical presentation is consistent with an insult to the spinal cord below the level of the lesion (eg, motor and sensory changes, autonomic dysfunction, bowel and bladder changes). Pain and paresthesias are frequent complaints, and many patients will exhibit a clear sensory line. MRI typically shows T2 hyperintense signal change at the segment(s) of the lesion, without evidence of compressive lesion. CSF may be abnormal including pleocytosis and elevated IgG. Treatment for TM includes high-dose steroids with plasma exchange in therapy-refractory cases, as well as treatment of any other associated diseases. Most patients show signs of improvement by 3 months, although recovery is frequently incomplete. Rapid onset with complete motor loss and the presence of spinal shock have been associated with worse functional outcomes.

Patients undergoing surgery to repair the thoracoabdominal aorta are at risk for spinal cord ischemia in the setting of decreased perfusion to the cord, to the anterior spinal artery (ASA), with 2% to 10% of patients sustaining injury. When the insult is to the ASA, the corticospinal and spinothalamic tracts are impacted, resulting in weakness and initially hyporeflexia, as well as impaired pain and temperature detection below the level of the insult, with preservation of touch, vibratory, and position senses. Bowel and bladder dysfunction may be present. Onset of neurologic deficits may be immediate or delayed by hours or even weeks, and the extent of impairment varies depending on the degree of insult. Deficits may be temporary when in the setting of transient hypoperfusion, in which case treatment should be aimed at maximizing cord perfusion as possible (including targeting higher mean arterial pressures and insertion of a lumbar drain to reduce intraspinal pressure).

Selected Readings

Awad H, Ramadan ME, El Sayed HF et al. Spinal cord injury after thoracic endovascular aortic aneurysm repair. *J Can Anesth.* 2017;64:1218-1235.

Beh SC, Greenberg BM, Frohman T, et al. Transverse myelitis. *Neurol Clin.* 2013;31:79-138.

Dowell VR Jr. Botulism and tetanus: selected epidemiologic and microbiologic aspects. *Rev Infect Dis.* 1984;6(suppl 1):S202-S207.

Drachman DB. Myasthenia gravis. *N Engl J Med.* 1994;330:1797-1810.

Elmqvist D, Lambert EH. Detailed analysis of neuromuscular transmission in a patient with the myasthenic syndrome sometimes associated with bronchogenic carcinoma. *Mayo Clin Proc.* 1968;43:689-713.

Gwathmey KG, Grogan J. Nutritional neuropathies. *Muscles Nerve.* 2020;62:13-29.

Kress JP, Hall JB. ICU-acquired weakness and recovery from critical illness. *N Engl J Med.* 2014;370:1626-1635.

Schweickert WD, Hall J. ICU-acquired weakness. *Chest.* 2007;131:1541-1549.

Tanskisi H, de Carvalho M, Z'Graggen WJ. Critical illness neuropathy. *J Clin Neurophysiol.* 2020;37:205-207.

Vanhorebeek I, Latronico N, Van den Berghe G. ICU-acquired weakness. *Intensive Care Med.* 2020;46:637-653.

West TW. Transverse myelitis—a review of the presentation, diagnosis and initial management. *Discov Med.* 2013;16(88):167-177.

Yuki N, Hartung H-P. Guillain-Barré syndrome. *N Engl J Med.* 2012;336:2294-2304.

31 Drug Overdose, Poisoning, and Adverse Drug Reactions

Michael O'Brien and Bryan D. Hayes

I. INTRODUCTION

A. Overdoses, poisonings, and adverse drug reactions are common diagnoses treated by intensivists. Deaths secondary to drug overdose have increased in recent years, primarily driven by opioid overdoses. Many of these poisonings rapidly deteriorate requiring intensive care unit (ICU) admission.

B. The initial approach to a patient with an overdose, poisoning, or adverse drug reaction varies. The American Association of Poison Control Centers is available 24 hours a day to assist—1-800-222-1222. In addition to pertinent labs and a thorough history and physical exam, it is imperative to know:

1. Which substance(s) the patient may have been exposed to.
2. The time, amount, and route (eg, ingestion, inhalation, injection) of the exposure.
3. Treatment(s) already provided.

C. Initiation of supportive care and stabilization should begin immediately upon patient presentation. Following identification of the substance and after consulting local experts (as necessary), additional treatments such as an antidote, enhancing elimination, or decreasing absorption may begin. Activated charcoal in doses of 25 to 100 g for adults may be effective for certain substances if given within the first few hours of ingestion. The benefits of activated charcoal must be weighed against the known risks (eg, aspiration pneumonitis and bowel obstructions), and the poison control center should be consulted if this is unclear. Contraindications to activated charcoal include:

1. Patients with a high risk of aspirating gastric contents without a secured airway
2. GI perforation or hemorrhage
3. Intestinal obstruction
4. Plan for endoscopy
5. Ingestion of a substance to which activated charcoal does not bind

D. Traditional treatment methods designed to minimize absorption through the GI tract, such as inducing emesis with syrup of ipecac or whole bowel irrigation, are no longer recommended except in specific situations. Similarly, gastric lavage is not routinely recommended but can be considered when a known lethal dose of a substance that does not have an antidote or bind activated charcoal was ingested within an hour of presentation and after consultation with the poison control center.

II. DRUG OVERDOSE

A. Drug overdoses can present in a variety of settings, from intentional (eg, suicide or recreational) to unintentional (eg, child ingesting pills), iatrogenic (eg, unintentional overdose of acetaminophen from multiple products), and work related (eg, chemical plant exposures).

B. **Acetaminophen (APAP)** is the leading cause of acute liver failure (ALF) in the United States and was associated with more than 100 deaths in 2019. APAP ingestion should be suspected in all patients being evaluated for suspected overdose, given its wide availability and the large number of combination products that contain APAP.

1. The majority of damage occurs when CYP2E1 metabolizes APAP to the active metabolite, *N*-acetyl-p-benzoquinone-imine (NAPQI). NAPQI is normally neutralized by glutathione; however, toxicity ensues when NAPQI depletes endogenous glutathione stores. Excess NAPQI binds mitochondrial proteins in hepatocytes, which inhibits cellular respiration. This leads to necrosis and apoptosis, ultimately causing ALF.
2. Patients may present without obvious illness, but then rapidly deteriorate to fulminant liver failure within 24 to 96 hours of ingestion. Initial symptoms can include nausea, vomiting, malaise, and anorexia. If untreated, these symptoms may progress to right upper quadrant abdominal pain, profound encephalopathy, hepatorenal syndrome, and metabolic acidosis. Lab abnormalities typically correlate with the severity of the ingestion and may include elevated AST/ALT, elevated PT/INR, and elevated bilirubin. The King's College Criteria can be used to help predict the need for liver transplantation among patients with ALF from both APAP overdoses and non-APAP ALF as shown in Table 31.1. Please note that there is a modified King's College Criteria that incorporates lactate and phosphate to increase the sensitivity (not shown).
3. To determine whether patients require treatment for their APAP ingestion, serum APAP levels are plotted on the Rumack-Matthew nomogram (see Figure 31.1). This nomogram should only be used following an acute, single ingestion of immediate-release APAP. The APAP level should be plotted on the nomogram as early as possible, but at least 4 hours postingestion. There is minimal utility in obtaining APAP levels between 0- and 4-hour postingestion, aside from confirming if APAP was the substance ingested. Because absorption and distribution are still occurring, this level cannot reliably predict which patients will need to be treated.
4. *N*-acetylcysteine (NAC) should be administered in the following circumstances:
   a. An APAP level above the treatment line on the Rumack-Matthew nomogram
   b. Unknown time of APAP ingestion with an APAP level greater than 10 μg/mL or evidence of liver injury
   c. History of chronic supratherapeutic APAP ingestion and evidence of liver injury
5. Administration of IV NAC is generally well tolerated by most patients, although adverse effects include nausea, vomiting, flushing, and anaphylactoid reactions. Anaphylactoid reactions are significantly more common in patients without a toxic APAP level. Despite the risks, it is generally better

TABLE 31.1 King's College Criteria for Need for Liver Transplantation

Acetaminophen-associated acute liver failure	Other causes of acute liver failure
pH <7.3	INR >6.5
or all of the following:	or three of the following:
INR >6.5	Age <10 yr or >40 yr
Creatinine >3.4 mg/dL	Non-A or non-B hepatitis or drug induced
Grade III-IV encephalopathy	>7 d of jaundice before encephalopathy
	INR >3.5
	Serum bilirubin >17.5 mg/dL

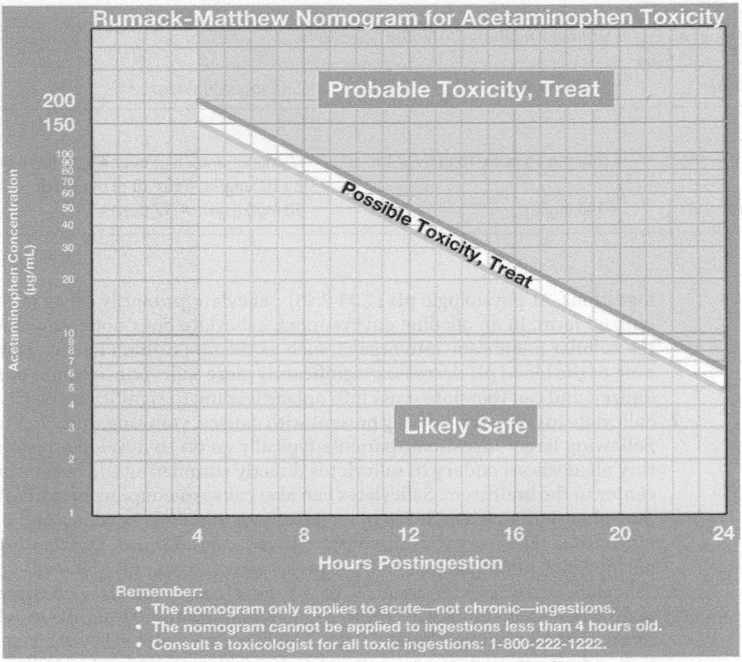

FIGURE 31.1 The Rumack-Matthew nomogram is designed to help determine the risk of hepatotoxicity based on hours since ingestion (*x*-axis) versus the serum acetaminophen level in µg/mL (*y*-axis). Any acetaminophen level greater than the "150-line" at any time since ingestion should be treated with NAC. (Courtesy Graham Walker, MD, Emergency Physician, Kaiser San Francisco, Assistant Clinical Professor, UCSF and MDCalc.com)

to overtreat with NAC and discontinue the infusion if it is not indicated. If administered within 8 hours postingestion, NAC is nearly 100% effective in avoiding liver transplantation. This is because the body's glutathione stores can last approximately 6 to 8 hours following a toxic ingestion. Therefore, waiting for the results of an APAP level between the 4- to 8-hour time frame before starting NAC won't change a patient's outcome. The use of IV NAC is far more common than PO NAC, given its ease of administration, potentially shorter treatment course, and increased tolerability. Discontinuation of NAC is typically recommended when the APAP level is undetectable, AST/ALT has significantly decreased for at least two consecutive draws, metabolic acidosis is resolved, serum creatinine is at baseline, and the INR is less than 2.0. Dosing can be found in Table 31.2.

C. Salicylates are available in many over-the-counter products. The most commonly encountered agent is aspirin, which is used for the prevention and treatment of cardiovascular disease, as well as many other conditions.

1. Salicylates are primarily absorbed in the stomach. Absorption is variable and can be delayed due to the formation of a bezoar, delayed release formulations, or salicylate-induced pylorospasm. The half-life is 2 to 4 hours, but this is prolonged up to 20 hours or longer with high doses or enteric-coated formulations. The volume of distribution is 0.2 to 0.3 L/kg and it is normally 90% protein bound, but this decreases to less than 75% following toxic

TABLE 31.2 Dosing Regimen for *N*-acetylcysteine

Route	Loading dose	Subsequent doses
Intravenous	150 mg/kg (max 15 g) over 1 h	50 mg/kg (max 5 g) over 4 h, followed by 100 mg/kg (max 10 g) over 16 h
Oral	140 mg/kg	70 mg/kg q4h × 17 doses

ingestions. At physiologic pH (7.35-7.45), salicylate primarily exists in the ionized form. In an alkaline environment, salicylate does not easily cross the cellular membrane into organs, such as the blood-brain barrier. However, as the blood pH decreases, significantly more salicylate becomes nonionized and can therefore cross into organs leading to significant toxicity.

2. Salicylate toxicity may initially present with nausea, vomiting, and tinnitus. Following larger ingestions, patients typically go on to develop a respiratory alkalosis secondary to salicylates directly stimulating the respiratory center in the brainstem. Salicylates can also cause uncoupling of oxidative phosphorylation, which leads to an anion gap metabolic acidosis and hyperthermia refractory to antipyretics. Altered mental status, gastrointestinal bleeding, pulmonary edema, seizures, and coma may also be seen.
3. Salicylate levels greater than 30 to 40 mg/dL are typically considered toxic whereas patients with levels greater than 90 to 100 mg/dL should receive emergent hemodialysis (HD). Following an acute salicylate ingestion, administration of oral activated charcoal may prevent significant absorption and avoid more invasive therapies. Multidose activated charcoal may also be considered if there is a concern for bezoar formation or if an extended-release formulation was ingested. Practically, each time a serum concentration is higher (or the same) as the previous one, another dose of activated charcoal may be considered, if safe to do so, as this likely represents continued absorption. It is recommended that pertinent labs, such as salicylate concentrations and blood gases (venous or arterial), be monitored at least every 2 to 4 hours until salicylate levels are decreasing on two sequential lab draws. For patients who develop symptoms of salicylate toxicity, alkalinization of blood and urine via administration of IV sodium bicarbonate should be considered. The typical alkalinization regimen includes a 1 to 2 mEq/kg bolus of IV sodium bicarbonate followed by an isotonic sodium bicarbonate infusion titrated to a urine pH greater than or equal to 7.5 and a blood pH 7.45 to 7.55. Alkalinization of the urine increases salicylate excretion by decreasing the relative concentration of nonionized salicylate to the blood and trapping the ionized salicylate in the urine. Patients critically ill secondary to salicylate ingestion should be discussed with a toxicologist and nephrologist and may require immediate HD. Potential indications for HD include:
   - **a.** Blood pH less than 7.2 despite aggressive alkalinization therapy
   - **b.** Altered mental status, seizures, persistent central nervous system (CNS) disturbances
   - **c.** Pulmonary edema or acute lung injury
   - **d.** Acute renal failure
   - **e.** Coagulopathy
   - **f.** Serum salicylate level greater than 100 mg/dL
   - **g.** Serum salicylate level greater than 90 mg/dL with impaired renal function

D. Cardiovascular medications, such as β-blockers (BB), calcium-channel blockers (CCB), and cardiac glycosides (eg, digoxin), can lead to significant morbidity and mortality when ingested in toxic amounts. With an aging population and the associated increases in prescriptions for cardiovascular drugs, overdoses of these medications are expected to increase in the United States.

1. BBs are used for a variety of medical conditions. They work by blocking β-adrenergic receptors, thus antagonizing catecholamines and decreasing intracellular cAMP. Across the BB class, the β-receptor-binding affinity and selectivity vary significantly. Drugs blocking β1 receptors reduce the inotropic and chronotropic effects on the heart, whereas drugs blocking β2 receptors reduce bronchodilatation and gluconeogenesis. However, in cases of overdose, BBs may lose β-receptor selectivity. Drugs such as labetalol and carvedilol also block α1 receptors, leading to a decrease in blood pressure.

a. Overdose can result in severe bradycardia and hypotension (cardiogenic shock) as well as hypoglycemia, atrioventricular (AV) block, bronchospasm, and seizures (eg, propranolol). Following ingestion of an immediate-release BB, symptoms should develop within 6 hours and if patients are still asymptomatic at that time then the patient can be medically cleared. Patients who ingest an extended-release formulation or sotalol require a longer period of observation (12-24 hours).

b. Initial treatment in overdose may include charcoal, IV fluids, and supporting the heart rate with the use of atropine or electrical pacing. Depending on the quantity of BB ingested, catecholamines (eg, epinephrine, norepinephrine) may be beneficial and sufficient to support patients until they recover without needing additional treatments. Glucagon is traditionally considered the first-line antidote for BB toxicity, though high-dose insulin is becoming increasingly popular and preferred. Glucagon increases intracellular cAMP and may be administered as a bolus of 3 to 5 mg IV push followed by an infusion at 3 to 5 mg/h. Patients frequently develop nausea and vomiting so care should be taken to prevent aspiration; ondansetron is often coadministered. Data increasingly support the use of high-dose insulin therapy for BB toxicity. Care should be taken when implementing this regimen, especially in BB overdose as these patients may already be hypoglycemic, so a concentrated dextrose solution should always be initiated concomitantly with the insulin bolus and infusion. Patients should receive an insulin bolus of 1 u/kg followed by an infusion of 1 u/kg/h, titrated to markers of organ perfusion. Doses up to 10 u/kg/h may be required. High-dose insulin improves cardiac function by improving cardiac myocyte glucose uptake and utilization. Venous-arterial extracorporeal membrane oxygenation (VA ECMO) may effectively be used for cardiac support if other treatment options are ineffective.

2. CCBs are used for numerous indications. CCBs antagonize L-type voltage-gated calcium channels in myocardial cells, smooth muscle cells, and β-islet cells in the pancreas, thus inhibiting calcium entry into the cells. Dihydropyridines (eg, amlodipine and nifedipine) act peripherally and cause systemic vasodilation, whereas nondihydropyridines (eg, verapamil and diltiazem) act primarily within the heart, reducing inotropy and chronotropy. In the pancreas, CCBs decrease insulin secretion, leading to hyperglycemia.

a. CCB overdoses present with hypotension (cardiogenic shock), sinus bradycardia, AV block, and hyperglycemia. As in BB overdose, CCBs may lose their selectivity and all agents may lead to hypotension and bradycardia.

b. The treatment of CCB toxicity is similar to a BB overdose. Initial treatment may include activated charcoal, IV fluids, atropine, and IV calcium. Catecholamines, such as epinephrine or norepinephrine, may also be used to improve perfusion. High-dose insulin therapy is typically the first-line therapy for CCB toxicity causing significant hemodynamic compromise. Initial insulin dosing is a bolus of 1 u/kg followed by an infusion at 1 u/kg/h titrated up to a maximum of 10 u/kg/h based on markers of organ perfusion. A concentrated dextrose solution should be initiated concomitantly to avoid hypoglycemia, but the dextrose requirement is likely to be lower than with a BB overdose as patients with CCB toxicity are frequently already hyperglycemic.

3. Digoxin is still used for the treatment of atrial fibrillation and congestive heart failure. Digoxin is a sodium-potassium ATPase inhibitor that increases intracellular sodium, leading to increased calcium and improved inotropy. It also stimulates the vagus nerve which causes decreased cardiac conduction velocity. Toxicity can occur with normal serum digoxin levels in the setting of hypokalemia, hypomagnesemia, or hypothyroidism. Conversely, serum digoxin levels can increase while on a stable dose if drugs such as amiodarone, verapamil, or erythromycin are coadministered or if renal elimination is decreased secondary to dehydration or other causes.

a. Toxicity leads to increased automaticity and dysrhythmias, including frequent premature ventricular contractions (PVCs), atrial fibrillation with a slow ventricular response, bidirectional ventricular tachycardia, or complete AV block. Scooping of the ST segment may be seen on an ECG but is not indicative of toxicity. Other symptoms include nausea, vomiting, abdominal pain, altered mental status, and visual disturbances, including the classic yellow halos around sources of light. Hyperkalemia is present in acute overdoses and is correlated to mortality. Digoxin's distribution in the body is bimodal; therefore, serum concentrations obtained less than 6 hours after ingestion may overestimate the severity of the overdose. Additionally, following the administration of digoxin immune antigen-binding fragments (Fab), digoxin is pulled from the tissue into the circulation and bound to the antidote. This may cause total digoxin serum concentrations to appear higher after administering this treatment, but this does not signal worsening toxicity. Therefore, we do not recommend following digoxin serum concentrations after antidote administration.

b. Treatment of acute or chronic digoxin toxicity typically begins with supportive care, atropine for bradydysrhythmias, and potentially multidose activated charcoal, as dioxin undergoes enterohepatic recirculation. Both hypokalemia and hyperkalemia can worsen toxicity. Patients with hypokalemia should receive IV potassium repletion until their potassium is within the normal range, and digoxin immune Fab should not be administered until the hypokalemia is corrected. Similarly, hyperkalemia should be corrected by the usual means. IV calcium in the context of hyperkalemia associated with digoxin toxicity is controversial, but recent data do not support the universal avoidance of IV calcium. Hypomagnesemia may also occur with digoxin toxicity, and correction may temporarily help stabilize the patients; therefore, it is generally recommended to administer 2 g of IV magnesium sulfate and give additional magnesium as needed based on the patient's magnesium concentration. Tachydysrhythmias may be managed with IV lidocaine; all Class IA antidysrhythmics are contraindicated. Ultimately, the administration of IV digoxin immune Fab is necessary for life-threatening toxicity.

The dose may be calculated based on either the reported amount of digoxin ingested or on the digoxin serum concentration. Additionally, empiric doses may be given if this information cannot be obtained. Indications for digoxin immune Fab include:

a. Life-threatening dysrhythmias secondary to digoxin

b. Potassium level greater than 5 mEq/L following an acute digoxin ingestion

c. Chronic ingestion of digoxin associated with dysrhythmias, significant GI symptoms, or altered mental status

d. Total digoxin level greater than 15 ng/mL at any point or greater than 10 ng/mL at least 6 hours postingestion

e. Ingestion of 10 mg of digoxin in adults or 4 mg of digoxin in children

E. Antipsychotics and Antidepressants

1. Antipsychotics include traditional (aka "typical antipsychotics") medications, such as haloperidol and chlorpromazine, and newer classes (aka "atypical antipsychotics") of antipsychotics such as quetiapine, olanzapine, and risperidone, which have less antidopaminergic effects. All antipsychotics can produce adverse reactions such as neuroleptic malignant syndrome (see **Section IV**), extrapyramidal side effects (ie, parkinsonism and dystonia), and tardive dyskinesia (irreversible, purposeless movements of the face and neck), though atypical antipsychotics produce these less frequently. In overdose, patients develop stupor and hypotension with reflex tachycardia, prolongation of the QT interval on electrocardiogram (ECG). Treatment of an antipsychotic overdose involves supportive care, IV benztropine or diphenhydramine if the patient develops extrapyramidal side effects, and IV magnesium for prolonged QTc.

2. Antidepressants include selective serotonin reuptake inhibitors (SSRIs), serotonin-norepinephrine reuptake inhibitors (SNRIs), atypical antidepressants (eg, bupropion), tricyclic antidepressants (TCAs), and monoamine oxidase inhibitors (MAOIs). Ingestion of SSRIs, SNRIs, and MAOIs may lead to serotonin toxicity (see **Section IV**). Bupropion overdose may be complicated by tachycardia, hypertension, agitation, seizures, and QRS prolongation. Bupropion-related seizures should be treated with IV benzodiazepines. Patients with a prolonged QRS should receive IV sodium bicarbonate. TCAs block cardiac sodium channels causing a prolonged QRS and lead to dysrhythmias such as wide-complex ventricular tachycardia and ventricular fibrillation. Treatment of a QRS greater than 100 ms or hypotension secondary to a TCA ingestion should include administration of a 1 to 2 mEq/kg sodium bicarbonate bolus repeated every 3 to 5 minutes until symptoms improve. Hypertonic saline (3%) may also be used in place of sodium bicarbonate if the latter is not available. TCA toxicity may also include the development of delirium, agitation, and seizures, which should be treated initially with IV benzodiazepines.

F. Lithium is used for the long-term treatment of bipolar disorder but has a narrow therapeutic window with several adverse side effects.

1. Acute lithium ingestions can present with nausea, vomiting, and diarrhea initially, and progress to the development of CNS depression and cardiac manifestations (eg, T-wave flattening and QTc prolongation). Early management includes aggressive fluid hydration with normal saline; activated charcoal does not bind lithium and should be avoided unless other medications are also ingested. Serum lithium levels should be obtained upon presentation and regularly every few hours to monitor absorption and elimination. In severe cases of lithium toxicity, emergent hemodialysis may be required. Initiation of hemodialysis should be discussed with a toxicologist and potential indications include:

a. Impaired renal function with lithium level greater than 4 mEq/L
b. Decreased level of consciousness, confusion, seizures, or life-threatening dysrhythmias
c. Lithium level greater than 5 mEq/L
d. Expected time to reach lithium level less than 1 mEq/L of more than 36 hours

2. Chronic lithium toxicity results in significantly different symptoms than those associated with acute ingestions. These symptoms include tremor, hyperreflexia, clonus, dysarthria, nystagmus, ataxia, altered mental status, and seizure. These symptoms occur because lithium is directly neurotoxic. Treatment is limited to discontinuation of lithium, and many of these symptoms may be irreversible.

III. POISONINGS

A. **Carbon Monoxide (CO)** is a colorless, odorless gas produced by incomplete combustion of organic compounds, such as in house fires or the operation of motor vehicles without proper ventilation.

1. CO avidly binds heme (>200 times stronger than oxygen), thus displacing oxygen and causing hypoxia. CO also causes direct cellular damage through both immunologic and inflammatory processes.
2. The symptoms of CO poisoning do not directly correlate with carboxyhemoglobin (COHgb) levels. Patients may present with dizziness, headaches, fatigue, confusion, chest pain, and/or shortness of breath. These symptoms may progress to include hypotension, dysrhythmias, reduced left ventricular ejection fraction, stroke-like symptoms, unresponsiveness, metabolic acidosis, and pulmonary edema following prolonged or higher levels of exposure. A traditional presentation of "cherry red skin" is rare and should not be relied upon for diagnosis. Oxyhemoglobin and COHgb absorb light at the same wavelength, and therefore pulse oximetry may be normal despite severe hypoxemia. COHgb levels of greater than 3% in nonsmokers and greater than 10% in smokers should raise suspicion for exposure. Diagnosis requires a high index of suspicion, given the typically nonspecific nature of initial presentation.
3. Treatment should be continued until COHgb levels are less than 3% and the patient is symptom free for a minimum of 6 hours. Initial therapy typically involves removing the patient from the source of CO, instituting 100% oxygen therapy, and providing standard supportive measures. Increasing the FIO_2 enhances the removal of CO from heme; at 21% FIO_2, the half-life of COHgb is 5 hours, versus approximately 1 hour in patients receiving 100% FIO_2 via a non-rebreathing mask. Further accelerations in reducing CO levels are seen with 100% FIO_2 via endotracheal tube and with hyperbaric oxygen (HBO). HBO does not improve short-term survival but is associated with less long-term neurologic sequelae in some studies. Patients with CO poisoning should be discussed with a toxicologist or HBO expert before initiation of HBO. Potential indications for HBO include:
   a. Syncope, coma, seizure, altered mental status (GCS <15), confusion, or abnormal cerebellar function
   b. COHgb greater than 25%
   c. Age greater than or equal to 36 years
   d. Prolonged CO exposure (≥24 hours)
   e. Pregnancy with fetal distress or COHgb greater than 20%
   f. Refractory metabolic acidosis
   g. Cardiac ischemia

B. **Cyanide** exposures may come from multiple different sources. Hydrogen cyanide is a by-product from the combustion of nitrogen-containing products (eg, plastics, wool, silk). Additionally, cyanide exposures may be secondary to numerous workplace exposures (eg, metallurgy, photography, manufacturing) or via ingestion of certain foods (eg, bitter almonds, cassava). Iatrogenic cyanide toxicity may occur in patients receiving IV nitroprusside.

1. Cyanide inhibits numerous enzymes; most notably cytochrome oxidase, which is necessary for aerobic metabolism to occur. Inhibition of cytochrome oxidase disrupts the electron transport chain leading to the accumulation of hydrogen ions and acidosis. Additionally, given the lack of aerobic metabolism, lactate is generated and builds up in the body. Cyanide also causes neurotoxicity via multiple pathways.
2. Early signs and symptoms of cyanide toxicity include tachypnea, confusion, agitation, dizziness, headaches, nausea, and vomiting. More serious findings include severe cardiac effects (eg, hypotension, bradycardia, heart failure with preservation of inotropy) and neurologic manifestations (eg, seizures, lethargy, and coma). Laboratory finds such as anion gap metabolic acidosis with elevated lactate and narrow arteriovenous oxygen gradient are highly suggestive of cyanide toxicity in the appropriate context.
3. Treatment consists of administering 100% oxygen and usually supportive measures as necessary. Hydroxocobalamin (Cyanokit) is commonly the preferred antidote as it complexes with cyanide to form cyanocobalamin (Vitamin B_{12}), which is easily excreted by the kidneys. Hydroxocobalamin also has the beneficial effect of scavenging nitric oxide, which raises blood pressure. However, it is important to note that hydroxocobalamin is a deep red color that can alter colorimetric lab tests and discolor body fluids. For adults, the dose is 5 g IV over 15 minutes and this may be repeated if needed based on the severity of toxicity and clinical response. An alternative and rarely used antidote is the combination of amyl nitrite, sodium nitrite, and sodium thiosulfate, which works by inducing methemoglobinemia and helps convert cyanide to thiocyanate. This combination antidote is less commonly used due to the potential for excessive methemoglobin generation and hypotension. Additionally, hydroxocobalamin is preferred over nitrite therapy in patients with suspected cyanide toxicity secondary to house fires due to the potential for concomitant CO poisoning and additional worsening in oxygen-carrying capacity when methemoglobinemia is induced. (Dosing for both regimens is found in Table 31.3.)

IV. ADVERSE DRUG REACTIONS

A. Hyperthermia-Related Drug Reactions are a broad category that often results in patients being admitted to the ICU. These are hyperthermic states and not the result of hypothalamic dysregulation as seen in infections, and therefore antipyretics are not indicated nor effective.

1. **Malignant hyperthermia** is caused by an autosomal dominant trait which, when exposed to certain provoking agents (succinylcholine or inhaled

TABLE 31.3 Hunter Serotonin Toxicity Criteria

Patient with exposure to at least one serotonergic agent and one of the following:
Spontaneous clonus
Inducible clonus + (agitation or diaphoresis)
Ocular clonus + (agitation or diaphoresis)
Tremor + hyperreflexia
Hypertonia + hyperthermia + (ocular clonus or inducible clonus)

volatile anesthetics), leads to a systemic hypermetabolic state in skeletal muscle due to excessive calcium release. This may result in increased oxygen utilization and CO_2 production, lactic acidosis, hyperthermia, and/or disseminated intravascular coagulation (DIC). Early presentation includes spasm of masseter muscles, tachypnea, and rigidity, while diagnostic testing will commonly show elevated end-tidal CO_2, hyperkalemia, and evidence of rhabdomyolysis. Hyperthermia is a late finding. Death is typically from cardiac dysrhythmias and multi-organ failure. Immediate administration of dantrolene has reduced the mortality rate to less than 5%. Dantrolene should be administered as an initial IV bolus of 2.5 mg/kg, doses of 1 to 2.5 mg/kg may be repeated until signs of hypermetabolism resolve or until a total of 10 mg/kg of dantrolene has been administered. Following clinical stabilization, dantrolene 1 mg/kg every 6 hours should be given for 24 hours. Additional supportive therapy to address hyperkalemia, bleeding, and prevent kidney damage is also indicated. Further information and 24-hour support are provided by the Malignant Hyperthermia Association of the United States (Website: www.mhaus.org; US Phone Number: 1-800-644-9737; International Phone Number: 001-209-417-3722).

2. **Neuroleptic malignant syndrome (NMS)** is an uncommon but serious condition that occurs in patients taking antidopaminergic drugs, most frequently antipsychotics. This syndrome can also present after the abrupt discontinuation of dopamine agonists. The mechanism for NMS is believed to be related to an acute decrease in dopaminergic activity in the hypothalamus and striatum leading to impaired thermoregulation and muscle rigidity. This is typically a diagnosis of exclusion; patients present initially with muscle rigidity and altered mental status, later developing hyperthermia and autonomic instability. NMS typically develops insidiously over days to weeks. Treatment includes supportive care, active cooling, and benzodiazepines for agitation and decreasing sympathetic outflow. Administration of either bromocriptine and/or dantrolene may be considered in severe cases, but these interventions should be discussed with a toxicologist.
3. **Serotonin syndrome (SS)** results from the increased serotonergic activity, predominantly at central 5-HT2A receptors. Drugs and substances associated with the development of SS include serotonin agonists (eg, triptans, buspirone, and LSD); serotonin reuptake inhibitors (eg, SSRIs, SNRIs, tramadol, and St. John's wort); MAOIs (eg, selegiline, phenelzine, linezolid, and methylene blue); and drugs that increase serotonin release (eg, MDMA, dextromethorphan, and methadone). SS typically starts within 6 hours of exposure to the causative agent(s) and most commonly occurs in patients taking two or more serotonergic agents but can occur with exposure to a single agent. Patients may present with symptoms ranging from mild to life-threatening. Mild or early symptoms may include akathisia, nausea/vomiting, diarrhea, tremor, and/or diaphoresis. Patients may go on to develop hyperreflexia, altered mental status, inducible or sustained clonus, muscle rigidity, and hyperthermia. Serotonin syndrome is a clinical diagnosis based on signs/symptoms and exposure to at least one serotonergic agent. The Hunter Serotonin Toxicity Criteria (Table 31.3) have largely replaced the Sternbach Criteria in clinical practice to aid in the diagnosis of SS. Treatment includes the removal of offending agent(s), supportive care, benzodiazepines for agitation, and active cooling. Although supportive care is the mainstay of treatment, cyproheptadine, chlorpromazine, and dantrolene can be considered in refractory cases.
4. **Anticholinergic syndrome** results from exposure to excessive amounts of drugs with anticholinergic properties (eg, antihistamines, TCAs,

neuroleptics, atropine, scopolamine, and antispasmodics). Symptoms include agitation, confusion, hyperthermia, dry mouth, blurred vision, tachycardia, flushing, and urinary retention. Toxicity occurs secondary to antagonism of peripheral and/or central muscarinic receptors. Initial treatment is primarily supportive, consisting of active cooling and benzodiazepines. Physostigmine is an acetylcholinesterase inhibitor that crosses the blood-brain barrier and helps increase acetylcholine levels centrally and peripherally. Studies have shown that it is more effective than benzodiazepines at treating delirium and agitation due to anticholinergic toxicity. The starting dose is typically 1 mg over 5 minutes, which may be repeated every 10 minutes as needed. Physostigmine is relatively short acting, and its effects may diminish over time. Some medications, specifically TCAs, may cause ECG changes (ie, QRS or QTc prolongation) and physostigmine should typically be avoided until these alterations have resolved.

5. **Drug fevers** are not uncommon in the ICU. They have a typical onset of 7 to 10 days after exposure. Many antimicrobials, antineoplastics, nonsteroidal anti-inflammatory drugs, and immunosuppressants are known causative agents, and symptoms resolve soon after the drug is discontinued.

B. Propofol-Related Infusion Syndrome (PRIS) was first defined in 1998 in the pediatric population as refractory bradycardia progressing to asystole with any of the following: severe metabolic acidosis, rhabdomyolysis, lipemia, or fatty liver. The specific mechanism of how PRIS develops is not clear, though it is believed to be due to defects in the mitochondrial respiratory chain. Cardiac dysfunction or Brugada-like ECG changes may be seen and may indicate impending instability. Treatment includes stopping propofol, supportive care, and HD. Inotropes demonstrate little benefit, though pacing and extracorporeal membrane oxygenation has been used in case reports. Ultimately, prevention is the best measure by limiting prolonged propofol use and utilizing high-carbohydrate, low-fat nutrition. Monitoring serum triglycerides may allow for early detection of patients at risk of developing PRIS. In order to minimize the risk of developing PRIS, it is generally recommended to keep doses less than 80 μg/kg/min.

C. Anaphylaxis and Anaphylactoid Reactions are indistinguishable in presentation, differing only in that anaphylactoid reactions are not IgE mediated. The incidence of anaphylaxis and related hospitalizations have increased globally for many years. Overall, foods and stinging insects represent the most frequent causes of anaphylaxis in children, whereas medications and stinging insects are the most common triggers in adults.

1. The most common presenting signs and symptoms are urticaria and angioedema (88%), followed by dyspnea and wheezing (47%), whereas dizziness, syncope, and hypotension (33%) are less commonly seen. Gastrointestinal complaints such as nausea, vomiting, diarrhea, and abdominal pain are important to identify,but are only present in 30% of patients.
2. Early identification of anaphylaxis is critical, and the National Institute of Allergy and Infectious Diseases (NIAID) diagnostic criteria are highly sensitive. Cardiac and respiratory arrest can occur within 5 minutes of onset, and nearly 50% of deaths occur in the first hour. Immediate administration of epinephrine (0.3 mg or 0.01 mg/kg up to 0.5 mg IM) is the most effective and life-saving intervention. Some patients may require repeated dosing of IM epinephrine and ultimately a continuous infusion. Antihistamines and steroids are frequently used in clinical practice, but these medications should not be used in place of epinephrine as they are slower acting and there is no strong evidence to support their use in the management of anaphylaxis. If possible, obtain a serum tryptase within 2 hours of symptom onset (Table 31.4).

TABLE 31.4 NIAID Criteria for Anaphylaxis

Anaphylaxis is likely when any one of these three criteria is fulfilled:

1. Acute onset of illness (minutes to several hours) with involvement of the skin, mucosal tissue, or both (eg, generalized hives, pruritus or flushing, swollen lips, tongue, or uvula) and at least one of the following:
   a. Respiratory compromise (eg, dyspnea, wheeze or bronchospasm, stridor, reduced peak expiratory flow, hypoxemia)
   b. Reduced blood pressure or associated symptoms of end-organ dysfunction (eg, hypotonia [collapse], syncope, incontinence)
2. Two or more of the following that occur rapidly after exposure to a likely allergen for that patient (minutes to several hours):
   a. Involvement of the skin or mucosal tissue (eg, generalized hives, itch or flush, swollen lips, tongue, or uvula)
   b. Respiratory compromise (eg, dyspnea, wheeze or bronchospasm, stridor, reduced peak expiratory flow, hypoxemia)
   c. Reduced blood pressure or associated symptoms (eg, hypotonia [collapse], syncope, incontinence)
   d. Persistent gastrointestinal tract symptoms (eg, crampy abdominal pain, vomiting)
3. Reduced blood pressure after exposure to known allergen for that patient (minutes to several hours):
   a. Infants and children: low systolic blood pressure (age specific) or >30% decrease in systolic blood pressure
   b. Adults: systolic blood pressure <90 mm Hg or >30% decrease from that person's baseline

V. SUBSTANCES OF ABUSE AND ADDICTION

A. Alcohols are in many common household products. Ethanol is one of the most used and abused substances in the world. Methanol, ethylene glycol, and isopropyl alcohol are more toxic and can require ICU level of care.

1. Ethanol accounts for nearly 100 000 deaths each year in the United States alone. Up to 40% of patients admitted to the hospital have alcohol use disorder and approximately half of these patients will experience alcohol withdrawal.

a. Ethanol is metabolized in the liver, first by alcohol dehydrogenase and then by acetaldehyde dehydrogenase, yielding acetate. In acute intoxication, the effects of ethanol are exerted on γ-aminobutyric acid type A ($GABA_A$) receptors by limiting glutamate activation of N-methyl-D-aspartate (NMDA) receptors. In chronic use, there is a downregulation of $GABA_A$ responses and upregulation of NMDA subtype glutamate receptors. In chronic ingestion, liver dysfunction and cirrhosis develop, leading to impaired hepatic function and portal hypertension. *Wernicke* (ophthalmoplegia, dementia, and ataxia)-*Korsakoff* (amnesia and aphasia, agnosia, or apraxia) syndrome can develop long term due to lack of thiamine.

b. Acute intoxication typically presents with CNS depression and dehydration, though at higher blood alcohol concentrations, cardiopulmonary dysfunction or collapse can occur. Hypoglycemia is common in small children. Acute intoxication is generally treated with supportive care. Alcoholic ketoacidosis can develop secondary to decreased intake of proteins and carbohydrates during alcohol binges, along with other metabolic changes that favor the conversion to free fatty acids and ketogenesis.

c. Alcohol withdrawal symptoms may occur following abrupt discontinuation in chronic users and can include tremors, irritability, and anxiety. Seizures and delirium tremens usually present 72 to 96 hours after the last drink. Withdrawal from chronic alcohol abuse can be lethal if not treated appropriately. Monitoring tools such as the Clinical Institute Withdrawal Assessment (CIWA) in patients who are awake or the Sedation Agitation Scale (SAS) in patients who are sedated or intubated have been developed to recognize and treat withdrawal. Benzodiazepines can lessen symptoms and prevent progression to severe symptoms via their effect on $GABA_A$ receptors. Phenobarbital is another treatment option that affects $GABA_A$ receptors as well but also acts as a direct GABA agonist and blocks glutamate activity at the α-amino-3-hydroxy-5-methyl-4-isoxazolepropionic acid (AMPA) receptor. Clonidine and haloperidol are sometimes used as adjuncts. Propofol, dexmedetomidine, and ketamine may also be effective for patients with more severe symptoms.

2. Methanol and ethylene glycol are both common solvents found in household and industrial materials. They can be ingested recreationally for their sedating and euphoric properties, unintentionally (eg, children drinking antifreeze), or intentionally (eg, attempts at self-harm). Common sources of exposure are antifreeze (ethylene glycol) and windshield wiper fluid (methanol). Methanol is also a potential by-product of ethanol distillation, such as in "moonshine."

a. Both methanol and ethylene glycol are readily absorbed through the GI tract. Methanol is initially metabolized by alcohol dehydrogenase into formaldehyde, which is further metabolized into formate. Ethylene glycol is also metabolized by alcohol dehydrogenase into glycolaldehyde which is then metabolized into glycolic, glyoxylic, and oxalic acids.

b. Both methanol and ethylene glycol produce sedation, stupor, and gastrointestinal distress, akin to early ethanol intoxication. Later, methanol can lead to bright-visual-field or total blindness described as "snow-field blindness." Formate, produced from methanol metabolism, is toxic to the mitochondria and interrupts oxidative phosphorylation. Neurons in the basal ganglia are most sensitive to these effects and may lead to lesions identifiable on CT or MRI. Oxalic acid from ethylene glycol metabolism can lead to acute kidney injury secondary to precipitation of calcium oxalate crystals in the kidneys. Ethylene glycol toxicity can also lead to cardiopulmonary compromise and failure.

c. Diagnosis is typically based on a suspected or reported ingestion of either substance because toxic alcohol serum concentrations are not immediately available. An elevated osmolar gap is evident early after ingestion for both toxic alcohols; however, over time, this normalizes while the anion gap increases from metabolite accumulation. A serum ethanol concentration should also be obtained, as a level greater than 100 mg/dL nearly completely excludes toxicity from toxic alcohols as this ethanol concentration would inhibit metabolism to the toxic metabolites. Calcium oxalate crystals may be seen upon analysis of the urine. Neither methanol nor ethylene glycol poisoning directly leads to significant lactate generation. However, some analyzers mistake glycolic acid and/or glyoxylic acid from ethylene glycol as lactate, thereby reporting a falsely high lactate.

d. Follow stabilization and initiation of supportive care, treatment of methanol and ethylene glycol toxicities typically involves the administration of fomepizole. Both fomepizole and ethanol act as competitive inhibitors of alcohol dehydrogenase, which significantly limits the breakdown of both ethylene glycol and methanol to their toxic metabolites (see dosing in Table 31.5). Fomepizole should typically be given

TABLE 31.5 Dosing Regimen for Ethanol and Fomepizole

Medication	Dose
Ethanol: goal blood alcohol concentration (BAC) of 100-150 mg/dL	Use 10% ethanol in sterile water w/ dextrose: load 7.6 mL/kg over 1 h Maintenance of 0.83 mL/kg/h for nondrinkers and 1.96 mL/kg/h for chronic ethanol users
Fomepizole	Load 15 mg/kg over 30 min Maintenance of 10 mg/kg over 30 min every 12 h for 4 doses[a]

[a]Dosing adjustments based on serum level/pH and if HD has been initiated.

for all suspected or confirmed methanol or ethylene glycol ingestions until confirmatory toxic alcohol concentrations can be obtained. Fomepizole should be continued until the toxic alcohol concentration is predicted or measured to be below 20 mg/dL. Hemodialysis is the definitive treatment for patients who are symptomatic with end-organ toxicity or persistent metabolic acidosis following ingestion of a toxic alcohol. For patients with blood pH less than 7.2, a bolus of sodium bicarbonate followed by an infusion may be considered.

3. **Isopropyl alcohol** is a common household product and key component in antiseptic hand sanitizer. Unlike ethylene glycol and methanol, isopropyl alcohol is the toxic substance instead of metabolites. Isopropyl alcohol is metabolized by alcohol dehydrogenase into acetone. Symptoms include mild GI upset, hemorrhagic gastritis, hypotension, seizures, and coma. Unlike methanol/ethylene glycol poisoning, isopropyl alcohol causes an osmolar gap *without* metabolic acidosis. Treatment is generally supportive.

B. **Opioid** overdoses, including both illegal and prescription opioids, are rapidly increasing. Over 100 000 people die worldwide every year from an opioid overdose, with a majority of those overdoses due to recreational use of synthetic opioids (eg, fentanyl).

1. Many opioids are metabolized in the liver by CYP2D6 and CYP3A4, with some having active metabolites. Opioid overdoses present with somnolence, sedation, respiratory depression, and decreased central response to increasing Pa_{CO_2}. Constricted pupils are a classic finding that does not dissipate with chronic use. Always maintain a high index of suspicion for other coingestants, such as benzodiazepines, sleep aides, acetaminophen, or alcohol. Treatment of opioid overdose includes naloxone to reverse respiratory depression, though the dose selected depends on the patient's history and current condition. Close monitoring is needed as the half-life of naloxone may be shorter than the opioid ingested (eg, methadone), in which case a naloxone infusion may be necessary. Watch for noncardiogenic pulmonary edema when treating with naloxone.
2. Naloxone administration may precipitate acute withdrawal. Opioid withdrawal symptoms may also present while the patient is in the ICU. Withdrawal symptoms are the result of a reflexive increase in sympathetic outflow, resulting in tachycardia, hypertension, diaphoresis, nausea, vomiting, and abdominal pain. Effective treatments include reinstituting low-dose opioids, initiating methadone or buprenorphine, clonidine, and symptomatic treatment.

C. **Benzodiazepines** are used frequently for anxiety, spasms, and sedation in both the inpatient and outpatient settings. Although this class of medications is generally safe, when combined with other substances that have sedative properties (eg, opioids, antidepressants, alcohol), their toxicity is additive.

1. Benzodiazepines provide sedative hypnosis, anterograde amnesia, muscle relaxation, and anxiolysis through their actions on $GABA_A$ receptors. Within the class, there is significant variation between their onset, duration of action, metabolism, and excretion. Symptoms of benzodiazepine overdose are nondescript but include neurologic and respiratory depression. Downtitration or discontinuation of the agent is the primary treatment, aside from traditional supportive care. Flumazenil can be considered, but there is a potential for it to induce acute benzodiazepine withdrawal resulting in seizures. Because its half-life is short, observe the patient closely if long-acting benzodiazepines were ingested.

2. Withdrawal from benzodiazepines occurs after chronic use. Symptoms include anxiety, irritability, sleep disturbances, hallucinations, vomiting, diarrhea, tachycardia, tachypnea, and seizures. Treatment typically consists of supportive care and a prolonged benzodiazepine taper or symptom-triggered management, similar to the treatment of alcohol withdrawal.

VI. NERVE AGENT TOXICITY

A. Nerve agents were first synthesized in the 1930s and are organophosphate (OP) compounds. The three main classes are the G-agents, V-agents, and Novichok agents. The G-agents include GA (tabun), GB (sarin), and GD (soman). V-agents were developed in England and include agents such as VX and VR. The Novichok agents were developed in Russia and are significantly more potent than the other classes. These agents and many others can lead to cholinergic toxicity. The toxic effects of OPs are due to their ability to irreversibly bind and inhibit acetylcholinesterase, thus drastically increasing acetylcholine within nerve synapses at skeletal muscle motor endplates and within the autonomic nervous system. In the central nervous system, OPs cause a release of glutamate which results in seizures. Additionally, with prolonged and uninterrupted exposure to OPs, "aging" occurs whereby the phosphorous moiety on the OP becomes more resistant to displacement by oxime antidotes.

1. Symptoms occur within seconds to minutes of exposure and may include miosis, hypersecretion, fasciculations, convulsions, coma, and death by cardiac and respiratory arrest. Diagnosis is usually clinical but may be aided by confirmatory sampling at the site of exposure. Commonly used memory aids to assist in identifying cholinergic toxicity are SLUDGE (salivation, lacrimation, urination, defecation, gastrointestinal upset, and emesis), DUMBBELLS (diarrhea, urination, miosis, bradycardia, bronchorrhea/bronchospasm, emesis, lacrimation, lethargy, and salivation), and Killer B's (bradycardia, bronchorrhea, and bronchospasm).

2. The first goal of treatment is to ensure the patient is properly decontaminated by removing the patient from the scene of exposure, removing all clothing, and washing them with soap and water. This helps stop the topical absorption of the chemical and prevents exposure to other bystanders and health care workers. For treatment, start with atropine 1 to 3 mg IM or IV along with pralidoxime 2 g IV over 20 to 30 minutes, followed by a pralidoxime infusion of 0.5 g/h. The patient should be frequently reassessed and if symptoms have not resolved, the dose of atropine should be doubled every 5 to 10 minutes until the therapeutic effect is reached. An atropine infusion may be considered for patients with persistent symptoms at a rate of 10% to 20% of the total dose that was needed to reach stability. Titrate atropine off slowly until symptoms remain controlled and continue the pralidoxime infusion for 12 to 24 hours after atropine is complete. Lastly, use benzodiazepines as needed for agitation and seizures.

Selected Readings

Brown CH. Drug-induced serotonin syndrome. *US Pharm.* 2010;35(11):HS-16-HS-21.

Campbell RL, Li JTC, Nicklas RA, Sadosty AT, Members of the Joint Task Force, Practice Parameter Workgroup. Emergency department diagnosis and treatment of anaphylaxis: a practice parameter. *Ann Allergy Asthma Immunol.* 2014;113(6):599-608.

Decker BS, Goldfarb DS, Dargan PI, et al. Extracorporeal treatment for lithium poisoning: systematic review and recommendations from the EXTRIP workgroup. *Clin J Am Soc Nephrol.* 2015;10(5):875-887.

Esser MB, Sherk A, Liu Y, et al. Deaths and years of potential life lost from excessive alcohol use—United States, 2011-2015. *MMWR Morb Mortal Wkly Rep.* 2020;69:981-987.

Goodson CM, Clark BJ, Douglas IS. Predictors of severe alcohol withdrawal syndrome: a systematic review and meta-analysis. *Alcohol Clin Exp Res.* 2014;38(10):2664-2677.

Hampson NB, Piantadosi CA, Thom SR, Weaver LK. Practice recommendations in the diagnosis, management, and prevention of carbon monoxide poisoning. *Am J Respir Crit Care Med.* 2012;186(11):1095-1101.

Juurlink DN, Gosselin S, Kielstein JT, et al. Extracorporeal treatment for salicylate poisoning: systematic review and recommendations from the EXTRIP workgroup. *Ann Emerg Med.* 2015;66(2):165-181.

Krenzelok EP, McGuigan M, Lheur P. Position statement: ipecac syrup. American Academy of Clinical Toxicology; European Association of Poisons Centres and Clinical Toxicologists. *J Toxicol Clin Toxicol.* 1997;35(7):699-709.

Lieberman P, Nicklas RA, Randolph C, et al. Anaphylaxis—a practice parameter update 2015. *Ann Allergy Asthma Immunol.* 2015;115(5):341-384.

Maldonado JR, Sher Y, Ashouri JF, et al. The "Prediction of Alcohol Withdrawal Severity Scale" (PAWSS): systematic literature review and pilot study of a new scale for the prediction of complicated alcohol withdrawal syndrome. *Alcohol.* 2014;48(4):375-390.

Mattson CL, Tanz LJ, Quinn K, Kariisa M, Patel P, Davis NL. Trends and geographic patterns in drug and synthetic opioid overdose deaths—United States, 2013-2019. *MMWR Morb Mortal Wkly Rep.* 2021;70:202–207. doi:10.15585/mmwr.mm7006a4

Nelson L, ed. *Goldfrank's Toxicologic Emergencies.* 11th ed. McGraw-Hill Education; 2019.

Palmer BF, Clegg DJ. Salicylate toxicity. *N Engl J Med.* 2020;382(26):2544-2555.

Schuckit MA, Danko GP, Smith TL, Hesselbrock V, Kramer J, Bucholz K. A 5-year prospective evaluation of DSM-IV alcohol dependence with and without a physiological component. *Alcohol Clin Exp Res.* 2003;27(5):818-825.

Shaker MS, Wallace DV, Golden DBK, et al. Anaphylaxis-a 2020 practice parameter update, systematic review, and Grading of Recommendations, Assessment, Development and Evaluation (GRADE) analysis. *J Allergy Clin Immunol.* 2020;145(4):1082-1123.

Tang A. A practical guide to anaphylaxis. *Am Fam Physician.* 2003;68(7):1325-1332.

Thanacoody R, Caravati EM, Troutman B, et al. Position paper update: whole bowel irrigation for gastrointestinal decontamination of overdose patients. *Clin Toxicol (Phila).* 2015;53(1):5-12.

Turner PJ, Campbell DE, Motosue MS, Campbell RL. Global trends in anaphylaxis epidemiology and clinical implications. *J Allergy Clin Immunol Pract.* 2020;8(4):1169-1176.

32

Adult Resuscitation

Paul S. Jansson

I. OVERVIEW

Cardiopulmonary resuscitation (CPR) is a fundamental skill for the intensivist, who will often be called to manage patients in cardiac arrest as well as in the immediate postresuscitation phase. The algorithms and protocols presented here are based on the American Heart Association 2020 Guidelines for Cardiopulmonary Resuscitation and Emergency Cardiovascular Care. These guidelines represent a set of recommendations for common cardiac arrest scenarios and form the foundation of the team-based approach to resuscitation practiced in the modern critical care unit. In addition to adherence to the routine recertification process, continued multidisciplinary training and frequent simulation of cardiac arrest scenarios in the clinical environment can solidify knowledge, processes, and teamwork, and can identify possible errors and opportunities for improvement.

II. RECOGNITION

Of the many possible interventions in CPR, among the most valuable are the most basic: the provision of **immediate, high-quality CPR** and the **early defibrillation of shockable dysrhythmias.** These interventions are most effective when provided immediately after the arrest. Therefore, **prompt recognition** of cardiac arrest is paramount to ensuring optimal outcomes. Although recognition of cardiac arrest in the ICU may be rapid, due to advanced physiologic monitoring and low nurse-to-patient ratios, the intensivist may be called to lead resuscitation in areas of the hospital with lower intensity of patient monitoring, or even in public areas. **Agonal breathing** represents ineffective ventilation, is present in many patients in cardiac arrest, and may delay the diagnosis of cardiac arrest. Additionally, a peripheral pulse is not reliably identified in many patients, even by health care professionals. Therefore, for the patient who is unresponsive with ineffective respirations, **cardiac arrest should be presumed** and CPR should be initiated along with the activation of the resuscitation team.

III. BASIC LIFE SUPPORT (BLS)

The single most important aspect of resuscitation is the provision of high-quality chest compressions. Although interventions such as advanced airway management and pharmacologic therapy have been integrated into advanced cardiovascular life support (ACLS) and may increase the chances of return of spontaneous circulation (ROSC), they have not been shown to improve survival to hospital discharge or neurologic function. Therefore, the fundamentals of BLS are critical for high-quality resuscitation and **should not be interrupted or delayed for ACLS interventions.**

A. Circulation: Assessment for a **carotid or femoral pulse** should take place immediately and for **at least five and not more than 10 seconds.** If the patient does not definitively have a pulse, chest compressions should be started. **High-quality chest compressions** are performed with the rescuer's hands at the lower half of the sternum at a rate of **100 to 120 compressions per minute.** The chest should be compressed to a **depth of at least 2 inches** and allowed to **completely recoil**

between compressions. Compressions are continued in cycles of **30 compressions to 2 rescue breaths** for the patient receiving facemask ventilation, or **continuously** for the patient with an advanced airway in place. Assessment for high-quality compressions may include the palpation of a pulse, observation of intra-arterial pressure monitoring pulsatility, utilization of a commercial feedback device, transesophageal echocardiography, and observation of quantitative waveform capnography. A firm surface behind the patient is critical to ensure effective compressions and may include deflation of the hospital mattress or placement of a hard backboard. Compressions are **briefly paused every 2 minutes** to allow for evaluation of shockable dysrhythmias or ROSC and should be immediately resumed after defibrillation or return to a perfusing rhythm for additional 2 minutes. Fatigue is common for the individual performing chest compressions; **the compressor should be switched every 2 minutes** in concert with the brief pause, and every effort should be made to minimize the time the patient is not receiving chest compressions. As the team leader, the intensivist should pay close attention to the quality of chest compressions and be ready to **provide constructive feedback** or arrange for a change in the chest compressor if the quality of compressions is not sufficient. **Commercial chest compression devices** are available; they have the advantage of providing fatigue-free and consistent chest compression depth, but their disadvantages include the cost of the device, need for training, and the length of chest compression-free time that may be required to set up the device.

B. Airway: Many patients in the ICU may already have a definitive airway in place. However, for those who do not, assessment and management of the airway are critical. The airway should be opened via the **head tilt-chin lift** maneuver or a **jaw thrust** in a patient for whom cervical spine immobilization must be preserved. An **airway adjunct** such as a nasopharyngeal or oropharyngeal airway may be placed to optimize bag-valve mask ventilation. If resources and training allow, the intensivist may elect to perform **advanced airway maneuvers** including the placement of a supraglottic airway device (such as a laryngeal mask airway) or endotracheal intubation. However, **it is critical that advanced airway maneuvers do not interfere with or distract from the performance of high-quality chest compressions.** Proper placement of the endotracheal tube is confirmed by direct visualization of the endotracheal tube passing between the cords and colorimetric (qualitative) or continuous waveform (quantitative) end-tidal CO_2 measurement. Other methods of confirmation include auscultation of the chest and epigastrium, bronchoscopy, and point-of-care tracheal or lung ultrasonography. More on airway management can be found in **Chapter 4.**

C. Breathing: Adequate ventilation is obtained by a bag-valve mask (BVM) ventilator using 100% inspired oxygen. Patients in the ICU who were receiving mechanical ventilation prior to the cardiac arrest should be disconnected from the mechanical ventilator and ventilated by hand using a BVM device. In the absence of an advanced airway, BVM ventilation should be delivered over one second each in **a ratio of two breaths to every 30 chest compressions** during a brief pause in compressions. When an advanced airway is in place, BVM ventilation should be delivered at a rate of **one breath every 6 seconds or 10 breaths per minute** during continuous compressions. A tidal volume of **500 to 600 mL** should be targeted or be enough to produce visible chest rise. **Excessive ventilation volumes and rates are harmful** during cardiac arrest because of the potential for gastric distension and aspiration in the patient who is nonintubated; additionally, the increase in intrathoracic pressure decreases venous return (preload) to the heart and decreases cardiac output, leading to decreased survival. Excessive ventilation is common in cardiac arrest due to the excitement of the situation, and the team leader must monitor the rate and volume of ventilations to optimize outcomes. Quantitative end-tidal CO_2 ($ETCO_2$) monitoring should be used during ventilation to ensure proper placement of the endotracheal tube, monitor adequacy of ventilation, and guide the quality of chest compressions. Because depth of compressions correlates with an increase in $ETCO_2$, values of less than 10 mm Hg should prompt improvements in the quality of compressions (such as increased depth or rate), until the $ETCO_2$ is above at least 10 mm Hg or ideally greater than 20 mm Hg. $ETCO_2$ may also predict ROSC, with persistent values of less than 10 mm Hg suggesting that ROSC is unlikely and an abrupt increase to 35 to 40 mm Hg suggesting that ROSC has been achieved.

D. **Defibrillation:** Along with high-quality chest compressions, **early defibrillation** for shockable rhythms remains one of the most valuable techniques in CPR. Early defibrillation of ventricular fibrillation (VF) or pulseless ventricular tachycardia (pVT) is highly effective in terminating the malignant rhythm; as time progresses without a shock, efficacy of defibrillation is decreased. Rhythm analysis is typically performed every 2 minutes during a pause in chest compressions; assessment for ROSC is typically performed contemporaneously. The entire process of rhythm analysis should take **less than 10 seconds** and should be followed by the immediate resumption of chest compressions.

1. **Automated External Defibrillators (AEDs)** have become prevalent in many public spaces and may be the first defibrillator available to the intensivist responding to a cardiac arrest outside of the intensive care unit. AEDs utilize a propriety algorithmic software to analyze the native cardiac rhythm, determine whether ventricular tachycardia (VT) or VF exists in the patient, and deliver a defibrillation dose of electricity. Although they have the advantage of being widely available and easily portable, analysis of the rhythm and delivery of the shock often takes longer than that of an experienced intensivist and may increase the time without compressions, which decreases the odds of ROSC.
2. **Manual defibrillators** are universal in the intensive care unit, and the intensivist should be thoroughly experienced and comfortable with the function of the defibrillator utilized at the institution. Most modern defibrillators are **biphasic**, which utilize electrical discharges of opposite polarity, allowing for the delivery of lower doses of electricity and with greater success in terminating dysrhythmias when compared to older **monophasic** defibrillators.
3. **Defibrillation** is performed after the recognition of VT or VF in the rhythm analysis during a brief pause in compressions. Most institutions have replaced hand-held paddles with self-adhesive pads to deliver electricity. The pads should be placed on the bare skin in an **anterolateral** or **anteroposterior** position to allow the electricity to traverse the heart. **Chest compressions should be resumed** while charging the machine, and **clear communication is essential** to ensure that all members of the team are "clear" from the patient before delivering the charge. Chest compressions should resume immediately after defibrillation. In the absence of a clear manufacturer recommendation, **200 J** is commonly used for the initial adult defibrillation dose. Reanalysis of the heart rhythm and repeat defibrillation, if necessary, should occur 2 minutes later at the next pulse/rhythm check. Subsequent defibrillations should utilize the **maximum electrical dose** available from the defibrillator.
4. **Controversial issues**: Some defibrillator manufacturers have created **artifact-filtering algorithms** to attempt to display the underlying cardiac rhythm, which is often obscured by the artifact of chest compressions. Although this may be of value in shortening the rhythm check period, these algorithms have yet to be proven in clinical practice. Case reports have

described the use of two defibrillators simultaneously to deliver **double sequential defibrillation** in refractory VT/VF. However, such techniques may damage the defibrillator and have not been shown to improve survival and so remain experimental at this point.

IV. ALGORITHM

An algorithm for the management of pulseless arrest is given in Figure 32.1.

V. VASCULAR ACCESS

Peripheral intravenous access is important for effective medication administration and is typically the first-line approach, but may be difficult to obtain under emergent conditions or low-flow states. **Intraosseous (IO) access** may be swiftly achieved, typically at the anterior tibia or proximal humeral sites, and has the advantage of reliable external landmarks and a noncollapsible insertion site. In the absence of reliable intravenous access, IO placement is a reasonable first-line approach for medication delivery during CPR. For the patient in the ICU with preexisting **central venous access**, this route provides rapid circulation time and peak concentrations of medications but can be difficult and time-consuming to obtain during chest compressions. **Endotracheal** administration of medications can be used, but due to the erratic medication absorption and ready availability of superior options, its use is discouraged. **Regardless of the route of vascular access chosen, obtaining access should not interfere with the provision of high-quality chest compressions and early defibrillation.**

VI. MEDICATIONS

A. Epinephrine remains the most important medication in ACLS, although the evidence to support its use is limited. Although the α-adrenergic effects are beneficial and **increase coronary and cerebral perfusion pressures,** the β-adrenergic effects may be harmful and include an increase in myocardial oxygen demand and ischemia, proarrhythmic effects, and a decrease in subendocardial perfusion. Epinephrine increases survival to hospitalization in the prehospital setting and rates of ROSC, but there is no neurologic benefit to survivors. Epinephrine is administered as a **1-mg bolus IV/IO** (of the 1:10 000 concentration) every 3 to 5 minutes until ROSC is achieved. It should be given **as early as possible in nonshockable arrests** and **after the first defibrillation in shockable arrest.**

B. Amiodarone is a class III antiarrhythmic that blocks sodium, potassium, and calcium channels as well as β-adrenergic receptors to decrease myocardial excitability and prolong the cardiac refractory period. It is used **for VF or pulseless ventricular tachycardia (pVT) at a dose of 300 mg.** Amiodarone may be redosed two cycles later **if the VF/pVT persists at a dose of 150 mg.** When given for stable VT or atrial fibrillation with rapid ventricular response, a loading protocol of 150 mg over 10 minutes followed by an infusion of 1 mg/min for 6 hours and then 0.5 mg/min for 18 hours is used.

C. Lidocaine is a local anesthetic which is a class Ib antiarrhythmic with sodium channel-blocking properties. It is a second-line agent for VF/pVT after amiodarone due to inferior rates of ROSC and higher rates of asystole. If chosen in place of amiodarone, the initial dose is 1 to 1.5 mg/kg IV/IO whereas a secondary dose is given approximately 5 minutes later at a dose of 0.5 to 0.75 mg/kg.

D. Sodium bicarbonate should not be routinely used during cardiac arrest due to its harmful effects, including paradoxical worsening of intracellular acidosis. It is best reserved for specific scenarios where it may be of benefit, such as hyperkalemia, tricyclic antidepressant overdose, or severe metabolic acidosis. The initial sodium bicarbonate dose is 1 mEq/kg, with a repeat dose of 0.5 mEq/kg given at subsequent 10-minute intervals.

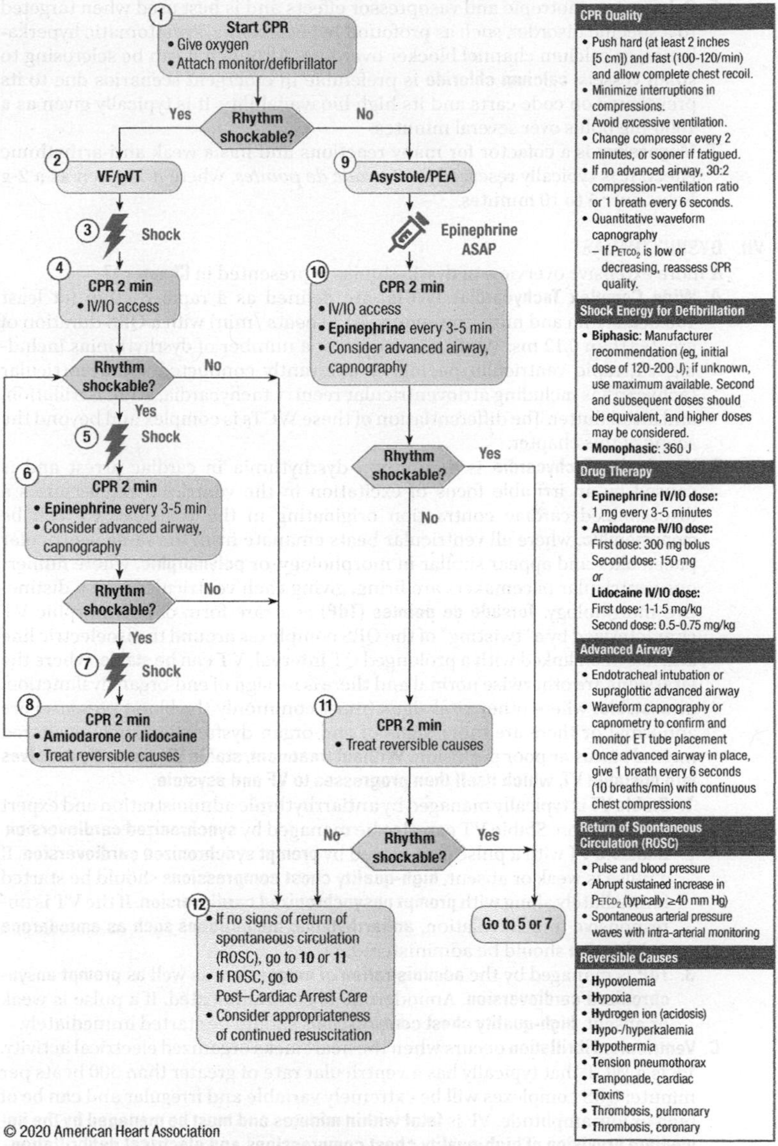

FIGURE 32.1 Adult cardiac arrest algorithm. CPR, cardiopulmonary resuscitation; ET, endotracheal; IO, intraosseous; IV, intravenous; PEA, pulseless electrical activity; pVT, pulseless ventricular tachycardia; VF, ventricular fibrillation. (From Panchal AR, Bartos JA, Cabañas JG, et al. Part 3: adult basic and advanced life support: 2020 American Heart Association guidelines for cardiopulmonary resuscitation and emergency cardiovascular care. *Circulation.* 2020;142(suppl 2):S366-S468.)

E. **Calcium** has inotropic and vasopressor effects and is best used when targeted to a specific disorder, such as profound hypocalcemia, symptomatic hyperkalemia, or calcium channel blocker overdose. Although it can be sclerosing to small vessels, **calcium chloride** is preferable in emergent scenarios due to its prevalence on code carts and its high bioavailability. It is typically given as a 1000-mg bolus over several minutes.

F. **Magnesium** is a cofactor for many reactions and has a weak anti-arrhythmic effect. It is typically reserved for *torsade de pointes*, where it is given as a 2-g bolus over 5 to 10 minutes.

VII. DYSRHYTHMIAS

A more extensive overview of dysrhythmias is presented in **Chapter 17**.

A. **Wide Complex Tachycardias (WCTs)** are defined as a rapid rhythm (at least 100 beats/min and most commonly >150 beats /min) with a QRS duration of greater than 0.12 ms. WCTs can represent a number of dysrhythmias including VT, rapid ventricular pacing, or aberrantly conducted supraventricular tachycardias including atrioventricular reentry tachycardia, atrial fibrillation, and atrial flutter. The differentiation of these WCTs is complex and beyond the scope of this chapter.

B. **Ventricular Tachycardia** is a common dysrhythmia in cardiac arrest and is caused by an irritable focus of excitation in the ventricle, which causes a disorganized cardiac contraction originating in the ventricle. VT can be **monomorphic**, where all ventricular beats emanate from the same ventricular pacemaker and appear similar in morphology, or **polymorphic**, where numerous ventricular pacemakers are firing, giving each ventricular beat a distinctive morphology. **Torsade de pointes (TdP)** is a rare form of polymorphic VT characterized by a "twisting" of the QRS complexes around the isoelectric line and has been linked with a prolonged QT interval. VT can be **stable**, where the vital signs are otherwise normal and there is no sign of end-organ dysfunction, or **unstable**, where other vital signs (most commonly the blood pressure) are abnormal or there are other signs of end-organ dysfunction such as altered mental status or poor perfusion. **Without treatment, stable VT generally devolves into unstable VT, which itself then progresses to VF and asystole.**

1. **Stable VT** is typically managed by antiarrhythmic administration and expert consultation. Stable VT can also be managed by **synchronized cardioversion.**
2. **Unstable VT** with a pulse is managed by **prompt synchronized cardioversion.** If a pulse is weak or absent, **high-quality chest compressions** should be started immediately along with **prompt unsynchronized cardioversion.** If the VT is unresponsive to defibrillation, **antiarrhythmic medications such as amiodarone or lidocaine** should be administered.
3. **TdP** is managed by the **administration of magnesium** as well as **prompt unsynchronized cardioversion.** Amiodarone is contraindicated. If a pulse is weak or absent, **high-quality chest compressions** should be started immediately.

C. **Ventricular Fibrillation** occurs when the heart lacks organized electrical activity. VF is a WCT that typically has a ventricular rate of greater than 300 beats per minute; QRS complexes will be extremely variable and irregular and can be of high or low amplitude. VF is **fatal within minutes and must be managed by the immediate provision of high-quality chest compressions and electrical defibrillation.**

D. **Pulseless Electrical Activity (PEA)** occurs when an electrical tracing (typically of a narrow complex rhythm) is noted on monitoring equipment without a corresponding mechanical contraction of the heart. Although some cardiac movement may be visible on ultrasound, any cardiac output is insufficient and should be **managed with high-quality chest compressions and epinephrine** while the underlying cause of the PEA is sought.

E. **Asystole** occurs when there is a lack of both electrical activity in the heart and mechanical contraction of the heart. Management of asystole is the **same as PEA.**

VIII. **CAUSES OF CARDIAC ARREST** are complex and numerous, but are classically taught and remembered as the **H's and T's.** During a cardiac arrest, a focused search for the cause of the arrest should be undertaken with concurrent management. As laboratory testing and imaging may not yield results in the appropriate time frame, empirical management of suspected conditions may need to be pursued. **Point-of-care ultrasonography** or other focused testing can be helpful in identifying reversible causes, but **should not be performed at the expense of high-quality chest compressions.**

A. **Hypovolemia** is a common cause of arrest in the patient undergoing trauma. Administration of blood (for hemorrhagic shock) and control of the bleeding should be identified. More on trauma can be found in **Chapter 9.** For nontraumatic hypovolemic shock, bolus crystalloid fluids should be administered.

B. **Hypoxia** is the most common cause of cardiac arrest. Airway management with attention to oxygenation and ventilation is prioritized for these patients. More on airway management can be found in **Chapter 4.**

C. **Hydrogen Ion** excess (acidosis) can be difficult to correct in cardiac arrest. Attention should be paid to the underlying cause of the acidosis. Sodium bicarbonate or tromethamine (THAM) can be used as temporizing measures. More on acid-base management can be found in **Chapter 8.**

D. **Hyperkalemia** is more commonly encountered in cardiac arrest than hypokalemia. It is managed by the administration of intravenous calcium, insulin with glucose, albuterol, and sodium bicarbonate. **Hypokalemia** is managed by potassium infusion. **Hypermagnesemia** is typically only seen in the obstetric setting and rarely causes cardiac arrest. **Hypomagnesemia** is managed by magnesium infusion. More on electrolytes can be found in **Chapter 8.**

E. **Hypothermia** can cause profound bradycardia and cardiovascular collapse. Because complete neurologic recovery can occur even with profound hypothermia and asystole, resuscitative efforts should be pursued in concert with active rewarming of the patient until the patient approaches euthermia. In contrast to standard resuscitation, defibrillation and epinephrine are typically used more sparingly due to the impaired metabolism of the patient.

F. **Tension pneumothorax** can be identified by physical examination or lack of lung sliding on point-of-care ultrasound in the appropriate clinical setting and is managed by prompt needle decompression of the affected side of the thorax, followed by tube thoracostomy.

G. **Tamponade (Cardiac)** is managed by infusion of fluids to augment preload of the heart and emergent pericardiocentesis.

H. **Toxins** are common causes of cardiac arrest and could fill an entire toxicology textbook. Management is focused on the offending agent. Toxins are discussed more in **Chapter 30.**

I. **Thrombosis (Coronary)** is a common cause of cardiac arrest, particularly in the subset of patients with shockable rhythms. Postarrest management of these patients focuses on prompt coronary angiography and percutaneous coronary intervention (PCI) of the culprit lesion. Coronary disease is further discussed in **Chapter 15.**

J. **Thrombosis (Pulmonary)** occurs with fulminant, massive pulmonary embolism. If traditional resuscitative efforts have not led to ROSC, emergent thrombolysis can be considered a salvage maneuver. Embolectomy is typically pursued after cardiac arrest if ROSC is achieved. Pulmonary embolism is covered more in **Chapter 22.**

IX. POSTRESUSCITATION CARE

Postresuscitation care is a critical aspect of resuscitation and attempts to avoid ischemia-reperfusion injury caused by cardiac arrest. After a cardiac arrest, the patient is often critically ill with **multiple organ system failure.** Close attention must be paid to identifying the cause of cardiac arrest, hemodynamics, mechanical ventilation and critical care, temperature management, and neuroprognostication.

A. **Identification and management of the underlying cause is critical** to the management of the patient after cardiac arrest. A 12-lead electrocardiogram (EKG) should be obtained after ROSC, and PCI should be pursued if signs of **acute ST-segment elevation** are noted or if the patient exhibits unstable cardiogenic shock or requires mechanical circulatory support.
B. **Hemodynamics** should be closely managed, **targeting a systolic blood pressure greater than 90 mm Hg** or a **mean arterial pressure greater than 65 mm Hg.** More on hemodynamic monitoring and management can be found in **Chapters 2** and **6**, respectively.
C. **Mechanical Ventilation** should target a **normal oxygen saturation** (92%-98%) while **avoiding hypoxia or hyperoxia. $Paco_2$ levels** should be kept in the normal range (35-45 mm Hg). More on mechanical ventilation can be found in **Chapter 5.**
D. **Targeted Temperature Management (TTM)** should be pursued if the patient is **comatose** after cardiac arrest. CT of the head and EEG should be obtained. Although the specific temperature and duration is controversial, most institutions **target a core temperature of 32°C to 36°C for 24 hours,** followed by a several-day period of normothermia. Clinically apparent seizures should be treated with antiepileptics.
E. **Neuroprognostication** becomes important for the patient after arrest who is comatose because hypoxic-ischemic brain injury can be devastating after cardiac arrest. Tools for neuroprognostication include **imaging** (typically MRI), **electrophysiology** (including EEG), **clinical examination** (including reflex testing), and **serum biomarkers.** Because its utility is limited in the immediate postarrest period, **neuroprognostication should be delayed until at least 72 hours after normothermia is achieved,** in the absence of other compelling reasons to withdraw life-sustaining treatments.

X. SPECIAL SCENARIOS

A. **Postcardiac Surgery** patients have unique anatomy and physiology. Because of the high rate of VT and VF in the immediate postoperative period and the risk of damage to the surgical site, **sequential defibrillation should be pursued for up to 1 minute before initiating chest compressions.** As most of these patients will have pacing leads in place, **temporary pacing should be attempted before chest compressions for symptomatic bradycardia or asystole** in the immediate postoperative period. Even small amounts of blood in the pericardium can cause tamponade, therefore **emergency resternotomy with open cardiac massage and defibrillation** should be pursued if qualified staff are available.
B. **Pregnancy** requires several modifications to standard resuscitation. In addition to high-quality chest compressions, the **uterus should be manually displaced to the left** to avoid compression of the vena cava and decreasing venous return. **Oxygenation and ventilation** should be prioritized as well, given the increased maternal metabolism and the sensitivity of the fetus to hypoxia. **Resuscitation of the mother should take priority** over monitoring or management of the fetus. However, if ROSC is not achieved within 5 minutes and the fetus is of a survivable gestational age, **preparations should be made for an emergent perimortem cesarean delivery.** More on critical care of the pregnant patient can be found in **Chapter 34.**
C. **Extracorporeal CPR (ECPR)** involves the **initiation of veno-arterial extracorporeal membrane oxygenation (VA-ECMO)** to the patient during resuscitative efforts. ECPR can provide cardiac output, ventilation, and oxygenation support to the patient **while the underlying condition is addressed.** VA-ECMO is an extremely resource-intensive intervention and so appropriate patient selection is key for optimal outcomes. More on ECMO can be found in **Chapter 19.**
D. **Do Not Resuscitate (DNR) orders** are advance directives by the patient that express the patient's wishes in the event that they should require CPR. Careful identification of the patient's advanced directives should be made to provide

care that is consistent with the patient's wishes. For patients without a DNR order who are at high risk for poor outcomes after CPR, the intensivist should consider **prompt and candid discussions with the patient's health care proxy** about those outcomes to ensure that continued resuscitative efforts are within the patient's goals of care. More on ethics and recovery after critical illness can be found in **Chapters 36** and **40**, respectively.

XI. **TERMINATION OF RESUSCITATION (TOR)** is an integral aspect of CPR and recognizes that CPR is a resource-intensive treatment with low rates of survival. Prehospital criteria for TOR have been developed and typically recommend TOR for **unwitnessed arrest, lack of shockable rhythm, and lack of ROSC in the field.** Although there is no absolute rule to suggest TOR in the hospital, **$ETCO_2$ of less than 10 mm Hg after 20 minutes of resuscitation in the patient who is intubated is strongly suggestive of futility.** Lack of any cardiac motion on point-of-care ultrasound can support the decision to terminate prolonged resuscitative efforts and the patient's comorbidities, premorbid functional status, and goals of care should all be considered in determining the appropriate duration of resuscitative efforts.

XII. **TEAMWORK AND LEADERSHIP**

CPR is an intensive treatment that requires a multidisciplinary team to seamlessly and rapidly collaborate in a high-stakes, high-stress environment. Some teams may be highly practiced at CPR whereas others may have never worked together. The intensivist is commonly the leader of this team and must act to **ensure roles are clear.** Specific roles in CPR include but are not limited to the compressor, airway manager, medication administration, documentation, quality control, proceduralist, and pharmacist. The team leader should use **clear, directed communication** and team members should utilize **closed-loop communication.** All nonessential communications should be kept to a minimum. After the termination of the resuscitation, a team **debrief** can be useful to reinforce successes and to identify opportunities for future improvement. Simulated resuscitations can also be helpful in recognizing system errors and potential solutions before they reach the patient.

Selected Readings

American Heart Association. 2020 American Heart Association guidelines for cardiopulmonary resuscitation and emergency cardiovascular care. *Circulation.* 2020;142(suppl 2):S366-S468.

Anderson LW, Holmberg MJ, Berg KM, et al. In-hospital cardiac arrest: a review. *JAMA.* 2019;321(12):1200-1210.

Bergum D, Haugen BO, Nordseth T, et al. Recognizing the causes of in-hospital cardiac arrest—a survival benefit. *Resuscitation.* 2015;97:91-96.

Cunningham LM, Mattu A, O'Connor RE, et al. Cardiopulmonary resuscitation for cardiac arrest: the importance of uninterrupted chest compressions in cardiac arrest resuscitation. *Am J Emerg Med.* 2012;30(8):1630-1638.

Dankiewicz J, Crongerg T, Lilja G, et al. Hypothermia versus normothermia after out-of-hospital cardiac arrest. *N Engl J Med.* 2021;384(24):2283-2294.

Hosseini M, Wilson RH, Crouzet C, et al. Resuscitating the globally ischemic brain: TTM and beyond. *Neurotherapeutics.* 2020;17(2):539-562.

Hunziker S, Johansson AC, Tschan F, et al. Teamwork and leadership in cardiopulmonary resuscitation. *J Am Coll Cardiol.* 2011;57(24):2381-2388.

Johnson NJ, Carlbom DJ, Gaiesky DF. Ventilator management and respiratory care after cardiac arrest: oxygenation, ventilation, infection, and injury. *Chest.* 2018;153(6):1477-1477.

Lascarrou J-B, Merdji H, Le Gouge A, et al. Targeted temperature management for cardiac arrest with nonshockable rhythm. *N Engl J Med.* 2019;381(24):2327-2337.

Perkins GD, Ji C, Deakin CD. A Randomized trial of epinephrine in out-of-hospital cardiac arrest. *N Engl J Med.* 2018;379:711-721.

33 Burn Critical Care

Chiaka O. V. Akarichi, Benjamin Levi, Victor W. Wong, and Robert Sheridan

I. INTRODUCTION

A. Scope of the Problem in the United States

1. Burns are a major source of morbidity: approximately 2 million burns occur per year. Burns result in approximately 40 000 hospitalizations and over 3000 deaths per year. Total health care expenditures approach 4 billion dollars per year. Recent reports demonstrate a 50% decline in burn-related deaths and hospital admissions over the past 30 years.
2. Patients with large burns should be cared for as are other critical care cases—providers should make sure to assess all organ systems. Although formulas for fluid resuscitation are well known, it is important to assess the resuscitative progress similar to the resuscitative efforts of other patients who are critically ill. Critical illness in patients with burns is most often caused by sepsis, and burn wound sepsis is no longer seen as frequently because of aggressive early debridement. In fact, pneumonia is the most common cause of sepsis in such patients.

B. The First Steps of the Overall Critical Care Management Plan are the initial assessment and resuscitation, followed by early wound excision and biologic closure either with autograft (if available) or allograft within 96 hours. Although rehabilitation occurs almost immediately, once definitive wound closure is achieved, aggressive rehabilitation can begin. Throughout the execution of this plan, the physiologic effects of burn injury must also be kept in mind. They are as follows:

1. Early hypodynamic "ebb" phase: early hours after injury with low cardiac output, hypodynamic state requiring aggressive critical support
2. Hyperdynamic "flow" phase: After the first few hours, the patient will develop increased cardiac output, increased muscle catabolism, and decreased peripheral vascular resistance.
3. Massive capillary leak: This is thought to result from burn wound inflammatory mediators.
4. Postresuscitative phase: Volume requirements often decline after the first 24 hours and capillary leak decreases. Patient then has a hyperdynamic phase with fever and increased protein catabolism. Inflammatory mediators such as tumor necrosis factor-α (TNF-α), interferon-γ (IFN-γ), and interleukin (IL)-6 and IL-10 are released.

II. COMPONENTS OF PRIMARY SURVEY IN PATIENTS WITH BURNS

During their initial evaluation, patients with burns should have a primary survey according to the advanced burn life support guidelines. The components of this are the following:

A. Airway: Signs and symptoms of airway compromise include inability to phonate, hoarseness, gurgling sounds, stridor, and difficulty swallowing. An airway assessment should include an intraoral and intranasal examination for soot and mucosal inflammation. The assessment should also include assessment for concomitant facial or neck injury. A cervical collar should be placed to protect the cervical spine if concomitant trauma cannot be ruled out. It is important to establish definitive airway before transport, especially if large fluid requirements are estimated (>30% total body surface area [TBSA]). Even without airway injury, patients develop progressive mucosal edema from massive inflammation and fluid requirements. For airway burns, it is crucial to evaluate for deep burns of the face, eyes, neck, and nasopharynx, including soot in these regions. Get a detailed history of where the patient sustained the burn because inhalation injuries rarely occur in nonenclosed spaces. Assess whether patient was exposed to chemicals or carbon monoxide. If carboxyhemoglobin levels are elevated, administer 100% humidified oxygen. In accordance with the advanced trauma life support guidelines, intubate for Glasgow Coma Score that is less than 8. When intubating, make sure an airway assessment is performed initially. If patient has a difficult anatomy, it is important to have fiberoptic setup, bougie, and surgical consultation in case a surgical airway is necessary. The patient's hemodynamics should be assessed before intubation. Typical induction medications can include propofol (make sure patient is not hypotensive) or etomidate (may get delayed adrenal insufficiency) and rocuronium as the paralytic. Avoid succinylcholine because this can result in lethal levels of hyperkalemia. All the aforementioned induction agents cause hypotension, so providers should be prepared with a vasopressor such as intravenous (IV) phenylephrine. Studies demonstrate that ketamine might represent an alternative with less hypotensive effects.

B. Breathing: Once a patient is intubated, it is crucial to assess the location of the tube through visualization of moisture in the endotracheal tube, bilateral chest rise, auscultation of bilateral lung fields, and end-tidal CO_2 capnography. A chest radiograph should be obtained to confirm that the endotracheal tube tip is 3 to 5 cm above the carina. Take care when securing the endotracheal tube around the head to prevent a potential tourniquet effect because the patient becomes edematous during resuscitation. If carbon monoxide poisoning is of concern, the patient should be given 100% FIO_2 to decrease the half-life of circulating carbon monoxide. It is important to note that patients with circumferential or near-circumferential, deep chest burns may have decreased respiratory excursions secondary to the constrictive burn eschar. This will present with increased rapid, shallow breaths, and increased peak airway pressures on the ventilator, resulting in respiratory embarrassment. These patients will require chest escharotomy.

C. Circulation: Assess the heart rate and blood pressure. It is important to obtain two large-bore IV accesses with 16 or 18G peripheral IVs. It is better to place the access in nonburned areas, although this is not always possible. If the patient is going to require invasive monitoring, a central line should be placed under sterile conditions. Blood pressure cuffs can be difficult to obtain an accurate read, making arterial lines useful. If a PiCCO® device (PULSION Medical Systems SE, Feldkirchen, Germany) is used to monitor the patient, it is best to have the central line in the internal jugular vein and the arterial line in the femoral artery. This technology uses thermodilution to determine cardiac performance. A FloTrac® system (Edwards Lifesciences, Irvine, CA), which uses only the arterial pressure waveform from an existing arterial line, can be used to monitor advanced hemodynamic parameters. Studies have demonstrated the feasibility of these technologies compared to the pulmonary artery (PA) catheter. It is during this part in the primary survey that peripheral circulation of burned extremities is assessed. Limb escharotomies may be necessary for limbs with circumferential or near-circumferential deep burns to prevent limb compartment syndrome.

D. Disability/Neurologic Assessment: Using the "AVPU" mnemonic, evaluate whether the patient is **A**lert, responsive to **V**erbal stimuli, responsive to **P**ainful stimuli only, or **U**nresponsive, which might help assess whether the patient is hypoxic, hypercarbic, or altered. Obtain a baseline Glasgow Coma Scale score by assessing eye opening, best verbal response, and best motor response. The neurologic assessment should include a pupillary examination and gross motor function. Make sure that there are no other injuries.

E. Exposure and Environmental Control: It is important to remove all clothing, especially if a chemical injury is sustained. This includes all jewelry (eg, rings, watches, piercings), contacts, undergarments, and diapers. Jewelry left in place can create a tourniquet effect once swelling begins. It is necessary to decontaminate with copious water irrigation before transport.

III. BURN-SPECIFIC SECONDARY SURVEY

The secondary survey is in accordance with the advanced burn life support guidelines.

A. History: mechanism and timing of injury. Was there chemical exposure and, if so, what are the side effects of this chemical; was the patient inside or outside; was there any risk of inhalation injury; neurologic status; extrication time; fluids and medications given on scene and during transport; tetanus status; code status; and decision-makers?

The mnemonic "AMPLET" should be used with history taking: **A**, allergies; **M**, medications; **P**, past medical history; **L**, last meal; **E**, events leading to injury/mechanism/timing; and **T**, tetanus status.

B. Weight: the patient's weight (in kilograms) before the burn

C. "Head-to-Toe" Physical Examination

1. **Head/face:** detailed orbital and periorbital exam. Electrical injury increases the risk of glaucoma. Massive fluid resuscitation can cause intraocular compartment syndrome. Ophthalmology consult should be obtained if there is concern about corneal injury, and they should perform a fluorescein dye test. If there is conjunctival swelling, the patient may not be able to close the eyelids. If this is the case, consider temporary tarsorrhaphy. Large-volume irrigation of globes with neutral pH solution is required, especially if it is a chemical injury. Examine the nose for singed vibrissae. Perform an intraoral exam to look for swelling and carbonaceous sputum.
2. **Neck:** cervical spine assessment. Leave cervical collar and proceed with cervical spine imaging if cervical spine cannot be cleared clinically. Assess for signs of injury to the soft tissues of the neck or other important structures within the neck (ie, carotid artery, jugular vein, and tracheal or esophageal injury).
3. **Chest:** Assess chest compliance and whether eschar is limiting chest excursion and decreasing compliance.
4. **Abdomen:** Patient may require abdominal escharotomy for large-volume resuscitation to avoid abdominal compartment syndrome. If patient develops abdominal compartment syndrome, it should be addressed by making sure adequate escharotomy is done, laying the patient supine, making sure the patient has a nasogastric tube, treating pain, and starting a paralytic (not succinylcholine) if needed. If these measures fail, the patient will need a laparotomy, which has extremely high mortality in patients with burns.
5. **Perineum:** Early Foley catheter placement allows for close monitoring of urine output and, therefore, of kidney perfusion. Deeply burned foreskin may affect penile perfusion.
6. **Musculoskeletal:** important to examine all extremities (proximal and distal) for compartment syndrome. Unlike crush injury or electrical injury (caused by immobile fascia), flame and scald burns cause compartment syndrome by creating an immobile skin layer. The most sensitive exam finding for compartment syndrome is pain with passive movement; however, this may not be possible in a patient who is intubated. Important

to assess distal two-point discrimination (normal <6 mm) and arterial pulses. By the time there is a change in neurologic or vascular exam of the extremity, it is usually too late. If it is an electrical injury, it is important to monitor serum creatine kinase (CK), and, in addition to escharotomy, the patient will require fasciotomy to release deeper compartments.

7. **Back/buttock:** Assess via log roll for obvious injuries, deformities, and burns.
8. **Vascular:** Assess for the presence and quality of pulses in all four limbs, as well as capillary refill in digits.
9. **Neurologic:** Abnormal neurologic exam may indicate carbon monoxide exposure.

D. **Burn Severity:** crucial to assess TBSA and depth of all burns. A burn wound can be characterized by three zones of injury (Figure 33.1). The zone of coagulation has undergone direct injury. The zone of stasis can go on to heal or progress to become a part of the zone of coagulation. The zone of hyperemia has been injured the least and will typically go on to heal.

1. **Total body surface area:** This can be done using a Lund and Browder burn diagram. "Rule of 9's" estimates that surface area for each upper extremity is 9%, lower extremity 18%, anterior chest/abdomen 18%, back 18%, and head 9% (Figure 33.2). In children, the head is 18% and the lower extremities are each 14%. Alternatively, one can use the "palmar method" to estimate the burn area. This method assigns 1% TBSA to the patient's palm.

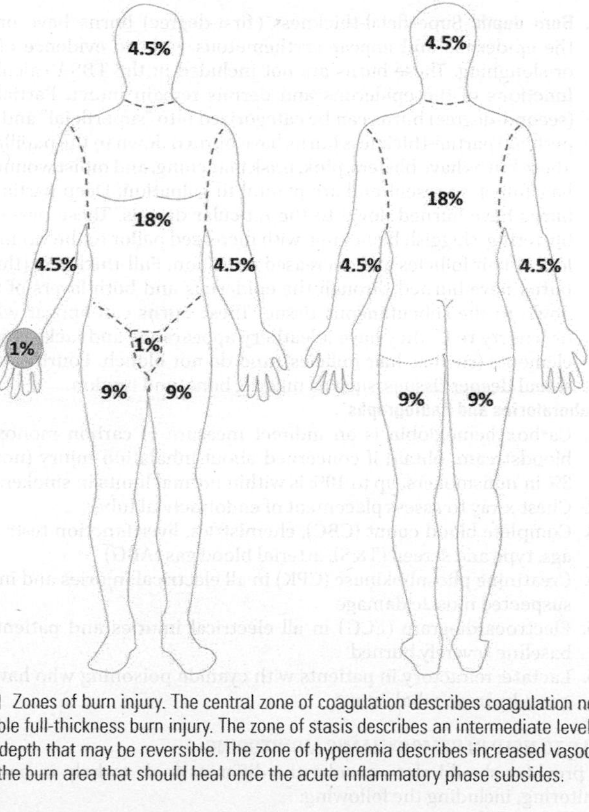

FIGURE 33.1 Zones of burn injury. The central zone of coagulation describes coagulation necrosis and irreversible full-thickness burn injury. The zone of stasis describes an intermediate level of injury severity and depth that may be reversible. The zone of hyperemia describes increased vasodilation surrounding the burn area that should heal once the acute inflammatory phase subsides.

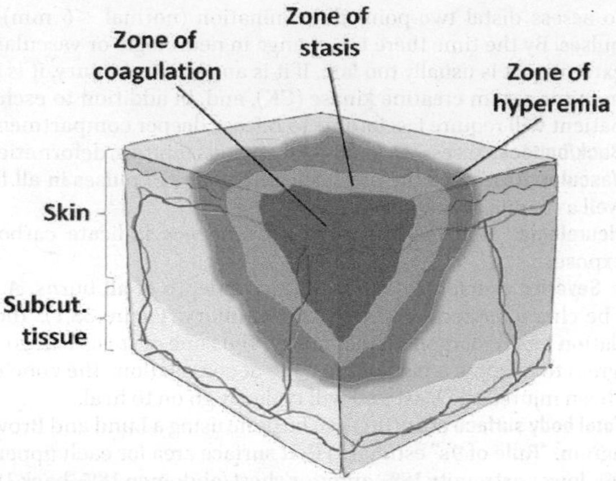

FIGURE 33.2 Schematic of "Rule of 9's" to estimate burn surface area in adults. Anterior (left panel) and posterior (right panel) views of body. Area of palm approximates 1% total body surface area.

2. **Burn depth:** Superficial-thickness (first-degree) burns have only burned the epidermis and appear erythematous with no evidence of blistering or sloughing. These burns are not included in the TBSA calculation. The functions of the epidermis and dermis remain intact. Partial-thickness (second-degree) burns can be categorized into "superficial" and "deep." Superficial partial-thickness burns have burned down to the papillary dermis. These burns have blisters, pink, brisk blanching, and moist wound base with hair follicles present and are painful to palpation. Deep partial-thickness burns have burned down to the reticular dermis. These burns may have blistering, sluggish blanching, with increased pallor to the wound base and loss of hair follicles and decreased sensation. Full-thickness (third-degree) burns have burned through the epidermis and both layers of the dermis down to the subcutaneous tissue. These burns can appear white, black, or "cherry red." They have a leathery appearance and lack sensation, skin elements (such as hair follicles), and do not blanch. Fourth-degree burns reveal deeper tissues, such as muscle, bone, and tendon.

E. Laboratories and Radiographs

1. Carboxyhemoglobin is an indirect measure of carbon monoxide in the bloodstream; obtain if concerned about inhalation injury (normal up to 3% in nonsmokers, up to 10% is within normal limits in smokers).
2. Chest x-ray to assess placement of endotracheal tube
3. Complete blood count (CBC), chemistries, liver function tests (LFTs), coags, type and screen (T&S), arterial blood gas (ABG)
4. Creatinine phosphokinase (CPK) in all electrical injuries and injuries with suspected muscle damage
5. Electrocardiogram (ECG) in all electrical injuries and patients who are baseline severely burned
6. Lactate: refractory in patients with cyanide poisoning who have not been given hydroxocobalamin

IV. TOOLS TO HELP IN HEMODYNAMIC MONITORING

The provider should also consider the different tools to help in hemodynamic monitoring, including the following:

A. Central venous pressure trend can be used to assess progress of resuscitation, although the absolute numbers have limited value.

B. Arterial lines can be helpful given difficulty using cuff pressures in very edematous extremities.

1. The FloTrak® system uses the arterial waveform obtained from an arterial catheter and may be used to obtain advanced hemodynamic parameters, such as cardiac output, cardiac index, stroke volume, and stroke volume variation. Systemic vascular resistance can be calculated when central venous pressure that is transduced from a central line is entered.
2. The arterial line with central venous catheter can also be used to assess cardiac output when using the PiCCO® system. This allows the provider to trend values, which may be more valuable than are absolute numbers.

C. Pulmonary Artery Catheters: As in other areas of critical care, the PA catheter allows for goal-directed therapy. Studies have failed to show improvements in outcomes using PA catheters. They may be more useful in older patients with histories of cardiac disease. Overall, PA catheters have largely been replaced by the abovementioned less invasive monitoring systems and point-of-care bedside ultrasound, which uses direct visualization of the heart to evaluate cardiac function and estimates volume status by assessing inferior vena cava (IVC) compressibility.

V. MECHANICAL VENTILATION

Similarly, mechanical ventilation can be employed with the following considerations:

A. Early endotracheal intubation is important in patients with inhalation injury or who have burns with significant TBSA involvement. Airway protection is needed in patients requiring large-volume resuscitation. Other common indications for intubation include hypoxia and hypercarbia with or without inhalation injury.

B. Follow ARDSNet protocol recommendations of lung-protective ventilation with low-volume protective lung ventilation: 4 to 6 mL/kg; plateau airway pressures should not exceed 30 cm H_2O. Positive end-expiratory pressure (PEEP) of at least 5 cm H_2O should be used to avoid derecruitment. Recruitment maneuvers may be needed (eg, 30 mm Hg for 30 seconds). Permissive hypercapnia is preferred over large tidal volumes. The use of high-frequency percussive ventilation (HFPV) remains controversial. However, there are some studies that report improvement in oxygenation, ventilation, and mortality with the use of HFPV in patients with inhalation injury. Keep head of bed (HOB) 30° to decrease swelling and to prevent aspiration and ventilator-associated pneumonia (VAP) in all patients who are on ventilation. Daily mouth care with chlorhexidine should be used for patients who are on ventilation. Spontaneous breathing trials and cuff leak assessment should be done when considering extubation.

C. When there is evidence or concern of carbon monoxide poisoning, fraction of inspired oxygen (FIO_2) should be set at 100% for the initial 6 hours to decrease the half-life of circulating carbon monoxide.

VI. CONSIDERATIONS SURROUNDING RESUSCITATIVE STRATEGIES

Similarly, the following considerations surrounding resuscitative strategies should be employed and are temporally bound:

A. First 24 Hours: Expect massive fluid shifts in both burned and nonburned tissues in patients with more than 20% TBSA burns. Release of proinflammatory mediators such as TNF-α, histamine, and leukotrienes leads to increased microvascular permeability, edema, and shock. In general, resuscitation should be considered in adult patients who have greater than or equal to 20% TBSA burns and pediatric patients who have greater than or equal to 15% TBSA burns. It is important to begin resuscitation via two large-bore peripheral IVs. The initial adjusted fluid rate includes lactated Ringer at 2 to 4 mL × kg × %TBSA (dependent on mechanism) burn with half the volume given in the first 8 hours of injury (not arrival) and the second half given in the subsequent 16 hours. Adult, nonelectrical injury burns should be given 2 mL × kg × % TBSA and pediatric (<14 years old), nonelectrical injury burns should be given 3 mL × kg × % TBSA. All patients, regardless of age, should be given 4 mL × kg × % TBSA burns. Children weighing less than 30 kg do not have large liver glycogen stores and should receive 0.45% saline with 5% dextrose at maintenance rate in addition to resuscitative fluid (Table 33.1). Colloid (5% albumin) can be added to the resuscitation fluids if the resuscitation rate approaches 6 mL/kg/%TBSA. This can be done by adding albumin in a 3:1, 2:1, or 1:1 ratio of colloid:crystalloid to equal the total adjusted fluid volume.

1. During resuscitation, it is imperative to follow the clinical response by monitoring urine output, lactate, base deficit, and, perhaps, cardiac output/index and stroke volume variation if using PiCCO® or FloTrac®. It is recommended to maintain urine output of 0.5 mL/kg/h in adults and 1.0 mL/kg/h in kids. However, urine output can lag behind resuscitation and care must be taken not to overresuscitate. IV fluid adjustments are made by increasing the rate by one-third if the urine output is below the calculated goal urine output by more than one-third. The IV fluid rate should be decreased by one-third if the urine output is above the calculated goal urine output by more than one-third. Studies do not necessarily demonstrate improved outcomes with either of these devices. PA catheters may lead to overresuscitation in healthy patients but are helpful in patients with cardiac diseases and those at risk for cardiac shock and congestive heart failure.
2. It is important to assess for the presence of compartment syndrome of the extremities. This is done by serial neurovascular examinations. Monitoring for abdominal compartment syndrome should also be done. This is performed by transducing bladder pressures. There should be heightened suspicion for abdominal compartment syndrome if there is increased difficulty ventilating and oxygenating, hypotension, and oliguria (due to decreased venous return). Ocular compartment syndrome can be assessed using a tonometer.

B. Second 24 Hours: All patients should receive crystalloid to maintain urine output and to maintain parameters of perfusion. Monitoring for adequacy of perfusion can be done by measuring lactate, pulse or stroke volume variation, and cardiac outputs. Nutritional support should be started, usually by employing

TABLE 33.1 Adjusted Fluid Calculations

Category	Age and weight	Adjusted fluid rate
Flame or scald	Adults and older children (≥14 yr old)	**2** mL LR × kg × % TBSA
	Children (<14 yr old)	**3** mL LR × kg × % TBSA
	Infants and young children (≤30 kg)	**3** mL LR × kg × % TBSA Plus D5LR at maintenance rate
Electrical injury	All ages	**4** mL LR × kg × % TBSA Plus D5LR at maintenance rate for infants and young children

LR, lactated Ringer; TBSA, total body surface area. Derived from *Advanced Burn Life Support Course Manual.*

enteral nutrition as soon as possible; ideally within 6 hours of injury. After 24 to 36 hours, IV fluids can be decreased by one-third, as long as the patient continues to produce adequate urine. IV fluids can again be decreased by one-third for hours 36 to 48 (as long as urine output is maintained). Colloids can be given after initial crystalloid resuscitation (5% albumin at 0.3-0.5 mL/kg/%TBSA over 24 hours) if blood pressure or urine output is not adequate.

C. After 48 Hours, IV fluid should be administered to maintain urine output at 0.5 to 1 mL/kg body weight/h. Insensible losses and hyperthermia are associated with a hyperdynamic state. Daily weights can be helpful to determine insensible fluid loss or fluid retention.

D. Overresuscitation: If during the first 24 hours, resuscitation exceeds 6 mL/kg/%TBSA burn/24 h, the physician should reassess the clinical picture. An exuberant administration of IV fluid can lead to abdominal or extremity compartment syndrome with decreased chest wall compliance leading to elevated peak airway pressures. Hourly neurovascular exams should be performed of all extremities at risk. Because patients are frequently intubated, physical exams can be limited. However, capillary refills can be assessed, as can pulse oximetry and compartment pressures with a Stryker needle or arterial line setup. If circumferential eschar is causing concern about compartment syndrome, extremity escharotomy should be performed. This includes making an incision along the lateral and medial aspects of the affected extremities. These incisions are down through the dermis only, exposing the underlying subcutaneous fat (Figure 33.3). Avoid incisions into the subcutaneous tissue and do not cut through the muscle or muscular fascia (Figure 33.4).

1. **Chest compartment syndromes:** The diagnosis is based on decreased chest wall compliance and increased peak airway pressures in the presence of circumferential or near-circumferential deep burns about the chest. Chest escharotomy should be performed along the anterior axillary line and connected at the subcostal lines.
2. **Abdominal compartment syndrome:** The diagnosis is based on exam and bladder pressure greater than 30 mm Hg. Patients may have hypotension, oliguria, and/or increased minute ventilation. Escharotomies laterally can also help prevent abdominal compartment syndrome. Once present, however, a bedside decompressive laparotomy may be needed, especially if high bladder pressures and high peak airway pressures remain after completion of the escharotomy.
3. **Orbital** compartment syndrome is relieved with lateral canthotomy.

VII. INHALATION INJURY AND CARBON MONOXIDE POISONING

A. Inhalation injury is divided into (i) upper airway (above the glottis [nasopharynx, oropharynx, larynx]), (ii) lower airway (below the glottis), and (iii) toxicity due to toxic gases.

1. **Upper airway:** swelling maximal at 12 to 24 hours. It can be diagnosed at the time of direct laryngoscopy. The upper airway has large absorptive capacity and prevents most burns to the lower airway. Decision to intubate should be based on patient exam. Signs of upper airway injury include pharyngeal swelling, carbonaceous sputum, hoarseness, stridor, and mucosal swelling. Treatment of upper airway burns includes admission to hospital, humidified oxygen, general pulmonary toilet, and bronchodilators if indicated. Intubation should be done by an experienced provider with access to fiberoptic technology and surgical intervention. If intubated, a larger tube allows for better bronchoscopy and pulmonary toilet.
2. **Lower airway:** caused by smoke combustion products and inhaled steam. It results in loss of ciliary clearance of damaged mucosa and debris, leading to a high incidence of pneumonia (50%). The initial chest radiograph will

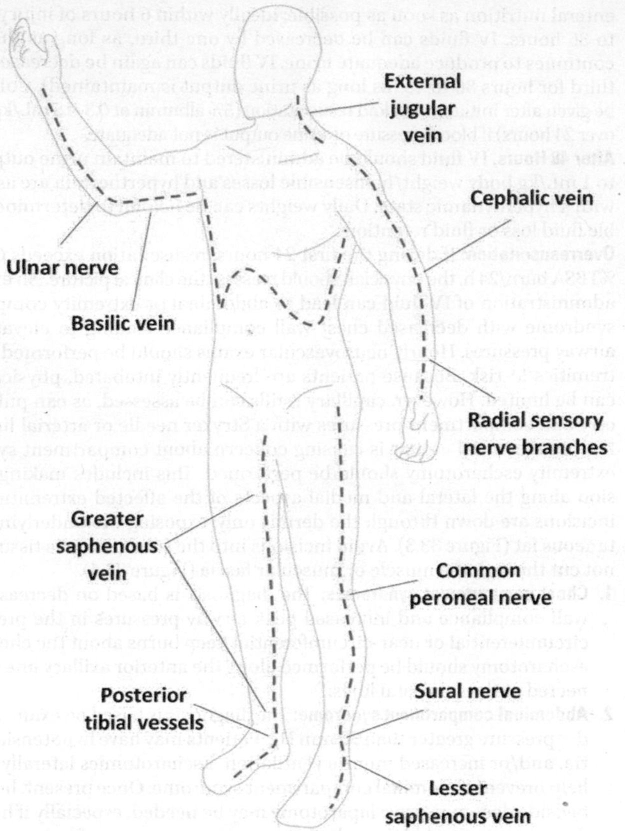

FIGURE 33.3 Schematic of burn escharotomy incisions. Dashed red lines depict full-thickness incisions through burned skin down to subcutaneous fat. Labels point to key anatomic structures that should be preserved whenever possible when performing escharotomies.

often appear normal because it typically takes 48 to 72 hours for the inflammatory response to blossom.

3. **Toxic gases**

   a. **Carbon monoxide:** Increased carbon monoxide is found commonly in fires occurring in enclosed settings. It results from incomplete combustion. Injury occurs from a combination of increased concentrations of carbon monoxide, the presence of both anoxia and hypotension. Carbon monoxide binds to heme-containing enzymes, such as hemoglobin, 200 times more avidly than does oxygen, resulting in a left shift in the oxygen dissociation curve. This makes tissue oxygenation more difficult. The half-life of carbon monoxide is 4 to 5 hours. This is reduced to 90 minutes when the patient is administered 100% oxygen and 30 minutes while breathing 100% hyperbaric oxygen. Patients start to become symptomatic at carboxyhemoglobin levels of 15% with vague

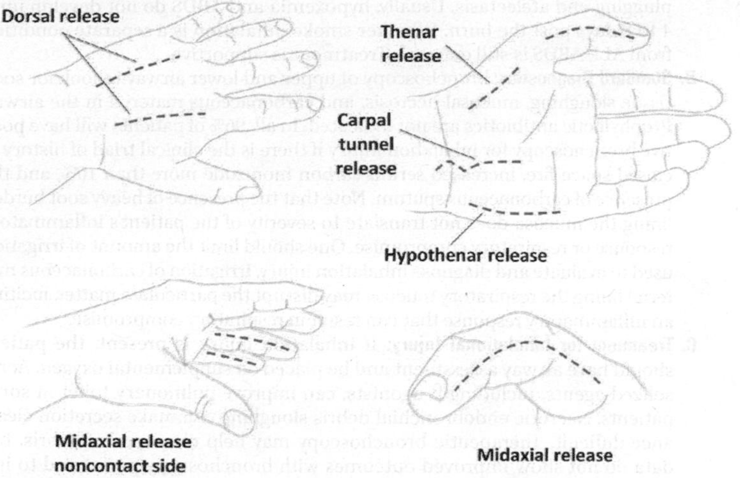

FIGURE 33.4 Schematic of burn escharotomy incisions for hand burns. Because these incisions are identical to those performed for hand compartment release, dissection should proceed bluntly through the muscular fascia if there is concern about hand compartment syndrome. Dorsal incisions should overlie the second and fourth metacarpals. Midaxial incisions should be on noncontact digit surfaces and avoid the volarly positioned neurovascular bundle.

complaints of headache, nausea, and vomiting. More severe symptoms of seizures and loss of consciousness occur at carboxyhemoglobin levels of more than 40%. The treatment is supportive care.

b. Hydrogen cyanide: another toxin inhaled commonly found in fires in enclosed spaces. It, too, is a product of incomplete combustion. Cyanide disrupts cellular oxidative phosphorylation resulting in the ability to produce adenosine triphosphate (ATP). This results in an increase in anaerobic metabolism. Symptoms of cyanide poisoning are nonspecific, such as headache, confusion, and shortness of breath. However, cyanide poisoning can progress to hypotension, bradycardia, and cardiac failure. Some patients may have a flush appearance or "almond" smell to the breath. A lactate acidosis that is refractory to resuscitation suggests cyanide poison. Cyanide levels do not return fast enough through hospital laboratories to be clinically meaningful. As a result, if cyanide exposure is of concern, cyanokit (hydroxocobalamin) should be given immediately to react with hydrogen cyanide producing the nontoxic cyanocobalamin. Hydroxocobalamin has a deep red color that will alter the color of the urine as it is excreted. This will make the assessment for red-pigmented urine found in rhabdomyolysis impossible.

VIII. SIGNIFICANT MORBIDITY AND MORTALITY ASSOCIATED WITH THERMAL BURNS WITH INHALATIONAL INJURIES

A. Mortality for patients with burns on the ventilator for more than 1 week is similar to that of acute respiratory distress syndrome (ARDS). Patients with burns are unique in their development of acute liver injury (ALI) and ARDS because they suffer smoke inhalation, causing respiratory insufficiency, hypoxia by increased capillary permeability, ciliary dysfunction, and interstitial edema. Damaged necrotic respiratory mucosa will slough, causing bronchial plugging and atelectasis. Usually, hypoxemia and ARDS do not develop until 4 to 8 days post the burn. Whether smoke inhalation is a separate condition from ALI/ARDS is still debated. Treatment is supportive.

B. Standard Diagnostics: bronchoscopy of upper and lower airway to look for soot, tissue sloughing, mucosal necrosis, and carbonaceous material in the airway. Prophylactic antibiotics are not indicated. In all, 96% of patients will have positive bronchoscopy for inhalation injury if there is the clinical triad of history of closed-space fire, increased serum carbon monoxide more than 10%, and the presence of carbonaceous sputum. Note that the presence of heavy soot burden lining the mucosa does not translate to severity of the patient's inflammatory response or respiratory compromise. One should limit the amount of irrigation used to evaluate and diagnose inhalation injury. Irrigation of carbonaceous material lining the respiratory mucosa may disrupt the particulate matter, inciting an inflammatory response that can result in respiratory compromise.

C. Treatment for Inhalational Injury: If inhalation injury is present, the patient should have airway assessment and be placed on supplemental oxygen. Aerosolized agents, including β-agonists, can improve pulmonary toilet in some patients. Necrotic endobronchial debris sloughing can make secretion clearance difficult. Therapeutic bronchoscopy may help clearance of debris, but data do not show improved outcomes with bronchoscopy performed to improve pulmonary toilet. Alternating every 4 hours nebulized heparin (10 000 U in 3 mL of normal saline), nebulized *N*-acetylcysteine (3 mL of 20%), and nebulized albuterol sulfate (0.5 mL) has shown to decrease mortality in children with inhalation injury. There is literature that suggests that this same regimen may reduce lung injury and decrease the progression to ARDS. Mechanical ventilation should deliver low tidal volume ventilation (4-6 mL/kg) to prevent volutrauma, increased levels of PEEP to support oxygenation, and keep plateau pressures less than 30 mm Hg to decrease barotrauma. Prophylactic systemic antibiotics and systemic steroids are to be avoided.

D. Pulmonary Infection: occurs in 30% to 50% of patients. Patients with purulent sputum, fever, and impaired gas exchange should be treated for pneumonia. Chest radiographic findings and leukocytosis should make the provider suspicious that the patient has pneumonia. If the patients have pneumonia and have been hospitalized for more than 48 hours, they should be treated for hospital-acquired pneumonia. Sputum should be sent for aerobic, anaerobic, and quantitative cultures. Empiric antibiotics include coverage of *Pseudomonas* and methicillin-resistant *Staphylococcus aureus* (MRSA). This should include vancomycin or linezolid. If vancomycin is used, it is important to check vancomycin trough levels to avoid renal toxicity. De-escalate antibiotics once cultures speciate and the sensitivity profile results.

E. Ventilator-Associated Pneumonia: *Staphylococcus aureus* and *Streptococcus* are common causes of early VAP. *Pseudomonas aeruginosa* is the most common cause of late VAP. The normal diagnosis of pneumonia (fever, purulent sputum, or leukocytosis) may not be helpful in patients with burns because almost all patients are febrile, tachypneic, and have elevated white blood cell counts. The best diagnostic test in this situation is probably a bronchial alveolar lavage sample with quantification of the bacteria. Bacterial growth greater than 10^3 colony-forming units (CFU) is indicative of infection. This level of bacteria is considered significant, as per American Burn Association (ABA) recommendations for VAP treatment. Antibiotic treatment duration is 7 days.

IX. METABOLIC RESPONSE AND NUTRITION

A. Metabolic rates in patients with burns are significantly greater than that of other patients who are critically ill, leading to lean body mass wasting. Positive nitrogen balance is the key to prevent skeletal muscle breakdown.

B. General composition of the enteral feeding should include at least 50% calories from carbohydrates, less than 30% lipids and essential fatty acids, and 20% to 25% protein. Enteral nutrition should be initiated within 6 hours of injury for adult patients with burns who are critically ill, as long as they are hemodynamically stable. It is expected that 80% of energy and protein goals are met by 48 to 72 hours. Failure to meet large energy and protein requirements can impair wound healing and alter organ function. Adequate nutrition is crucial and overfeeding must be avoided. Previously, a randomized, double-blind, prospective study demonstrated that aggressive high-calorie feeding with enteral and parenteral nutrition was associated with increased mortality. The daily caloric requirements should be calculated using 30% to 35% kcal/kg if ideal body weight (Hamwi equation) is less than 20%; 35 to 40 kcal/kg if ideal body weight is greater than 20%. An estimated 1.5 to 2 g/kg/d of protein is needed for the synthetic needs of the patient. Patients with burns should receive less percentage calorie requirements from fat than do other patients in the intensive care unit (ICU). Livers in patients with burns have less very low-density lipoprotein (VLDL), causing hepatic triglyceride (TG) elevation. Increased fat consumption leads to increased complications including fatty liver, infection, hyperlipidemia, hypoxia, and mortality.

C. Micronutrients: There is decreased gastrointestinal absorption and increased urinary losses of micronutrients. Thus, patients with burns can develop deficiencies in vitamin C, vitamin E, zinc, iron, and selenium. Patients with burns have been shown to benefit from glutamine supplementation. It has been found to boost gut integrity and immune function.

D. Acute response to thermal injury is biphasic, with the hypodynamic shock state at 24 to 72 hours and hyperdynamic catabolic state that plateaus by the fifth postburn day. Patients have supraphysiologic cardiac outputs, elevated body temperatures, supranormal oxygen consumption, supranormal glucose consumption, altered glucose metabolism, and increased CO_2 production due to accelerated tissue catabolism. This hyperdynamic catabolic state is thought to be caused by an excessive release of catabolic hormones, including catecholamines, glucagon, and cortisol. A shift from an anabolic-catabolic homeostasis to this hypercatabolic state leads to an increased need for energy. This leads to loss of skeletal muscle, which is broken down to maintain a sufficient supply of glucose and amino acids. The increased resting metabolic rate is directly related to the severity of the burn injury. A persistent hypermetabolic state is unsustainable. To decrease this hypermetabolic state, the provider should attempt to decrease the catabolic response by treating sepsis, performing early excision and skin grafting, and maintaining the core body temperature between 3.33 and 3.61 °C. A nonselective β-blocker, such as propranolol, can also be used because it inhibits the effect of catecholamines and slows muscle catabolism. Herndon et al demonstrated that the usage of propranolol for the treatment of acute burns in the pediatric population improved net muscle synthesis and increased lean body mass.

E. Other medications to consider include pharmacologic agents that convert catabolism to anabolism: oxandrolone (a testosterone analog given 0.1 mg/kg q12h) improves muscle synthetic activity, increases expression of muscle anabolic genes, and increases net muscle protein synthesis. These effects improve lean body mass composition and have reduced weight loss. This also improves donor site wound healing and decreases the duration of the hospital stay. The provider needs to check LFTs weekly because of the risk of transaminitis when receiving anabolic steroids. The practice has been to continue oxandrolone for 6 months. Human growth hormone and insulin-like growth factors have also been investigated but the results of their administration have been mixed.

F. Glucose Control: Increase in hepatic gluconeogenesis and impaired insulin-mediated glucose transport into skeletal and cardiac muscle and adipose tissue occur regularly in patients with burns. Hypermetabolism leads to hyperglycemia and insulin resistance. Data do not support strict glucose control (<110 mg/dL), but moderate blood glucose control is recommended (blood glucose <180 mg/dL).

X. ELECTROLYTE ABNORMALITIES AND ACUTE RENAL FAILURE

A. The immediate effect of burn injury on kidney function occurs when there is hypovolemia (see earlier text) and because of the release of cytokines.

B. A diuretic phase is seen at 48 to 72 hours after "third-space" fluid is reabsorbed.

C. Hyponatremia is often seen because of large-volume resuscitation with hypotonic IV fluids. This will self-correct. Open burn wounds or use of topical silver nitrate can also cause hyponatremia. Be aware that renal hypoperfusion exacerbates hyponatremia by decreasing glomerular filtration.

D. Hypernatremia is due to insensible and evaporative water losses.

E. Providers should monitor patients for hyperkalemia and hypokalemia.

F. Hypophosphatemia can result from dilution or when a refeeding syndrome occurs.

G. Hypocalcemia can result from the use of silver nitrate.

H. Acute Kidney Injury: Risk factors for acute kidney injury include sepsis, TBSA burns, organ failure, and antibiotic administration. Physiologically in burns, there is a decrease in renal perfusion, glomerular filtration rate, and renal plasma flow. The renal medulla is the most sensitive to hypoxia and the renal tubular cells are the most vulnerable.

1. **Presentation:** oliguria and decreased creatinine clearance
2. **Early renal failure:** often results from hypovolemia-induced ischemic injury. Early fluid resuscitation is important to prevent this. Overresuscitation can cause abdominal compartment syndrome, which will also compromise renal perfusion. Renal failure can also be caused by rhabdomyolysis, most commonly seen in burns due to electrical injury.
3. **Late renal failure:** occurs after the fifth postburn day. It can be caused by sepsis and nephrotoxic antibiotics. Continuous renal replacement therapy (CRRT) has been shown to improve outcomes in patients with burns who have acute kidney injury and require vasopressors.
4. **Pharmacologic treatments:** Dopamine has **not** been shown to improve outcomes. However, the dopamine-1 receptor agonist, fenoldopam, at low doses has been shown to increase urine output and decrease serum creatinine without decreasing blood pressure. Lasix and mannitol will improve urine output but have not been shown to improve outcomes in patients with burns.
5. Initial care of patients with acute renal failure (ARF) should focus on reversing the underlying cause, as well as correcting any fluid and electrolyte imbalances. Ensure adequate volume status, avoid nephrotoxins, and dose medications appropriately. A high aldosterone response often necessitates potassium supplementation.

XI. CHEMICAL BURNS

A. General Approach to Chemical Burn Treatment: Protect yourself with personal protective equipment—always consider that the chemicals are still present and must be neutralized or temporized. With few exceptions (see subsequent text), all chemical burns should be copiously irrigated with water. Water dilutes (but does not neutralize the chemical) and cools the burning area. Neutralization of chemical burns is generally contraindicated because neutralization may induce a hyperthermic reaction. Water irrigation is contraindicated or ineffective in several scenarios, including the following:

1. Elemental sodium, potassium, and lithium: these may precipitate an explosion.
2. Dry lime: should be brushed off and not irrigated
3. Phenol: water insoluble and should be wiped from the skin with polyethylene glycol-soaked sponges or ethyl alcohol

B. Types of Chemical Burns

1. **Alkali:** causes liquefaction necrosis and protein denaturation. Found in oven and drain cleaning products, fertilizers, and industrial cleaners. Alkali injuries extend deeper into tissues until the source is removed or diluted and are especially disruptive to the eye.
2. **Acids:** damage tissue via coagulation necrosis and protein precipitation
3. **Organic compounds (phenol and petroleum):** cause damage via cutaneous damage because of fat solvent action (cell membrane solvent action) and systematic absorption with toxic effects on the liver and kidneys. These can also cause significant erythema in the surrounding areas that may be mistaken for cellulitis.

C. Specific Types of Chemical Burns

1. **Hydrofluoric acid:** potent and corrosive acid used as a rust remover, in glass etching, and to clean semiconductors. Although a weak acid, the fluoride ion is toxic. It causes severe pain and local necrosis. Treatment is copious water irrigation. Fluoride ion is neutralized with topical calcium gel (one ampoule calcium gluconate in 100 g lubricating jelly). If symptoms persist, intra-arterial calcium infusion (10 mL calcium gluconate diluted in 80 mL of saline, infused over 4 hours) and/or subeschar injection of dilute (10%) calcium gluconate solution is recommended. Fluoride ion binds free serum calcium; make sure to check the serum calcium and replace with IV calcium as needed.
2. **Phenol:** commonly used in disinfectants and chemical solvents. Phenol is an acidic alcohol with poor water solubility and causes protein disruption and denaturation, resulting in coagulation necrosis. It is responsible for cardiac arrhythmia and liver toxicity. Cardiac and liver function should be monitored. It is cleared by the kidneys. Phenol causes demyelination and has a local anesthetic effect, and thus pain is not a reliable indicator of injury. Recommended treatment is copious water irrigation and cleansing with 30% polyethylene glycol or ethyl alcohol. ECG monitoring is required.
3. **Tar:** used in the paving and roofing industry. It can be heated to 260 °C before application and causes thermal injury. Tar solidifies as it cools and will become enmeshed with hair and skin. It should be cooled with copious water irrigation to stop the burning process. Tar removers promote micelle formation to break the tar-skin bond. Sterile surfactant mixture (De-Solv-it® or Shur-Clens®) and mineral oil allow tar to be wiped away in real time. Applying wet dressings using polysorbate (Tween 80), neomycin cream, or bacitracin for 6 hours before tar removal can also be effective.
4. **White phosphorus:** used to manufacture military explosives, fireworks, and methamphetamine. Obvious particles should be brushed off. Skin should be irrigated with a 1% to 3% copper sulfate solution. Copper sulfate stains the particles black for identification. Copper sulfate will also prevent ignition when particles are submerged in water. After copper sulfate irrigation, the exposed area should be placed in a water bath and the white phosphorous should be removed.
5. **Anhydrous ammonia:** alkali used in fertilizer. Skin exposure is treated with irrigation and local wound care. Exposure is associated with rapid airway edema, pulmonary edema, and pneumonia. Always consider early intubation for airway protection.

6. **Methamphetamine:** causes tachycardia (greater than expected with a similar size burn), hyperthermia, agitation, and paranoia

D. **Injury to Eyes:** Treat with prolonged irrigation with Morgan lenses. Eyelids may need to be forced open because of edema or spasm. Utilize a topical ophthalmic analgesic and consult an ophthalmologist.

XII. ELECTRICAL INJURY

A. Unlike other burns, TBSA is not necessarily associated with prognosis; the TBSA does not quantify damage to deeper tissues. It is difficult to determine the type and severity of damage between contact points because the direction through the tissues cannot be determined. The tissue resistance in decreasing order is bone, fat, tendon, skin, muscle, vessel, and nerve. The bone heats to a high temperature and burns surrounding structures. The higher the resistance, the more the heat is emitted.

B. Mechanism of injury
   1. Thermal: can generate temperatures above 100 °C
   2. Electroporation: Electrical force drives water into lipid membrane, causing cell rupture.
   3. Conduction: when a piece of metal (eg, watch band or ring) conducts current via direct contact with the energy source (ie, car battery)
   4. Contact: The heat that is generated from the passage of current through the tissues also heats metal that may be in direct contact with the skin (ie, belt buckle or necklace)
   5. Secondary ignition: The heat that is generated from the passage of current through the tissues heats clothing and nearby items past their flashpoints, resulting in flames.
   6. Concomitant trauma: Electrical injuries can be associated with the victim being thrown or falling a distance, which results in concomitant traumatic injuries.

C. **Injury Severity:** determined by voltage, current type, and resistance. High-voltage burns are those involving more than 1000 volts. Alternating current causes tetanic muscle contraction and the "no let-go" phenomenon. This occurs because of simultaneous contraction of (stronger) forearm flexors and (weaker) forearm extensors. Low-voltage electrical injuries are a result of less than 1000 voltage. This would include injuries from most home appliances.

D. Current flow through tissue can cause burns at contact points and burns to deep tissue. A current will preferentially travel along low-resistance pathways. Current will commonly pass through soft tissue, contact high-resistance bone, and travel along bone until it exits to the ground. However, the direction of the current through the tissue is unknown, especially with alternating current sources. Vascular injury to nutrient arteries through damage to their intima and media leads to thrombosis.

E. **Cardiac Effects:** All patients being evaluated for electrical injury should undergo a 12-lead ECG to identify arrhythmias. Telemetry monitoring for at least 24 hours is recommended to watch for coronary artery spasm, myocardial injury, and infarction in victims who have demonstrated arrhythmia on ECG and endorsed loss of consciousness or cardiac arrest.

F. **Gastrointestinal Effects:** injury to solid organs, acute bowel perforation, and gallstones after myoglobinuria

G. **Initial Monitoring**
   1. Airway maintenance: C-collar until c-spine cleared
   2. Breathing and ventilation—100% oxygen
   3. Circulation and cardiac status: cardiac monitor, two large-bore IVs, assess peripheral perfusion, 12-lead ECG
   4. 24-hour monitoring indicated if any of these is present—ectopy or dysrhythmia, loss of consciousness, cardiac arrest, or abnormal rate or rhythm.

5. Disability, neurologic deficit, and gross deformity: Assess level of consciousness, note any neurologic deficit, and note any gross deformity.
6. Exposure and environmental control: Stop the burning process, then remove clothes and avoid hypothermia.
7. Perform renal function analysis, urine myoglobin, and CPK levels to assess for evidence of rhabdomyolysis.

H. Fluid Resuscitation: TBSA provides inadequate estimation of electrical burn severity. Unlike thermal injury, electrical injury often occurs deep to the skin and is not visible. According to the consensus formula, 4 mL × kg × %TBSA should be used in all patients who have undergone electrical injury and have more than 20% TBSA (in adults) or more than 15% TBSA (pediatric). If no urine pigmentation is present, the minimum acceptable urine output is 0.5 mL/kg/h in adults. Pigmented urine can be caused by myoglobin (secondary to rhabdomyolysis) and/or free hemoglobin (from damaged red blood cells [RBCs]). For myoglobinuria, the urine dipstick test finding will be positive for blood and microscopy will not demonstrate RBCs. The goal for urine outputs when rhabdomyolysis and myoglobinuria have occurred is 1.0 to 1.5 mL/kg/h or about 75 to 100 mL/h in adults or 1.5 mL/kg/h in pediatric patients. Insufficient volume resuscitation can predispose to myoglobin-induced acute tubular necrosis.

I. Compartment Syndrome can occur after high-voltage electrical injury to an extremity. Current travels along bone, which has high resistance. The bone serves as a conductor and "cooks" adjacent tissue from deep to superficial. In the upper extremity, flexor digitorum profundus and flexor pollicis longus will be most severely affected because they are closest to bone. Overaggressive fluid resuscitation can worsen tissue edema, resulting in increased tissue pressures and exacerbating raised compartment pressures, and typically occurs within 48 hours of injury. Clinical concern about raised compartment pressures mandates an evaluation of compartment pressures or exploration and release of compartments in the operating room. The 6 "P" signs/symptoms include pain out of proportion, paresthesia, pallor, paralysis, pulselessness, and poikilothermia. Elevated compartment pressures can be used as an adjunct to clinical diagnosis or for cases where the patient is unable to participate in a clinical exam. Absolute pressure greater than or equal to 30 mm Hg or elevated pressure within 20 mm Hg of the diastolic blood pressure is also diagnostic of compartment syndrome. Forearm compartment syndrome is managed via surgical release of volar and extensor compartments and the mobile wad. In the hand, release carpal tunnel, the Guyon canal, and the nine compartments of the hand. Lower extremity compartment syndrome is managed with fasciotomies of the anterior, lateral, superficial posterior, and deep posterior compartments.

XIII. BURN WOUND MANAGEMENT

A. Topical Antimicrobials

1. **Silver sulfadiazine:** broad-spectrum antimicrobial activity due to silver ion. Soothing sensation that does not cause significant metabolic or electrolyte complications. Does not penetrate eschar. Can cause neutropenia but this is often self-limited. Assess whether patient has sulfa allergy.
2. **Sulfamylon (mafenide acetate):** penetrates eschar and is useful on ears to prevent suppurative chondritis. Can be used as a cream or as a soak (2.5% or 5%). It does not stop fungi, which silver nitrate does. Can also cause metabolic acidosis because of its inhibition of carbonic anhydrase. Can be painful on partial-thickness burns
3. **Silver nitrate:** offers broad-spectrum antimicrobial coverage against gram-positive and gram-negative bacteria and fungal coverage. Delivered

as an aqueous 0.5% solution every 4 hours to keep dressing moist and prevent precipitation of the silver nitrate. Side effects include staining skin (and anything it contacts) black, hyponatremia, and hypomagnesemia. Rare instances of methemoglobinemia necessitating methylene blue treatment

4. **Santyl (collagenase):** enzymatic debriding cream that can assist with debridement of burn eschar throughout a wound. No antimicrobial properties. Recommend supplementing this cream with another salve that has antimicrobial properties.
5. **Amphotericin B:** has fungicidal properties when used directly on the wound as topical irrigation
6. **Dakins:** diluted bleach that is used to irrigate wounds containing resistant microbes and tenacious fungi
7. **Mupirocin:** effective against MRSA and can be used in addition to other topicals to expand coverage

XIV. COLD INJURY

A. Frostbite occurs in response to a slow rate of cooling with ice crystal formation in tissue when tissue temperature is less than 28 °F.

B. Concentrated solutes draw fluid out of cells and ice crystals subsequently cause cell membrane puncture.

C. Intravascular ice crystals cause direct vascular damage and indirect vascular sludging.

D. With rewarming in a circulating 40 to 42 °C water bath, tissue thaws from the blood vessels outward.

E. Freeze-induced endothelial damage allows capillary leaking to occur. This allows extravasation of polymorphonuclear leukocytes (PMNs) and mast cells, causing inflammation, edema, microvascular stasis, and occlusion.

F. Blisters will form at 6 to 24 hours when extravasated fluid collects beneath the detached epidermal sheet. If the dermal vascular plexus is disrupted, hemorrhagic blisters will be present.

G. Stages of Frostbite

1. **First degree:** hyperemia, intact sensation, no blisters on rewarming, no tissue loss expected
2. **Second degree:** blisters containing clear or milky fluid, local edema, no tissue loss expected
3. **Third degree:** hemorrhagic blisters, edematous tissue, shooting or throbbing pain, and likely tissue loss
4. **Fourth degree:** mottled or cyanotic skin, hemorrhagic blisters, and frozen deeper structures. Mummification occurs over several weeks.

H. Treatment

Multiple freeze-thaw cycles cause multiplicative, not additive, damage to the affected tissues. Intact blisters should be left alone. Debride ruptured blisters and apply bacitracin ointment or Silvadene. Beware of the "afterdrop" phenomenon during rewarming, where central rewarming results in peripheral vasodilation. This returns cold blood from the extremities to the central circulation and can result in systemic hypothermia. Rapid rewarming of affected area in 40 to 42 °C circulating water bath, not radiant heat. Additional strategies include ibuprofen 400 mg po every 12 hours; penicillin 600 mg every 6 hours × 48 to 72 hours; elevation of limb with splinting to decrease movement; no smoking, caffeine, or chocolate; and tetanus prophylaxis. Three-phase bone scan may identify "at-risk" tissue. There is evidence that single-photon emission computed tomography (SPECT)/CT can be used to accurately predict the need for amputation early in the patient's care and maximizing limb length when considering amputation.

I. Acute Interventions After Warming

1. For patients with severe frostbite who are stable, rapid extrication to a center with interventional radiology capabilities within 12 hours is indicated. Arterial catheterization can identify and treat vasospasm and microvascular thrombosis with tissue plasminogen activator (tPA) or heparin. Catheter-directed tPA should be given for 24 hours and then the patient should be placed on a heparin gtt.
2. Reversal of local microvascular thrombosis may restore perfusion before irreversible necrosis and ischemia occur.
3. Several studies have shown significant decrease in amputation rates and tissue loss with this aggressive protocol.
4. Early regional sympathectomy of an affected extremity is controversial.

XV. STEVENS-JOHNSON SYNDROME AND TOXIC EPIDERMAL NECROLYSIS

A. Steven-Johnson syndrome (SJS) and toxic epidermal necrolysis (TEN) are immunologically mediated exfoliating disorders along the same spectrum of disease. They are characterized by sloughing of the skin secondary to disruption of the epidermis and dermal junction. Both SJS and TEN have widespread necrosis of the superficial portion of the epidermis.

B. Steven-Johnson Syndrome: total involvement less than 10% TBSA. Widespread erythematous or purpuric macules or flat atypical targets are present.

C. Toxic Epidermal Necrolysis With Spots: total cutaneous involvement of greater than 30% TBSA. Widespread purpuric macules or flat atypical targets are present.

D. Toxic Epidermal Necrolysis Without Spots: total cutaneous involvement greater than 10% TBSA. Large epidermal sheets present. No purpuric macules or targets

E. Overlap Steven-Johnson Syndrome-Toxic Epidermal Necrolysis: total cutaneous involvement of 10% to 30%. Widespread purpuric macules or flat atypical targets are present.

F. Steven-Johnson Syndrome-Toxic Epidermal Necrolysis is commonly associated with sulfonamides, trimethoprim-sulfamethoxazole, oxicam NSAIDs, chlormezanone, and carbamazepine. A single offending drug is identified in less than 50% of cases. Antibiotic-associated SJS/TEN presents approximately 7 days after the drug is first taken. Anticonvulsant-associated SJS/TEN can present up to 2 months after the drug is first taken.

G. Initial symptoms can be a 2- to 3-day prodrome of nonspecific findings such as fevers, headaches, and chills. Symptoms of mucosal irritation such as conjunctivitis, dysuria, and/or dysphagia may be present. These symptoms are followed by mucosal and cutaneous lesions.

H. Mucosal irritation typically occurs at two or more sites. Involved sites may include vaginal, urinary, respiratory, gastrointestinal, oral, and/or conjunctival. Consultation with dermatology, gynecology, urology, gastroenterology, and/or ophthalmology may be necessary.

I. Skin lesions are diffusely present. Lesions are typically erythematous macules with purple, possibly necrotic, centers. Nikolsky sign is typically positive (rubbing the skin causes exfoliation of outermost layers and/or a new blister to form).

J. Differential diagnosis of acute, diffuse blistering includes staphylococcal-scalded skin syndrome, pemphigus vulgaris, pemphigus foliaceus, paraneoplastic pemphigus, bullous pemphigoid, acute graft-versus-host disease, and linear immunoglobulin A (IgA) dermatosis.

K. Diagnosis of SJS/TEN is largely clinical and can be confirmed by both skin biopsy and histology.

L. Treatment: Discontinue all potentially offending drugs and change out all indwelling central venous catheters while evaluating all potential septic sources. Transfer to a burn ICU for fluid/electrolyte monitoring and dressing changes/wound care, and temperature regulation is recommended. Remove areas of necrotic epidermis to reduce bacterial growth. Otherwise, minimize debriding sloughing skin. To prevent inadvertent debridement of fragile epidermis, minimize dressing changes using long-acting silver-based dressings, such as ACTICOAT or Mepilex®Ag, which remain in place for 7 days. Steroid creams (eg, triamcinolone) may be applied directly to the wound and covered with a clear, nonadherent, breathable primary dressing, such as N-TERFACE® or Telfa™ Clear. These dressings will allow for visualization of the skin without disturbing the dressing. They can also be removed without causing inadvertent debridement. Empiric systemic antibiotics have been associated with increased mortality and are not indicated. Consider hemodialysis to remove potentially offending drugs with long half-lives. Early ophthalmology consultation is recommended. More than 50% of patients with SJS/TEN can develop symblepharon or entropion. Treatment can involve other consultant services (pulmonary, urology, gynecology, gastroenterology) as needed. Currently, there is no standard immunomodulating therapy for this immunologically mediated condition. Administration of steroids and intravenous immunoglobulin (IVIG) has shown no benefit over supportive care alone. Cyclosporin A has been shown to decrease disease progression and lower mortality. Studies, such as the North American Therapeutics In Epidermal Necrolysis Syndrome (NATIENS) trial, are ongoing to determine the optimal treatment regimen for SJS/TEN. This particular trial is using a phase III randomized multicenter study to determine the efficacy of a TNF blocker in treating SJS/TEN.

Selected Readings

Allan PF, Osborn EC, Chung KK, Wanek SM. High-frequency percussive ventilation revisited. *J Burn Care Res.* 2010;31(4):510-520. doi:10.1097/BCR.0b013e3181e4d605

Branski LK, Mecott GA, Herndon DN, et al. The use of exenatide in severely burned pediatric patients. *Crit Care.* 2010;14(4):R153. doi:10.1186/cc9222

Herndon DN, Hart DW, Wolf SE, et al. Reversal of catabolism by beta-blockade after severe burns. *N Engl J Med.* 2001;345(17):1223-1229.

Hill DM, Rizzo JA, Aden JK, Hickerson WL, Chung KK; RESCUE Investigators. Continuous venovenous hemofiltration is associated with improved survival in burn patients with shock: a subset analysis of a multicenter observational study. *Blood Purif.* 2021;50(4-5): 473-480. doi:10.1159/000512101

Kraft C, Millet JD, Agarwal S, et al. SPECT/CT in the evaluation of frostbite. *J Burn Care Res.* 2017;38(1):e227-e234. doi:10.1097/BCR.0000000000000359

Mosier MJ, Pham TN. American Burn Association practice guidelines for prevention, diagnosis and treatment of VAP in burn patients. *J Burn Care Res.* 2009;30:910-928.

Priuitt BA, Ciofi WG. Thermal injuries. In: Davis JH, Sheldon GF, eds. *Surgery: A Problem Solving Approach.* 2nd ed. Mosby; 1995:643-720.

Simmons JW, Chung KK, Renz EM, et al. Fenoldopam use in a burn intensive care unit: a retrospective study. *BMC Anesthesiol.* 2010;10:9. doi:10.1186/1471-2253-10-9

Sharer SR, Heimbach DM. Management of inhalation injury in patients with and without burns. In: Haponik EF, Munster AM, eds. *Respiratory Injury—Smoke Inhalation and Burns.* McGraw-Hill; 1990:195–215.

Wischmeyer PE. Glutamine in burn injury. *Nutr Clin Pract.* 2019;34(5):681-687. doi:10.1002/ncp.10362

Zimmermann S, Sekula P, Venhoff M, et al. Systemic immunomodulating therapies for Stevens-Johnson syndrome and toxic epidermal necrolysis: a systematic review and meta-analysis. *JAMA Dermatol.* 2017;153(6):514-522. doi:10.1001/jamadermatol.2016.5668

34 Transfusion Medicine

Walter (Sunny) Dzik and Robert S. Makar

I. INDICATIONS FOR TRANSFUSION THERAPY

Blood component transfusion is usually performed because of decreased production, increased utilization/destruction or loss, or dysfunction of a specific blood component (red cells, platelets, or coagulation factors).

A. Anemia

1. **Red cell mass:** The primary reason for red blood cell (RBC) transfusion is to maintain an adequate oxygen-carrying capacity of the blood. Healthy individuals or individuals with chronic anemia can usually tolerate a hematocrit (Hct) of 20% to 25%, assuming normal intravascular volume. The measured values for the Hct and hemoglobin (Hgb) are roughly in a 3:1 numerical ratio. Modern analyzers directly measure the Hgb concentration by light absorbance and calculate the Hct depending on the product of the mean corpuscular volume and the red cell count.
2. Anemia may be caused by **decreased production** (marrow suppression), **increased loss** (hemorrhage and diagnostic phlebotomy), **destruction** (hemolysis), or dilution. Acute blood loss generally does not change the relative concentration of RBCs immediately (because other intravascular volume is lost at the same rate) but the infusion of intravenous (IV) fluid may contribute to a dilutional effect.
3. Anemia in the critically ill is common. The exact Hgb level that should prompt RBC transfusion remains controversial and should be individualized to the patient. Multiple large randomized trials conducted among patients who are critically ill suggest that a "restrictive" transfusion policy (maintaining Hgb 7-9 g/dL) is as good as a "liberal" strategy (10-12 g/dL). For an individual patient, the decision to transfuse should take into consideration oxygen delivery to tissues rather than be based exclusively on Hgb or Hct values.
4. For a patient who is not bleeding, each unit of packed RBCs is expected to raise the Hct by 3% and the Hgb by 1 g/dL. The volume of RBCs to transfuse can also be estimated depending on desired change in RBC volume as follows:

$$\text{Red cell volume (mL)} = \text{BV (mL)} \times (\text{Hematocrit}/100)$$

where BV is blood volume, which may be estimated at 70 mL/kg actual body weight in male adults and 65 mL/kg in female adults. Higher values may be used in infants (80 mL/kg) and neonates (85 mL/kg). The Hct of transfused blood is approximately 55 ± 5%.

B. **Thrombocytopenia:** Spontaneous bleeding is unusual with platelet counts more than 10 000/μL, but in the immediate postoperative period, platelet counts of more than 20 000 to 50 000/μL are sometimes recommended. Thrombocytopenia may be due to decreased bone marrow production (eg, chemotherapy, tumor infiltration, liver disease) or increased consumption (eg, trauma, sepsis, medications, autoantibodies, inflammatory disorders), sequestration in the spleen, or dilution.

II. PRETRANSFUSION TESTING

Before elective RBC transfusion, **recipient blood** is routinely typed for **ABO antigens** and the **Rh(D)** antigen, tested for the presence of antibodies against ABO antigens, and "screened" for the presence of antibodies to blood groups other than ABO. Patients found to have a negative "antibody screen" can safely receive donor RBCs of compatible ABO group. **Crossmatching** involves directly mixing the patient's plasma with the donor's red cells to establish that agglutination does not occur.

A. ABO Genes are codominant. The antigens are histoantigens found on all cells. Individuals have naturally occurring antibodies directed against the antigens they lack:

ABO genes	ABO antigens on tissue	ABO antibodies in plasma
A/A; A/0	A	Anti-B
B/B; B/0	B	Anti-A
A/B	AB	neither
0/0	0	Anti-A, anti-B, anti-A/B

B. The Rh Blood Group is a large family of protein antigens with expression restricted to red cells. The Rh(D) antigen is the most clinically important member of the Rh system of antigens and its presence or absence is commonly referred to as Rh-positive or Rh-negative. Antibodies to the Rh antigens do not occur naturally. However, individuals who are Rh(D)-negative may develop antibodies to the Rh(D) antigen when exposed by pregnancy, transfusion, or transplantation. Antibodies to Rh antigens are generally immunoglobulin (Ig) G, do not fix complement, but can cause hemolysis of transfused Rh-positive cells and can cross the placenta to cause hemolytic disease of the fetus and newborn. **Rh-immune globulin**, an Rh(D)-blocking antibody, prevents primary sensitization of the patient who is Rh(D) negative after exposure to low volumes of Rh(D)-positive red cells. Rh-immune globulin cannot address an antibody response that has already occurred, nor does it block the immune response to Rh antigens other than Rh(D). Rh-immune globulin is routinely administered to Rh(D)-negative women during the last trimester of pregnancy when small volumes of fetal blood enter the maternal circulation. The standard dose is one vial (~300 μg) for every 15 mL of Rh-positive blood transfused.

III. BLOOD COMPONENT THERAPY

A. Whole Blood

1. Whole blood was used before the development of blood component therapy. Whole blood is currently under investigation as an alternative to components for emergency transfusion. There is no evidence of the superiority of whole blood in trauma or cardiovascular surgery.
2. Whole blood is most safely given when ABO identical with the recipient because transfusion includes both red cell antigens and plasma antibodies from the donor.

B. Red Blood Cells

1. Packed red blood cells (pRBCs) contain concentrated RBCs from a single donor. One unit (typically 250-300 mL) can be expected to raise the Hgb of a euvolemic adult by approximately 1 g/dL once equilibration has taken place.
2. pRBCs must be ABO compatible (Table 34.1). For urgent transfusion, ABO identical or compatible pRBCs can usually be obtained within

TABLE 34.1 Transfusion Compatibility

	Donor					
	A	**B**	**O**	**AB**	**Rh(D)+**	**Rh(D)–**
Recipient						
1. Red blood cells						
A	OK		OK			
B		OK	OK			
O			OK			
AB	OK	OK	OK	OK		
Rh+					OK	OK
Rh–						OK
2. Plasma						
A	OK			OK		
B		OK		OK		
O	OK	OK	OK	OK		
AB				OK		
Rh+					OK	OK
Rh–					OK	OK

minutes if the patient's blood type is known. In emergencies, before determining the patient's ABO type, group O pRBCs (either Rh(D)-positive or Rh(D)-negative) may be transfused. Type-specific blood should be substituted as soon as possible to conserve group O resources and to minimize the amount of type O plasma (containing anti-A and anti-B antibodies) transfused (Table 34.1).

C. Platelets

1. One adult dose of platelets contains at least 3×10^{11} platelets suspended in donor plasma at a concentration of 1 000 000/µL in approximately 300 mL of plasma. An adult dose represents the platelets obtained from approximately 6 units of whole blood. An adult dose can be obtained either by pooling platelets made from six individual whole blood donations or by collecting platelets from one donor using an apheresis machine. In the absence of clinical factors that impair transfusion increments, an adult dose will raise the recipient platelet count by 30 000 to 60 000/µL. A posttransfusion platelet count drawn 5 to 60 minutes after completion of platelet transfusion can confirm a successful increment or demonstrate platelet refractoriness if the count fails to increase following transfusion.
2. **ABO-compatible platelets** are not required for transfusion, although platelet products contain a considerable volume of donor plasma that carries donor ABO antibodies. Platelets obtained by apheresis (single-donor platelets) are not superior to whole-blood derived platelets (pooled platelets). Platelets are leukoreduced before storage, which reduces recipient sensitization to donor human leukocyte antigen (HLA) antigens. In cases where HLA alloimmunization has already occurred because of prior pregnancy, transfusion, or transplantation, platelet donor selection based on HLA compatibility may be required for effective platelet transfusion. Platelets from Rh(D)-negative donors are preferred but not required for transfusion to Rh(D)-negative women of childbearing age because of the very low possibility of Rh(D) sensitization by residual donor red cells in platelet components.

D. **Plasma** is the liquid portion of blood after the RBCs and platelets have been removed by centrifugation. It contains primarily coagulation factors and Igs. One unit is approximately 200 to 250 mL.
   1. A typical dose of 10 to 20 mL/kg will increase plasma coagulation factors by about 20%. Fibrinogen levels increase by approximately 8 mg/dL for each bag (200 mL) of plasma transfused. By definition, 1 mL of normal human plasma contains 1 IU of each clotting factor. The concentration of electrolytes and proteins in plasma is that of normal human blood.
   2. Acute reversal of warfarin can be obtained by transfusion of approximately 5 to 10 mL/kg of fresh frozen plasma (FFP) or the equivalent of four-factor prothrombin complex concentrate. The international normalized ratio (INR) of plasma averages 1.1 (0.9-1.3) because of dilution of donor blood with citrate and dextrose.
   3. Plasma transfers donor ABO antibodies to the recipient and should be ABO compatible with the recipient (Table 34.1).
   4. Patients who are Rh(D)-negative may receive Rh(D)-positive plasma. An adult dose of platelets contains the equivalent of one unit of plasma.

E. **Cryoprecipitate** is formed by cold precipitation and centrifugation of previously frozen plasma. Each unit is approximately 15 mL, is typically prepared for transfusion as a pool of 5 units, and is transfused to an adult as 5 to 10 units (1-2 pools).
   1. Each unit of cryoprecipitate typically contains 80 IU of factor VIII and approximately 200 to 300 mg of fibrinogen. It also contains factor XIII, von Willebrand factor, and fibronectin.
   2. **Indications for cryoprecipitate** include hypofibrinogenemia, von Willebrand disease, hemophilia A (when factor VIII is unavailable), and preparation of topical fibrin glue (although commercially available virally inactivated concentrates have a higher fibrinogen concentration and are preferred for this purpose). One unit per 7 to 10 kg raises the plasma fibrinogen concentration by approximately 50 to 80 mg/dL in a patient without ongoing consumption. Plasma-derived fibrinogen concentrates contain the same amount of fibrinogen as cryoprecipitate but do not contain the von Willebrand factor.
   3. ABO compatibility is not required for transfusion of cryoprecipitate but it is preferred because of the presence of 10 to 20 mL of plasma per unit.

F. **Factor Concentrates:** Human plasma–derived or monoclonal coagulation factor concentrates are available for patients with specific factor deficiencies.
   1. **Four-factor prothrombin complex concentrate** is a human plasma–derived concentrate approved for the reversal of anticoagulation by vitamin K antagonists. For acute reversal of Coumadin in an adult, doses of 1000 to 3000 IU can be used.
   2. **Antithrombin III (AT-III) concentrate** is a human plasma–derived concentrate that can be used in the treatment of heparin resistance caused by congenital or acquired AT-III deficiency. Plasma transfusions contain all natural anticoagulants, including AT-III, protein C, and protein S. Human plasma transfusion provides a source of AT-III to overcome heparin resistance. Human plasma augments heparin and does not reverse heparin.

G. **Technical Considerations**
   1. **Compatible infusions:** Because red cells undergo metabolic stress during storage, it is not recommended to directly inject into a blood bag any medication or solution other than normal saline or albumin. IV coadministration of transfused blood with medications or IV fluids at the point of entry into the vein or through multilumen catheters is safe and commonly done. Dextrose-containing solutions in tubing sets will cause agglomeration of pRBCs into clumps. Direct injection of calcium-containing fluids or

medications into blood bags accompanied by prolonged dwell time before transfusion risks activation of clotting in the bag. Sodium chloride, albumin, and FFP are all compatible with pRBCs.

2. **Blood filters** (~170-270 µm clot screen filters) should be used for all blood components to remove debris and clots that may have formed during storage.
3. **Leukocyte removal filters** are commonly used to remove donor white blood cells to reduce transmission of cytomegalovirus (CMV), to reduce alloimmunization to donor HLA antigens, and to reduce the incidence of febrile reactions.

IV. SYNTHETIC BLOOD SUBSTITUTES

Blood product availability is limited and stored products maintain their integrity for a limited time. They continue to carry risks of infection and other adverse events (see **Section VII**), and some individuals have religious beliefs that prohibit allogeneic blood transfusion (eg, Jehovah's Witnesses). Despite decades of research, safe and effective **oxygen-carrying blood substitutes** have not been developed and no licensed product is available in the United States.

V. PHARMACOLOGIC THERAPY

A. **Erythropoietin** is an endogenous hormone produced in the kidneys that stimulates proliferation and development of erythroid precursor cells. Exogenous administration has been used to correct anemia in patients with chronic renal failure and to increase red cell mass before preoperative autologous donation. Excess administration is associated with thrombotic complications. Current evidence does not support the routine administration of erythropoietin for the critically ill. It may be used for anemia due to renal failure, for patients who refuse blood transfusion, and for patients with specific hematologic conditions. Iron and folate supplementation is also recommended for patients receiving erythropoietin. Initial recommended doses in patients with renal failure range from 50 to 100 units/kg IV or SC tid a week. Longer acting preparations given monthly are also available.

B. **Thrombopoietin** is an endogenous hormone produced in the liver that stimulates megakaryocyte proliferation and platelet production. It is principally used in the treatment of patients with immune thrombocytopenic purpura.

C. **Granulocyte Colony-Stimulating Factor (GCSF) and Granulocyte-Macrophage Colony-Stimulating Factor (GMCSF)** are myeloid growth factors useful for shortening the duration of neutropenia induced by chemotherapy. GCSF is specific for neutrophils, and GMCSF increases the production of neutrophils, macrophages, and eosinophils. Administration of these drugs enhances both neutrophil count and function. As such, they are frequently used for the treatment of infection in the setting of reversible transient severe neutropenia. Treatment results in an initial brief decrease in the neutrophil count (owing to endothelial adherence) and then in a rapid (usually after 24 hours) sustained leukocytosis that is dose dependent. Recommended doses are GCSF 5 µg/kg/d or GMCSF 250 µg/m^2/d and should be individualized for the patient.

D. Other interventions to enhance hemostasis are discussed in **Chapter 27.**

VI. BLOOD CONSERVATION AND SALVAGE TECHNIQUES

Blood transfusion of the critically ill is common, with approximately 40% of patients being transfused during an intensive care unit (ICU) stay. Those patients who are older and stay longer in the ICU are more likely to receive a transfusion.

A. **Losses From Diagnostic Phlebotomy** among the critically ill can be significant, ranging from 40 to 400 mL/d. Patients with more severe illness and a greater number of dysfunctional organs suffer higher phlebotomy losses because of a greater number of blood draws. Techniques demonstrated to reduce phlebotomy losses include (a) a **"closed" system** of blood sampling where the initial aspirated blood is reinjected into the patient instead of discarded, (b) use of **small-volume phlebotomy tubes**, and (c) **"point-of-care" testing** at the bedside, which frequently requires less blood than the clinical laboratory. Finally, the presence of both arterial and central venous catheters in patients who are critically ill is correlated with higher phlebotomy losses, suggesting another reason to repeatedly evaluate the need for such catheters with respect to hemodynamic monitoring or medication/nutritional support administration.

B. Surgical Drain Salvage Devices allow the reinfusion of shed blood. They are most commonly used in the immediate postoperative period to recover blood collected from chest tubes. Use of these devices requires a skilled operator for safe administration and sterile technique. They are contraindicated in conditions where the drained cavity is infected. Side effects result from reinfusion of multiple by-products of hemolyzed cells including life-threatening hyperkalemia. Systems designed to wash shed blood before infusion overcome these side effects.

VII. COMPLICATIONS OF BLOOD TRANSFUSION THERAPY

A. Transfusion Reactions

1. **Acute hemolytic transfusion reactions** are estimated to occur in 1 in 250 000 transfusions and are usually due to a label or clerical error at the time of sample collection, bag labeling, or bedside infusion. Symptoms include anxiety, agitation, chest pain, flank pain, headache, dyspnea, and chills. Nonspecific signs include fever, hypotension (or cardiovascular collapse), unexplained bleeding (or disseminated intravascular coagulation [DIC]), and hemoglobinuria (or renal failure). Fatal reactions are estimated at 1 in 1 250 000 units. Table 34.2 describes the steps to be taken if a transfusion reaction is suspected.
2. **Nonhemolytic transfusion reactions** are usually due to antibodies against donor white cells or plasma proteins. These patients may complain of anxiety, pruritus, or mild dyspnea. Signs may include fever, rigors, flushing, hives, tachycardia, tachypnea, and hypertension. The transfusion should be stopped and the possibility of a hemolytic transfusion reaction evaluated (see earlier text).
   a. If the reaction is *only* urticaria, the transfusion should be slowed and may be continued. Antihistamines (eg, **diphenhydramine**, 25-50 mg IV)

TABLE 34.2 Treatment of Suspected Acute Hemolytic Transfusion Reaction

1. Stop transfusion, check label on blood bag with patient wristband, and frequently monitor patient's vital signs.
2. Send remaining donor blood and fresh patient sample to the blood bank for analysis.
3. Send patient sample to laboratory for CBC, LDH, and DIC screen.
4. Treat hypotension with fluids and/or vasopressors as necessary.
5. Consider use of corticosteroids.
6. Consider measures to preserve renal function and maintain brisk urine output (intravenous fluid, furosemide).
7. Monitor patient for DIC.

CBC, complete blood count; DIC, disseminated intravascular coagulation; LDH, lactate dehydrogenase.

are not required but may be given for symptomatic relief of itching. There is no role for antipyretics such as acetaminophen in allergic transfusion reactions. Urticarial reactions are usually not reproducible in subsequent transfusions. Routine pretransfusion use of antihistamines or antipyretics is not recommended.

b. Patients with a prior history of febrile transfusion reactions should be transfused with leukoreduced pRBCs and platelets. Premedication is not recommended.

c. Anaphylactic reactions occur rarely and have been associated in some studies with high-titer antibodies to IgA among patients with undetectable IgA. Transfusion of patients with a documented history of transfusion anaphylaxis should be undertaken in consultation with a transfusion medicine physician. Because there is very poor correlation between IgA deficiency and anaphylactic reactions, prophylactic use of washed RBCs in patients with IgA deficiency without a history of prior anaphylaxis is not recommended.

B. Metabolic Complications of Blood Transfusions

1. Potassium (K^+) concentration changes are common with rapid blood transfusion but seldom of clinical importance. Although red cells leak K^+ into the extracellular storage fluid during storage, red cells rapidly take back the K^+ after transfusion. Large-volume transfusion results in recipient *hypokalemia*.

2. Calcium (Ca^{2+}) is bound by citrate, which is present in excess concentration as the anticoagulant in stored blood products. Rapid transfusion causes direct citrate infusion. Citrate is metabolized in all mitochondria and is excreted unchanged in the urine. Rapid infusion of citrate by transfusion may bind blood Ca^{2+} and decrease the *ionized* calcium level. Because citrate in blood components partitions with the plasma, plasma transfusions given rapidly are more likely than are pRBCs to induce citrate toxicity in the recipient. Severe hypocalcemia, manifested as tetany in the patient who is not anesthetized, hypotension, QT-segment prolongation on the electrocardiogram, and narrowed pulse pressure may occur. Citrate toxicity only occurs in rapid transfusion and is exacerbated by hypothermia, hyperkalemia, and impaired hepatic or renal perfusion. Ionized calcium levels should be monitored during rapid transfusions and aggressively repleted before development of signs or symptoms of severe hypocalcemia.

3. Acid-base status: Although banked blood is acidic because of the metabolic effects of storage, the clinical effect on the patient is minimal. Citrate metabolism following transfusion induces a metabolic alkalosis. Acidosis in the setting of ongoing transfusion is more likely due to hypoperfusion and recipient lactic acidosis and will improve with volume resuscitation and tissue oxygenation.

4. Other analytes: Blood storage solutions are hypernatremic and hyperglycemic. Transient disturbance of Na^+ and glucose can be seen after large-volume transfusion. There is no evidence that the ammonia content of stored blood is of any clinical consequence. The level of free Hgb in RBCs due to storage hemolysis is less than 1%. Routine stored blood transfusions do not result in elevation of bilirubin or lactate dehydrogenase (LDH) or depression of haptoglobin in normal recipients.

C. Infectious Complications of blood transfusions have been markedly reduced because of improved testing of donated blood. Recent changes to U.S. blood bank screening for viral pathogens include addition of specific nucleic acid testing of small pooled donated samples to enhance detection of hepatitis C virus (HCV) and HIV before serologic antibody conversion has occurred. Pooled products (eg, cryoprecipitate) have an increased risk of infection proportional to the number of donors.

1. **Hepatitis B:** The current risk of HBV transmission is estimated to be 1 in 220 000 units transfused. Although the majority of infections are asymptomatic (only 35% of infected individuals demonstrate acute disease), approximately 1% to 10% become chronically infected with potentially significant long-term morbidity.
2. **Hepatitis C:** The risk of transfusion-related HCV is approximately 1 in 1 935 000 units. Risks of HCV infection are more serious than those with HBV, however, because 85% of patients suffer chronic infection, 20% develop cirrhosis, and 1% to 5% of infections cause hepatocellular carcinoma.
3. **HIV:** Because of improved screening and testing, the risk of transfusion-associated HIV has been estimated to be approximately 1 in 2.1 million units transfused in the United States.
4. **Cytomegalovirus (CMV):** The prevalence of antibodies to CMV in the general population is approximately 70% by adulthood. The incidence of transfusion-associated CMV infection in patients who are previously uninfected is quite low following the use of leukoreduced blood.
5. **West Nile virus** is a seasonal epidemic causing febrile and neurologic illnesses including meningoencephalitis and acute flaccid paralysis. Transfusion transmission was first documented in 2002 and blood donors are routinely screened for infection. The current risk in these areas is estimated at 1 in 1 million units transfused.
6. **Bacterial infections:** Exclusion of donors with evidence of infectious disease and the storage of blood at 4 °C reduces the risk of transmitted bacterial infection. However, the necessity of room-temperature storage of platelets to maintain functional integrity creates a favorable medium for bacterial growth. Infection rates for platelets are estimated at 1 in 1000 to 2000 units and rates of septic reactions are on the order of 1 in 100 000 platelet doses transfused. Organisms likely to infect platelet concentrates include *Staphylococcus aureus*, coagulase-negative *Staphylococcus*, and diphtheroids. All platelet products are now screened for bacterial contamination during storage. RBCs are much less likely to become contaminated with bacteria, but the most commonly cultured organism is *Yersinia enterocolitica*, and the mortality rate from transfusion-acquired sepsis is approximately 60%.

D. Transfusion-Related Acute Lung Injury (TRALI) is a syndrome of acute lung injury (see **Chapter 19**) after blood product transfusion. Symptoms may include severe hypoxemia, dyspnea, frothy sputum, and noncardiogenic pulmonary edema, sometimes accompanied by fever and hypotension, and usually occurring 4 to 6 hours after transfusion. The pathophysiology is incompletely understood but includes recipient exposure to HLA or granulocyte antibodies present in donor plasma. Mild forms are likely to go underrecognized.

The incidence of TRALI has decreased over the past several years largely due to reduction in collections from multiparous donors and screening other at-risk donors for HLA antibodies. Any transfused product that contains plasma may cause TRALI. Mortality from TRALI is approximately 5%. Treatment is similar to that of other forms of acute lung injury and frequently requires mechanical ventilation. Most patients show dramatic clinical improvement within 48 hours and radiographic clearing of edema within a few days.

E. Transfusion-Associated Circulatory Overload (TACO) is the most common serious noninfectious hazard of transfusion. TACO is associated with transfusion of multiple units of blood, older recipients, renal impairment, and cardiopulmonary disease. TACO commonly is associated with hypertension, tachypnea, venous engorgement, and signs of right or left heart volume overload.

VIII. MASSIVE TRANSFUSIONS (SEE TABLE 34.3)

A. Massive Transfusion was previously arbitrarily defined as the administration of 10 units of blood transfused within a 24-hour period. Modern definitions focus more on critical bleeding defined by the rate of transfusion over shorter time intervals.

TABLE 34.3 Abridged Massive Transfusion Protocol of the Massachusetts General Hospital

1. The protocol can be initiated at any time during the patient's hospitalization, including before arrival to the Massachusetts General Hospital (MGH).
2. Appropriate candidates include the following:
   a. Any patient with an initial blood loss of at least 40% of blood volume or in whom it is judged that at least 10 units of blood replacement is immediately required
   b. Any patient with a continuing hemorrhage of at least 250 mL/h
   c. Any patient, when clinical judgment is made such that blood loss as identified in "A" and "B" is imminent
3. Once the decision is made to initiate this protocol, the appropriate physician needs to do the following:
   a. Notify the blood bank with the age and gender of the patient.
   b. Ensure that a properly labeled blood bank sample is obtained and sent to the blood bank.
4. A transfusion medicine faculty member is on call at all times to assist in transfusion support.
5. RBC selection
   a. 4 units of emergency-release, uncrossmatched group O whole blood will be released for all emergency transfusion requests. After the initial 4 units of whole blood, group O pRBCs or ABO compatible pRBCs will be used.
6. Blood component requests After the initial assessment, if >10 total units are expected to be needed, the clinical team should request pRBCs and components according to the anticipated needs of the patient and guided by laboratory testing.
7. It is essential that the clinical team communicates to the blood bank when the patient is being moved to a different location.
8. Laboratory monitoring for ongoing blood support in cases requiring >10 units of RBCs:
   a. Transfusion support should be individualized for each patient.
   b. The following general guidelines apply:
      1. Check Hgb, platelet count, INR, and fibrinogen after each blood volume lost/infused.
      2. Include the number of "cell saver" units in the tally of pRBCs.
      3. Target a ratio of 2 pRBCs to 1 FFP during the course of acute bleeding.
      4. Anticipate fibrinolysis and treat with antifibrinolytics if there is ongoing diffuse bleeding.
      5. Verify that the INR is <2.5 and fibrinogen >100. Values outside these ranges may indicate systemic fibrinogenolysis, DIC, or hemodilution.
      6. In the absence of platelet transfusion, anticipate a halving of the platelet count with each blood volume resuscitation. Transfuse platelets to maintain an anticipated platelet count >50 000 μL.
      7. A stat AST or ALT can be used to document shock liver (values >800 IU/mL), which is an independent indication for antifibrinolytic therapy; and if accompanied by ongoing shock, may indicate futility of resuscitation.
   c. Monitor and treat abnormalities of ionized Ca^{2+}, K^{+}, pH, and temperature.
9. Not all patients with massive injuries can be saved. The decision to withdraw support for these patients should be made by consensus of the treating team and the available resources.

ALT, alanine aminotransferase; AST, aspartate aminotransferase; DIC, disseminated intravascular coagulation; FFP, fresh frozen plasma, INR, international normalized ratio; pRBCs, packed red blood cells; RBC, red blood cell.

1. Transfusion of RBCs equal to one recipient blood volume can cause a 50% drop in the platelet count and produce a **dilutional thrombocytopenia** that, if progressive and uncorrected, can result in diffuse oozing and failure to form a clot.
2. Adequate hemostasis may occur with plasma clotting factor concentrations as low as 30% of normal. There is approximately a 10% decrease in clotting factor concentration for each 500 mL of replaced blood loss. Bleeding from factor deficiency during a massive transfusion is usually due to diminished levels of fibrinogen and labile factors (V, VIII, and IX), which may be replaced with FFP. Bleeding from hypofibrinogenemia is unusual unless the fibrinogen level is less than 75 mg/dL.
3. Shock and acidosis can precipitate the release of tissue plasminogen activator from blood vessels with consequent increased **fibrinolysis** and **fibrinogenolysis**. Antifibrinolytic agents (epsilon aminocaproic acid or tranexamic acid, see **Chapter 27**) will improve local hemostasis and reduce blood loss in the setting of hyperfibrinolysis.
4. **Additional complications** of massive transfusion include **hypothermia** from the rapid infusion of refrigerated blood, **citrate toxicity** (see **Section VII.B.2**), and dysrhythmias secondary to **electrolyte abnormalities** (hypocalcemia and hypomagnesemia).
5. Once bleeding has begun from extreme **dilutional coagulopathy** and thrombocytopenia, it can be very **difficult to control**. Therefore, some form of balanced blood resuscitation is recommended (eg, 1 unit of FFP for every 2 units of pRBCs). Randomized trial data showed equivalent survival for patients undergoing trauma treated with 1:1:2 versus 1:1:1 blood ratios. In addition, 1 adult dose of platelets should be administered if the circulating platelet count is observed to be or expected to be less than 50 000/μL. When using intraoperative blood salvage, reinfused salvage units should be included as part of the tabulation of pRBCs. Washed salvaged blood does not contain coagulation factors or platelets.
6. In addition to transfusion of appropriate blood products, the strategy for massive transfusion includes **maintaining intravascular volume**, administering **calcium** as needed to offset the effects of citrate, and the consideration of **vasopressors with inotropic properties** to support adequate perfusion until resolution of the underlying pathology can be established. Strict attention of **topical hemostasis** is essential. Use of packing with or without topical antifibrinolytics, topical thrombin-soaked gauze, and combat dressings, cautery, and sutures may be critical to successful hemostasis. Frequent laboratory measures of coagulation status may be needed because these parameters change rapidly in the setting of massive hemorrhage and transfusion. Finally, direct **communication with the blood bank** and a transfusion medicine specialist is fundamental to expedite component preparation.
7. Currently, there are no reliable markers that accurately predict when further transfusion and resuscitation is futile.

Selected Readings

American Society of Anesthesiologists Task Force on Blood Component Therapy. Practice guidelines for perioperative blood transfusion and adjuvant therapies. *Anesthesiology.* 2006;105(1):198-208.

Bosboom JJ, Klanderman RB, Migdady Y, et al. Transfusion-associated circulatory overload: a clinical perspective. *Transfus Med Rev.* 2019;33(2):69-77.

Callum J, Farkouh ME, Scales DC, et al. Effect of fibrinogen concentrate vs cryoprecipitate on blood component transfusion after cardiac surgery: the FIBRES trial. *JAMA.* 2019;322(20):1966-1976. doi:10.1001/jama.2019.17312

Carson JL, Stanworth SJ, Alexander JH, et al. Clinical trials evaluating RBC thresholds. *Am Heart J.* 2018;200:96-101.

Carson JL, Terrin ML, Noveck H, et al; FOCUS Investigators. Liberal or restrictive transfusion in high-risk patients after hip surgery. *N Engl J Med.* 2011;365(26):2453-2462.

Carson J, Triulzi DJ, Ness PM. Indications for and adverse effects of RBC transfusion. *N Engl J Med.* 2017;377(13):1261-1272.

Chang TM. From artificial red blood cells, oxygen carriers, and oxygen therapeutics to artificial cells, nanomedicine, and beyond. *Artif Cells Blood Substit Immobil Biotechnol.* 2012;40(3):197-199.

Corwin HL, Gettinger A, Fabian TC, et al. Efficacy and safety of epoetin alfa in critically ill patients. *N Engl J Med.* 2002;357(10):965-976.

CRASH-2 Trial Collaborators; Shakur H, Roberts I, et al. Effects of tranexamic acid on death, vascular occlusive events, and blood transfusion in trauma patients with significant haemorrhage (CRASH-2): a randomized, placebo-controlled trial. *Lancet.* 2010;376(9734):23-32.

Dutton RP, Shih D, Edelman BB, et al. Safety of uncrossmatched type-O red cells for resuscitation from hemorrhagic shock. *J Trauma.* 2005;59(6):1445-1449.

Finfer S, Bellomo R, Boyce N, et al; SAFE Study Investigators. A comparison of albumin and saline for fluid resuscitation in the intensive care unit. *N Engl J Med.* 2004;350(22):2247-2256.

Gunter OL, Au BK, Isbell JM, et al. Optimizing outcomes in damage control resuscitation: identifying blood product ratios associated with improved survival. *J Trauma.* 2008;65(3):527-534.

Hajjar LA, Vincent JL, Galas FR, et al. Transfusion requirements after cardiac surgery: the TRACS randomized controlled trial. *JAMA.* 2010;304(14):1559-1567.

Holcomb JB, Tilley BC, Baraniuk S, et al. Transfusion of plasma, platelets and red cells in a 1:1:1 vs a 1:1:2 ratio. *JAMA.* 2015;313(5):471-482.

Holland LL, Brooks JP. Toward rational fresh frozen plasma transfusion: the effect of plasma transfusion on coagulation test results. *Am J Clin Pathol.* 2006;126(1):133-139.

Keir AK, Hansen AL, Callum J, et al. Coinfusion of dextrose-containing fluids and red blood cells does not adversely affect in vitro red blood cell quality. *Transfusion.* 2014;54(8):2068-2076.

Looney MR, Roubinian N, Gajic O, et al. Prospective study on the clinical course and outcomes in transfusion-related acute lung injury. *Crit Care Med.* 2014;42(7):1676-1687.

McQuilten Z, Crighton G, Brunskill S, et al. Optimal dose, timing and ratio of blood products in massive transfusion. *Transfus Med Rev.* 2018;32(1):6-15.

Mesar T, Larentzakis A, Dzik W, Chang Y, Velmahos G, Yeh DD. Association between ratio of FFP to RBCs during massive transfusion and survival among patients without traumatic injury. *JAMA Surg.* 2017;152(6):574-580.

Perel P, Roberts I, Ker K. Colloids versus crystalloids for fluid resuscitation in critically ill patients. *Cochrane Database Syst Rev.* 2013;2:CD000567.

Roubinian JJ, Hendrickson JE, Triulzi DJ, et al. Contemporary risk factors and outcomes of transfusion-associated circulatory overload. *Crit Care Med.* 2018;46(4):577-585.

Stainsby D, MacLennan S, Thomas D, et al. Guidelines on the management of massive blood loss. *Br J Haematol.* 2006;135(5):634-641.

Zarychanski R, Turgeon AF, McIntyre L, et al. Erythropoietin-receptor agonists in critically ill patients: a meta-analysis of randomized controlled trials. *CMAJ.* 2007;177(7):725-734.

35 Obstetric Critical Care

Emily E. Naoum and Elisa C. Walsh

I. INTRODUCTION

Despite a historical perception of the obstetric patient population as being overall healthy, the past several decades have seen a rise in preexisting comorbidities and diseases of pregnancy with a coincident increase in maternal morbidity and mortality. The incidence of intensive care unit (ICU) admission for pregnant and postpartum women ranges from 0.7 to 32.1 per 1000 deliveries, with the majority of admissions occurring in the postpartum period (Figure 35.1). Regionalization of perinatal care classifies institutions depending on capabilities and personnel to provide care for peripartum women, and the American College of Obstetricians and Gynecologists (ACOG) defines four levels of maternal care. All facilities should be able to stabilize patients and accommodate transfer; centers at Level 3 and Level 4 are those capable of providing ICU level of care. (See also Video 35.1: Fetal Heart Rate Monitoring.)

A. When caring for the pregnant woman who is critically ill, it is important to consider how management may affect the fetus.

B. Any pregnant patient admitted to the ICU should prompt multidisciplinary care plan formation, including the need for fetal monitoring and a potential labor and delivery plan. Preterm labor and delivery are common in the setting of critical illness.

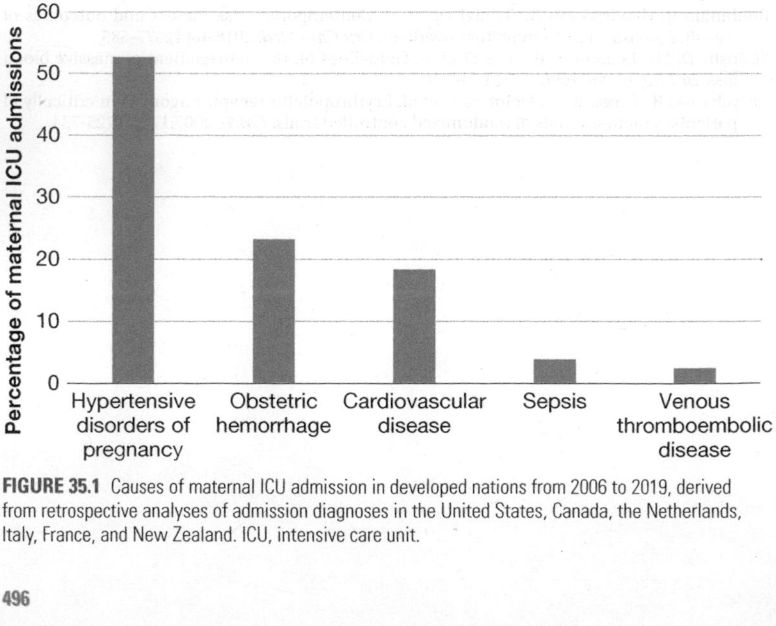

FIGURE 35.1 Causes of maternal ICU admission in developed nations from 2006 to 2019, derived from retrospective analyses of admission diagnoses in the United States, Canada, the Netherlands, Italy, France, and New Zealand. ICU, intensive care unit.

II. GENERAL CONSIDERATIONS RELEVANT TO THE OBSTETRIC, CRITICALLY ILL POPULATION

A. Physiologic Changes of Pregnancy

1. Pregnant women undergo normal physiologic changes associated with pregnancy, labor, and delivery (see Table 35.1 for details). Maintenance of these physiologic changes is critical for placental perfusion and fetal oxygenation. Thus, common treatments in the ICU such as high levels of positive end-expiratory pressure (PEEP), diuretics, and vasopressors must be weighed against the risk of decreased venous return, decreased cardiac output, and changes in maternal blood flow distribution—all of which may affect placental perfusion and fetal oxygenation.
2. After 20 weeks' gestation (uterus palpable above the umbilicus), patients should be positioned with left uterine displacement or in the lateral position to minimize aortocaval compression and resultant hypotension.
3. Physiologic changes of pregnancy can alter the pharmacokinetics and pharmacodynamics for many medications used in the ICU.

B. Viability of the Fetus and Fetal Heart Rate Monitoring (refer Video 35.1)

1. Most sources define the age of fetal viability as being about 24 weeks of gestation. After 24 weeks, fetal heart rate monitoring is recommended to evaluate fetal well-being. Normal fetal heart rate varies between 110 and 160 beats/min. A fetal heart rate outside of these parameters or with minimal variability may signal a potential problem with the fetus and should prompt consultation with an obstetrician and/or a neonatologist.

C. Teratogenic Agents

1. **Teratogens** are substances that act to irreversibly alter growth, structure, or function of the developing fetus.

TABLE 35.1 Physiologic Changes of Pregnancy

Parameter	Change (relative to nonpregnant state)
Blood volume	+45%
Plasma volume	+55%
Red blood cell volume	+30%
Tidal volume	+45%
Cardiac output	+50%
Stroke volume	+25%
Heart rate	+25%
Systemic vascular resistance	−20%
Left ventricular end-diastolic volume	↑
Ejection fraction	↑
Left ventricular stroke work index	No change
Central venous pressure	No change
Pulmonary capillary wedge pressure	No change
Maternal oxygen consumption	+20%
Inspiratory reserve volume	+5%
Expiratory reserve volume	−25%
Residual volume	−15%
Vital capacity	No change
Total lung capacity	−5%
Inspiratory capacity	+15%
Functional residual capacity	−20%
Minute ventilation	+45%
Alveolar ventilation	+45%

↑, increase.

2. Timing of exposure and the drug-dosing regimen can influence teratogenicity. The classic period of susceptibility to teratogenic agents is between 2.5 and 8 weeks after conception, during the period of organogenesis. Later effects are more prominent on growth and/or nervous system and gonadal tissue. The U.S. Food and Drug Administration (FDA) issued a drug classification system with five categories (A-D and X) implying a progressive fetal risk from Category A to X. Category X drugs are contraindicated in pregnancy.
3. Medications commonly encountered in the ICU setting and have known teratogenic properties include antiepileptics (phenytoin, carbamazepine, phenobarbital, valproic acid, topiramate), lithium, statins, angiotensin-converting enzyme (ACE) inhibitors, amiodarone, warfarin, tetracyclines, and ribavirin.
4. Multiple internet resources are available for further drug and teratogen information, including the websites of the ACOG and the Centers for Disease Control and Prevention (CDC).
5. Most drugs are safe for use during lactation. Typically, only 1% to 2% of the maternal dose appears in breast milk. The Drugs and Lactation database (LactMed) of the National Library of Medicine's Toxicology Data Network is a resource for further information.

D. Vasopressor Use and Potential Effects on the Fetus

1. Little data exist regarding vasopressor use for maternal hypotension or shock due to critical illness. Traditionally, there have been concerns with vasopressor use during pregnancy regarding the potential adverse effects on uterine blood vessels and fetal blood flow; however, maintaining adequate systemic perfusion is imperative to maintain placental perfusion because it is not autoregulated.
2. When managing hypotension, it is reasonable to attempt other interventions initially, such as administering intravenous (IV) fluids and placing the patient in the left lateral decubitus position to prevent aortocaval compression by the gravid uterus.
3. In the setting of persistent hypotension, restoring maternal perfusion pressure is of paramount importance, and it should override any theoretical concerns of vasopressor-induced uterine vasculature constriction. Increasing the mean arterial pressure (MAP) will improve perfusion pressure to the organs, including the gravid uterus. Norepinephrine, an endogenous catecholamine that crosses the placenta, is often used as a first-line vasopressor. Second-line vasopressors such as epinephrine or vasopressin may be considered. No good data exist regarding the use of vasopressin in pregnant women and it is considered a Category C medication. Therefore, caution is recommended if this agent is used because it may theoretically activate uterine V1a receptors, leading to uterine contractions.

E. Ventilation and Blood Gases (Table 35.2)

1. Most aspects of mechanical ventilation are the same for pregnant and nonpregnant women with the exception of the target arterial carbon dioxide tension ($PaCO_2$). Ventilator settings should be adjusted to maintain mild respiratory alkalosis with $PaCO_2$ between 30 and 32 mm Hg and arterial pH between 7.40 and 7.47. This replicates normal pregnancy physiology due to progesterone-induced respiratory stimulation resulting in an increased minute ventilation and an increased sensitivity to CO_2 by the end of the first trimester.
2. Maternal hypercapnia ($PaCO_2$ >40 mm Hg) may result in decreased removal of CO_2 from the fetus, causing fetal acidosis, in addition to increased fetal breathing movements, which may increase fetal oxygen consumption. Thus, it seems prudent to avoid maternal hypercapnia even though studies have not identified any adverse sequelae in fetuses that were exposed to

TABLE 35.2 Blood Gas Measurements During Pregnancy

		Trimester		
Parameter	**Nonpregnant**	**First**	**Second**	**Third**
$Paco_2$ (mm Hg)	40	30	30	30
Pao_2 (mm Hg)	100	107	105	103
pH	7.40	7.44	7.44	7.44
$[HCO_3^-]$ (mEq/L)	24	21	20	20

$Paco_2$ levels as high as 60 mm Hg during permissive hypercapnia. Significant maternal hypocapnia ($Paco_2$ <30 mm Hg) should also be avoided because it may decrease uteroplacental perfusion and contribute to fetal hypoxia. Maternal oxygen consumption increases in pregnancy by 20% to 30% at term, largely because of increased consumption by the fetus and placenta. To minimize fetal effects, the maternal Pao_2 should be maintained at greater than 65 mm Hg.

III. PREECLAMPSIA

Preeclampsia is part of a spectrum of hypertensive disorders specific to pregnancy. Although the precise etiology of preeclampsia remains unknown, it is a disease that occurs only in the presence of placental tissue. A combination of chronic uteroplacental ischemia, immune maladaptation, lipoprotein toxicity, genetic predisposition, and an exaggerated maternal inflammatory response likely play a role in disease progression, which is characterized by abnormal vasospasm and ischemia. Hypertensive disorders of pregnancy account for 25% to 60% of ICU admissions in developed nations and are a major contributor to maternal morbidity.

Preeclampsia complicates 2% to 8% of pregnancies globally and around 5% of all pregnancies in the United States, and the incidence has been rising over the past three decades. Hypertensive disorders of pregnancy contribute to 16% of maternal deaths. Risk factors for preeclampsia include nulliparity, multifetal gestation, history of preeclampsia in prior pregnancies, gestational diabetes, maternal age older than 35, and maternal pre-pregnancy body mass index (BMI) greater than 30. A patient meets the criteria for a diagnosis of preeclampsia if she has persistently elevated blood pressure after 20 weeks' gestation in the setting of previously normal blood pressure, and proteinuria of greater than 300 mg in 24 hours or signs of end-organ dysfunction. The diagnosis of preeclampsia is divided into preeclampsia and preeclampsia with severe features based on the presence or absence of specific signs, symptoms, and abnormal laboratory values (Table 35.3).

A. Two additional diagnoses, **eclampsia and HELLP syndrome**, are a part of this spectrum of disease.

1. Eclampsia is defined as the occurrence of **seizures or coma** in a woman with preeclampsia that cannot be attributed to other causes. Eclamptic seizures may occur antepartum, intrapartum, or postpartum. Eclampsia is a cause of significant maternal and fetal morbidity, and mortality ranges from 0% to 14%. However, in high-resource countries where patients are managed in tertiary care centers with experienced providers, the mortality is closer to 1% to 2%. Eclamptic seizures are usually preceded by headache and visual disturbances. The pathophysiology remains unknown but may be related to failure of cerebral autoregulation, endothelial dysfunction, and/or cerebral vessel vasoconstriction. Seizures are generally abrupt and self-limited, but may be complicated by cardiopulmonary arrest or pulmonary aspiration of gastric contents.

TABLE 35.3 Diagnostic Criteria for Preeclampsia and Preeclampsia With Severe Features

Blood pressure	≥140 mm Hg systolic or ≥90 mm Hg diastolic on two occasions at least 4 h apart after 20 wk of gestation in a woman with a previously normal blood pressure ≥160 mm Hg systolic or ≥110 mm Hg diastolic, hypertension can be confirmed within a short interval (minutes) to facilitate timely antihypertensive therapy
and	
Proteinuria	≥300 mg per 24-h urine collection (or this amount extrapolated from a timed collection) or Protein-creatinine ratio ≥0.3 (each measured by mg/dL) Dipstick reading of 1+ (used only if other quantitative methods are not available)
Or in the absence of proteinuria, new-onset hypertension with the new onset of any of the following:	
Thrombocytopenia	Platelet count <100 000/μL
Renal insufficiency	Serum creatinine concentrations >1.1 mg/dL or a doubling of the serum creatinine concentration in the absence of other renal disease
Impaired liver function	Elevated blood concentrations of liver transaminases to twice normal concentration
Pulmonary edema	
Cerebral or visual symptoms	New-onset headache unresponsive to medication and not accounted for by alternative diagnoses or visual symptoms
Severe Features	
Blood pressure	SBP >160 mm Hg or DBP ≥110 mm Hg on two or more occasions at least 4 h apart (unless antihypertensive therapy is initiated before this time)
Thrombocytopenia	Platelet count <100 000/μL
Impaired liver function	Elevated blood concentrations of liver enzymes to twice the upper limit of normal or severe, persistent RUQ or epigastric pain unresponsive to medications that is not accounted for by alternative diagnoses
Renal insufficiency	Serum creatinine concentrations >1.1 mg/dL or a doubling of the serum creatinine concentration in the absence of other renal disease
Pulmonary edema	
Cerebral or visual disturbances	New-onset headache unresponsive to medication and not accounted for by alternative diagnoses or visual symptoms

DBP, diastolic blood pressure; SBP, systolic blood pressure; RUQ, right upper quadrant. Adapted from Gestational hypertension and preeclampsia: ACOG Practice Bulletin, Number 222. *Obstet Gynecol.* 2020;135(6):e237-e260.

2. **HELLP** (**h**emolysis, **e**levated **l**iver enzymes, and **l**ow **p**latelets) **syndrome** is characterized by a constellation of laboratory abnormalities and was previously regarded as a subset of severe preeclampsia; however, it is now recognized as a potentially distinct clinical entity because 15% to 20% of cases do not have hypertension or proteinuria. The diagnosis of HELLP syndrome is also associated with an increased risk of adverse outcomes including placental abruption, renal failure, hepatic subcapsular hematoma, hepatic rupture, and fetal and maternal death. Management entails administering magnesium, supportive care with normalizing blood pressure in the face of severe hypertension, and delivery of the fetus with recognition of the increased risk of hemorrhage in this population. Platelet

counts can fall precipitously, and platelet transfusions are indicated in any parturient with significant bleeding or with a platelet count of less than 20 000/mm^3. Subcapsular hematoma, if it occurs, is an emergency and can result in shock and fulminant hepatic failure. Death is typically due to exsanguination and coagulopathy. Prompt surgical intervention and resuscitative measures have led to improvement in maternal survival.

B. Management

1. **Delivery:** The only definitive treatment for preeclampsia, eclampsia, or HELLP syndrome is delivery of the fetus and placenta. The decision of when to deliver is made on the basis of the gestational age and the severity of the disease. Each patient and clinical situation should be individualized with a management strategy that seeks to balance and minimize both maternal and fetal morbidity. If needed, maternal stabilization should precede delivery to reduce morbidity.

2. **Pharmacologic therapy**

   a. **Seizure prophylaxis:** Although the mechanism of action is unknown, **magnesium sulfate** is the medication of choice for prophylactic prevention and treatment of eclamptic seizures. Dosage of magnesium is 4 to 6 g IV bolus over 30 minutes followed by 2 g/h IV, but because it is renally cleared, this may need to be adjusted if severe renal dysfunction is present. The drug is administered during active labor, delivery, and for 24 to 48 hours postdelivery. Because of its relaxant effect on vascular and visceral smooth muscle, magnesium may decrease maternal blood pressure and predispose to postpartum atony and hemorrhage. It also inhibits acetylcholine release at the motor endplate, leading to potentiation of neuromuscular blocking agents. Finally, magnesium therapy increases the risk of pulmonary edema.

   b. **Antihypertensive medications** such as **labetalol** (IV), **hydralazine** (IV), and **calcium channel blockers** (po) are frequently administered for control of blood pressure. The goal is not to normalize blood pressure but to keep patients from progressing to a hypertensive crisis, encephalopathy, or stroke with a goal systolic blood pressure (SBP) less than 160 mm Hg. When administering antihypertensive medications, it is important to remember that the placenta has no ability to autoregulate flow. Thus, a sudden drop in maternal blood pressure may decrease placental perfusion and result in significant compromise to the fetus. In cases of refractory hypertension, continuous infusions of nicardipine, esmolol, sodium nitroprusside, or nitroglycerin may be indicated.

IV. ACUTE FATTY LIVER OF PREGNANCY

Acute fatty liver of pregnancy (AFLP) is a rare but potentially fatal complication of pregnancy, involving microvesicular fat deposition in the liver and characterized by liver dysfunction, disseminated intravascular coagulation (DIC), severe and refractory hypoglycemia, encephalopathy, and renal insufficiency. The incidence ranges from 1 to 3 cases per 10 000 deliveries and patients usually present in the third trimester, although the disease has been described as early as 23 weeks' gestation. There is a significant concurrence of AFLP and preeclampsia and differentiating the two conditions can be challenging. Some authors consider AFLP and HELLP to be part of a spectrum of a single disease, but AFLP can be distinguished from HELLP on the basis of severe hepatic synthetic dysfunction, rather than merely elevated liver transaminases (as occurs in HELLP) with coagulopathy and hypoglycemia. The precise pathogenesis of AFLP is believed to be due to defective mitochondrial β-oxidation of fat either in the fetus and/or the mother, which results in multi-organ fatty infiltration, impaired liver function and clearance, and placental and endothelial dysfunction. Maternal mortality rates have dropped significantly in the past two decades from as high as 70% to now around 2% because of improved recognition, early intervention, and aggressive management of critical illness. Perinatal mortality is reported to be around 10% to 20% because of fetal acidosis and prematurity.

A. Clinical Manifestations: Patients frequently present with nonspecific symptoms such as malaise, nausea and emesis, jaundice, epigastric or right upper quadrant pain, headache, and anorexia. Severe symptoms such as jaundice, ascites, encephalopathy, and hypoglycemia may be present.

B. Diagnosis and Laboratory Findings: One distinct laboratory finding of AFLP is hyperbilirubinemia with serum levels of 3 to 40 mg/dL reported. Antithrombin III level is often decreased in AFLP and elevated ammonia, elevated urate, and renal impairment may also be present. Patients also have profound elevation of alkaline phosphatase with mild to moderate transaminase elevations, and progression to hepatic failure can be rapid. In addition to hepatic dysfunction, renal failure, **coagulopathy, profound hypoglycemia**, and metabolic acidosis are early complications. The Swansea criteria have been prospectively validated for the diagnosis and comprise clinical symptoms, laboratory abnormalities, ultrasound, and pathologic findings. A score of 6 or more of these features in the absence of another explanation is used to make the diagnosis of AFLP.

1. Hyponatremia from diabetes insipidus can be present in up to 10% of patients.
2. Pancreatitis is a rare complication that typically develops after renal and hepatic dysfunction and is associated with poorer outcomes when present.
3. Liver biopsy is rarely required and should be performed only when absolutely necessary because of the concomitant coagulopathy.

C. Management: Hepatic failure associated with AFLP is reversible in most patients, and **supportive care** and **expeditious delivery** are the mainstays of treatment. AFLP is a medical emergency that requires immediate evaluation. The most important component of treatment is the delivery of the fetus. Careful attention to **fluid balance** is crucial because of the increased risk of pulmonary and cerebral edema secondary to low colloid osmotic pressure. There is frequently comorbid **acute renal dysfunction** (90%), which is usually reversible, but temporary renal support may be required. Worsening liver failure may be accompanied by cerebral edema, circulatory dysfunction, persistent coagulopathy, infection, and renal failure. Transplantation is generally not required for AFLP but may be necessary in severe cases.

1. **Serum glucose levels** should be checked every 1 to 2 hours and hypoglycemia aggressively treated; all patients should receive an infusion of at least 5% dextrose, and many will require higher concentrations with intermittent boluses to maintain normoglycemia.
2. **Coagulation studies** should be followed at regular intervals and postpartum hemorrhage anticipated. Regardless of the mode of delivery, patients should have adequate IV access and cross-matched blood products available. If the patient requires a cesarean delivery, coagulopathy should be improved or corrected before incision when possible.
3. ***N*-acetylcysteine** may be considered in patients with moderate to severe AFLP.
4. There is often a worsening of liver function, renal function, and coagulopathy for 48 hours after delivery, but then improvement should be expected.

V. NEUROLOGIC DISEASE

A. Stroke: Pregnant women are at higher risk than are nonpregnant women for stroke, with an incidence of 5 to 15 per 100 000 deliveries and cerebrovascular events accounting for 5% of maternal deaths. A significant proportion of strokes occur late in pregnancy, with the highest incidence in the peripartum period. **Ischemic strokes** appear to account for one-half to two-thirds of cerebrovascular events in pregnancy, whereas **hemorrhagic strokes** are less common.

1. **Etiologies: Ischemic stroke** may be divided into arterial or venous etiologies. **Arterial etiologies** include vasculopathies, dissections, and embolic events; **venous infarctions** may result from hypercoagulable states, dehydration, or infections. **Hemorrhagic events** are largely a result of aneurysms, vascular malformations, preeclampsia, or trauma.
2. **Clinical manifestations** are similar to those in nonpregnant women. **Headache** is the most common presenting symptom. Other symptoms include focal neurologic deficits and seizures.
3. **Diagnosis:** In addition to physical examination, neurologic imaging is critical for establishing the diagnosis and etiology. Attempts should be made to minimize fetal exposure to radiation, but appropriate diagnostic imaging should not be avoided. The fetal radiation exposure from noncontrast computed tomography (CT) scan is less than 1 rad.
4. **Management** in the pregnant patient resembles treatment in nonpregnant patients. Care is supportive, and thrombolytic therapy should be considered if indicated for ischemic stroke. Thrombolysis with recombinant tissue plasminogen activator (r-tPA) has been reported during pregnancy and appears to be safe for the fetus; there is minimal transplacental passage of r-tPA. However, retroplacental bleeding with pregnancy loss has been reported. The therapeutic window for r-TPA (ie, time from onset of symptoms to administration of the agent) is 4.5 hours.
   a. Goals to preserve fetal well-being include adequate oxygenation, maintaining euvolemia, and avoidance of hypotension, hyperglycemia, and fever. Delivery of the fetus may be complicated by the risk of aneurysm or arteriovenous malformation (AVM) rupture, thrombolytic therapy, or anticoagulation; both the route of delivery and anesthetic management should be tailored to each individual patient.

B. **Epilepsy** affects approximately 1 in 200 parturients. A third of women will experience an increase in their seizure frequency during pregnancy, which is likely multifactorial but may be secondary to increases in plasma volume, higher drug clearance, decreased gastrointestinal absorption, and stress. Monitoring of antiepileptic levels may be beneficial to ensure therapeutic levels. In addition, many antiepileptic medications carry an elevated risk of teratogenicity to the fetus. Patients and providers must weigh the risks and benefits of continuing these medications in pregnancy. Whenever possible, it is recommended to pursue monotherapy with the agent with the lowest teratogenic potential and folate supplementation. Valproate is associated with the highest risk of major malformations, whereas newer agents such as lamotrigine and levetiracetam have the lowest risk. Uncontrolled generalized seizures pose a serious risk to both mother and fetus.

1. **Status epilepticus** (also see **Chapter 10**). Although the frequency of seizure activity is increased in a significant portion of parturients, pregnancy itself does not increase the likelihood of status epilepticus.
   a. Should status epilepticus occur in a pregnant patient, **treatment goals** include (a) maintaining an adequate airway, (b) ensuring adequate oxygenation, (c) addressing any precipitant for the seizure, and (d) aborting the seizure. The patient should be placed in full lateral position and supplemental oxygen administered, in addition to receiving advanced airway support if needed.
   b. **Pharmacologic therapy** should be initiated after 2 to 5 minutes of prolonged seizure activity with benzodiazepines or propofol.
   c. For **intractable seizure activity**, pharmacologic suppression of seizure activity, tracheal intubation, and mechanical ventilation may be necessary. Fetal bradycardia may occur and necessitate prompt delivery.

2. **Eclampsia:** The diagnosis of eclampsia should be ruled out in any pregnant woman who presents with a new-onset seizure disorder after 20 weeks' gestation. Management of eclamptic seizures includes magnesium sulfate and prompt delivery. See **Section III** for further discussion.

VI. ACUTE RESPIRATORY DISTRESS SYNDROME

Acute respiratory distress syndrome (**ARDS**, also see **Chapter 20**) is a rare but serious complication in pregnancy and, when present, may result in significant maternal and fetal mortality. The incidence of ARDS in pregnancy ranges from 17 to 130 per 100 000 deliveries, or 0.013% to 0.13%. No large studies are available, but data from the past several decades place maternal mortality rates in the range of 25% to 40% and fetal mortality over 20%.

A. **Risk Factors Specific to Pregnancy** include gastric aspiration, medications used for tocolysis, preeclampsia, amniotic fluid or trophoblastic embolism, and abruption. The physiologic changes of pregnancy that may increase the risk of ARDS include decreased lower esophageal sphincter tone, increased intra-abdominal pressure, increased circulating blood volume, decreased serum albumin, a possible upregulation of acute inflammatory response components, and increased capillary leak.

B. **Management:** As in the nonpregnant population, the mainstay of treatment is supportive care. However, the following should be considered when managing a pregnant patient with ARDS.
   1. **Ventilation:** Goals of ventilation should strive to maintain physiologic alterations of pregnancy (see **Section II.E**).
   2. **Maintenance of maternal cardiac output** is critical for placental perfusion and fetal oxygenation. Thus, standard treatments in ARDS therapy such as high levels of PEEP, diuretics, and vasopressors must be weighed against the risk of decreased venous return, decreased cardiac output, and changes in maternal blood flow distribution—all of which may decrease placental perfusion and fetal oxygenation. In addition, after 20 weeks' gestation (uterus palpable above the umbilicus), patients should be positioned with left uterine displacement or in the lateral position to minimize aortocaval compression.
   3. **Rescue therapies** can be considered for pregnant patients. Literature from the hemagglutinin type 1 and neuraminidase type 1 (H1N1) and COVID-19 pandemics provide substantial evidence to support the use of prone positioning, neuromuscular blockade, inhaled vasodilators, and even extracorporeal membrane oxygenation (ECMO) for pregnant patients with refractory hypoxemia.

C. **Obstetric Considerations:** Fetal assessment should be performed at regular intervals to evaluate fetal well-being. Historically, it was advocated to deliver the preterm fetus after 28 weeks' gestation in patients with ARDS for maternal benefit; however, improvement in respiratory parameters from delivery is purely theoretical, and mechanical restriction is not significant until later in the third trimester. Pregnant patients at or after 32 weeks of gestation with refractory hypoxemia may be considered for delivery if it will allow further optimization of care and there may be a benefit in reducing the physiologic demands. The decision to deliver should be made in a multidisciplinary team with critical care physicians, obstetricians, and neonatologist involvement.

VII. CARDIOVASCULAR DISORDERS

Cardiovascular disorders are a rising cause of maternal mortality in the United States because of increasing adult survivors of congenital heart disease and intolerance of the physiologic changes of pregnancy with preexisting maternal heart disease. Preconception counseling is crucial for patients with a history of cardiac disease desiring pregnancy. Several tools have been developed to assess maternal cardiac risk during pregnancy including the ZAHARA-I risk score, CARPREG-1/2 risk score, and the modified World Health Organization (WHO) classification. The ZAHARA risk score predicts the risk for cardiac events based on the weighted presence of various underlying conditions. The CARPREG-2 risk score identifies 10 predictors of maternal cardiac complications: 5 general predictors (prior cardiac events or arrhythmias, poor functional class or cyanosis, high-risk valve disease/left ventricular (LV) outflow tract obstruction, systemic ventricular dysfunction, no prior cardiac interventions); 4 lesion-specific predictors (mechanical valves, high-risk aortopathies, pulmonary hypertension (pHTN), coronary artery disease); and 1 delivery of care predictor (late pregnancy assessment). The Modified WHO Pregnancy Risk Classification is broken into four classes based on the presumptive risk of maternal morbidity and mortality related to underlying cardiac comorbidities.

A. Valvular Heart Disease (also see **Chapter 16**)

1. Chronic **regurgitant lesions** are well tolerated with the normal physiologic changes of pregnancy. A decrease in systemic vascular resistance, reduced LV afterload, and a modest increase in heart rate all lead to a reduction in regurgitant flow. However, in the immediate postpartum period, the sudden increase in venous return and vascular resistance may lead to decompensation, and patients should be carefully monitored for the first 24 to 48 hours.
   a. **Aortic regurgitation (AR)** with preserved LV function is well tolerated in pregnancy. In symptomatic, severe AR, the treatment is **salt restriction and diuretics.** Vasodilators such as **hydralazine** and **nitrates** may be used as substitutes to ACE inhibitors, which are contraindicated in pregnancy.
   b. **Mitral regurgitation (MR)** during pregnancy is usually due to rheumatic valvular disease or the myxomatous degeneration of mitral valve prolapse. Patients with MR in pregnancy will rarely become symptomatic, but if decompensation occurs, medical management with **vasodilators** and **diuretics** may be helpful.
   c. As in the nonpregnant population, **acute regurgitant lesions** are poorly tolerated and constitute a medical and surgical emergency.
2. In contrast to regurgitant lesions, **stenotic lesions** are not well tolerated in pregnancy. Increased intravascular volume, increased heart rate, and decreased systemic vascular resistance in pregnancy adversely affect these patients. The autotransfusion and increased venous return associated with delivery and the immediate postpartum period (where cardiac output is highest) may lead to further decompensation, and patients should be closely monitored for the first 24 to 48 hours postpartum. Considerations for invasive blood pressure monitoring using arterial lines, continuous electrocardiogram (ECG) to evaluate for arrhythmias, and central venous access (via a central venous line or a peripherally inserted central catheter) for central venous pressure (CVP) monitoring and potential vasopressor administration should be part of the multidisciplinary planning discussion regarding these patients.
   a. **Aortic stenosis (AS)** is most often associated with a congenital bicuspid valve. Women with mild to moderate disease will tolerate pregnancy provided they are followed up closely and managed appropriately. In contrast, women with severe AS (transvalvular gradient >40 mm Hg, valve area <1 cm^2, and impaired LV function) are at risk for deterioration with development of heart failure and preterm delivery.
      1. **Medical management** consists of **maintenance of preload, afterload, relative bradycardia, and normal sinus rhythm.**
      2. If possible, patients with severe disease should undergo preconceptual valve replacement or valvuloplasty. In the setting of an established pregnancy, valvuloplasty is the procedure of choice to minimize the risk of fetal loss.
      3. For **delivery**, hemodynamic monitoring, early neuraxial anesthesia, and an assisted second stage (which may require a dense sacral

block if forceps delivery is attempted) are recommended for mild and moderate cases. Patients with severe AS may be managed with low-concentration local anesthetic epidural mixes for labor analgesia or sequential combined spinal epidural (CSE) technique with vasopressor support for cesarean delivery. Even in a controlled setting, there is a risk of decompensation because of the hemodynamic effects of neuraxial medications, and patients with severe disease may require general anesthesia for cesarean delivery.

b. **Mitral stenosis (MS)** is most commonly associated with rheumatic heart disease. Increased stroke volume and heart rate during pregnancy in the setting of a significantly narrowed valve leads to increased left atrial pressure, arrhythmias, and worsened symptoms.

1. Patients with severe MS contemplating pregnancy (valve area <1.5 cm^2, pHTN) should be offered valvuloplasty or replacement; in patients who are already pregnant, valvuloplasty is preferred.
2. Optimal **medical management** of the pregnant patient involves administration of **β_1-blockers** for decreasing heart rate, maintaining sinus rhythm, and reducing left atrial pressure. **Diuretics** and **salt restriction** may also be necessary to avoid rapid changes in preload. **Anticoagulation** should be considered in patients with severe MS and an enlarged left atrium, even in the absence of atrial fibrillation.
3. Hemodynamic monitoring, early epidural anesthesia, and an assisted second stage are recommended for delivery. Patients frequently require admission and monitoring in an intensive care setting following delivery because they are particularly vulnerable to heart failure and pulmonary edema.

3. **Prosthetic cardiac valves:** Patients may present with either mechanical or bioprosthetic valves. For women who desire children, the bioprosthetic valve is often selected because they do not require long-term systemic anticoagulation (in the absence of arrhythmias) and carry a lower thromboembolic risk. However, they deteriorate at a more rapid rate.

a. **Anticoagulation:** Thromboembolic events are of particular concern in pregnancy, and all obstetric patients with mechanical valves or bioprosthetic valves in atrial fibrillation should receive anticoagulation. Anticoagulation in pregnancy is usually accomplished with **unfractionated heparin (UFH)** or **low-molecular-weight heparin (LMWH)** because warfarin is Category D for women with a mechanical heart valve and Category X for all other indications in pregnant women. **Endocarditis prophylaxis** is recommended in this patient population.

B. **Congenital Heart Disease:** Pregnant women with a history of repaired congenital disease are becoming increasingly common as more patients survive to childbearing age, and congenital heart lesions are now the most common cause of cardiac disease in the pregnant population. Some patients **present with a partially repaired or completely uncorrected lesion**, making management considerably more complex. Predictors of poor maternal-fetal outcome include the following: use of cardiac medication before pregnancy, elevated pulmonary artery pressure (PAP), depressed right ventricular (RV) or LV function, cyanosis, and impaired New York Heart Association functional class. **Endocarditis prophylaxis** should be given to patients with unrepaired cyanotic heart disease, repaired disease with residual defects adjacent to prosthetic material, or a repair involving placement of prosthetic material within the previous 6 months. Essentially, all parturients with congenital heart disease require multidisciplinary discussion with their cardiology team to understand their anatomy (because corrections of the lesions may differ) and the best course of management. A detailed discussion of specific disorders is beyond the scope of this book but may be found in resources such as *Chestnut's Obstetric Anesthesia: Principles and Practice.*

C. Myocardial Infarction is uncommon in pregnancy, with an estimated incidence of 6.2 to 6.5 per 100 000 deliveries and a maternal mortality rate of 5%. Possible etiologies include atherosclerotic disease with or without acute plaque rupture, coronary artery dissection, and coronary vasospasm. Risk factors for myocardial infarction (MI) in pregnancy include advanced maternal age, hypertension, diabetes, thrombophilia, smoking, cocaine abuse, and diabetes.

1. The balance between **myocardial oxygen supply and demand** is affected by the physiologic changes of pregnancy with increased myocardial mass, heart rate, contractility, and wall tension. In addition, labor and delivery are associated with a significant increase in cardiac output, myocardial oxygen consumption, and elevated levels of circulating catecholamines. Although pregnancy itself is not thought to be a risk factor for MI, the changes associated with pregnancy may place high-risk individuals at even greater risk.
2. **Diagnosis:** As in nonpregnant individuals, the diagnosis of MI is made by history, examination, and appropriate diagnostic tests. **Troponins** remain sensitive and relatively specific in the pregnant population (although they are elevated at baseline in patients with preeclampsia), whereas minor **ECG** changes such as T-wave inversions and ST-segment depressions are common in pregnancy and thus less specific for myocardial ischemia.
3. **Management** of an acute MI in pregnancy is guided by the same principles as in the nonpregnant population, with several important considerations.
   a. **Medical management: β_1-blockers, low-dose aspirin**, and **nitrates** may be used safely in pregnancy. Conversely, ACE inhibitors and statins are contraindicated in pregnancy and both should be avoided.
   b. **Anticoagulation** may be safely achieved with **UFH** or **LMWH.** There is very limited information about the safety and efficacy of **thrombolytic therapy** in pregnancy; although successful use has been reported, there is an increased risk of puerperal hemorrhage and placental abruption.
   c. **Revascularization: Percutaneous coronary intervention (PCI)** is the preferred modality for treatment of pregnancy-associated acute MI. Typically, a bare metal stent is placed to minimize the amount of time on dual antiplatelet therapy to avoid risk of intrapartum and postpartum hemorrhage. The fetal effects of clopidogrel are unknown.
   d. **Obstetric management:** The fetus should be carefully monitored and, if viable, a plan for delivery established in the event of sudden maternal or fetal decompensation. Patients receiving dual antiplatelet therapy may not receive neuraxial analgesia.

D. Peripartum Cardiomyopathy (PPCM) is a rare form of dilated cardiomyopathy with an estimated incidence of 1 in 300 to 3000 live births with significant regional variation. The etiology remains unclear, although risk factors include multiple gestation, advanced maternal age, obesity, African race, gestational hypertension, cocaine abuse, and preeclampsia.

1. **Clinical presentation and diagnosis:** Patients present with symptoms of heart failure such as dyspnea, fatigue, and edema that may be difficult to distinguish from normal changes in pregnancy. The diagnosis requires echocardiographic evidence of cardiomyopathy and three criteria: (i) onset within a 6-month period, from the last month of pregnancy to 5 months postpartum; (ii) no prior history of cardiomyopathy or preexisting heart failure; and (iii) exclusion of all other identifiable causes of cardiomyopathy. Echocardiographic criteria include left ventricular ejection fraction (LVEF) less than 45% and end-diastolic LV dimension greater than 27 mm/m^2 body surface area (BSA).
2. **Medical management** is the same as that in other patients with congestive heart failure. Patients may benefit from **inotropic support, diuretics**, and **ventricular afterload reduction.** Patients with PPCM are at high risk for thromboembolism, and **anticoagulation** should be considered. Pregnant patients

should not receive ACE inhibitors, and nitroprusside should be used cautiously because of the risk of fetal cyanide toxicity with prolonged use. Finally, mechanical support with a **ventricular assist device** or **intra-aortic balloon pump** should be considered as a bridge to transplant in patients who fail to respond to medical management.

3. **Obstetric management:** Delivery should be strongly considered in pregnant patients diagnosed with PPCM, particularly if the fetus is at risk or the patient is not responding to medical management, or if the patient also has preeclampsia. Neuraxial anesthesia is ideal because of the reduction in both preload and afterload.
4. **Prognosis and recurrence:** The all-cause 5-year survival rate is greater than 95% in the United States. There is no clear consensus on the recurrence of PPCM in subsequent pregnancies, but the data would suggest that patients with residual LV impairment at the time of conception have an increased risk of recurrence and mortality.

E. Pulmonary Hypertension (pHTN) is defined as mean PAP greater than or equal to 20 mm Hg at rest with normal pulmonary artery occlusion pressure less than 15 mm Hg assessed by right heart catheterization. Etiologies include primary pulmonary arterial hypertension, left-sided heart disease or congenital heart disease, pulmonary disease, thromboembolic disease, or idiopathic disease. The pathophysiology involves pulmonary vasoconstriction, which leads to RV overload, vascular wall remodeling, and RV hypertrophy and later dilation leading to RV failure and death. Pregnancy should be discouraged in this population because of significantly elevated maternal mortality, with most recent estimates of 16% to 33% despite modern treatment modalities.

1. **Medical management** should be individualized in each case, and a multidisciplinary team approach adopted. **Oxygen,** either continuous or for several hours each day, reduces PAP and improves cardiac output. **Anticoagulation** with UFH or LMWH is often recommended to prevent pulmonary emboli, which may be fatal. **Specific pulmonary vasodilator therapy** includes **inhaled nitric oxide**; inhaled, subcutaneous, or IV **prostaglandins**; and **phosphodiesterase-5 (PDE-5) inhibitors.** Use of **endothelin receptor antagonists** is contraindicated in pregnancy because of teratogenicity.
2. Throughout pregnancy and delivery, the hemodynamic goals should be (i) to avoid pain, hypoxemia, acidosis, and hypercarbia; (ii) to maintain intravascular volume and preload, but with careful monitoring to avoid volume overload and RV failure in the peripartum period; (iii) to maintain SBP greater than PAP to ensure adequate coronary perfusion of the RV; (iv) to augment cardiac output as needed; and (v) to avoid tachydysrhythmias. Intensive care monitoring is generally indicated postpartum.

VIII. VENOUS THROMBOEMBOLISM

Venous thromboembolism (VTE) accounts for almost one-sixth of all maternal mortality in the United States. Several normal physiologic changes of pregnancy increase the risk of VTE, including venous stasis in the lower extremities from mechanical compression of the uterus, hypercoagulability of pregnancy, placental delivery leading to endometrial trauma, and increased platelet activation.

A. Incidence: VTE has an event rate of 1.99 per 1000 pregnancies, with 1.26 deep venous thrombosis (DVT) and 0.73 pulmonary embolism (PE) events. Compared with nonpregnant patients, pregnant women have 5-fold greater odds of VTE during pregnancy and 60-fold greater odds of VTE postpartum, particularly the first week postpartum but persisting up to 12 weeks postpartum. VTE-related maternal mortality in the United States is approximately 1.49 deaths per 100 000 births. There is an increased risk of iliac or femoral DVTs compared to the nonpregnant population, and a higher incidence of left-sided DVTs presumably due to uterine compression of the left iliac vein.

B. Risk Factors: In addition to the factors listed, obesity, increased age and parity, prior VTE, postpartum hemorrhage and infections, cesarean delivery (particularly emergent), and acquired or congenital hypercoagulable states are associated with an increased risk of VTE.

C. Diagnosis: Pregnant patients present with the same signs and symptoms as the nonpregnant population. However, confirming the diagnosis may be more complex. **Compression ultrasonography** of the lower extremities may be used safely in pregnancy. If negative but symptoms persist, it is recommended to perform further imaging. Although the imaging studies commonly used to diagnose PE (**spiral computerized tomography and ventilation-perfusion [V/Q] scanning**) do expose the fetus to radiation, both expose the fetus to less than 1 mGy of radiation.

D. Management: Therapeutic anticoagulation should be initiated with LMWH (guided by anti-factor Xa activity) or UFH (guided by activated partial thromboplastin time [aPTT] monitoring). In the event of a massive PE resulting in hemodynamic instability, thrombolytic therapy may be considered but a thrombectomy is preferred because of the significant risk of hemorrhage.

IX. HEMORRHAGE

Obstetric hemorrhage is a leading cause of maternal morbidity and mortality worldwide, particularly in developing nations. The majority of adverse outcomes in hemorrhage are likely preventable and are due to factors such as failure to recognize risk factors, inaccurate estimation of blood loss, and delays in resuscitation. One statewide review of maternal mortality found that 40% of cases were deemed potentially preventable with improved medical care, particularly in hemorrhage (93%).

A. Antepartum Hemorrhage occurs in approximately 25% of pregnancies but is infrequently life-threatening to the parturient; the fetus is at the highest risk. Most commonly, it arises from abnormal placentation.

1. **Etiologies** include the following:

   a. **Placenta previa** is defined as a placenta that partially or completely covers the internal cervical os. Risk factors include prior previa, uterine scar from a previous surgery or procedure, increasing multiparity, and advanced maternal age. The classic presentation is painless vaginal bleeding during the second or third trimester. Ultrasound confirms the diagnosis. Of note, the presence of a placenta previa increases the risk of placenta accreta spectrum disorders, particularly in women with prior cesarean delivery.

   b. **Placental abruption** is defined as complete or partial premature separation of the placenta from the uterus. Bleeding occurs because of the exposed vessels, and fetal distress may ensue from a loss of placental surface for oxygen and nutrient exchange. The etiology remains unclear, but **risk factors** are hypertension, advanced maternal age, increasing multiparity, trauma, prior history of abruption, tobacco and cocaine use, and preterm premature rupture of membranes. The classic presentation is vaginal bleeding, uterine tenderness, and painful, frequent contractions. The diagnosis is largely clinical because ultrasonography is specific (96%) but not sensitive (24%) for placental abruption. Of note, a significant amount of bleeding may be concealed in the retroplacental space. Placental abruption results in exposure of tissue factor and other factors that can result in consumptive coagulopathy and DIC. Other complications include hemorrhagic shock and fetal demise, with a perinatal mortality rate of 12%.

   c. **Uterine rupture** is a rare complication of pregnancy with potential for significant maternal and fetal morbidity. The major **risk factor** is a previous uterine scar; in patients with a previous lower uterine segment incision, the incidence is less than 1%. The incidence is higher in patients with a history of a classical uterine incision; in these patients, rupture is associated with greater morbidity because of the vascularity of the anterior uterine wall and the possible disruption of the placental bed. Presentation is variable. The most common signs are abdominal pain (including breakthrough pain with neuraxial analgesia) and abnormal fetal heart tone (FHT).

2. **Management:** In all cases of antepartum bleeding, the first steps are maternal stabilization and assessment of fetal status. Providers should obtain **large-bore IV access** and blood for a type and screen and assess coagulation status and hemoglobin/hematocrit. Placental abruption and previa may be expectantly managed, depending on the degree of bleeding and gestational age. If preterm with minimal abruption and no evidence of compromise, delivery may be delayed for corticosteroid treatment. For a patient who is normovolemic and noncoagulopathic, labor and vaginal delivery may be considered. For significant bleeding, prompt delivery and aggressive volume resuscitation are critical. Previa and abruption place patients at increased risk for atony and development of coagulopathy, which should be anticipated and aggressively treated. Uterine rupture requires immediate delivery of the fetus, most commonly with general anesthesia to facilitate an exploratory laparotomy. The uterus may be repaired, but hysterectomy is sometimes required.

B. **Postpartum Hemorrhage:** The average blood loss for vaginal delivery and cesarean delivery is less than 500 and 1000 mL, respectively. Postpartum hemorrhage (PPH) may be defined as blood loss in excess of the level mentioned, or clinically as a 10% decrease in hematocrit from admission to the postpartum period. Primary PPH occurs within 24 hours, whereas secondary PPH occurs between 24 hours and 6 weeks postpartum.

1. **Significant etiologies** include the following:

   a. **Uterine atony** is the most common cause of primary postpartum hemorrhage accounting for 80% of cases. Typically, uterine contraction (mediated by endogenous oxytocin) leads to constriction of spiral arteries, which contributes to hemostasis during delivery. **Risk factors** include prolonged labor, multiple gestations, high parity, chorioamnionitis, augmented labor, cesarean delivery, precipitous labor, tocolytic agents, and use of volatile anesthetics. Given the frequency of uterine atony, the ACOG recommends prophylactic treatment with uterotonics for all deliveries. Initial treatment should include bimanual massage, placement of large-bore IV access, volume resuscitation, and **oxytocin** infusion (0.3-0.6 IU/min). Further pharmacologic therapy may include administration of uterotonic medications such as **methergine 0.2 mg intramuscular (IM), misoprostol 600 to 1000 µg buccal or per rectum (PR)**, and **15-methyl prostaglandin F2a 250 µg IM.** Surgical intervention may be required, including a peripartum hysterectomy.

   b. **Placenta accreta** occurs in three subtypes: **placenta accreta**, defined as adherence of the placenta to the myometrium without a decidual layer, **placenta increta**, defined as invasion into the myometrium, and **placenta percreta**, defined as invasion through the uterine serosa.

      1. **Risk factors** for placenta accreta include a previous uterine incision or instrumentation, advanced maternal age, multiparity, assisted reproductive techniques, and a low-lying placenta or placenta previa. The incidence of accreta rises significantly when placenta previa is present in a patient with one or more previous uterine incisions, with an incidence of greater than 60% in women with placenta previa and three or more prior cesarean deliveries.

      2. **Diagnosis** is usually made antenatally with ultrasonography and occasionally magnetic resonance imaging (MRI).

3. **Management** is typically planned preterm cesarean delivery with peripartum hysterectomy with the placenta left in situ. Internal iliac artery balloon catheters may be considered to decrease blood loss after delivery. Estimated blood loss exceeds 2 L in two-thirds of cases and may be precipitous; **large-bore access** and **rapid volume resuscitation** are essential.

c. **Uterine inversion** is a rare event that may cause significant hemorrhage because of ischemia of the fundus, precipitating uterine atony. The first-line treatment is manual replacement of the uterus, which is facilitated by discontinuation of uterotonic agents and administration of uterine relaxants (eg, nitroglycerin IV or sublingual, terbutaline, magnesium). This is followed by aggressive medical management (readministration of uterotonic medications) to improve uterine tone and limit further hemorrhage.

d. **Retained placenta** is defined as failure of placental separation within 30 minutes of delivery. Management involves the removal of the placenta manually or with curettage and may require uterine relaxation through additional neuraxial analgesia or IV nitroglycerin.

2. **Invasive treatment options** to control PPH include intrauterine balloon placement, uterine compression (B-Lynch) sutures, uterine artery embolization or ligation, and perioperative hysterectomy.

3. **Chapter 34** discusses optimal resuscitation and transfusion in hemorrhagic shock in nonpregnant patients. Tranexamic acid (TXA) reduces the risk of death due to bleeding in the setting of PPH without increasing the risk of thrombotic events (1 g IV plus an additional 1 g IV if bleeding continues after 30 minutes). Traditional, trauma-based resuscitation with 1:1:1 product transfusion is often used in the peripartum period despite the hematologic changes of pregnancy that may not warrant such aggressive factor replacement. The use of rotational thromboelastometry (ROTEM) and thromboelastography (TEG) has expanded over the past decade and there are pregnancy-specific resuscitation algorithms that have been developed targeting higher fibrinogen levels in this population. Studies have shown that viscoelastic-guided resuscitation reduces the number of blood products transfused and may reduce the need for hysterectomy and ICU admission in the peripartum population.

X. SEPSIS

Sepsis (see **Chapter 12**) remains a leading cause of maternal morbidity and mortality. In the United States, sepsis complicates approximately 0.04% of deliveries and contributes to an estimated 12% to 23% of maternal deaths.

A. **Causes:** Obstetric sepsis primarily arises from chorioamnionitis, endometritis, urologic infections, septic abortions, wound infections, and pneumonia. Most obstetric infections are polymicrobial. Common pathogens implicated with maternal sepsis are *Escherichia coli*, staphylococcus, streptococcus, and gram-negative and anaerobic organisms.

B. **Risk Factors** for maternal sepsis can be subdivided into demographic, obstetric, and comorbidity factors. Known risk factors include cesarean delivery, Medicaid insurance, multiple gestation, postpartum hemorrhage, preterm delivery, and retained products of conception.

C. **Diagnosis** of maternal sepsis can be challenging. Pregnancy is associated with an increase in heart rate, a decrease in blood pressure, and an increase in cardiac output. These changes may mask some early signs of sepsis because of their overlap with systemic inflammatory response syndrome (SIRS) and may further compromise organ perfusion in the patient with sepsis. **Obstetric early warning systems** (eg, maternal early warning criteria [MEWC] and modified early warning score [MEOWS]) are highly sensitive and reasonably specific in predicting maternal morbidity and the need for ICU care, including in maternal sepsis. In a multicenter case-control study of maternal sepsis screening tools, the authors identified the highest to lowest sensitivity in the SIRS, MEW, and quick Sequential Organ Failure Assessment (qSOFA) criteria, and the highest to lowest specificity in the qSOFA, MEW, and SIRS criteria. The sepsis in obstetrics score (SOS) is a highly specific and reasonably sensitive scoring tool to predict women at risk for ICU admission from sepsis.

D. Management: Early diagnosis with prompt and aggressive treatment is critical for minimizing morbidity and mortality. Patients with a positive screen for maternal sepsis should be urgently evaluated by a physician to determine potential obstetric and nonobstetric causes, have diagnostics ordered to assess end-organ injury, and initiated on treatment with **source-directed broad-spectrum antibiotics within 1 hour, 30 mL/kg fluid resuscitation within 3 hours**, and additional vasopressor support with norepinephrine to maintain a MAP greater than 65 mm Hg. The antibiotic regimen chosen should provide empiric coverage for the common obstetric infections and should include either a combination of gentamycin, clindamycin, and ampicillin or a combination of vancomycin and piperacillin/tazobactam. Fetal status is best managed by optimizing maternal treatment, but nonreassuring FHT may prompt delivery.

XI. ENDOCRINE DISORDERS (also see **Chapter 28**)

A. Diabetic Ketoacidosis (DKA) is infrequent in pregnancy, with an estimated incidence between 0.5% and 3% in pregnancies complicated by preexisting or gestational diabetes. In recent years, maternal mortality associated with DKA has improved, but fetal loss remains high, with estimates ranging from 10% to 35% in affected pregnancies and morbidity includes preterm delivery, hypoxia, and acidosis.

1. **Clinical presentation** and **laboratory abnormalities** may be identical to those in the nonpregnant population; however, studies have shown that pregnant women are more likely to present with much lower glucose values, including normoglycemia, than their nonpregnant counterparts, making this a diagnostically challenging situation. More rapid development in the pregnant patient may also lead to a delayed diagnosis and treatment, necessitating a raised awareness of this condition. In addition, evidence of fetal compromise is frequently present.
2. **Risk factors** for DKA in pregnancy include emesis of any cause, use of ß-sympathomimetics, starvation, infection, previously undiagnosed diabetes, and poor patient compliance with using insulin.
3. Several **physiologic changes of pregnancy** predispose patients to developing DKA. Pregnancy is a state of relative insulin resistance and increased lipolysis, with a tendency toward ketone body formation. In addition, increases in minute ventilation cause a mild respiratory alkalosis that is compensated by increased renal excretion of bicarbonate; this compensated respiratory alkalosis leaves patients less capable of buffering serum ketone acids. Accelerated starvation, dehydration, reduced caloric intake, and stress are additional risk factors unique to the pregnant state.
4. **Fetal concerns:** Maternal acidosis decreases uterine blood flow and causes a leftward shift in the maternal oxyhemoglobin dissociation curve, both of which compromise fetal oxygenation. Ketoacids dissociate and cross the placenta, contributing to a metabolic acidosis in the fetus. Lastly, glucose readily crosses the placenta, causing fetal hyperglycemia, osmotic diuresis, and hypovolemia.
5. **Medical management** is unchanged from that for the nonpregnant population. Aggressive fluid resuscitation, glucose control with insulin, search for

and treatment of the underlying etiology, and control of electrolyte abnormalities are the mainstays of treatment.

6. **Obstetric management.** Fetal status may be measured indirectly by fetal heart rate tracings or biophysical profile. Maternal resuscitation is imperative to improving the fetal outcome, and delivery for fetal indications should be reserved for fetal compromise that continues after appropriate maternal stabilization. Nonreassuring fetal heart tracings may revert to normal within hours of correction of the maternal acidemic and hypovolemic state.

B. Ovarian Hyperstimulation Syndrome (OHSS) is a rare, iatrogenic complication of ovulation induction in fertility treatments. It usually occurs in the luteal phase or within the first week post conception. The seminal event in the genesis of OHSS is ovarian enlargement, with an acute fluid shift out of the intravascular space, resulting in ascites and intravascular hypovolemia.

1. The reported **prevalence** of the most severe form is 0.5% to 5%, with an estimated mortality of 1 per 450 000 to 1 per 50 000 patients.
2. **Clinical presentation:** Signs and symptoms result from an overproduction of inflammatory and vasoactive cytokines that lead to increased capillary permeability and arteriolar vasodilation, which leads to intravascular volume shifting into the extravascular spaces. Patients may present with ascites, oliguria, renal failure, hydrothorax, pericardial effusion, or ARDS. Laboratory abnormalities include **electrolyte imbalances** (hyponatremia and hyperkalemia), elevated liver enzymes, metabolic acidosis, elevated creatinine, **hemoconcentration**, leukocytosis, and thrombocytosis.
3. **Management:** Treatment of OHSS is supportive. Patients should be carefully monitored, administered isotonic fluids to restore intravascular volume, and treated for electrolyte disturbances. Increased intra-abdominal pressure from ascites may result in poor pulmonary function and impaired renal perfusion and may have significant deleterious effects on maternal circulation. **Ultrasound-guided paracentesis** has been shown to improve creatinine clearance, urine output, dyspnea, and osmolarity, but care must be taken to avoid inadvertent puncture of ovarian cysts with subsequent intraperitoneal hemorrhage. Pulmonary support may include thoracentesis, oxygen supplementation, or even mechanical ventilation. These patients are also at risk for developing thrombosis in either the arterial (20%) or venous (80%) circulations, and prophylactic **anticoagulation** should be initiated.
4. **Resolution:** After a period of several days, patients begin to mobilize the extravascular fluid and a natural diuresis occurs. Complete resolution typically takes 2 weeks from the onset of symptoms.

XII. AMNIOTIC FLUID EMBOLISM

Amniotic fluid embolism (AFE) is a rare but possibly catastrophic complication of pregnancy. Because AFE remains a diagnosis of exclusion, the true incidence is unknown but is estimated to be between 2 and 8 per 100 000 live births. The mortality rate among affected parturients is as high as 80%, and the disease accounts for up 5% to 10% of maternal deaths overall. Among survivors, significant and permanent neurologic sequelae are common. Approximately 50% of patients who have an AFE are at risk for cardiac arrest, according to one epidemiologic study.

A. Clinical Presentation: Classically, up to 70% of patients present during labor or delivery and the remaining 30% in the immediate postpartum period (up to 4 hours after delivery in some case reports), with acute hypoxia and hypotension that rapidly deteriorates to cardiovascular collapse, dysrhythmias, coagulopathy, and death. In the initial phase, systemic hypertension and pHTN are present along with profound hypoxemia and are then followed by LV dysfunction and coagulopathy.

B. **Pathophysiology:** The etiology is likely multifactorial and is poorly understood. Although some believe the inciting event is a breach in the barrier between the maternal and fetal compartments leading to the presence of fetal cells, amniotic fluid, and inflammatory mediators in the maternal circulation, others hypothesize that there may be a humoral response to an unknown instigator because many asymptomatic pregnant women have fetal cells present in their blood. The pathophysiology is likely an overexaggerated response to endogenous inflammatory mediators. Although an effort was made to change the term to "anaphylactoid syndrome of pregnancy" given that it is not truly embolic in nature and thus "amniotic fluid embolus" is a misnomer, the name persists. **Risk factors** for AFE include cesarean delivery, instrumental delivery, placental previa, and placental abruption.

C. **Manifestations** affect multiple organ systems, and presentation may vary depending on the predominant physiologic change.

1. **Cardiovascular:** Hypotension is a hallmark feature, present in 100% of patients with severe disease. A biphasic model of shock has been proposed to explain the findings seen in patients with AFE. The initial transient response is systemic hypertension and pHTN, likely from the release of vasoactive substances, causing hypoxia and right heart failure. Patients who survive the initial insult develop a second phase of left heart failure and pulmonary edema.
2. **Pulmonary:** Hypoxia is an early manifestation, arising from acute pHTN with subsequent $\dot{V}/Q$ mismatch and shunting. Later, pulmonary edema develops in association with LV dysfunction. A substantial portion of patients will also manifest noncardiogenic pulmonary edema after LV function improves.
3. **Coagulation:** Disruption of the normal clotting cascade occurs in up to 85% of patients. It remains unclear whether the coagulopathy is the result of a consumptive process or from massive fibrinolysis, and is postulated to be due to the release of fetal/placental thromboplastic material into the maternal circulation. Patients may experience significant bleeding, massive hemorrhage, and DIC and it can be extremely challenging to control.

D. **Management** involves aggressive resuscitation; supportive care is aimed at minimizing additional hypoxia and subsequent end-organ damage. Goals of therapy include maintenance of oxygenation, circulatory support, and correction of the coagulopathy.

1. Most patients will require intubation and mechanical ventilation.
2. Hemodynamic instability should be corrected with fluid resuscitation and vasopressor support as needed.
3. **Lines and monitors** should include central and peripheral large-bore IV access, continuous pulse oximetry, invasive blood pressure monitoring, and, possibly, a pulmonary artery catheter and/or transesophageal echocardiography to assess ventricular function.
4. **Laboratory studies** should be sent at regular intervals and coagulopathy aggressively treated.
5. If the event occurs before delivery, the fetus should be delivered as quickly as possible to minimize fetal hypoxia and to aid maternal resuscitation.
6. Rescue therapies such as cardiopulmonary bypass, ECMO, and intra-aortic balloon counterpulsation have been described in the literature as successful options for the treatment of refractory AFE and should be considered. ECMO may improve neurologically intact survival compared to standard resuscitation in peripartum patients. An area of future study appears to be

the role of inflammatory cytokines in the pathophysiology of this disease, which may be targeted for treatment strategies to improve survival.

XIII. TRAUMA

Trauma (see **Chapter 9**) is the leading cause of nonobstetric mortality and morbidity in pregnancy, accounting for 45% to 50% of all maternal deaths in the United States and complicates 5% to 7% pregnancies. Common causes include motor vehicle accidents (49%-70%), domestic violence (11%-25%), and falls (9%-23%). Hemorrhagic shock and brain injury are the most frequent mechanisms of death. Blunt trauma is more common than is penetrating trauma. Owing to increased vascularity and shifting of abdominal contents by the gravid uterus, splenic and retroperitoneal injury is more common in pregnant women, whereas bowel injury is less frequent. Risk factors for maternal trauma include age younger than 25 years, low socioeconomic status, minority race, use of illicit drugs or alcohol, and history of domestic violence. It is important to remember that any female of reproductive age who undergoes trauma could be pregnant at the time of injury.

A. Complications will vary based on the mechanism and severity of injury. Concerns specific to maternal trauma include the following:

1. **Placental abruption** complicates 20% to 60% of cases of severe maternal trauma, most commonly after 16 weeks' gestation. It can cause occult hemorrhage and coagulopathy and should be considered a source of bleeding in cases of unstable pregnant trauma. Early, frequent contractions are a sensitive indicator of abruption. The period of monitoring and observation should be increased in women with contractions, abdominal tenderness, or significant maternal injury.
2. **Uterine rupture** is a rare complication of trauma (0.6%) but presents a major threat to the mother (10% mortality) and fetus (nearly 100% mortality).
3. **Preterm labor** is a common complication of trauma (up to 25%), even with minor trauma.
4. **Amniotic fluid embolism** is an uncommon complication of trauma but should be considered if resuscitation is refractory.
5. **Direct fetal injury** increases in risk after 13 weeks' gestation as the uterus elevates from the bony pelvis.

B. Management: Standard guidelines for care of patients undergoing general trauma apply to pregnant patients, with several important modifications:

1. Patients at 20 weeks' gestation or more who are placed on a backboard should be placed in left uterine displacement, to minimize aortocaval compression.
2. Owing to increased blood volume during pregnancy, signs of cardiovascular deterioration in hemorrhage may be delayed compared to a nonpregnant patient.
3. Efforts should be made to transfuse only O-negative blood in the event that transfusion is required before a type and cross can be performed to avoid maternal isoimmunization to Rh.
4. It is crucial to preserve maternal cardiac output, blood pressure, and oxygen delivery to optimize maternal recovery and protect fetal well-being.

C. Testing: Beyond standard workup for trauma, additional testing specific to pregnancy may include a **Kleihauer-Betke test**, which can indicate the severity of uterine-placental trauma by measuring fetal blood in the maternal circulation. All patients should have a type and screen, and Rh-negative patients with a positive Kleihauer-Betke test result should be given **Rh-immune globulin**. Early evaluation for pregnancy complications and assessment of fetal well-being should be performed. If greater than 20 weeks' gestation, **fetal heart rate monitoring** should be initiated for at least 4 hours and **ultrasonography** may also be considered.

D. Fetal Outcome is dependent on maternal outcome and the mechanism of injury. Maternal death is the most common cause of fetal death, and severe maternal injuries result in fetal death in 20% to 40% of cases. In significant penetrating abdominal trauma, fetal injuries are common with fetal mortality ranging from 40% to 70% because of direct fetal injury or premature delivery. Even after maternal discharge from the hospital, a 2-fold risk for preterm delivery and 9-fold risk for fetal demise persist.

XIV. LOCAL ANESTHETIC SYSTEMIC TOXICITY

Systemic absorption or inadvertent intravascular injection of local anesthetics may result in toxicity that is typically manifested by central nervous system (CNS) symptoms and cardiovascular compromise. The reported incidence of local anesthetic systemic toxicity (LAST) with epidural anesthesia ranges from 1.2 to 11 per 10 000; however, more recent studies suggest that the incidence of LAST has decreased over the past decade. Toxicity of local anesthetics is correlated with potency and their rank in order of **increasing** toxicity is as follows: 2-chloroprocaine, mepivacaine, lidocaine, tetracaine, and bupivacaine.

A. CNS Symptoms reported by patients correlate with increased plasma concentrations of local anesthetics. At lower levels, **perioral numbness, metallic taste,** and **tinnitus** are reported. As the serum concentration increases, muscle twitching, **loss of consciousness, seizures,** and **respiratory arrest** may occur.

B. Cardiovascular Manifestations occur at much higher serum concentrations than do CNS symptoms. They may progress from **increased blood pressure to bradycardia, ventricular dysfunction, ventricular tachycardia, and fibrillation.** As in nonpregnant patients, the more potent amide local anesthetics such as bupivacaine have a smaller margin of safety and may cause refractory arrhythmias. Despite this, bupivacaine remains the most common local anesthetic in obstetric anesthesia.

C. Pregnancy increases the risk of adverse outcomes from local anesthetic toxicity by several mechanisms: Decreased concentrations of plasma proteins result in a higher free serum concentration, progesterone may increase the sensitivity of nerve axons to neural blockade, and vascular engorgement may increase the risk of epidural catheter placement into an epidural vein. In addition, resuscitation is more difficult because of unclear symptomatology, rapid development of hypoxemia, and the technical difficulty of performing effective chest compressions in pregnant patients.

D. Management is largely supportive. Seizures should be terminated with **benzodiazepines** or **propofol.** In addition, resuscitation with **intralipid therapy** should be considered standard practice with an initial bolus followed by an infusion. All patients should be given supplemental oxygenation, and tracheal intubation should be considered early because acidemia may worsen the outcome. Monitoring should include the fetal heart rate. Blood pressure should be supported with fluids, vasoactive medications, and, if needed, advanced cardiac life support (ACLS). If LAST is suspected, **epinephrine dose** should be **reduced to 1 μg/kg** (a significantly smaller dose than usual) and vasopressin should be avoided on the basis of small but compelling animal studies. Calcium channel blockers and β-blockers should also be avoided. If ventricular arrhythmias develop, **amiodarone** is recommended and local anesthetics should not be administered. See **Section XV** for additional critical modifications to ACLS in the obstetric patient.

XV. CARDIOPULMONARY RESUSCITATION

Cardiac arrest complicates roughly 1 in 12 000 pregnancies, with a higher incidence in women with underlying cardiopulmonary disease. In a recent study, the most common precipitating cause of cardiac arrest in pregnant patients is hemorrhage. Overall, outcomes are better in pregnant patients than in nonpregnant patients, with up to 58% survival to discharge. Etiologies include anesthetic complications, trauma, bleeding, dysrhythmias, cardiomyopathy, drugs, and embolic events. In general, cardiopulmonary resuscitation (CPR) algorithms are unchanged for pregnant women because maternal resuscitation is the best therapy for the fetus. However, there are a few critical modifications that must be performed such as **continuous manual left uterine displacement** and consideration of perimortem cesarean delivery if gestational age is greater than or equal to 24 weeks. Prior guidelines had advocated for a higher hand position on the sternum for chest compressions; however, the most recent recommendations do not support this practice. **Vasoactive medications** and **defibrillation** should be administered as in the nonpregnant population. There are some important differences, as follows:

A. Airway: The pregnant patient should be intubated soon after initiation of CPR to protect the airway from aspiration and facilitate oxygenation and ventilation. A difficult airway should be anticipated.

B. Circulation: Cardiac output is significantly affected by patient positioning after approximately 20 weeks' gestation due to uterine compression of the inferior vena cava (IVC) and aorta that can considerably compromise preload and cardiac output. A critical component of resuscitation in the obstetric population involves manual left uterine displacement, or, if this cannot be performed, left uterine displacement accomplished with a wedge or pillow under the patient's right hip.

C. Delivery: If cardiac arrest occurs before 24 weeks' gestation (age of fetal viability), the rescuer's efforts should be directed exclusively toward the mother. If arrest occurs after 24 weeks, the fetus should be delivered within 5 minutes if CPR has not been successful in achieving return of spontaneous circulation, to optimize both maternal and fetal outcomes. A review of perimortem cesarean delivery led to clear maternal survival benefit in almost one-third of cases. Prompt delivery of the fetus minimizes the risk of hypoxic insult to the mother and improves maternal cardiac output by relieving aortocaval compression, decreasing metabolic demands, and allowing for more effective chest compressions. Delivery may be considered even in a nonviable pregnancy to improve resuscitation of the mother.

D. Venous Access should be secured in the upper extremities above the level of the diaphragm given the concern for aortocaval compression. If no venous access is obtainable after attempts, intraosseous line placement in the humeral heads should be considered.

E. Cardiopulmonary Bypass, ECMO, and Open Cardiac Massage have been advocated if closed-chest resuscitative efforts are unsuccessful.

Selected Readings

American College of Obstetricians and Gynecologists. *ACOG Practice Bulletin No. 183: Postpartum Hemorrhage.* American College of Obstetricians and Gynecologists; 2017.

American College of Obstetricians and Gynecologists. *ACOG Committee Opinion No. 793: Guidelines for Diagnostic Imaging During Pregnancy.* American College of Obstetricians and Gynecologists; 2017.

American College of Obstetricians and Gynecologists. ACOG Practice Bulletin No. 211: critical care in pregnancy. *Obstet Gynecol.* 2019;133(5):e303-e319.

Bauer ME, Housey M, Bauer ST, et al. Risk factors, etiologies, and screening tools for sepsis in pregnant women: a multicenter case-control study. *Anesth Analg.* 2019;129(6):1613-1620. doi:10.1213/ANE.0000000000003709

Budev MM, Arroliga AC, Falcone T. Ovarian hyperstimulation syndrome. *Crit Care Med.* 2005;33:S301-S306.

Creanga AA, Syverson C, Seed K, Callaghan WM. Pregnancy-related mortality in the United States, 2011-2013. *Obstet Gynecol.* 2017;130(2):366-373.

Gestational hypertension and preeclampsia: ACOG Practice Bulletin, Number 222. *Obstet Gynecol.* 2020;135(6):e237-e260.

Hensley MK, Bauer ME, Admon LK, Prescott HC. Incidence of maternal sepsis and sepsis-related maternal deaths in the United States. *JAMA*. 2019;322(9):890-892.

Jeejeebhoy FM, Zelop CM, Lipman S, et al; American Heart Association Emergency Cardiovascular Care Committee, Council on Cardiopulmonary, Critical Care, Perioperative and Resuscitation, Council on Cardiovascular Diseases in the Young, and Council on Clinical Cardiology. Cardiac arrest in pregnancy: a scientific statement from the American Heart Association. *Circulation*. 2015;132(18):1747-1773.

Lapinsky SE. Acute respiratory failure in pregnancy. *Obstet Med*. 2015;8(3):126-132.

Leffert L, Butwick A, Carvalho B, et al. The Society for Obstetric Anesthesia and Perinatology consensus statement on the anesthetic management of pregnant and postpartum women receiving thromboprophylaxis or higher dose anticoagulants. *Anesth Analg*. 2018; 126(3):928-944.

Mendez-Figueroa H, Dahlke JD, Vrees RA, et al. Trauma in pregnancy: an updated systematic review. *Am J Obstet Gynecol*. 2013;209(1):1-10.

Mhyre JM, D'Oria R, Hameed AB, et al. The maternal early warning criteria: a proposal from the national partnership for maternal safety. *Obstet Gynecol*. 2014;124(4):782-786. doi:10.1097/AOG.0000000000000480

Naoum EE, Leffert LR, Chitilian HV, et al. Acute fatty liver of pregnancy: pathophysiology, anesthetic implications, and obstetrical management. *Anesthesiology*. 2019;130(3):446-461.

Neal JM, Barrington MJ, Fettiplace MR, et al. The Third American Society of Regional Anesthesia and Pain Medicine Practice Advisory on Local Anesthetic Systemic Toxicity: executive summary 2017. *Reg Anesth Pain Med*. 2018;43(2):113-123.

Oud L. Epidemiology of pregnancy-associated ICU utilization in Texas: 2001-2010. *J Clin Med Res*. 2017;9(2):143-153.

Ramanathan K, Tan CS, Rycus P, et al. Extracorporeal membrane oxygenation in pregnancy: an analysis of the extracorporeal life support organization registry. *Crit Care Med*. 2020;48(5):696-703.

Shamshirsaz AA, Clark SL. Amniotic fluid embolism. *Obstet Gynecol Clin North Am*. 2016;43(4): 779-790.

Sibai BM, Viteri OA. Diabetic ketoacidosis in pregnancy. *Obstet Gynecol*. 2014;123(1):167-178.

Silversides CK, Grewal J, Mason J, et al. Pregnancy outcomes in women with heart disease: the CARPREG II study. *J Am Coll Cardiol*. 2018;71(21):2419-2430.

Singh A, Guleria K, Vaid NB, Jain S. Evaluation of maternal early obstetric warning system (MEOWS chart) as a predictor of obstetric morbidity: a prospective observational study. *Eur J Obstet Gynecol Reprod Biol*. 2016;207:11-17. doi:10.1016/j.ejogrb.2016.09.014

Thorne S, MacGregor A, Nelson-Piercy C. Risks of contraception and pregnancy in heart disease. *Heart*. 2006;92:1520-1525.

Wanderer JP, Leffert LR, Mhyre JM, et al. Epidemiology of obstetric-related ICU admissions in Maryland: 1999-2008. *Crit Care Med*. 2013;41(8):1844-1852.

WOMAN Trial Collaborators. Effect of early tranexamic acid administration on mortality, hysterectomy, and other morbidities in women with post-partum haemorrhage (WOMAN): an international, randomised, double-blind, placebo-controlled trial. *Lancet*. 2017;389(10084): 2105-2116.

36 Intensive Care Unit Handoffs and Transitions

Clíodhna Ashe and Jamie L. Sparling

I. HANDOFFS DEFINED

A handoff is defined by The Joint Commission as "the process of transferring primary authority and responsibility for providing clinical care to a patient from one departing caregiver to one oncoming caregiver."

A. In the intensive care unit (ICU) setting, caregivers include, but are not limited to, attending, fellow, and resident physicians; nurse practitioners; physician assistants; nurses; respiratory therapists; physical therapists; occupational therapists; speech-language pathologists; dieticians; and pharmacists.

II. ESSENTIAL ROLE OF COMMUNICATION IN ADVERSE EVENTS

Communication is frequently recognized as a primary contributor to preventable adverse events, as illustrated by these examples:

A. The Joint Commission Sentinel Event Alerts: The Joint Commission collects voluntarily submitted sentinel event reports from hospitals nationwide. Communication is among the top three root causes of sentinel events resulting in patient harm or death each year. A 2020 review of the most common sentinel event types cited communication failures as contributing to wrong site surgery, patient falls, and delays in treatment.

B. Closed Malpractice Claims: Analysis of closed malpractice claims has identified communication as a significant factor in adverse patient events leading to litigation.

1. **Obstetric anesthesia:** Communication failures contributed to 26% of cases of maternal injury.
2. **Surgical cases:** Communication breakdown contributed to error in 24% of malpractice cases.
3. **Cases involving trainees:** Teamwork breakdowns contributed to 70% of malpractice cases, with handoff problems being a leading cause.

III. COMMUNICATION AND TEAMWORK STRATEGIES IN OTHER INDUSTRIES

Many high-risk industries have realized the importance of standardized communication and have devised strategies for structuring communication between team members. Notable examples include the aviation industry, the nuclear power industry, and the military.

A. Airline Industry

1. **Sterile cockpit rule**
   a. In the early 1980s, the Federal Aviation Administration (FAA) identified that crew distractions by non-flight-related activities contributed significantly to a large number of air accidents and incidents.
   b. A review of the aviation safety reporting system database demonstrated incidents related to extraneous conversation (including with the control

tower), distractions from the flight attendants, nonpertinent radio calls and public announcement (PA) announcements, and sightseeing. Some of these incidents resulted in fatalities.

c. These incidents led directly to the implementation of the Sterile Cockpit Rule in 1981. This rule states that during "critical phases of the flight" (ground operations, takeoff, landing, and all flight operations below 10 000 feet), crew are prohibited from performing duties other than those required for safe operation of the aircraft.

2. **Crew resource management**

a. Root cause analysis of plane crashes in the 1970s revealed that failures of communication and teamwork resulted in significant risk. These investigations resulted in teamwork training programs for flight crews.

b. The program is designed to enhance team situational awareness and communication using standardized techniques called "inquiry and advocacy" and fosters a questioning attitude among team members. Standardized communication, outlined here, is used to escalate concerns or questions:

1. Get the person's attention.
2. State your concern.
3. State the problem as you see it.
4. State a solution.
5. Obtain agreement.

IV. COMMUNICATION STRATEGIES ADAPTED FOR HEALTH CARE: TEAMSTEPPS

This evidence-based program for improving teamwork in hospitals was developed and distributed by the Agency for Healthcare Research and Quality (AHRQ) and the Department of Defense (DoD). With the goal of enhancing team situational awareness, AHRQ provides materials to support readiness assessment, implementation, and sustainment. The program was field tested and then fully implemented at many hospitals throughout the country, with plans to disseminate to all hospitals nationwide. TeamSTEPPS is based on team structure and four teachable-learnable skills (Figure 36.1):

A. Team leadership
B. Situation monitoring
C. Mutual support
D. Communication

TeamSTEPPS promotes an environment of open communication and candor, where everyone on the team feels comfortable "speaking up."

V. TYPES OF HANDOFFS IN THE INTENSIVE CARE UNIT

Critical care medicine involves a variety of different types of handoffs, and each member of the ICU team may participate jointly or in parallel (eg, nursing handoff, physician handoff). Examples of major categories in which an effective and efficient transfer of patient responsibility is necessary include the following:

A. **Shift-to-Shift Handoff:** This is a direct transfer of responsibility for the patient from one clinician to another for a defined period. Provision of 24/7 care requires that clinicians sign out to oncoming teams at the end of their shifts. The departing clinician must deliver an efficient and informative overview of the patient's clinical condition over the preceding shift and provide anticipatory guidance for events for the following shift.

B. **Permanent Unit-to-Unit Handoff:** This is a permanent (or a semipermanent) change in location of a patient within the hospital. Examples include emergency room or operating room (OR) to ICU and ICU to floor.

C. **Temporary Unit-to-Unit Handoff:** This is a temporary transfer of clinical responsibility for a patient for a short length of time, typically for a procedure or

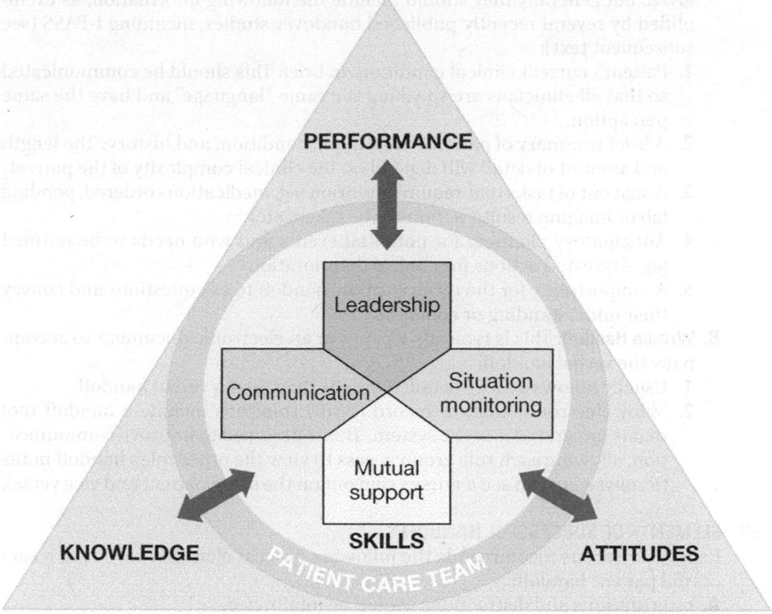

FIGURE 36.1 TeamSTEPPS 2.0 framework and competencies. (From Agency for Healthcare Research and Quality. Pocket Guide TeamSTEPPS 2.0: team strategies & tools to enhance performance and patient safety. Published December 2013. Accessed September 30, 2022. https://www.ahrq.gov/teamstepps/instructor/essentials/pocketguide.html)

diagnostic test at locations such as interventional radiology, imaging, or the OR with plans to return to the ICU.

D. External Transfer: This is a handoff between the referring facility and the accepting facility when a patient is being transferred between institutions. It should cover all of the same information as an internal handoff, plus additional information that will not be available to the receiving clinician (such as copies of reports for procedures, tests, etc). In addition, clinicians responsible for transporting the patient (eg, emergency medical services [EMS], MedFlight) must receive pertinent information to ensure a safe transport (see **Chapter 14**).

E. Escalating an Acute Situation: If there is a rapid and significant change in a patient's clinical condition, it is paramount that this information be efficiently and effectively communicated up the chain of command.

F. Medical Record: Included as part of written sign-out only, the background and history of the patient's hospital course should be updated at least daily and can reside in the electronic record.

VI. WRITTEN AND VERBAL HANDOFFS

In both the written and verbal handoffs, it is important that the clinician handing off dedicate time to prepare a comprehensive, well-organized synopsis of the patient being transferred to the receiving clinician.

A. Verbal Handoff: This should include an efficient summary of the patient's clinical condition. There are several different styles by which verbal handoffs are given, but generally they should include the following information, as exemplified by several recently published handover studies, including I-PASS (see subsequent text):

1. Patient's current clinical condition, in brief: This should be communicated so that all clinicians are speaking the same "language" and have the same perception.
2. A brief summary of patient's treatment, condition, and history: The length and amount of detail will depend on the clinical complexity of the patient.
3. A sign out of tasks that require attention (eg, medications ordered, pending lab or imaging results, actions to be taken, etc)
4. Anticipatory planning for potential events and who needs to be notified (eg, suggested actions for clinical deterioration)
5. An opportunity for the receiver of the handoff to ask questions and convey their understanding or concerns

B. **Written Handoff**: This is typically a paper or an electronic document to accompany the verbal handoff.

1. Usually follows a more detailed format than does a verbal handoff
2. Many electronic medical record (EMR) solutions include a handoff tool that is integrated into the system. This is designed to improve communication, allowing each role group access to view the other role's handoff notes (ie, physician can see a nurse's sign out on the same patient and vice versa).

VII. ELEMENTS OF SUCCESSFUL HANDOFFS

Expert consensus recommends the following process elements to ensure a successful patient handoff:

A. Interruptions and distractions should be minimized.
B. Adequate time should be allotted, with an explicit expectation for the participants to ask questions and raise concerns.
C. Information transfer should be thorough yet concise.
D. Communication should be clear, concise, consistent, and interactive.
E. All participants should act with mutual respect and practice positive teamwork, establishing role clarity, willingness to collaborate, and equality of value of others' information.
F. The handoff should have a structured or standardized process.
G. One person should speak at a time.
H. All participants should have had handoff education and training.
I. A setting-specific checklist or cognitive aid should be used.
J. The quality of the handoff process should be assessed periodically with feedback for clinicians.
K. The receiving clinician should summarize critical information to establish a mutually shared understanding.
L. The handoff should include anticipatory guidance and contingency planning for events that may occur.
M. Participants should plan and prepare for the handoff before its commencement.
N. The handoff should be documented, with the use of an EMR, if available.
O. All relevant team members should be present at the bedside when appropriate with introductions and clear roles.

VIII. COMMONLY USED HANDOFF TOOLS

There are a variety of tools available for handoffs. Two commonly used tools are as follows:

A. **SBAR**

1. Components and mnemonic
    a. **S = Situation**: a concise statement of the problem
    b. **B = Background**: pertinent and brief information related to the situation

   - **c. A = Assessment**: analysis and considerations of options—what you found/think
   - **d. R = Recommendation**: action requested/recommended—what you want to happen
2. This tool was developed by the Navy and it is not health care specific.
3. Intended for unexpected or escalation situations but has been adapted successfully for other scenarios as well
4. Provides clinicians with a predictable and structured framework for communication that is standardized across settings

B. I-PASS

1. Components and mnemonic (Figure 36.2)
   - **a. I = Illness Severity:** standard language of "stable," "watcher," or "unstable"
   - **b. P = Patient Summary:** statement of events leading up to admission, the hospital course, ongoing assessment, and the plan of care
   - **c. A = Action List:** a "to-do" list with timeline and assigned ownership
   - **d. S = Situational Awareness/Contingency Planning:** high-level context of patient care and plans for potential complications or events (ie, if "X" happens, do "Y")
   - **e. S = Synthesis by Receiver:** receiver recaps handoff, restating key items and asking questions; encourages active listening and participation of receiver
2. Two multisite studies published the following:
   - **a.** Ten-site study with approximately 50% reduction in medical errors

I-PASS
BETTER HANDOFFS. SAFER CARE.

I	Illness Severity	• Stable, "watcher," unstable
P	Patient Summary	• Summary statement • Events leading up to admission • Hospital course • Ongoing assessment • Plan
A	Action List	• To do list • Time line and ownership
S	Situation Awareness and Contingency Planning	• Know what's going on • Plan for what might happen
S	Synthesis by Receiver	• Receiver summarizes what was heard • Asks questions • Restates key action/to do items

FIGURE 36.2 I-PASS framework. (Reproduced with permission from Starmer A, Spector N, Srivastava R, et al. I-PASS, a mnemonic to standardize verbal handoffs. *Pediatrics*. 2012;129:201-204. © 2012 by the AAP.)

b. Twenty-three-site study in children showing approximately 30% reduction in medical errors

3. Originally created for physicians but may be implemented by all disciplines

4. May be adapted to institutions' and units' specific handoff needs; one example is shown in Figure 36.3.

IX. IMPLEMENTING HANDOFF TOOLS IN THE INTENSIVE CARE UNIT

A. Implementation science provides a framework for understanding the institutional context, assessing a team's performance, informing project implementation, and facilitating the adoption of a new practice.

ICU ↔ OR HANDOFF GUIDE

HUDDLE SHOULD INCLUDE ANESTHETIST, ICU RN, ICU CLINICIAN, AND RT (IF APPLICABLE)

- ❑ **Illness & Patient Summary**
  - One-liner (active issues & procedure)
  - Vitals and physical exam
  - Latest labs, active T&S
  - Allergies
  - Precautions (contact, positioning)
  - NPO Status
  - Code Status, Consents, HCP
- ❑ **Access & Airway**
  - Line types & locations (PIV, A-line, CVL, PICC, etc.)
  - Any restricted use lines? All CVL lumens patent?
  - Drains & tubes (foley catheter, epiduraa, spinal, chest, etc.)
  - Trach/ETT details
  - Vent settings
- ❑ **Bleeding, Blood Products & Fluid Balance**
- ❑ **Medications**
  - Vasoactives
  - Sedation/Pain
  - High-risk (anticoag, insulin, KCl, etc.)
  - Antibiotics
  - Neuro (AED/brain relaxation)
- ❑ **Relevant ICU/OR Course**
- ❑ **Action List** (meds due soon, pending labs, etc.)
- ❑ **Situation-Specific Planning**
  - What has or hasn't worked for this patient
  - Extubation goal or other concerns
- ❑ **Receiver Read-Back/Synthesis**
  - Big-picture summary. Ask any remaining questions.

FIGURE 36.3 Example of institution-specific implementation of I-PASS framework for transitions of care between the ICU and the OR. AED, anti-epileptic drug; CVL, central venous line; ETT, endotracheal tube; HCP, health care proxy; ICU, intensive care unit; NPO, nothing by mouth; OR, operating room; PICC, peripherally inserted central catheter; PIV, peripheral intravenous line; T&S, type and screen. (Courtesy of Dr. Aalok Agarwala.)

B. Successful implementation of best practices is a multistep process involving planning, engaging, executing, and evaluating. Research on other patient safety priorities (eg, safe surgery checklists, emergency manuals) has demonstrated the need for a well-defined implementation process when attempting widespread adoption.

C. Figure 36.4 outlines questions that should be addressed from the outset in approaching handoff redesign.

D. Steps in implementation include the following:

1. Identify and recruit a multidisciplinary team consisting of all stakeholders involved in the handoff process (eg, attending intensivist, resident and/or fellow, ICU nurse, respiratory therapist, surgeon, anesthesiologist, and OR nurse may all participate in OR to ICU handoffs).
2. Set up frequent, regular meetings with the team to discuss project status and opportunities for improvement.
3. Agree on a set of values or guiding principles that describes the team's shared vision for an ideal handoff. Examples of guiding principles include the following:
   - **a.** Handoffs are documented electronically.
   - **b.** Include face-to-face communication.
   - **c.** Include all team members involved in the care of the patient.
   - **d.** Conducted efficiently
   - **e.** Include all pertinent information related to the patient's care.
4. Use process maps to develop a shared understanding of the existing handoff process. Mapping software or using sticky notes on a wall may be helpful to depict the process.
5. Compare the current process with values set forth by the team to determine whether there is alignment. Observe and audit key steps to assess reliability of current process and accuracy of the process map. Establish baseline metrics, for example:
   - **a.** Does the team actually meet to give handoff?
   - **b.** Are anesthesia and surgical reports given?
   - **c.** Does the receiving team ask questions and recap the plan?
6. For any gaps, perform a root cause analysis to assess why certain steps are not occurring. Use a fishbone diagram to help visualize the issues, as needed.

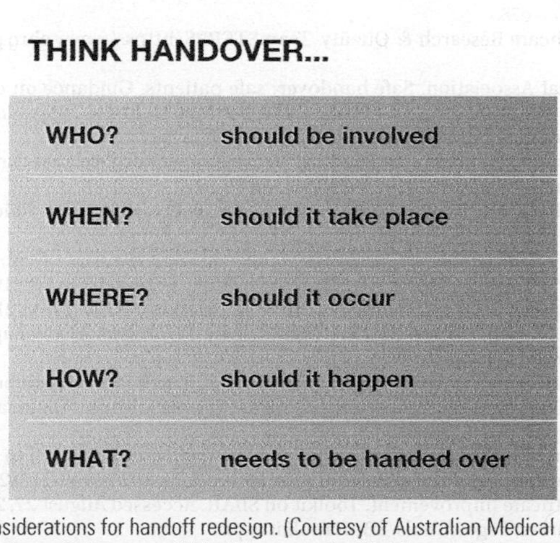
THINK HANDOVER...
WHO? should be involved
WHEN? should it take place
WHERE? should it occur
HOW? should it happen
WHAT? needs to be handed over

FIGURE 36.4 Considerations for handoff redesign. (Courtesy of Australian Medical Association Safe Handover: Safe Patients, Guidance on Clinical Handover for Clinicians and Managers.)

7. Brainstorm solutions to address root causes. Examples include the following:
   a. Implement a handoff tool, such as I-PASS, to standardize handoff content.
   b. Develop a communication process to alert senders and receivers of impending handoff time and location.
   c. Build an electronic template to capture handoff documentation.
   d. Create an education campaign to inform clinicians about the expectations for proper handoff.
8. Prioritize solutions based on ease of implementation and level of impact; use a prioritization matrix to visualize this exercise with the team.
9. Test solutions by implementing and measuring progress (eg, PDSA or "Plan-Do-Study-Act" cycle). Use "run" or "control" charts to help visualize progress over time.
10. Perform additional improvement cycles, repeating the abovementioned steps, as needed.

X. SUSTAINING IMPROVEMENTS

It is essential to sustain focus on handoffs even after an initial implementation, especially in high-turnover environments (such as teaching hospitals).

A. Incorporate handoff education materials into onboarding documents and orientation curriculum.
B. Establish regular auditing and reporting frequency on key measures in the handoff process; establish regular review frequency with ICU leadership.
C. Review handoff and communication-related safety reports, and share lessons learned with unit staff.
D. Conduct periodic safety culture surveys to assess staff perceptions on handoffs and communication, and discuss results with staff to understand how handoffs can be further improved.
E. Incorporate redundancies into handoff process to ensure that any missed steps do not hinder patient care.

Selected Readings

Agarwala AV, Lane-Fall MB, Greilich PE, et al. Consensus recommendations for the conduct, training, implementation, and research of perioperative handoffs. *Anesth Analg.* 2019;128(5):e71-e78.

Agency for Healthcare Research & Quality. TeamSTEPPS. https://www.ahrq.gov/teamstepps/index.html

Australian Medical Association. Safe handover: safe patients. Guidance on clinical handover for clinicians and managers. Accessed September 8, 2021. https://www.ama.com.au/sites/default/files/documents/Clinical_Handover_0.pdf

Bigham MT, Logsdon TR, Manicone PE, et al. Decreasing handoff-related care failures in children's hospitals. *Pediatrics.* 2014;134(2):e572-e579.

Clancy CM, Tornberg DN. TeamSTEPPS: assuring optimal teamwork in clinical settings. *Am J Med Qual.* 2007;22(3):214-217.

Cooper GE, White MD, Lauber JK. *Resource Management on the Flight Deck: Proceedings of a NASA/Industry Workshop. NASA CP-2120.* NASA-Ames Research Center; 1980.

Crewmember Duties. Code of Federal Aviation Regulations. Title 14. §121.542 (1981) and §135.100 (1981). https://www.ecfr.gov/current/title-14/chapter-I/subchapter-G/part-121/subpart-T/section-121.542

Flight Safety Foundation. Cockpit chatter leads to crash. Accident/incident briefs. *Flight Safety Digest.* Published August 1992. Accessed August 27, 2021. https://flightsafety.org/fsd/fsd_aug92.pdf

Geoffrion TR, Lynch IP, Hsu W, et al. An implementation science approach to handoff redesign in a cardiac surgery intensive care unit. *Ann Thorac Surg.* 2020;109(6):1782-1788.

Institute for Healthcare Improvement. Toolkit on SBAR. Accessed August 27, 2021. http://www.ihi.org/resources/Pages/Tools/SBARToolkit.aspx

Kovacheva VP, Brovman EY, Greenberg P, Song E, Palanisamy A, Urman RD. A contemporary analysis of medicolegal issues in obstetric anesthesia between 2005 and 2015. *Anesth Analg.* 2019;128(6):1199-1207.

Multi-Center Handoff Collaborative. Accessed September 5, 2021. www.handoffs.org

Rogers SO Jr, Gawande AA, Kwaan M, et al. Analysis of surgical errors in closed malpractice claims at 4 liability insurers. *Surgery.* 2006;140(1):25-33.

Singh H, Thomas EJ, Petersen LA, et al. Medical errors involving trainees: a study of closed malpractice claims from 5 insurers. *Arch Intern Med.* 2007;167(19):2030-2036.

Starmer AJ, O'Toole JK, Rosenbluth G, et al. Development, implementation, and dissemination of the I-PASS handoff curriculum: a multisite educational intervention to improve patient handoffs. *Acad Med.* 2014;89(6):876-884.

Starmer AJ, Spector ND, Srivastava R, et al. I-PASS, a mnemonic to standardize verbal handoffs. *Pediatrics.* 2012;129:201-204.

Sumwalt RL. The sterile cockpit. *ASRS Directline.* 1993;4. Accessed August 27, 2021. http://asrs.arc.nasa.gov/publications/directline/dl4_sterile.htm.

The Joint Commission Office of Quality Monitoring. Sentinel event data—event type by year. https://www.jointcommission.org/-/media/tjc/documents/resources/patient-safety-topics/sentinel-event/most-frequently-reviewed-event-types-2020.pdf

Timmel J, Kent PS, Holzmueller CG, et al. Impact of the comprehensive unit-based safety program (CUSP) on safety culture in a surgical inpatient unit. *Jt Comm J Qual Patient Saf.* 2010;36(6):252-260.

Wiener EL, Kanki BG, Helmreich RL. *Cockpit Resource Management.* Harcourt Brace; 1993.

37 Recovery After Critical Illness

Alan J. Sutton, Ronald E. Hirschberg, and Laurie O. Mark

I. LONG-TERM OUTCOMES OF PATIENTS IN THE INTENSIVE CARE UNIT

The intensive care unit (ICU) serves to provide acute care to patients with severe and life-threatening illnesses or injuries that require immediate care, as well as close and constant monitoring. Once the patient has recovered from the critically ill period, they are discharged to the floor and often lost to follow-up. The ICU treats various complicated conditions, but not much information is provided to clinicians in the ICU about the long-term outcomes of the patients. Over the past 50-plus years in trauma and ICU care, there has been a paradigm shift in outcome assessment from that of pure mortality-survival (ie, death or life), to specific morbidity for the survivors. Progress continues in this area as we attempt to show *functional gains and abilities* in the continuum of care, from ICU to community. This chapter serves to discuss the long-term outcomes of patients in the ICU who survive trauma, acute respiratory distress syndrome (ARDS), sepsis, and traumatic brain injury (TBI)—some of the most common conditions encountered in this setting.

II. TRAUMA

A. Trauma can range from blunt trauma (eg, motor vehicle accidents, falls) to penetrating trauma (eg, gunshot, stab wounds).

1. The established studies do not differentiate between blunt and penetrating trauma, but "major trauma in the ICU" is associated with the following:

a. Requiring urgent surgery

b. Admission to an ICU for more than 24 hours

c. Requiring mechanical ventilation

d. An injury severity score greater than 15

e. Death occurring after injury

B. The available data suggest that the trauma population is greatly affected in all aspects of life post discharge from the ICU, and in all measured dimensions the scores are lower than that of the general population. These effects are most pronounced within the first year, but scores remain consistently low even after several years.

1. One reason for such a drastic change is that trauma patients are usually previously healthy individuals (compared with, eg, patients with sepsis), so the changes in quality of life (QOL) do appear profound.

2. As a general rule, many of our trauma patients are of a younger age, with vocational and social expectations at prime time in their lives, and taking this into consideration with respect to return to work, pain issues, emotional and social health, and so forth is critical.

C. ICU survivors of trauma consistently have a lower health-related QOL in the years after ICU discharge. Although QOL is certainly subjective, the most common measurement tool for QOL is the Short Form 36 Health Survey (SF-36) questionnaire, which evaluates individual health status, enables comparison across diseases or injuries, and determines how QOL is affected by treatment.

1. The eight sections included (each with a score 0-100; the lower the score, the greater the disability) are vitality, physical functioning, bodily pain, general health perception, physical role functioning, emotional role functioning, social role functioning, and mental health.

2. In short-term follow-up (3-12 months after ICU discharge), an increase in physical function, bodily pain, and social functioning scores was observed in one study but the scores plateaued by 12 months, and, of note, were still consistently lower than that of the general population.
3. After 2 years of follow-up, a large decrease in health-related QOL was also evident, predominantly in the physical dimensions section, which was attributed to musculoskeletal effects and secondary pain. Extending the follow-up period even further to 7 years demonstrated the same results.
4. Demographics (age, area of the country, personal wealth), trauma characteristics (motor vehicle accident [MVA] vs violence related), the injury severity score, preexisting disease (especially psychological disorders and abuse problems), and pain issues were all shown to be predictors of poor QOL among trauma survivors.
5. Patients who obtained higher levels of education, had greater family and social support, and better material and housing conditions were perhaps predisposed to optimism and might "see the positive side of things after a severe illness."

D. ICU survivors of trauma had a lower incidence of returning to work and a higher incidence of early retirement compared with the nontrauma, non-ICU general population.

1. Only 52% of survivors returned to work (of the ~80% who survived after the ICU discharge) and 20% pursued an early retirement.
2. The odds of returning to work increased within the first year of ICU discharge but plateaued after 12 months. Again, pain and physical disability were the main reasons for a lower return-to-work rate.
3. Interestingly, spouses and close family members of survivors of trauma had a low rate of return to work. This may speak to the "outcome" of primary caregivers themselves in the home and caregiver burden.

E. Importantly, a common theme found between studies was an increased incidence of chronic pain after trauma. Pain scores were reported to be the highest during the 6- to 12-month period after ICU discharge, with mild improvement after 12 months. The only reliable predictor identified for the development of chronic pain was the prevalence of pain *before trauma*.

F. Physical and emotional recovery from a significant trauma can take multiple years. The vast majority of studies only looked at the first year post the injury. The trend of health-related QOL, return to work, and chronic pain within the first decade of injury might be more informative. However, such long-term follow-up is difficult to perform once the patient has been discharged.

III. ACUTE RESPIRATORY DISTRESS SYNDROME

ARDS is an inflammatory process in the lungs that significantly reduces gas exchange and can be triggered by infection, sepsis, or trauma. Recovery from ARDS can be more extensive than is recovery from sepsis or trauma in that patients must overcome the initial insult and then recover from the massive insult to their lungs, which includes mechanical ventilation in and of itself, excessive fluid requirements, and relative hypoxemia. As a result, patients can have significant impairment after discharge that can last for months to years.

A. Survivors of ARDS have poorer QOL compared with the general population. The main features affected are mobility, energy, social relationships, domestic tasks, and professional tasks. Mobility is greatly impaired in patients with long ICU and hospital courses, and especially in those who have had long intubation or sedation times. Although modern ICU treatment supports early mobilization, there is indeed significant relative immobilization, which quickly can lead to deconditioning of the muscle, bone and joints, soft tissue, skin, and cardiovascular systems, specifically. Overcoming ICU-acquired weakness after ARDS requires weeks to months of rehabilitation and, depending on the functional level of the patient post-ICU discharge, will require admission to a rehabilitation hospital or discharge home with planned outpatient therapies.

B. Fatigue and lack of energy are common long-term complaints experienced post-ARDS treatment that likely has multifactorial contributions (eg, direct sarcopenia, decreased sleep secondary to other impairments, low cardiopulmonary endurance, depression). Social and family relationships can be affected because patients in the acute care hospital and, potentially, in the rehabilitation hospital undergoing treatment are discharged to recuperate at home following weeks to months of relative isolation, and relationships can be strained. In addition, patients may feel they are a burden to their family, or caretakers may feel resentful for having to give up their time, job, and money to care for the patient.

C. The incidence of depressive symptoms in the population with ARDS is increased. Recovery is long and grueling, which can be a significant stressor or trigger for depression. Some patients lack the necessary social support to get through their recovery, which further compounds the problem.

D. ARDS causes significant damage to the lungs and adversely affects pulmonary physiology. Survivors typically can regain baseline or normal pulmonary function after 12 months, and strict follow-up with imaging and pulmonary function tests after discharge are needed. Follow-up studies and appointments are expensive, and the time and commitment required to make the appointments is significant, which may contribute to the lack of return to work.

E. Long-term neuropsychological impairment is *not* uncommon in survivors of ARDS. In addition to the psychological effects of the hospitalization and the "ICU delirium," physiologic repercussions from ARDS treatment have been documented. Hypoxemia and hypotension can be detrimental and have been associated with impaired executive function on follow-up examinations.

1. Poor fluid management can prolong a disease course, such as liberalizing fluid administration leading to pulmonary edema and worsening of ARDS, which in turn contributes to a prolonged intubation and hospitalization.
2. In patients in the ICU with hypoxemia and/or hypotension, the brain receives less oxygen than is needed and the effect on brain functioning can be apparent even in the long term.
3. Observational studies have demonstrated cognitive impairments at 1 year from ARDS from 30% to 55% prevalence. The cognitive changes (executive functioning, memory, attention, processing speed, etc) can impact further recovery of physical functioning because of the need for optimal mentation for the rehabilitation process.

F. Outcome studies for ARDS have several limitations, especially lack of emphasis on differences regarding age, patient comorbidities, demographics, and inciting event. Significant differences have been noted between survival and recovery between the young and previously healthy and the older adult with preexisting cardiac and pulmonary disease and should be considered for future outcome studies.

G. The novel COVID-19 virus pandemic from 2020 demonstrated a high incidence of ARDS among affected patients, and up to 23% of patients who were hospitalized required mechanical ventilation. Given the relatively high incidence of ARDS among patients with COVID-19, pulmonary fibrosis remains a concerning potential long-term outcome of COVID-19. Outside of COVID-19, there have been previous coronavirus SARS (severe acute respiratory syndrome) outbreaks with similar severity of disease. In these patients, studies have demonstrated mild or moderate restrictive pattern of pulmonary function consistent with muscle weakness in 6% to 20% of those affected, and persistent pulmonary function impairment in a third of patients after 1 year. The vast majority (up to 94%) of patients post COVID-19 experience at least one post-COVID-19 symptom, with 26% to 43% of patients reporting persistent symptoms 6 months after infection, worse with increasing age. The most common symptoms reported by such patients on follow-up after ICU hospitalization were fatigue and breathlessness, followed by psychological distress including posttraumatic stress and depression. Patients after ICU hospitalization also reported worse QOL measures compared to those hospitalized on the wards. Rehabilitation efforts aim to target symptomatic relief of dyspnea, psychological distress, and improving participation in exercise, mobility, activities of daily living (ADLs), and, of course, QOL.

IV. SEPSIS

Sepsis is one of the leading causes of death in the ICU. Over 1 665 000 cases of sepsis occur in the United States each year, and even with optimal treatment, mortality due to severe sepsis or septic shock is approximately 40% and can exceed 50% in patients who are extremely sick. Sepsis affects all organ systems, and recovery can be long and difficult. Much like trauma, patients who survive sepsis in the ICU demonstrate an impaired QOL, with continued reduction in scores as compared with the general population. Most of the studies available use mortality at 28 days as the clinical end point, but it is important to note that patients with varying comorbidities and degrees of sepsis die or decompensate in months and years after this; only 61% of all comers will survive to 5 years.

A. Morbidity: From a morbidity standpoint, the most common long-term adverse effects of sepsis are neurologic or cognitive impairment, psychological symptoms, and impaired physical or emotional QOL.

1. Survivors demonstrate deficits in attention, verbal fluency, executive function, and verbal memories, even in the absence of psychiatric disturbances. Many display significant exhaustion and fatigue, which can manifest as irritability, lack of concentration, and lack of stamina to perform tasks they were previously able to perform.
2. Evidence suggests that patients who experience ICU delirium are at higher risk for cognitive dysfunction, and neuropsychological test scores are frequently low in these survivors.

B. Emotional disturbances were also commonly noted in survivors of sepsis in the ICU.

1. Patients can feel traumatized because their body is "failing" or when interventions are being performed. For example, they may feel a threat of suffocation when a central line is being placed, have a feeling of impending death when they are being induced for intubation, or feel frustrated when they cannot communicate with an endotracheal tube in place.
2. Memories of actual events from the ICU can have more of an effect on a patient in the long run than do episodes of delusion or hallucination they may have experienced during this time. These factual memories can lead to acute stress disorders or even posttraumatic stress disorder (PTSD).
3. Mood disruptions have been observed in survivors of sepsis, and premorbid anxiety and depression might play a part in this development, but further studies are needed to confirm this hypothesis.

C. The QOL dimensions most affected after sepsis are social functioning (ability to engage in old relationships, hobbies, or recreational activities), and physical functioning in ADLs. Much like trauma, the return-to-work rate of survivors of sepsis is relatively low because of physical and mental/cognitive limitations. One study reported a negative impact on employment of 33% by 6 months and 28% by 1 year.

D. As with patients with ARDS, considerable muscle wasting and weakness after surviving a sepsis syndrome in the ICU is common and places strain on the patient and family, and, given the extended recovery process, on the health care system as a whole, because patients require several months to years of rehabilitation to regain independent functioning.

1. Physical limitations are directly the result of impairments at the physiologic level, as well as the result of cognitive, psychological, and/or social stressors or limitations that affect the ability to rehabilitate optimally.
2. Conversely, emotional and social functioning typically are directly impacted upon by the physically functional level of the individual.
3. Lastly, and of key importance, is the introduction of emotional stress when patients become dependent on their spouses or primary caretakers, which can affect the overall outcome on both the patient and the family.

E. Of interest, the longest follow-up period of any study of patients with sepsis in the ICU was 1 year. Patients who show improvement or decline in multiple areas of their life in many years after discharge have not been studied. The data also fail to stratify patients related to both premorbid conditions and age. For example, an older patient with end-stage renal disease on hemodialysis 3 days a week who became sick in the ICU is different from a 30-year-old patient who developed an infection and multi-organ dysfunction after a routine gynecologic surgery.

V. TRAUMATIC BRAIN INJURY

TBI affects approximately 1.4 million people in the United States every year and is classified as mild, moderate, or severe. Outcomes after TBI can range from full functional recovery to death. The Glasgow Coma Scale (GCS) is the most commonly used scale to determine severity and is used along with adjunctive tests, such as computed tomography (CT) and magnetic resonance (MR) imaging studies. The severity is also determined by the nature, speed, and location of the injury and complicating factors, such as hypoxemia, hypotension, intracranial hemorrhage, or increased intracranial pressure. Many survivors will experience long-term disabilities, from the purely cognitive, to physical and psychosocial, and all of these.

A. Understanding outcomes in TBI includes knowledge of some of the expected neurologic and medical morbidities.

1. Seizures are common sequelae of most types of TBI. Within the first 24 hours of injury, 25% of patients with brain contusions or hematomas and 50% of patients with penetrating TBI will develop seizures. Injury severity is correlated with the chance of developing seizures, but no evidence suggests that these patients will develop epilepsy.
2. Development of neurodegenerative disorders (such as dementia of the Alzheimer type and Parkinson disease) is associated with mild to moderate TBI.
3. The risk of disease development is correlated with chronic damage to the brain, as is seen in professional boxers and more recently observed in the professional football player.
4. Other known sequelae of TBI include aphasia, dysarthria, dysphagia, incontinence, muscle pain and spasticity, deep vein thrombosis, heterotopic ossification, and PTSD.

B. Over decades, the majority of studies on outcome after TBI have focused on short-term outcomes, approximately 6 to 12 months after injury. Initial literature discusses mortality in these time intervals, and more recently there are more data on severe TBI outcome. Over the past 20 years, more effort has been made to examine outcomes several years after injury.

1. There is a 2-fold increased risk of mortality for patients with TBI compared with the general population, and studies have demonstrated evidence for risk factors that contribute to premature death in these patients post TBI.
   a. Head injury–associated deaths range from 15 to 30 per 100 000 population (the majority being young adults) and are associated with motor vehicle accidents and falls.
   b. Documented history of prior problems with alcohol or substance abuse, personal problems, and social/behavioral issues were found to contribute to mortality rates.
   c. People with disabilities post TBI have a higher risk of death after TBI than do able-bodied individuals, and not surprisingly significant functional limitations upon discharge from rehabilitation were also noted to correlate with increased mortality.
2. Overall, differentiating between death as a direct result and death as an indirect result of TBI is difficult. For example, patients with significant disability following TBI have prolonged hospitalizations and are prone to developing complications that include pneumonia, ICU-acquired weakness, and cognitive impairments. Interestingly, the cognitive impairments could contribute to accidents that would have otherwise not have occurred had the patients been in their preinjury state of health.

C. The most frequent complications seen after TBI are cognitive, such as memory loss, loss of reasoning ability and concentration, and various behavioral issues (depression, anxiety, personality changes, and lack of social situational awareness).

1. The severity of a patient's cognitive disability after TBI depends on the severity of the injury as well as preinjury characteristics (such as educational level, emotional variability, physical condition, and personality disorders, in addition to substance use). Preinjury intelligence, volume of brain tissue lost, and brain region injured also contribute to the severity of cognitive dysfunction.
2. Of note, in penetrating brain injury, the cognitive effects of *normal aging* are exacerbated.
3. TBI decreases the chance of returning to work and to the same position held preinjury.
   a. Long-term disability was predicted by older age, preinjury unemployment, substance abuse, and more severe disability upon discharge from a rehabilitation center.
   b. Long-term unproductivity was predicted by preinjury unemployment, longer posttraumatic amnesia, substance abuse, and more disability upon admission to a rehabilitation center.
4. TBI adversely affects recreational activities, social and familial relationships, functional status, and levels of independence.
5. Severity of injury is correlated to social outcome, but the evidence is insufficient to specify which type of injury will produce a specific adverse outcome.

D. Factors known to influence long-term survival include basic functional skills (such as mobility and the ability to feed oneself), the type and severity of injury, and specific neurofunctional impairments (cognitive changes, risk-taking behavior, and mood disorders).

1. The Community Integration Questionnaire (CIQ) is frequently used to assess long-term home and social integration and productivity after TBI.
   a. Three months post injury, a decline in CIQ score compared with preinjury condition with respect to home and social integration and productivity
   b. Maximal improvement was achieved within the first year but slight improvement continued up to 3 years following the injury.
   c. The major determinants of community integration were preinjury community integration, age, and destination after hospital discharge.
   d. Lower CIQ scores were found among males, older patients, those living with others preinjury, longer hospitalizations, abnormal CT scan findings, those who were more dependent on others, those with motor and

cognitive impairment, and those who were discharged to an inpatient rehabilitation center or nursing home.

E. It should be noted that the GCS as a single variable has been shown to have limited value as a predictor of functional outcome.

1. GCS assessment is not useful in day-to-day ICU assessment and neurologic change and has not been shown to predict longer term outcome.
2. The highly vetted Coma Recovery Scale–Revised (CRS-R) was established first in 1991 with the goal of tracking levels of consciousness over weeks to months following severe TBI. The scale incorporates detailed assessments of auditory, visual, motor, and verbal communication and level of arousal as patients emerge from vegetative state (VS) through the levels of minimally conscious state (MCS).
3. The standard in functional outcome assessment (as opposed to specific levels of consciousness) for moderate to severe TBI is the Disability Rating Scale (DRS), which was established to follow up patients "from coma to community." This scale incorporates visual, motoric, and verbal aspects of impairment akin to the GCS, in addition to level of functional limitation (ADLs, etc) as well as disability (employability, social integration). Both highly reliable and valid, the DRS demonstrates functional changes of survivors of TBI over months to years.

F. The most severe injuries result in prolonged (≥28 days) disorders of consciousness (DoC) including the VS, now referred to as the unresponsive wakefulness syndrome (UWS), and MCS.

1. Patients with DoC comprise a population at risk, vulnerable to misdiagnosis and medical mismanagement. Estimates of misdiagnosis among patients with DoC (eg, VS/UWS vs MCS) remain consistently high, approximating 40%. Of note, the cost of lifetime care for persons with prolonged DoC can exceed $1 000 000.
2. Recent guidelines recommend discontinuing the use of the term *permanent vegetative state* in favor of the term *chronic vegetative state* (*UWS*) based on the frequency of recovery of consciousness at 12 months in traumatic VS/UWS.
3. MCS has been dichotomized into MCS+ and MCS− based on the presence or absence, respectively, of signs of preserved language function such as command following or intelligible speech.
4. Clinicians should consider prescribing amantadine for adults with traumatic VS/UWS or MCS (4-16 weeks post injury) to hasten the rate of functional recovery and reduce disability early in recovery. This recommendation is based on a 4-week treatment result of a randomized clinical trial demonstrating faster recovery (measured by the DRS) in the amantadine group of patients with posttraumatic DoC (VS/UWS or MCS).

Selected Readings

Adhikari NK, Tansey CM, McAndrews MP, et al. Self-reported depressive symptoms and memory complaints in survivors five years after ARDS. *Chest.* 2011;140(6):1484-1493.

Barker-Davies RM, O'Sullivan O, Senaratne KPP, et al. The Stanford Hall consensus statement for post-COVID-19 rehabilitation. *Br J Sports Med.* 2020;54(16):949-959.

Bazarian JJ, Cernak I, Noble-Haeusslein L, et al. Long-term neurologic outcomes after traumatic brain injury. *J Head Trauma Rehabil.* 2009;24:439-451.

Carlson CG, Huang DT. The Adult Respiratory Distress Syndrome Cognitive Outcomes Study: long-term neuropsychological function in survivors of acute lung injury. *Crit Care.* 2013;17(3):317.

Chan KS, Zheng JP, Mok YW, et al. SARS: prognosis, outcome and sequelae. *Respirology.* 2003;8(suppl 1):S36-S40.

Gabbe BJ, Simpson PM, Sutherland AM, et al. Evaluating time points for measuring recovery after major trauma in adults. *Ann Surg.* 2013;257(1):166-172.

Giacino JT, Katz DI, Schiff ND, et al. Comprehensive systematic review update summary: disorders of consciousness: report of the Guideline Development, Dissemination, and Implementation Subcommittee of the American Academy of Neurology; the American Congress of Rehabilitation Medicine; and the National Institute on Disability, Independent Living, and Rehabilitation Research. *Neurology*. 2018;91(10):461-470.

Giacino JT, Katz DI, Schiff ND, et al. Practice guideline update recommendations summary: disorders of consciousness: report of the Guideline Development, Dissemination, and Implementation Subcommittee of the American Academy of Neurology; the American Congress of Rehabilitation Medicine; and the National Institute on Disability, Independent Living, and Rehabilitation Research. *Neurology*. 2018;91(10):450-460.

Giacino JT, Whyte J, Bagiella E, et al. Placebo-controlled trial of amantadine for severe traumatic brain injury. *N Engl J Med*. 2012;366(9):819-826.

Griffiths J, Hatch RA, Bishop J, et al. An exploration of social and economic outcome and associated health-related quality of life after critical illness in general intensive care unit survivors: a 12-month follow-up study. *Crit Care*. 2013;17(3):R100.

Halpin SJ, McIvor C, Whyatt G, et al. Postdischarge symptoms and rehabilitation needs in survivors of COVID-19 infection: a cross-sectional evaluation. *J Med Virol*. 2021;93(2):1013-1022.

Kalmar K, Giacino JT. The JFK coma recovery scale—revised. *Neuropsychol Rehabil*. 2005;15(3-4):454-460.

Korosec Jagodic H, Jagodic K, Podbregar M. Long-term outcome and quality of life of patients treated in surgical intensive care: a comparison between sepsis and trauma. *Crit Care*. 2006;10(5):R134.

Kowalczyk M, Nestorowicz A, Fijałkowska A, et al. Emotional sequelae among survivors of critical illness. *Eur J Anaesthesiol*. 2013;30(3):111-118.

Lazosky A, Young GB, Zirul S, et al. Quality of life after septic illness. *J Crit Care*. 2010;25(3): 406-412.

Logue JK, Franko NM, McCulloch DJ, et al. Sequelae in adults at 6 months after COVID-19 infection. *JAMA Netw Open*. 2021;4(2):e210830.

Mandal S, Barnett J, Brill SE, et al. "Long-COVID": a cross-sectional study of persisting symptoms, biomarker and imaging abnormalities following hospitalisation for COVID-19. *Thorax*. 2021;76(4):396-398.

McDonald LT. Healing after COVID-19: are survivors at risk for pulmonary fibrosis? *Am J Physiol Lung Cell Mol Physiol*. 2021;320(2):L257-L265.

Misak C. Cognitive dysfunction after critical illness: measurement, rehabilitation, and disclosure. *Crit Care*. 2009;13:312.

Neviere R. Sepsis and the systemic inflammatory response syndrome: definitions, epidemiology, and prognosis. *UpToDate*. Published May 2014. http://www.uptodate.com/contents/sepsis-and-the-systemic-inflammatory-response-syndrome-definitions-epidemiology-and-prognosis

Orwelius L, Bergkvist M, Nordlund A, et al. Physical effects of trauma and the psychological consequences of preexisting diseases account for a significant portion of the health-related quality of life patterns of former trauma patients. *J Trauma Acute Care Surg*. 2012;72(2):504-512.

Overgaard M, Hoyer CB, Christensen EF. Long-term survival and health-related quality of life 6 to 9 years after trauma. *J Trauma*. 2011;71(2):435-441.

Ribbers GM. Brain injury: long term outcome after traumatic brain injury. In: Stone JH, Blouin M, eds. *International Encyclopedia of Rehabilitation*. http://web.archive.org/web/20160324184413/http:/cirrie.buffalo.edu/encyclopedia/en/article/338/

Safaz I, Alaca R, Yasar E, et al. Medical complications, physical function and communication skills in patients with traumatic brain injury: a single centre 5-year experience. *Brain Inj*. 2008;22(10):733-739.

Toien K, Bredal I, Skogstad L, et al. Health related quality of life in trauma patients. Data from a one-year follow up study compared with the general population. *Scand J Trauma Resusc Emerg Med*. 2011;19-22. doi:10.1186/1757-7241-19-22

Ulvik K, Kvale R, Wentzel-Larsen T, et al. Quality of life 2-7 years after major trauma. *Acta Anaesthesiol Scand*. 2008;52(2):195-201.

Ware JE. SF-36 health survey update. In: Maruish M, ed. *The Use of Psychological Testing for Treatment Planning and Outcomes Assessment*. 3rd ed. Lawrence Erlbaum Associates; 2004:693-718.

Willemse-van Son AH, Ribbers GM, Hop WC, et al. Community integration following moderate to severe traumatic brain injury: a longitudinal investigation. *J Rehabil Med*. 2009;41: 521-527.

Willemse-van Son AH, Ribbers GM, Verhagen AP, et al. Prognostic factors of long-term functioning and productivity after traumatic brain injury: a systematic review of prospective cohort studies. *Clin Rehabil*. 2007;21:1024-1037.

Zafonte RD, Hammond FM, Mann NR, et al. Relationship between Glasgow Coma Scale and functional outcome. *Am J Phys Med Rehabil*. 1996;75(5):364-369.v

38 The Economics of Critical Care: Measuring and Improving Value in the Intensive Care Unit

Kyan C. Safavi

I. COSTS AND BURDEN OF CRITICAL CARE

A. Caring for the critically ill or injured is a complex and resource-intensive endeavor. There are roughly 5200 intensive care units (ICUs) in the United States, representing 14.3% of the total hospital beds but a disproportionate share of hospital operating costs—roughly one-third. Today's ICUs are highly specialized units dedicated to care for very specific populations of patients at risk for or experiencing overt, critical organ dysfunction. Many hospitals, typically in larger centers, further subdivide patients into cardiac, neurologic, burn, pediatric, neonatal, and other subspecialty ICUs. This increased specialization, coupled with the growing demand for intensive care services, presents challenges to hospitals seeking to control costs. Applying a family- and patient-oriented, value-based framework to intensive care helps practitioners focus on optimizing outcomes while simultaneously reducing costs.

B. Detailed analysis indicates that critical care represents 13.2% of hospital charges, 4.1% of U.S. health care expenditures, and 0.72% of U.S. gross domestic product (GDP). This is due in part to high overhead costs—on average, an ICU bed costs $4300 per day—together with the expense of high-intensity physician, nurse, and therapist staffing. Moreover, critical care expenditures in the United States are projected to increase as a proportion of total health care costs as the population ages, the prevalence of chronic disease increases, and technologic advances help people live longer following serious illness and injury. In the year 2000, for example, roughly 12% of the U.S. population was age 65 years or older; by 2050, persons age 65 years and older are projected to comprise roughly 22% of the U.S. population. More people are expected to live to advanced ages, with the percentage of U.S. adults age 85 and older projected to increase from less than 1% in the year 2000 to 5% in 2050. This growth in the older population will fuel demand for intensive care services, further straining resources. In addition, health care economists suggest that technologic advances, combined with greater access to health insurance, increased demand for critical care services in recent years, a trend that is likely to continue. Thus, for most hospitals with shrinking margins in a difficult policy environment, critical care represents a potential high-impact opportunity for focusing on efficiencies and improving care.

C. Multiple competing factors influence whether there is an adequate supply of intensivists to staff ICUs. There has been a general increase in the total number of ICU beds, suggesting an increase in demand for critical care services. As mentioned, longer life expectancy and the aging population are also key factors that are likely to increase this demand. Further, there is evidence to suggest that hospitals with 24/7 staffing by an intensivist have better patient outcomes. On the other hand, there are factors that potentially lead to an increased use of ICU beds when they may not be needed. These include the admission of patients to the ICU who do not require ICU-level care and those at the end of life (EOL) whose goals do not include intensive therapy. In some hospitals, relative shortages of general care beds for transfer or post–acute care rehabilitation beds for discharge can lead to extended ICU length of stay (LOS) and utilization when the patient no longer requires critical care.

D. All of these factors combine to create a challenging matrix for providing high-value, patient- and family-centered care to patients who are critically ill. Measuring the value of the care provided in our ICUs is an essential first step in addressing these challenges and can help identify opportunities to create efficiencies and improve clinical outcomes.

II. THE VALUE OF CRITICAL CARE EXPENDITURES

A. To evaluate the success of the health care system, health care policy makers, managers, and providers have increasingly shifted to a "value" framework, in which the outcomes experienced by the patient are divided by the cost of delivering those outcomes. Value can therefore be maximized by either improving quality outcomes and/or reducing costs. The value provided by ICUs can be considered at a hospital level and also at a broader population or societal level. Measuring hospital costs is challenging because health care costs are much less transparent than that in other industries. The prices charged by providers and the amounts reimbursed by insurers often do not reflect the actual cost of the care provided. In addition, high-margin treatments and procedures are used to subsidize other areas where reimbursements do not cover the costs. Determining costs for patients in the ICU is particularly challenging because of the interdisciplinary nature of the care provided and the heterogeneity of the patient population in the ICU. The value measurement framework includes equal emphasis on achieving goals for both quality outcomes and costs. The value of medical care can be improved either by reducing costs or improving quality. Ideally, both scenarios would be met to maximize value.

B. Quality Care: Traditionally, measures of quality for critical care were focused solely on the ICU portion of the patient's hospital stay, using metrics (such as LOS) that are easy to measure but less important to patients and families (functional status, long-term survival, and quality of life). The value framework provides a structure for measuring the impact and value of critical care services over the long term, using patient- and family-centered outcomes. One popular approach groups health outcomes into three tiers: health status achieved or retained, process of recovery, and sustainability of health (Table 38.1).

This approach provides a framework for measuring value for the patients who are critically ill that includes a continued focus on survival but also calls attention to duration of recovery and ultimate health obtained.

1. Measures of outcomes that drive up overall cost: hospital-acquired infection rates, pressure ulcer rates, falls and injury rates, readmissions to the ICU, and readmissions to the hospital post discharge (within specified time periods, typically 30 days). Measures of overall quality that are value producing: adherence to protocols for managing specific diseases such as sepsis, early mobilization, monitoring for delirium, and so on.

C. Costs: There are many different approaches to measuring health care costs, each with advantages and disadvantages. Many analyses of costs are completed retrospectively using **administrative (billing) data**. This approach is often used because data are readily available and in a structured format that lends itself to analysis. However, hospital billing data are complex, with many assumptions built in regarding direct, indirect, variable, and fixed costs. Direct costs are directly related to patient care (labor and supplies); indirect costs refer to shared resources that are allocated to individual patients on the basis of a set of assumptions (eg, salaries of administrators). Fixed costs are those that do not change with the volume of patients; these tend to represent the operational costs of the ICU, such as clinician salaries, or the purchase of specialized equipment. Variable costs will change with the volume of patients, such as the cost of mechanical ventilation or the cost of lab tests. Conventional wisdom is that roughly 80% of costs in the ICU are fixed costs, although new thinking on costing methodology for the health care industry

TABLE 38.1 Outcomes Hierarchy for Critical Care

Tier	Domain	Measure
1. Health status achieved or maintained	Survival	• In-hospital mortality • Postdischarge mortality (30 d, 6 mo, 1 yr)
	Degree of health or recovery	• Discharge location (LTACH, SNF, home) • Ability to live independently • Ability to return to work • Related readmissions • For end-of-life patients, ability to access palliative care and hospice services in accordance with patient/family goals
2. Process of recovery	Time to recovery	• Critical care unit length of stay • Overall hospital length of stay • Time to return of full functionality (reanimation)
	Disutility of Care	• Hospital-acquired infections (eg, CLABSI, CAUTI, MRSA, *C. difficile*, SSI) • Incidence of pressure ulcers • Delirium
3. Sustainability of Health	Sustainability of health recovery and nature of recurrences	• Quality of life years • Return to full functionality (reanimation)
	Long-term consequences of therapy	• Long-term cognitive deficits • Depression/anxiety/other mental health diagnoses

CAUTI, catheter-associated urinary tract infection; CLABSI, central line–associated bloodstream infection; LTACH, long-term acute care hospital; MRSA, methicillin-resistant *Staphylococcus aureus*; SNF, skilled nursing facility; SSI, surgical-site infection. Adapted from Porter ME, Teisberg EO. *Redefining Health Care.* Harvard Business School Press; 2006.

is challenging that notion. Alternatively, costs can be measured prospectively using a framework of **time-driven activity-based costing (TDABC)**, which involves tracking the amount of time it takes each clinician to conduct patient care tasks and then calculating the costs of the labor and supplies on the basis of the actual amount of time spent on each task. This approach is much more accurate in terms of determining the actual costs for a specific procedure or patient with a particular clinical condition because it views every resource as variable and fungible. However, TDABC is a more labor-intensive method that involves process mapping and time studies, which may not be practical in all situations. The approach to measuring costs will depend on the question of interest and the amount of time and resources available for the analysis. Administrative data are best suited to address basic questions of utilization (eg, number of central line days, number of computed tomography [CT] scans) and the associated labor and supply costs. This approach is a simple way to determine whether key metrics around resource utilization are trending in the desired direction and is therefore often used in ongoing monitoring. Yet, it is often challenging to disentangle the total costs of a particular patient's ICU stay using administrative data. Physician billing data are often located in a separate data system. Nursing costs are typically included in "room and board" charges, with no ability to track the actual costs of the time that providers spend with patients.

D. Cost-Effectiveness: Cost-effectiveness analysis (CEA) is a method of analysis that uses the value framework of health care to measure the outcomes of a health care program relative to its cost. These analyses can be used at a societal level to help guide the views of policy makers and the general public with regard to the benefits of health care for the populace relative to its cost. This is particularly relevant to ICUs where care is more expensive and the impact on patient survival and well-being may be significant. In CEA, accounting for cost includes not only the cost of the index critical care encounter but also ward care, post–acute facility use, home care, outpatient follow-up, readmissions, and income transfers borne by the patient and society (eg, sickness allowances, disability, lost economic productivity, etc). Thus, cost is considered not only to the payer (eg, government or insurance companies) but also to employers, patients, their families, and society itself. Outcomes are measured in terms of life-years or quality-adjusted life-years (QALYs) gained by the patient as well as their potential economic productivity. Benchmarks for what is considered "cost-effective" vary, but common approaches include measuring relative to the per-person GDP of a country or the cost-effectiveness of hemodialysis (roughly $50 000 per QALY). Studies applying CEA to the critical care setting have been limited, although they are growing in number. Systematic reviews demonstrate that most studies have shown favorable cost-effectiveness profiles of ICUs in general and in specific interventions offered to patients. Several of the specific interventions studied include sepsis goal-directed therapy, culture-guided antibiotics, short-term and long-term ventilatory support, and extracorporeal mechanical oxygenation (ECMO).

III. INFLUENCE OF POLICY ENVIRONMENT

A. Health care reform is redefining the way we think about and measure quality and costs in the ICU. Under a traditional fee-for-service model, ICU care was viewed as a distinct and separate part of the patient's hospital stay. As reimbursement policy evolves from fee-for-service to bundled payments for episodes of care and population health management, the care provided in the ICU must be measured in a broader context.

B. The Affordable Care Act (ACA) that was passed in 2010 is one of the most consequential (and controversial) pieces of health care legislation in decades. More than 10 years after its passage, the impact of the law and how it may influence critical care are still evolving. Broadly, the ACA has two areas of focus: (i) coverage and access to care and (ii) health care delivery systems and payment reform.

C. Coverage and Access to Care: The ACA extended health care coverage to millions of Americans through Medicaid expansion and subsidies as well as protections for people purchasing insurance in the individual marketplace. The effect of the law has been a dramatic decrease in the number of uninsured patients from approximately 48.6 million in 2010 to approximately 30.4 million in 2020. The impact of the increase in number of insured patients for ICUs is unclear. On the one hand, evidence has demonstrated that patients with insurance are more likely to seek acute care when needed, which may drive up ICU demand. Studies have also demonstrated that coverage can enable individuals to seek out preventative care and care earlier in their disease episode to reduce the likelihood of progression to severe disease that may require admission to the ICU.

D. Health care delivery systems and payment reform: The portion of the ACA dealing with delivery systems and payments aims to decrease cost and increase quality (value). This portion of the law set in motion a large variety of reforms in this space. It has been difficult to assess the impact of these given the multitude occurring often within the same time frame with few easy control comparisons. These reforms have garnered bipartisan support and have largely focused on expanding value-based purchasing initiatives that depart from traditional fee-for-service payment models. These initiatives can be categorized into two areas: (i) those that incentivize hospitals and health systems to shift toward global accountability for health care in the form of accountable care organizations (ACOs) and bundled payment care initiatives (BPCIs) and (ii) those that provide incentives (or levy penalties) to hospitals and health systems based on the quality of care targets.

1. **Global payment systems:** The ACA created incentives for providers to enter into payment models for their Medicare and Medicaid populations in which they are reimbursed for the care that they render based on a single lump sum of money for the entire care of the patient rather than for each service they provide, as is the case with traditional fee for service. These incentives have led to the formation of more than 500 Medicare ACOs by 2021 and approximately 1200 hospitals, physician groups, and health care organizations have participated in a Medicare ACO. Similarly, BPCI programs provide a single payment for care related to a particular episode, such as a knee replacement. This payment may cover prehospital, hospital, and posthospital care for up to 90 days. More than 1000 health care organizations have entered into BPCI contracts. How critical care will be impacted by these shifting incentives is still evolving. Of note, much of hospital-based care remains under the older fee-for-service model. Likely, however, these payment models will add focus to how the ICU is connected to the care of the patient in the pre-ICU and post-ICU setting. Key areas of focus will include greater coordination and communication of care to reduce ICU and hospital readmissions, careful avoidance of overuse of post–acute care facilities given their high cost, and thoughtful engagement with patients and families about their goals of care to avoid overly intense and costly interventions that are incongruous with these wishes.
2. **Value-based payments:** Value-based payment (VBP) is a Centers for Medicare & Medicaid Services (CMS) annual pay-for-performance program incenting optimized process of clinical care, patient experience, outcomes, and efficiency. Under this program, for example, hospitals have an opportunity to gain or lose up to 1.75% of their base diagnosis-related group (DRG) payments in fiscal year (FY) 2023 is 2%. Although process of care measures were initially 70% of the VBP program, by FY 2016 these measures will represent only 10% of the dollars at risk. Outcome and efficiency measures, in contrast, will comprise 65% of the dollars at risk in VBP by FY 2016. Outcome measures in the VBP program include many ICU-related phenotypes, such as mortality from heart failure, acute myocardial infarction (AMI), and pneumonia, hospital-acquired infections (central line–associated bloodstream infection [CLABSI] and catheter-associated urinary tract infection [CAUTI]), the Agency for Healthcare Research and Quality (AHRQ) composite patient safety indicator (PSI-90), and surgical-site infections. The efficiency score is based on Medicare Spend Per Beneficiary, a risk-adjusted measure of total expenditures for 3 days before and 30 days after an inpatient hospital stay.
3. **Hospital-acquired condition reduction program:** The CMS annual hospital-acquired condition reduction program (HACRP) is a payment penalty assessed on hospitals with poor performance (7th to 10th decile) on hospital-acquired infection rates; the penalty is currently 1% of base DRG payments. In the first year of the program, metrics included AHRQ PSI-90 (a composite score of several PSIs), CLABSI, and CAUTI (ICU rates only). In future years, the program will include surgical-site infection rates for hysterectomy and colon surgery, methicillin-resistant *Staphylococcus*

aureus (MRSA) bacteremia, and *Clostridium difficile*. Hospitals that work to reduce the rate of these potentially preventable, hospital-acquired conditions in the ICUs will have a competitive advantage in this performance program.

4. **Hospital readmission reduction program:** The CMS Hospital Readmissions Reduction Program (HRRP) represents another effort to incent efficiency and improve the value of care by reducing readmissions within 30 days of discharge for selected conditions and procedures. Up to 3% of the hospital's base DRG payments are at risk in this program. Conditions and procedures currently included in the program include AMI, heart failure, pneumonia, chronic obstructive pulmonary disease (COPD), and hip and knee arthroplasty (additional conditions and procedures will be added in the future). It is not uncommon for patients with these diagnoses and procedures to spend some portion of their inpatient stay in the ICU. Thus, care provided in the ICU has the potential to influence the trajectory of recovery and thereby the likelihood of readmission within 30 days.
5. **Additional areas of focus for health care policy with implications for critical care:**
   a. **End-of-life care:** EOL care is an important aspect of ICU medicine where critical care providers often have substantial influence. EOL care is expensive, with more than 25% of all Medicare spending occurring in the last year of life. In addition, studies have found wide variation in EOL spending, even within the same country. The combination of high cost and variability makes this an area of high focus for policy makers. Further, patients with advanced illness report often receiving care that is discordant with their personal goals at EOL. For example, the vast majority of patients report a preference to die at home but 20% die within the hospital. Addressing EOL is challenging. Studies have found that it is difficult for individual providers or even machine learning algorithms to predict who will die during their hospitalizations or when they will die. These factors make addressing EOL challenging. Initiatives, however, at the health care organizational level and within the ICU have focused on engaging patients who are at or nearing the EOL about their goals for the quality of their remaining time. This includes establishing advanced planning directives in which a patient can state these goals and increasing the awareness of all providers, including intensivists, about these documents.

   b. **Telehealth:** The realm of telehealth has been shifting substantially over the course of recent years. Tele-ICU has been implemented in various settings over the past decades, primarily motivated by data suggesting that ICUs staffed with or supported by intensivists achieve better outcomes than those staffed by non-intensivists. Tele-ICU programs range in terms of whether they offer continuous intensivist support versus as-needed consultative capability. Programs also vary in the amount of technology they employ, ranging from real-time remote monitoring systems and virtual video visitations with patients to simple remote electronic health record access. Thus, assessing the cost-effectiveness of such programs has been challenging, with evidence pointing in either direction. The expectation is, however, that telehealth in general and tele-ICU capacity is likely to expand in the coming years as hospitals, patients, and their families grow more comfortable with such interactions and the payment mechanisms evolve. Importantly, during 2020, Medicare rapidly expanded the number of covered telehealth services and moved toward making those changes permanent while continuing to evaluate their impact.

TABLE 38.2 Five Things Physicians and Patients Should Question: The Choosing Wisely Campaign

1. Don't retain catheters and drains in place without a clear indication.
2. Don't delay progress toward liberation from mechanical ventilation.
3. Don't continue antibiotic therapy without evidence of need.
4. Don't delay mobilizing patients in the ICU.
5. Don't provide care that is discordant with the patient's goals and values.

ICU, intensive care unit. Adapted from Society for Critical Care Medicine. Choosing Wisely©: five things physicians and patients should question. Accessed September 4, 2021. www.choosingwisely.org/societies/society-of-critical-care-medicine

E. Interventions That Affect Value: The Five Do's and Five Don'ts of Critical Care

1. The term post–intensive care unit syndrome (PICS) was coined recently to refer to phenotypes associated with survival after severe, debilitating, critical illness. PICS describes new or worsening problems for patients and/or their families during recovery from critical illness, including physical, cognitive, and/or mental health deterioration. Two recent, complementary, national campaigns illustrate how performance improvement interventions can be used to improve the value of care provided in ICUs and to potentially avoid the ravages of PICS. For example, both the American Association of Critical Care Nursing and the Society of Critical Care Medicine promote the ABCDE bundle, which couples five best-practice protocols into a coherent approach to care redesign: coordination of spontaneous awakening and spontaneous breathing trials, delirium assessment and management, and early mobilization. Use of this bundle in a study of patients in medical and surgical ICUs was associated with less time on the ventilator, less delirium, and less immobility. The cost-saving implications are therefore significant (and should be compelling to hospital administrators responsible for performance improvement). Similarly, the American Board of Internal Medicine, partnering with the Critical Care Societies Collaborative, identified by consensus five ICU care areas in which to "choose wisely": the ICU Choosing Wisely Campaign (Table 38.2). These items are intended to educate and to prompt discussions between ICU clinicians, patients, and their families to evaluate critically use of therapies that may not be helpful (and may even be harmful) under certain conditions. Lack of benefit and/or avoiding harm both increase quality and decrease costs, supporting the value proposition.

Selected Readings

Angus DC, Deutschman CS, Hall JB, et al. Choosing Wisely© in critical care: maximizing value in the intensive care unit. *Crit Care Med.* 2014;42(11):2437-2438.

Balas MC, Vasilevskis EE, Olsen KM, et al. Effectiveness and safety of the awakening and breathing coordination, delirium monitoring/management, and early exercise/mobility bundle. *Crit Care Med.* 2014;42(5):1024-1036.

Bloomfield EL. The impact of economics on changing medical technology with reference to critical care medicine in the United States. *Anesth Analg.* 2003;96(2):418-425.

Blumenthal D, Collins SR, Fowler EJ. The Affordable Care Act at 10 years—its coverage and access provisions. *N Engl J Med.* 2020;382(10):963-969.

Blumenthal D, Abrams M. The Affordable Care Act at 10 years—payment and delivery system reforms. *N Engl J Med.* 2020;382(11):1057-1063.

Centers for Medicare and Medicaid Services. Hospital-acquired condition (HAC) reduction program. Accessed September 5, 2021. https://www.cms.gov/Medicare/Medicare-Fee-for-Service-Payment/AcuteInpatientPPS/HAC-Reduction-Program

Centers for Medicare and Medicaid Services. Hospital value-based purchasing program. Accessed September 5, 2021. https://www.cms.gov/Medicare/Quality-Initiatives-Patient-Assessment-Instruments/Value-Based-Programs/HVBP/Hospital-Value-Based-Purchasing

Centers for Medicare and Medicaid Services. Hospital readmission reduction program. Accessed September 5, 2021. https://www.cms.gov/Medicare/Medicare-Fee-for-Service-Payment/AcuteInpatientPPS/Readmissions-Reduction-Program

Centers for Medicare and Medicaid Services. ACO participation and performance data. Accessed September 5, 2021. https://www.cms.gov/Medicare/Medicare-Fee-for-Service-Payment/sharedsavingsprogram/program-data

Centers for Medicare and Medicaid Services. Bundled payments for care improvement initiative: general information. Accessed September 5, 2021. https://innovation.cms.gov/innovation-models/bundled-payments

Centers for Medicare and Medicaid Services. Trump administration finalizes permanent expansion of Medicare telehealth services and improved payment for time doctors spend with patients. Accessed September 5, 2021. https://www.cms.gov/newsroom/press-releases/trump-administration-finalizes-permanent-expansion-medicare-telehealth-services-and-improved-payment

Franzini L, Sail KR, Thomas EJ, et al. Cost and cost-effectiveness of a telemedicine intensive care unit program in 6 intensive care units in a large health system. *J Crit Care.* 2011;26(3):329.e1-e6.

Jha AK. End of life care, not end of life spending. *JAMA.* 2018;320(7):631-632.

Kaplan RS. Improving value with TDABC. *Health Financ Manage.* 2014;68:76-83.

Kumar G, Falk DM, Bonello RS, et al. The costs of critical care telemedicine programs: a systematic review and analysis. *Chest* 2013;143(1):19-29.

Napolitano LM, Fulda GJ, Davis KA, et al. Challenging issues in surgical critical care, trauma, and acute care surgery: a report from the Critical Care Committee of the American Association for the Surgery of Trauma. *Trauma.* 2010;69:1619-1633.

Needham DM, Davidson J, Cohen H, et al. Improving long-term outcomes after discharge from intensive care unit: report from a stakeholders' conference. *Crit Care Med.* 2012;40(2):502-509.

Pandharipande P, Banerjee A, McGrane S, et al. Liberation and animation for ventilated ICU patients: the ABCDE bundle for the back-end of critical care. *Crit Care.* 2010;14(3):157.

Population Division, U.S. Census Bureau. Demographic turning points for the United States: population projections for 2020 to 2060 (NP2008-T12). Accessed September 5, 2021. https://www.census.gov/library/publications/2020/demo/p25-1146.html

Porter ME. What is value in healthcare? *N Engl J Med.* 2010;363:2477-2481.

Porter ME, Teisberg EO. *Redefining Health Care.* Harvard Business School Press; 2006.

Society of Critical Care Medicine. Critical care statistics. Accessed September 4, 2021. https://www.sccm.org/Communications/Critical-Care-Statistics

The American Association for the Surgery of Trauma. Critical care illness.

Wilcox ME, Vaughan K, Chong CA. Cost effectiveness studies in the ICU: a systematic review. *Crit Care Med.* 2019;47(8):1011-1017.

Wunsch H, Gershengorn H, Scales DC. Economics of ICU organization and management. *Crit Care Clin.* 2012;28:25-37.

Zimmerman JJ, Harmon LA, Smithburger PL, et al. Choosing Wisely for critical care: the next five. *Critical Care Med.* 2021;49(3):472-481.

39 Telemedicine and Remote Electronic Monitoring Systems in the Intensive Care Unit

Shu Yang Lu and Benjamin Christian Renne

I. INTRODUCTION

A. "Telemedicine," sometimes referred to as telehealth, as defined by the American Telemedicine Association, is the electronic exchange of medical information from one site to another via communication to improve a patient's clinical health status. Many forms of technology have been used to support telemedicine. Telemedicine is not a separate medical specialty but is meant to augment traditional models of health care as a delivery tool or system. Intensive care unit (ICU) telemedicine refers to the care of patients who are critically ill using telehealth. This paradigm can be an attractive strategy to mitigate the shortages of intensivists by improving access to trained intensivists, whose presence is associated with lower mortality, decreased ICU length of stay (LOS), and lower medical costs. The focus of telemedicine in the ICU ("Tele-ICU") is to supplement traditional ICU care by delivering collaborative physician oversight utilizing electronic medical records combined with audiovisual technologies to assist bedside nurses and clinicians in patient care activities. In this chapter, we describe the brief history of ICU telemedicine, different models of implementation, evidence for the effectiveness of ICU telemedicine, and barriers/challenges to its implementation.

II. HISTORY OF INTENSIVE CARE UNIT TELEMEDICINE/TELE-ICU

The initial concept of Tele-ICU was described by Grundy et al in 1982. This was a teleconsultative model providing intermittent consultative advice to an inner-city hospital via two-way video and telephones. The report concluded that patients were more likely to survive when intensivists' suggestions were implemented. In 1997, a team of investigators at an academic medical center demonstrated improved ICU and hospital mortality, ICU LOS, and hospital costs after using telemedicine to achieve 24-hour intensivist coverage of a 10-bed surgical ICU. The around-the-clock model whereby a remote intensivist provides telemedicine care to adult patients in the ICU was first reported in 2000 by Rosenfeld et al. Following these results, the United States saw a rapid growth in the number of Tele-ICU systems, averaging a 61% increase per year. Today, Tele-ICU programs cover at least 15% of ICU beds in the United States.

III. TELE-ICU MODELS AND ORGANIZATION OF SERVICE

A. Centralized (Hub-and-Spoke) Model

Despite a rapid growth in Tele-ICU, there is significant variation in its implementation. The centralized model, also known as the hub-and-spoke model, is the most commonly utilized model for Tele-ICU (Figure 39.1). In this model, Tele-ICU intensivists and support personnel are located in a central location in an urban hospital (the hub) and provide Tele-ICU interventions to several types of outlying units or rural/community hospitals (the spokes). The intensivists and support personnel work in shifts providing around-the-clock monitoring and recommend interventions for these patients. Recent reports

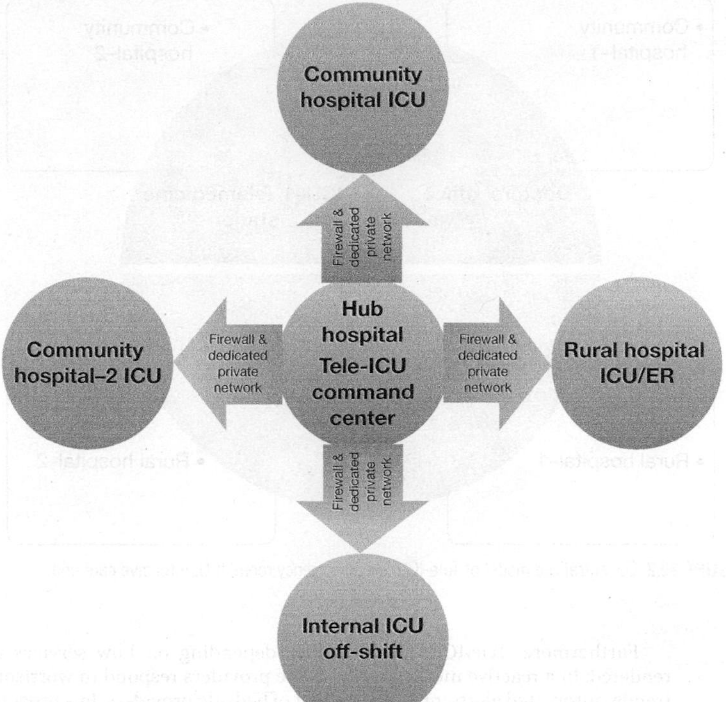

FIGURE 39.1 Centralized Tele-ICU model. ER, emergency room; ICU, intensive care unit.

suggest that compliance with evidence-based ICU protocols is improved with this centralized Tele-ICU care model. This model is typical with the commonly used term "electronic ICU" or "eICU care." This model typically has higher setup and operational costs (in thousands of dollars per bed).

B. Decentralized Model

Alternatively, the decentralized model allows intensivists in different locations to access the Tele-ICU via desktop or laptop without relying on a central hub from which to practice (Figure 39.2). In this model, computers equipped with audiovisual technology are located at sites of patient care, but the remote monitoring occurs from sites of convenience (decentralized) such as physician offices or homes. This is associated with significantly reduced start-up cost for both the consulting and receiving organizations.

C. Hybrid Model

This model combines features of both the centralized and decentralized models. The consulting intensivists are not located in one central location but may be in multiple facilities, and the model has the ability to provide Tele-ICU care to multiple facilities. Similar to the decentralized model, start-up and operational costs for the hub are typically lower with this model.

Similar to the diversity of Tele-ICU models, the intensity of interaction between Tele-ICU and bedside providers also varies widely. Some services entail 24 hours per day of Tele-ICU coverage, whereas others may provide services intermittently or during certain times of the day or days of the week.

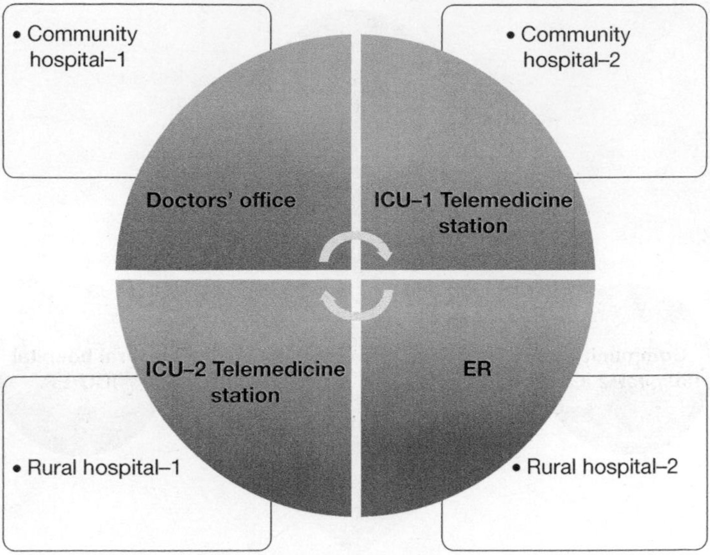

FIGURE 39.2 Decentralized model of Tele-ICU. ER, emergency room; ICU, intensive care unit.

Furthermore, Tele-ICU services differ depending on how services are rendered: In a reactive model, telemedicine providers respond to worrisome trends, automated alerts, or at the request of bedside providers. In a proactive model, Tele-ICU services provide continuous remote surveillance of patients including methodical review of patient data and ensuring adherence to best clinical practice such as lung-protective ventilation, antibiotic stewardship, and so on.

IV. ORGANIZATION OF TELE-ICU SERVICE

Successful organization of Tele-ICU service requires clinical, business/administrative, and legal collaboration between two or more health care facilities with the common goal of improving access to high-quality critical care. The collaborative domains include personnel, technology, and patient populations.

A. Personnel

Critical care clinicians and business administrators at both the consulting and receiving facility must collaborate for the service to work. Optimally, physician and business administration champions must be identified from each facility to facilitate discussions during the formative and implementation stages and to monitor the progress of the Tele-ICU service. All critical care physician consultants from the consulting organization must be fully licensed to practice their specialty in the state or province where the receiving facility is located. In addition, the critical care consultants must be credentialed by the receiving hospital's medical staff office. Typical care providers at the receiving facility include hospitalists, advanced care practitioners, critical care nurses, respiratory therapist, and/or emergency department physicians. Health care providers participating in Tele-ICU services should have appropriate orientation and education to ensure they possess necessary competencies in clinical care, communication, documentation, and safety protocols, consistent with the clinical environment encountered.

B. Technology

All components of Tele-ICU technology must comply with federal and state regulations to protect personal privacy, confidentiality, and health care-related patient information. Consent for Tele-ICU consultation should be included in the patient registration process at the consulting and receiving facility. Electronic and video connections between the two facilities should have multiple levels of security and a firewall built for transmission of encrypted information. Providers at both institutions should have full access to the electronic health record. The ideal hardware solution should be located on a mobile cart at the receiving facility. The institutional IT infrastructure on both ends must be committed to providing technical support for hardware and software.

C. Patient Population

Tele-ICU services may be provided to all types of patients at the receiving hospital, regardless of status. The patient may be located in the ICU, in the general care unit, or in the emergency room. Triage decisions—regarding transfer to the ICU or to another hospital—are often made during the Tele-ICU consult. Figure 39.3 is a schematic representation of the organizational flow required to set up Tele-ICU services.

V. TELE-ICU OUTCOMES AND QUALITY METRICS

There are many reports in the literature documenting the significant positive impact on outcomes of patients who are critically ill using intensivist-supported Tele-ICU service. Two recent meta-analyses concluded lower ICU mortality after implementation of Tele-ICU service, although the topic remains somewhat controversial because benefit of Tele-ICU-based care is dependent on both the patient phenotype and care environment. Besides the reported benefit to mortality, Tele-ICU has been shown to improve adherence to best practices, decreased medication errors, and foster early intervention and consultation by providing additional provider resources for critical care access. Additional potential benefits of implementing Tele-ICU include decreased LOS in the ICU, cost savings

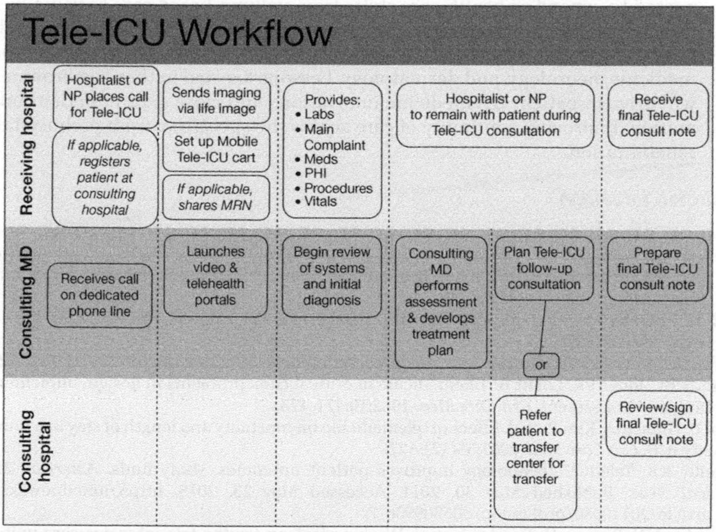

FIGURE 39.3 Tele-ICU workflow. ICU, intensive care unit; MRN, medical record number; NP, nurse practitioner; PHI, protected health information.

from decreases in transportation costs, and improved patient and family satisfaction with care provided "close to home" (ie, avoiding unnecessary transfers). In addition to standard ICU value measures, quality metrics for Tele-ICU service should also include the number of consults performed and transfer data, patient and family acceptance of Tele-ICU services, consultant provider response time, quality of audio and video transmissions, and reasons for patient transfers and their attendant costs.

VI. BARRIERS AND CHALLENGES TO TELE-ICU

The rapid expansion of ICU telemedicine in the early 2000s was based on its potential to improve patient outcomes and quality of care. However, despite its initial rapid expansion, the adoption of Tele-ICU has slowed in recent years. Several barriers to adoption of Tele-ICU technology may explain this trend. The start-up costs, both in terms of financial and human capital, may be substantial. This is particularly true if many ICU beds in different locations require Tele-ICU coverage. In addition, lack of provider experience with communication technology or unwillingness to change practice patterns and processes of care are major barriers to adoption of Tele-ICU technology. A range of options are available, from built-in, fixed systems for each bed added to existing hospital IT infrastructure (more expensive) to stand-alone, mobile carts using out-of-the-box computer video software and wireless communications (less expensive). Many third-party payers (insurance agencies) provide little to no reimbursement for Tele-ICU services, although the evidence for improved value is motivating change. Finally, ICU telemedicine also faces regulatory challenges. Some states require providers to have special license to deliver telemedicine and states vary in their policies for regulating these services.

VII. SUMMARY

Tele-ICU services accomplish the "triple aims" of reducing costs, improving access to quality care, and improving patient/family experiences, especially in rural areas. Despite the challenges described, Tele-ICU is here to stay and is expected to expand as health care shifts from volume-based care to value-based care for population management. In addition to Tele-ICU, telemedicine has been successfully applied in radiology, emergency medicine, psychiatry, pain medicine, neurology, and dermatology. Lessons learned in these environments will drive in-patient telemedicine innovations and close gaps in patient information, improving continuity of care across the spectrum, from prehospital to rehabilitation.

Selected Readings

American Telemedicine Association. Accessed May 22, 2015. http://www.atmeda.org

Breslow MJ, Rosenfeld BA, Doerfler M, et al. Effect of a multiple-site intensive care unit telemedicine program on clinical and economic outcomes: an alternative paradigm for intensivist staffing. *Crit Care Med.* 2004;32:31-38.

Krell K. Critical care workforce. *Crit Care Med.* 2008;36(4):1350-3. doi: 10.1097/CCM.0b013e31816 9ecee. PMID: 18379263.

Goran S. A new view: tele-intensive care unit competencies. *Crit Care Nurse.* 2011;31(5)17-29.

Grundy BL, Jones PK, Lovitt A. Telemedicine in critical care: problems in design, implementation, and assessment. *Crit Care Med.* 1982;10:471-475.

Kohl B, Gutsche J, Kim P, et al. Effect of telemedicine on mortality and length of stay in a university ICU. *Crit Care Med.* 2007;35(12):A22.

O'Reilly KB. Tele-ICU technology improves patient outcomes, study finds. *American Medical News.* Published May 30, 2011. Accessed May 23, 2015. http://amednews.com/article/20110530/profession/305309936/7/

Reynolds HN, Rogove H, Bander J, et al. Working lexicon for the tele-intensive care unit: we need to define for the tele-intensive care unit to grow and understand it. *Telemed J E Health.* 2011;17:773-783.

Rogove H. How to develop Tele-ICU model? *Crit Care Nurse Q.* 2012;35:357-363.

Rosenfeld BA, Dorman T, Breslow MJ, et al. ICU telemedicine: alternative paradigm for providing continuous intensivist care. *Crit Care Med.* 2000;28:1-7.

Rosenfeld BA, Dorman T, Breslow MJ, et al. Intensive care unit telemedicine: alternate paradigm for providing continuous intensivist care. *Crit Care Med.* 2000;28:3925-3931.

Shaffer JP, Breslow MJ, Johnson JW, et al. Remote ICU management improves outcomes in patients with cardio-pulmonary arrest. *Crit Care Med.* 2005;33(12):A5.

Wilcox ME, Adhikari NK. The effect of telemedicine in critically ill patients: systematic review and meta-analysis. *Crit Care.* 2012;16(4):R127.

Yeo W, Grass-Ahrens SL, Wright T. A new era in the ICU: the case for telemedicine. *Crit Care Nurse Q.* 2012;35:316-321.

Young LB, Chan PS, Lu X, et al. Impact of telemedicine intensive care unit coverage on patient outcomes: a systematic review and meta-analysis. *Arch Intern Med.* 2011;171(6):498-506.

Zawada ET, Herr P, Larson D, et al. Impact of an intensive care unit telemedicine program on a rural health care system. *Postgrad Med.* 2009;121:160-170.

40 Quality Improvement and Standardization of Practice

Lauren A. Sweetser and Brian M. Cummings

I. QUALITY IMPROVEMENT

A. Background: Ensuring optimal quality of health care delivery is an essential goal of clinicians, administrators, and payors. Many patients do not receive recommended care while hospitalized. This occurs for a variety of reasons—access to medications or equipment, cost, staffing, and knowledge gaps all contribute. In addition, the complexities of care delivery in the critical care environment make it particularly prone to medical error, with the patient population at risk for substantial morbidities related to their hospitalization. Advancing clinical knowledge, ongoing process improvement efforts, and a focus on quality and safety have improved intensive care unit (ICU) care. Despite increasing age and severity of illness, ICU mortality rates decreased 35% between 1988 and 2012, with adult ICUs reporting 10% to 30% overall mortality. Ensuring that all patients receive optimal evidence-based treatment, proactively preventing morbidity, and eliminating medical errors remains the goal. In brief, delivering safe, high-quality care remains a moral imperative.

B. Definition of Quality Care: The Institute of Medicine (IOM) describes quality using six metrics: care that is safe, timely, effective, efficient, equitable, and patient centered.

C. Financial Implications: Reimbursement for care is increasingly bundled and linked to performance using quality metrics and the prevention of patient harm. For example, Medicare does not reimburse hospitals for certain preventable, hospital-acquired infections (HAIs). Financial incentives are used as a tool to drive behavior and decrease unwanted practice variance.

D. Components: In the classic Donabedian framework, there are three quality of care components: structure, process, and outcome.

1. **Structure:** The structure of ICUs varies between individual units, hospitals, and regions. Elements of the structure of an ICU include the training and experience of care providers, staffing organization, and the diagnostic and treatment technology available. Changing unit structure is challenging and requires coordination with hospital and health care system infrastructure. There remains insufficient data to recommend the ideal structure given multiple variables.
2. **Process:** Process refers to both the actual care provided to patients (and how well this care complies with best practices) as well as administrative practices that have an indirect effect on patient care. Examples of processes of care include number of patients utilizing a central line and use of a checklist for line placement. Hundreds of process-based studies that inform ICU best practice are published annually.
3. **Outcome:** Outcome refers to patient results and has been the traditional metric to judge performance of critical care clinicians and researchers. The usual benchmark is 28-day, risk-adjusted mortality. Length of stay, length of ventilation, HAIs, and quality-adjusted life years (QALY) are other common outcome measures in clinical trials. However, advances in patient- and family-centered ICU care increasingly argue for use of patient-related outcome measures (PROMs), such as early, full functional recovery, and return to work.

4. **Focus on Process in Quality Improvement:** Although ultimately outcome measures are the goal, quality improvement (QI) that focuses on process measures has advantages. Clinicians have more control on process and aspects of care delivery. Process measures decrease the need for risk adjustment as with outcome measures, allow smaller sample sizes, and decrease time to see results and understand whether changes are resulting in improvement. In addition, these can be utilized to provide immediate direct feedback to providers. Regardless of outcome or process, the quality measures used in the ICU should be meaningful, scientifically sound, generalizable, and interpretable.

E. **Leadership and Culture:** To deliver quality ICU care, there must be an enthusiastic and motivated core of people dedicated to the hard work of sustained improvement. In the ICU, this requires a multidisciplinary team that brings insights from many different facets of care. A leader in QI fosters a culture of safety and constant learning and is willing to resist the argument "because we've always done it that way." An environment that empowers frontline providers or a "ground" team at the point of care is critical to understand issues and ultimately implement process improvement. Hospitals can perform annual safety culture surveys that provoke transparency and may form the groundwork for an improvement mindset. There are various available measures to assess the safety climate of a unit.

F. **Model Framework for Approaching Quality Improvement:** The Institute for Healthcare Improvement (IHI) recommends a model for improvement developed by the Associates in Process Improvement (see Figure 40.1).

1. **Formulate the right questions:** Three fundamental questions can focus on a QI effort, moving from a general issue to a specific target.
2. **Target measure and goal:** The target measure must be carefully defined and importantly followed over time. Measures easily extracted from databases to establish baseline performance and to allow easy monitoring over time are ideal. A specific improvement goal should be explicitly stated.
3. **Plan-Do-Study Act cycle:** The Plan-Do-Study Act (PDSA) cycle is a method to create a course for testing and measuring a change. Initial PDSA cycles start in a limited or test population. The first step is developing the approach to improvement (Plan)—ideally, a strategy tailored to the environment and the hopes for the improvement explicitly stated. Thus, the target measure needs to be defined. Interventions in the ICU often start with education—interactive teaching, informal discussion, and more structured lectures with dissemination of written information on whatever is planned. Audit and feedback of recent performance is also commonly employed. After an intervention is initiated (Do), the results on the target measure should be evaluated (Study), as well as reflection on what worked and what did not. This information is incorporated into the next improvement effort (Act) and the next intervention modified appropriately, restarting the PDSA cycle. Once an intervention has been optimized, it should be expanded and more universally applied.
4. **Impact of quality improvement:** The potential impact of a QI effort can be measured in terms of five dimensions. As individual providers, hospitals, and health care systems institute QI programs, they should address most, if not all, dimensions.
   a. **Reach:** How much of the target population participated?
   b. **Efficacy:** What is the success rate if implemented as intended?
   c. **Adoption:** What proportion of target institutions and practitioners adopt the intervention?
   d. **Implementation:** To what extent is it implemented as intended?
   e. **Maintenance:** How is the intervention sustained over time?

II. STANDARDIZATION

A. **Checklists:** As the number of QI initiatives increases, with both individual items and bundles, ensuring that each patient receives all appropriate interventions is a challenge. The use of checklists, often incorporated as part of

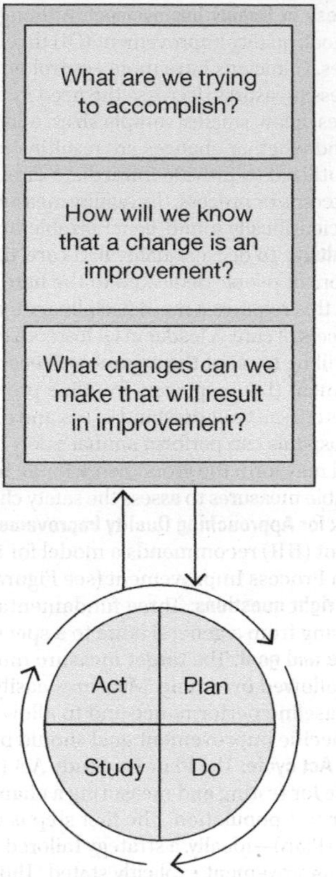
What are we trying to accomplish?
How will we know that a change is an improvement?
What changes can we make that will result in improvement?
Act
Plan
Study
Do

FIGURE 40.1 The Plan-Do-Study Act (PDSA) cycle.

daily rounds or procedures, brings attention to these interventions and helps coordinate care. Checklists increase implementation of best practices and are associated with improved outcomes. Checklists may also be used to ensure that all best practice elements in a particular process are completed, such as central line insertion. Figure 40.2 shows the central line infection prevention checklist at our hospital. Importantly, the existence of a checklist per se is not sufficient to ensure quality care; in most studies, compliance rates reported in ICUs are low (30%-70%), indicating opportunities for improvement.

B. Care Bundles: Care bundles are aggregated, evidence-based interventional practices designed to improve outcomes by delivering structured, measurable processes of care. Typically, bundles consist of three to six separate elements supported by evidence from clinical trials. These elements are more successful when implemented together rather than when used individually and should be delivered to every patient every time. Bundles should decrease unwanted practice variance while still allowing for individualized care when indicated.

1. **Compliance:** Measurement of compliance with bundles is integral to their success, and completion of a bundle is an all-or-nothing event. Bundles should be dynamic and evolve over time as new evidence changes best practice. The greatest effect on outcomes occurs when more than 90% bundle compliance is reached.

MASSACHUSETTS
GENERAL HOSPITAL

CENTRAL LINE INFECTION PREVENTION CHECK LIST

Goal	To decrease patient harm from catheter-related blood stream infections
Who	An operator & a monitor
What	Assure compliance with and documentation of checklist elements
Where	At the site of the procedure
When	During all central venous line insertions or rewires
How	The monitor verifies that the steps have occurred, immediately informs the operator/supervisor of deviations, & completes the checklist

Roles: _Operator:_ the clinician placing the central line
Supervisor: an experienced operator who is involved in training the operator in central line placement
Monitor: an individual who is qualified to observe the procedure and watch for breaks in sterile technique. If a break in sterile technique is observed, the monitor asks the operator to repeat a portion of the procedure after correcting the observed break. Please identify a monitor for this line placement prior to the time out.

Procedure Planning

Line Insertion Site: ❒ Subclavian ❒ Internal Jugular ❒ Femoral ❒ PICC ❒ UA/UV ❒ Other (specify)

	Yes	No	Comments/Reason
Emergent placement	❒	❒	
Timeout documented separately	❒	❒	
Consent documented separately	❒	❒	

If there is a deviation in any of the critical steps, immediately notify the operator and stop the procedure until corrected. If the step is completed properly, check the "Yes" box. If the step is not completed properly, check the "No" box and note the issue in the "Comments/Reason" section. Contact the Attending if any item on the checklist is not adhered to or with any concerns.

Critical Step for Line Insertion	Yes	No	Comments/Reason
Before the procedure, the operator will:			
Confirm hand sanitizing (Cal Stat) or antimicrobial soap immediately prior	❒	❒	
Disinfect procedure site (chlorhexidine) using a back & forth friction scrub for 30 seconds. In patients < 2 months of age, use povidone iodine instead of chlorhexidine.	❒	❒	
Allow site to dry for 30 seconds	❒	❒	
Operator(s): hat, mask, sterile gown/gloves, eye protection	❒	❒	
Assistant/Monitor: hat, mask & standard precautions (if at risk for entering sterile field use sterile gown/gloves)	❒	❒	
Use sterile technique to drape from head to toe; Pediatrics use judgment to determine extent of draping.	❒	❒	
During the procedure, the operator will:			
Maintain a sterile field	❒	❒	
Flush and cap line before removal of drapes	❒	❒	
After the procedure, the operator will:			
Remove blood with antiseptic agent (chlorhexidine), if present, before placement of sterile dressing. Use sterile water/saline for patients < 2 months of age.	❒	❒	
Apply appropriate (green = all "yes", red = 1 or more "no") dated sticker on patient's line	❒	❒	

Date & Time:		Unit:	
Operator:	MD/RN	Monitor:	Credentials

White - Medical Record Copy 85428 (12/08)

FIGURE 40.2 The Massachusetts General Hospital central line infection prevention checklist.

2. **Patient care:** Bundles have been shown to have success in reducing ventilator-associated pneumonia (VAP), reducing central line–associated bloodstream infections (CLABSIs), and improving the management of sepsis and septic shock. A frequent example in practice today is the ABCDE bundle, which links Awakening and Breathing Coordination of daily sedation and ventilator removal trials, Delirium monitoring and management, and Early exercise and mobility. ABCDE bundle use minimizes sedative exposure, reduces duration of mechanical ventilation, and decreases ICU-acquired delirium and weakness (see Figure 40.3). Patients cared for following implementation of this bundle spent 3 more days breathing without assistance,

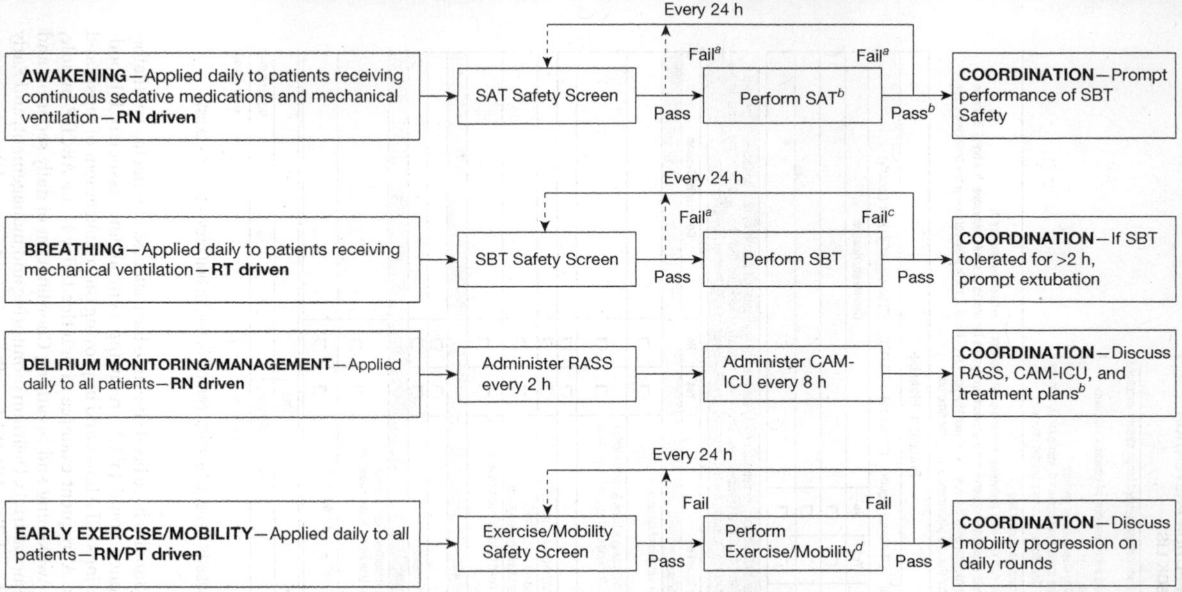

FIGURE 40.3 The ABCDE bundle. CAM-ICU, confusion assessment method-intensive care unit; PT, physical therapist; RASS, Richmond Agitation Sedation Scale; RN, registered nurse; RT, respiratory therapist; SAT, spontaneous awakening trial; SBT, spontaneous breathing trial. (From Balas MC, Vasilevskis EE, Olsen KM, et al. Effectiveness and safety of the awakening and breathing coordination, delirium monitoring/management, and early exercise/mobility bundle. *Crit Care Med.* 2014;42(5):1024-1036.)

[a]Continuous sedative medications maintained at previous rate if spontaneous awakening trial (SAT) safety screen failed. Mechanical ventilation continued, and continuous sedative medications restarted at half the previous dose only if needed because of spontaneous breathing trial (SBT) safety screen failure.

[b]Continuous sedative infusions stopped, and sedative boluses held. Bolus doses of opioid medications allowed for pain. Continuous opioid infusions maintained only if needed for active pain.

[c]Continuous sedative medications restarted at half the previous dose and then titrated to sedation target if spontaneous awakening trial (SAT) failed. Interdisciplinary team determines possible causes of SAT/spontaneous breathing trial (SBT) failure during rounds. Mechanical ventilation restarted at previous settings and continuous sedative medications restarted at half the previous dose only if needed if SBT failed.

[d]Spontaneous awakening trial (SAT) pass if the patient is able to open the eyes to verbal stimulation without failure criteria (regardless of trial length) or does not display any of the failure criteria after 4 hours of shutting off sedation.

experienced less delirium, and were more likely to be mobilized in their ICU stay. There were no significant differences in self-extubation and reintubation rates.

3. Multiple examples of checklists and care bundles are provided under **Section III.**

III. QUALITY METRICS, MORBIDITY, AND SAFETY IN THE INTENSIVE CARE UNIT

A. Background: The ICU is a high-stakes environment. Critical illness itself, the treatments provided, and the methods of monitoring can each be associated with significant morbidity and mortality. Common ICU-related harm measures are reviewed here.

B. Central Line–Associated Bloodstream Infection: Patients in the ICU often require central venous access to deliver certain medications or nutrition (eg, vasopressors, total parenteral nutrition [TPN]), for central monitoring, and for access stability. These benefits are balanced by risks, including issues during placement, CLABSIs, and thrombus formation. The high attributable costs of CLABSIs have led federal agencies to base a significant fraction of annual reimbursement on better outcomes (ie, low CLABSI rates compared with peer institutions).

1. **Costs:** Estimates vary from \$6000 to \$45 000 per CLABSI owing to attributed costs of care related to central line infections, with annual health care costs exceeding \$1 billion.
2. **Prevention:** The most direct way to reduce the occurrence of CLABSIs is to ensure that lines are necessary and to remove the line promptly.
3. **Infectious sources:** Line contamination can occur at the time of placement, either extraluminally or intraluminally. Therefore, strict sterile technique should be employed, using full-barrier precautions. Bacteria that enter extraluminally from the skin surface are often responsible for infections that occur with short-term use (3-7 days). Infection from intraluminal spread is increasingly being recognized as a continued cause of CLABSIs, especially with longer term use (>7 days).
4. **Central venous catheter bundle of care:** Certain process of care recommendations can reduce CLABSIs, frequently included in insertion bundles and checklists. Daily review of indications for continued catheter use is also indicated.
   - **a.** All associated equipment should be maintained in a central line cart.
   - **b.** Educate health care personnel on insertion, care, and maintenance of central venous catheters (CVCs), with periodic assessment of this knowledge.
   - **c.** Perform hand hygiene before insertion and any manipulation of CVCs.
   - **d.** Wear cap, mask, gown, and sterile gloves for insertion.
   - **e.** Use maximal sterile barrier precaution with drapes during CVC insertion.
   - **f.** Avoid the femoral vein as an access site in adult patients if able.
   - **g.** Use more than 0.5% chlorhexidine-based antiseptic skin preparation in patients older than 2 months of age.
   - **h.** Use ultrasound guidance to place catheters to reduce cannulation attempts and mechanical complications.
   - **i.** Use a chlorhexidine-impregnated sponge dressing if CLABSI rates remain high despite implementation of other guidelines.
   - **j.** Consider use of antimicrobial-impregnated catheters in high-risk populations or if CLABSI rates remain high despite instituting other guidelines.
   - **k.** Disinfect catheter hubs, needleless connectors, and injection ports before accessing catheters.

l. Change administration sets used for blood, blood products, or fat emulsions every 24 hours. Change other continuous-use administration sets no more frequently than every 96 hours but at least every 7 days.

m. Change dressings sterilely when soiled or loose, and at least every 7 days even if clean, dry, and intact.

n. Remove catheter as soon as clinically able. Any ongoing need should be discussed daily on interdisciplinary rounds.

o. Do not rewire lines if infection is the reason for a line change.

p. Consider addition of an auditing team to regularly monitor central lines.

C. Catheter-Associated Urinary Tract Infection: Indwelling urinary catheters are frequently used in the ICU for output monitoring and skin protection. However, as with intravenous (IV) catheters, urinary catheters carry significant risk of infection, including urinary tract infection (UTI) and urosepsis. Urinary catheters and the associated asymptomatic bacteriuria represent a significant reservoir for drug-resistant organisms.

1. **Costs:** The costs associated with catheter-associated urinary tract infection (CAUTI) is less than that with other health care–associated infections, although it has been reported to exceed $10 000 per Medicare patient in the ICU. As with CLABSI, CAUTI rates are reported nationally and factor into pay for performance by federal agencies.
2. **Causes:** Absence of sterile technique during insertion, retrograde flow of urine from urinary collection devices, and duration of catheter use all increase the risk of CAUTI and asymptomatic bacteriuria.
3. **Prevention and care bundle:** Given here are recommendations for avoiding CAUTI.

a. Use indwelling urinary catheters only for appropriate indications, such as the following:

1. Acute urinary retention or bladder outlet obstruction
2. Need for accurate measurement of urine output in patients who are critically ill hemodynamically unstable
3. Perioperative use for selected surgical procedures and/or epidural use
4. To assist healing in sacral or perineal wounds in patients who are incontinent
5. Patients requiring prolonged immobilization
6. To improve comfort in end-of-life care

b. Remove indwelling catheters as soon as clinically able (ie, when initial indication is no longer present). Any ongoing need should be discussed daily on interdisciplinary rounds.

c. Intermittent catheterization is preferable to indwelling catheters in patients with bladder-emptying dysfunction.

d. Perform hand hygiene immediately before and after inserting or manipulating indwelling urinary catheters.

e. Insert using aseptic technique and sterile equipment—sterile drapes, gloves, sponges, sterile antiseptic solution for periurethral cleaning, and single-use lubricant packets.

f. Choose appropriately sized catheter and properly secure after insertion to prevent movement and urethral traction.

g. Maintain a closed drainage system and replace catheter and system if breaks occur.

h. If urinary specimen is required, take specimen aseptically via a sampling port.

i. Maintain unobstructed flow, avoiding kinks and keeping collecting bag below the level of the bladder at all times to avoid retrograde flow.

j. Bladder irrigation is not recommended, including routine irrigation with antimicrobials. If required because of obstruction, use closed continuous irrigation.

k. Use antimicrobial-impregnated catheters if CAUTI rates remain high despite implementing other guidelines. They may be helpful in at-risk populations.

D. Ventilator-Associated Events: Mechanical ventilation is an essential and lifesaving therapy for patients who are critically ill and studies estimate that nearly 300 000 patients receive mechanical ventilation annually. However, mechanical ventilation presents a serious risk of complications (including death), and thus it is important to track and prevent these serious sequelae. Previous monitoring relied on the term "ventilator-associated pneumonia (VAP)," which was defined as a combination of three features of pulmonary infection in a patient who is mechanically ventilated: radiographic evidence, clinical signs, and laboratory and microbiologic results. However, some of these data are subjective (eg, new infiltrates on chest x-ray [CXR]), leading to variability in interpretation and weak interobserver concordance. In contrast, the surveillance definition of a ventilator-associated event (VAE) put forth by the Centers for Disease Control and Prevention (CDC) in 2013 (and continually updated) relies more on objective, streamlined, and potentially automatable data. A VAE is defined as any changes in ventilator settings made by bedside clinicians to optimize patient status. Event triggers include infectious and noninfectious complications of mechanical ventilation (such as barotrauma), pulmonary embolus, acute respiratory distress syndrome (ARDS), atelectasis, and pulmonary edema. There are three definition tiers within the VAE surveillance definition algorithm, and the CDC provides examples on their website as well as a calculator to help appropriately classify these events. These are surveillance definitions only and are not intended for clinical management of patients.

1. **Ventilator-associated condition:** The patient experiences worsening oxygenation following a period of stability or improvement on the ventilator (>2 calendar days of stable or decreasing daily minimum FIO_2 or positive end-expiratory pressure [PEEP] values). Worsening oxygenation is defined as increase in daily minimum FIO_2 of greater than 0.20 or daily minimum PEEP greater than 3 cm H_2O.
2. **Infection-related ventilator-associated complication:** After calendar day 3 of mechanical ventilation and in the 2 calendar days before or after the onset of worsening oxygenation as in ventilator-associated condition (VAC), the patient has both temperature greater than 100.4 °F (38 °C) or less than 96.8 °F (36 °C) or white blood cell (WBC) greater than 12 000 or less than 4000 cells/mm^3 *and* a new antimicrobial agent is started and continued for more than 4 calendar days.
3. **Possible and probable ventilator-associated pneumonia:** Both involve meeting the criteria for infection-related ventilator-associated complication (IVAC) with additional requirements.
   a. Possible VAP includes criteria for purulent respiratory secretions *or* positive culture of sputum, endotracheal aspirate, bronchoalveolar lavage, lung tissue, or protected specimen brushing (culture of normal respiratory flora and certain other microorganisms excluded).
   b. Probable VAP includes purulent respiratory secretions *and* a positive culture finding (cannot be from sputum and there are minimum quantitative requirements with the same microorganism exclusions). Probable VAP is also diagnosed if criteria for IVAC are met and there is a positive pleural fluid culture result, positive lung histopathology finding, positive diagnostic test result for *Legionella*, or a positive diagnostic test result for influenza virus, respiratory syncytial virus, adenovirus, parainfluenza virus, rhinovirus, human metapneumovirus, and coronavirus.
4. **Costs:** VAEs are associated with significant morbidity, including prolonged periods of mechanical ventilation, extended hospitalization, excess use of

antimicrobial medications, and increased mortality. Health care costs are estimated at $14 000 to $29 000 per occurrence and exceed $1 billion annually.

5. **Risk factors:** VAE risk factors include prolonged intubation, enteral feeding, witnessed aspiration, paralytic agents, underlying illness, and extremes of age. For example, pneumonia arises secondary to bacterial invasion of the formerly sterile lower respiratory tract from aspiration of secretions, colonization of the aerodigestive tract, or use of contaminated medications or equipment.
6. **Prevention and bundles of care:** Efforts should be directed toward these sources of infection and risk factors, similar to strategies for preventing CLABSI and CAUTI.
   - **a.** Maintain hand hygiene.
   - **b.** Minimize duration of ventilation.
     1. Use noninvasive ventilation to prevent intubation or to allow quicker extubation if indicated.
     2. Discuss daily assessment of readiness to wean ventilator.
   - **c.** Prevent aspiration.
     1. Maintain in semirecumbent position (35°-45°).
     2. Avoid gastric overdistension.
     3. Avoid unplanned extubation and reintubation.
     4. Use cuffed endotracheal tube (with cuff maintained at $\leq$20 cm H_2O) with in-line or subglottic suctioning.
   - **d.** Reduce colonization of aerodigestive tract.
     1. Prioritize orotracheal intubation over nasotracheal intubation when possible.
     2. Avoid H_2-blocking agents or proton-pump inhibitors (PPIs) in patients not at high risk for developing stress ulcers or stress gastritis.
     3. Perform regular oral care.
   - **e.** Minimize contamination of equipment.
     1. Use sterile water to rinse reusable ventilator equipment.
     2. Remove condensate from respiratory circuit, keeping circuit closed while removing condensate and avoiding retrograde flow of condensate.
     3. Change circuit only when visibly soiled or malfunctioning.
     4. Store and disinfect respiratory therapy equipment properly.

E. Antimicrobial Resistance

1. **Background:** Antimicrobial resistance rates continue to increase and impact the ICU. More than 2.8 million antibiotic-resistant infections occur in the United States each year, and more than 35 000 people die as a result. Dedicated prevention methods have helped but still these numbers are expected to increase (2019 CDC report).
2. **Risk factors:** Any antibiotic use (in humans, animals, or crops) can lead to resistance microbes, and this resistance can easily and rapidly spread between people, animals, and the environment.
3. **Prevention:** Three main goals are to prevent infection in the first place, slow the development of resistance through improved antibiotic use (use only when necessary and for appropriate duration), and stop the spread of resistance when it does occur. Moreover, hospitals should utilize an antimicrobial stewardship program with core elements including hospital leadership commitment, pharmacy expertise, education, accountability, tracking, and reporting. Finally, when appropriate, consider alternative approaches such as vaccines, antibody therapy, bacteriophages, and live biotherapeutics (such as fecal microbiota transplants).

F. Deep Venous Thrombosis and Venous Thromboembolism

1. **Background:** Pulmonary embolus remains a significant proximal cause of morbidity and mortality among patients who are critically ill. Preventing

the formation and mobilization of deep venous thrombi that can lead to pulmonary embolus is an important goal of critical care.

2. **Risk factors:** The risk of deep venous thrombosis (DVT) and pulmonary embolism (PE) varies among the heterogeneous populations in ICUs but exists for all patients. Some proportion (2%-10%) of patients admitted to adult medical-surgical ICUs already have DVTs. An additional 10% to 30% of patients develop DVTs within the first 7 days of ICU admission. It has been recently reported that patients in the ICU with SARS-CoV-2 have an increased cumulative incidence of venous thromboembolism (VTE) ranging from 11% to 70%.
3. **Medication thromboprophylaxis:** Unfractionated heparin thromboprophylaxis reduces acquired DVT rate by 50%. Low-molecular-weight heparin (LMWH) may have greater risk reduction of pulmonary embolus and DVT in some populations. The comparative bleeding risk is still being examined.
4. **Mechanical thromboprophylaxis:** Graduated compression stockings and pneumatic compression devices are not well studied in the population in the ICU, especially in comparison with heparin prophylaxis. Existing studies show mixed results with either no effect or up to 30% reduction in DVT risk. Mechanical devices should be utilized if there is a contraindication to medication-based prophylaxis but should not be used as a substitute for heparin.
5. **Screening:** Owing to increased risk of bleeding, anticoagulation may be withheld in some high-risk patients (eg, those with a traumatic brain, pelvis, or spinal cord injury). In these cases, it is recommended to perform periodic screening with venous duplex ultrasound.
6. **High risk for thrombosis with heparin contraindications:** Inferior vena cava filters do not prevent DVT but may be considered to prevent PE when medical prophylaxis is contraindicated.

G. Stress Ulcer Prophylaxis

1. **Background:** Gastrointestinal bleeding in patients who are critically ill has been documented since the 1800s. This is thought to be secondary to compromised mucosal perfusion and/or reperfusion injury that interferes with the normal protective mechanisms of the gastric mucosa. Endoscopic studies show that up to 75% to 100% of patients who are critically ill have gross gastric lesions in the first 1 to 3 days of illness. Determining the incidence and prevalence of clinically significant bleeding is more difficult to quantify; however, it is likely to be in the range of 1.5% to 4% of patients who are critically ill. The relative risk of mortality is approximately 2 to 4 times compared with those without clinically significant bleeding, controlling for other factors.
2. **Risk factors:** Includes respiratory failure, acute hepatic failure, coagulopathy, hypotension, chronic renal failure, prolonged duration of nasogastric (NG) tube, history of alcohol abuse, sepsis, *Helicobacter pylori*, and immunoglobulin A (IgA) greater than 1.
3. **Prevention:** To reduce morbidity and mortality, a variety of acid suppressors and mucosal protectants have been utilized. These include histamine 2 receptor antagonists (H2RA), PPIs, misoprostol, sucralfate, and antacids. PPIs allow greater acid suppression compared with H2RA and may provide better reduction in gastric bleeding. In addition, there may be rapid development of tolerance to H2RA. However, recent large-scale randomized control trials have demonstrated no clinically significant outcomes between the H2RAs and PPIs. Small studies have suggested decreased gastrointestinal bleeding with stress ulcer prophylaxis (SUP) compared to placebo, but high-quality data to reliably identify optimal therapy with minimal risk is lacking. Early enteral nutrition may help minimize gastric

ulceration and reduce the risk of bleeding. More information on which patients should receive SUP, which agents should be used, and how enteral feedings change these recommendations will hopefully be provided with future studies.

4. **Potential harm:** SUP has been shown to increase the risk of HAIs, including VAP and *Clostridium difficile* infection. Furthermore, recent studies propose that SUP may actually increase mortality in patients with high illness severity, and thus should be considered before initiation in all patients in the ICU.

H. Severe Sepsis and Septic Shock (SEP-1 Bundle)

1. **Background**: In 2004, the Surviving Sepsis Campaign released a one-hour bundle aimed at improving survival of sepsis and septic shock. Widespread approval of the SEP-1 measure led to its incorporation into the Centers for Medicare and Medicaid Services in 2015. Any hospital that receives funding from Medicare or Medicaid must measure and report their SEP-1 compliance. However, this bundle has been surrounded in controversy ever since its release.
2. **Hour-1 Bundle recommendations**
   - **a.** Obtain blood cultures before initiation of antibiotics.
   - **b.** Administer broad-spectrum antibiotics.
   - **c.** Rapidly administer 30 mL/kg crystalloid for hypotension or elevated lactate.
   - **d.** Apply vasopressors if patient is hypotensive during or after fluid resuscitation to maintain mean arterial pressure (MAP) greater than or equal to 65 mm Hg.
3. **The Controversy**
   - **a.** There is no clear consistently used definition of sepsis.
   - **b.** There are no definitive data to support that bundle compliance improves mortality in patients with sepsis, and the data are mixed regarding improved survival in patients with septic shock.
   - **c.** Time zero is defined as time of triage, but in reality it should be the time the physician suspects infection.
   - **d.** There is no clear data supporting a lactate cutoff of 2 mmol/L.
   - **e.** Fluid resuscitation should be considered carefully by a clinician for each individual patient and their comorbidities.
   - **f.** There is no strong evidence supporting the aggressive use of antibiotics within the first hour, and side effects of these antibiotics need to be considered when being given to all patients.

IV. INFECTION CONTROL AND THE INTENSIVE CARE UNIT

A. Background: As noted earlier, HAI is a potentially preventable, serious complication in patients in the ICU. These are associated with statistically significant worsening of important ICU quality measures, including morbidity, mortality, length of stay, and costs of care. Despite recent improvements in prevention strategies, there is significant variability in how hospitals perform in preventing these infections. An important element of delivering quality care is prevention of infections and further transmission.

B. Transmission: Transmission of infection requires three elements: a source or reservoir of infectious agents, a susceptible host with a portal of entry the infectious agent can access, and a mode of transmission for the agent. Patients admitted to the ICU are at particular risk for the acquisition of new infections while in the hospital. Critical illness itself increases susceptibility to new infections due to "immune paralysis" secondary to lymphocyte depletion and downregulation of adaptive immunity. In addition, many patients in the ICU have underlying risk factors for infection, such as extremes of age, diabetes, malignancy, and drug-induced immunosuppression. Medications delivered in the ICU such as antibiotics, gastric acid suppressants, and corticosteroids alter the patient's normal microbial flora and responses to microbes. Lastly, many devices used to monitor or treat patients breach the natural barriers to infection, including skin and mucosal surfaces, creating ports of entry for infectious agents. The source of the infectious agent transmission is usually other people (health care workers, other patients, visitors, etc). Health care providers are regularly exposed to multiple sources of infection; hence, strict hygiene is paramount, as described subsequently. Physical elements of the hospital environment may also participate in the transmission of infections and are minimized by contemporary methods of room cleaning and disinfection.

C. Standard Precautions

1. **Background:** Standard precautions against infection should be used with all patient interactions. They are based on the principle that all blood, body fluids, secretions, excretions (except sweat), nonintact skin, and mucous membranes may contain transmissible infectious agents.
2. **Standard precautions include the following:**
    a. **Hand hygiene:** Use of alcohol-based products or washing with soap and water after any contact with body fluids, after removing gloves, and between all patient contacts (ie, before entering and upon exiting each patient's room).
    b. **Personal protective equipment**
        1. **Nonsterile gloves:** Wear when touching body fluids, any mucous membrane, or nonintact skin.
        2. **Nonsterile gown:** Wear a single-use impermeable gown during procedures and during any patient interaction in which clothing or exposed skin may contact patient body fluids, mucous membranes, or nonintact skin.
        3. **Mask, eye protection (goggles), or face shield:** Wear during procedures and patient care activities that may generate a splash or spray of blood, body fluid, secretion, or excretion.
3. **Environmental surfaces and devices:** Soiled patient care equipment is handled with gloves or other personal protective equipment (PPE) until appropriately discarded or cleaned, followed by hand hygiene. Environmental surfaces are routinely cleaned and disinfected. Laundry and textiles are handled to prevent transmission of infection.
4. **Sharps injury prevention**
    a. **Background:** Injuries from needles and other sharps have been associated with the transmission of hepatitis B virus (HBV), hepatitis C virus (HCV), and HIV to health care providers. Direct costs associated with sharps injuries range from $71 to $5000 per incident. Six devices cause nearly 80% of injuries: disposable syringes, suture needles, winged steel needles, scalpel blades, IV catheter stylets, and phlebotomy needles. In one study, 56% of such injuries occur with hollow-bore needles, which are associated with the highest likelihood of HIV transmission to health care workers. Safe handling of these devices is an essential element of standard precautions. Hospital sharps injury prevention programs typically include a well-defined process for reporting sharps injuries as well as providing evaluation and potential infection prophylaxis for health care workers following a sharps injury. Education and intervention should be targeted to areas with prior incidents as well as those at high risk (eg, emergency and operating rooms).
    b. **Injury prevention strategies**
        1. Use needleless systems and devices when able.

2. Use needles and sharps engineered with safety devices.
3. During procedures:
   a. The user of the sharp should be in control of its location and ensure that others are aware a sharp is in use.
   b. Use instruments, not fingers, to grasp needles, retract tissues, and load/unload needles and scalpels.
   c. Do not directly pass sharps to another person; instead, pass through a preidentified neutral zone.
4. Avoid recapping needles and, if necessary, do so using a one-handed technique.
5. Avoid leaving sharps with sharp end exposed.
6. Ensure all sharps are appropriately disposed of immediately in designated and marked disposal containers.

D. Transmission-Based Precautions: These precautions are utilized when a specific infectious etiology is known or suspected. They are based on how that microorganism may be transmitted. They are used, singly or in combination, in addition to standard precautions. Recommendations change frequently, so practitioners should always reference the latest CDC guidelines.

1. **Contact transmission and precautions**
   a. Contact transmission can be separated into two types:
      1. Direct contact transmission occurs when microorganisms are transferred from one infected person to another, without an intermediate object or person. It includes passage of infectious agents through blood or body fluid that contacts mucous membranes or nonintact skin, or transfer from skin to skin.
      2. Indirect contact transmission involves transfer of an infectious agent using another person or object as an intermediary. It includes transfer by nondisinfected hands of health care professionals, common patient care devices or toys, or improperly sterilized surgical equipment.
   b. Contact precautions are utilized with a variety of conditions that are usually spread via direct contact transmission. These include infectious agents such as methicillin-resistant *Staphylococcus aureus* (MRSA), respiratory syncytial virus (RSV), parainfluenza, lice, rotavirus, vancomycin-resistant enterococcus, and *C. difficile*. They are also utilized with wound drainage or other excessive amounts of body fluid.
   c. Health care professionals should wear gown and gloves during all interactions with patients on contact precautions to prevent exposure from patients or their environment.
   d. Patients should be placed in single rooms or cohorted with other patients infected with the same microorganism.
2. **Droplet transmission and precautions:** Microorganisms that are transferred by droplet transmission travel in droplets directly from the infected person's respiratory tract to another person's susceptible mucosal surfaces over short distances (~3 feet). They may also be transferred by contact transmission.
   a. Infectious agents transmitted by droplet include *Bordetella pertussis*, influenza virus, adenovirus, rhinovirus, *Mycoplasma pneumonia*, group A strep, and *Neisseria meningitidis*.
   b. Health care professionals should wear a mask, usually in addition to contact precaution gear, when interacting with patients on droplet precautions.
   c. Patients should be placed in private rooms and they should also wear masks when outside of their room.
3. **Airborne transmission and precautions:** Airborne transmission occurs by airborne droplet nuclei and small particles that remain infective over time

and distance. They may traverse large distances and infect people who have not been in the same room with the patient.

a. Infectious agents transmitted by the airborne route include *Mycobacterium tuberculosis*, *Varicella zoster*, and rubeola.

b. Health care professionals should wear an N95 mask or a respirator during all interactions with the patient.

c. The patient should be placed in a private isolation room with special ventilator capacity ("negative pressure room") that allows 12 air exchanges per hour. The patient should wear a mask whenever out of the isolation room.

E. SARS-CoV-2 (COVID-19) Pandemic

1. Transmission reduction via enhanced respiratory precautions: The SARS-CoV-2 virus is thought to be transmitted via airborne respiratory particles as well as via contact transmission. Therefore, it is recommended that health care providers wear gown, gloves, and surgical masks during all patient interactions, as well as N95 respirators when in contact with a patient who is COVID-19 positive and receiving aerosol-generating procedures (eg, intubations, nebulized medications, etc). Eye protection is recommended to limit risk of droplets entering the exposed mucosal membrane.
2. Optimize TeleHealth services when possible to reduce overall exposure.
3. Screen and triage everyone entering a health care facility for signs and symptoms of COVID-19.
4. Implement universal source control measures (includes the wearing of a face covering at all times while in the hospital by staff, visitors, and patients when possible).
5. Encourage physical distancing whenever possible (maintaining at least 6 feet between people).
6. Consider performing targeted SARS-CoV-2 testing of patients who are asymptomatic as a screening tool before planned procedures.
7. Optimize the use of engineering controls (such as physical barriers) and indoor air quality control when possible.
8. Create a process to respond to SARS-CoV-2 exposures in health care providers and/or patients.
9. Follow CDC guidance for evolving recommendations and pay specific attention to how to optimize PPE supplies during a global pandemic.

F. Infection Control Surveillance Programs

1. It is essential for ICUs to have real-time tracking of HAIs to prevent further morbidity and mortality. A close working relationship with the hospital's infection control staff is required.
2. Weekly or monthly reports should be displayed for staff to promote accountability and a culture of safety. Practices adopted from industry such as prominent displays of "weeks from last infection," for example, are effective and increasingly popular.

Selected Readings

Alhazzani W, Lim W, Jaeschke RZ, et al. Heparin thromboprophylaxis in medical-surgical critically ill patients: a systematic review and meta-analysis of randomized trials. *Crit Care Med.* 2013;41:2088-2098.

Balas MC, Vasilevskis EE, Olsen KM, et al. Effectiveness and safety of the awakening and breathing coordination, delirium monitoring/management, and early exercise/mobility bundle. *Crit Care Med.* 2014;42(5):1024-1036.

Barbateskovic M, Marker S, Granholm, A, et al. Stress ulcer prophylaxis with proton pump inhibitors or histamin-2 receptor antagonists in adult intensive care patients: a systematic review with meta-analysis and trial sequential analysis. *Intensive Care Med.* 2019;45:143-158.

Byrnes MC, Schuerer DJE, Schallom ME, et al. Implementation of a mandatory checklist of protocols and objectives improves compliance with a wide range of evidence-based intensive care unit practices. *Crit Care Med.* 2009;37(10):2775-2781.

Centers for Disease Control and Prevention. Antibiotic Resistance Threats in the United States, 2019. https://www.cdc.gov/drugresistance/pdf/threats-report/2019-ar-threats-report-508.pdf.

Centers for Disease Control and Prevention. Ventilator-associated event protocol. Accessed June 17, 2015. http://www.cdc.gov/nhsn/acute-care-hospital/vae/

Centers for Disease Control and Prevention. Workbook for designing, implementing, and evaluating a sharp injury prevention program. Accessed June 17, 2015. http://www.cdc.gov/sharpssafety/pdf/sharpsworkbook_2008.pdf.

Chenoweth C, Saint S. Preventing catheter-associated urinary tract infections in the intensive care unit. *Crit Care Clin.* 2013;29:19-32.

Coffin SE, Klompas M, Classen D, et al. Strategies to prevent ventilator-associated pneumonia in acute care hospitals. *Infect Control Hosp Epidemiol.* 2008;29(S1):S31-S40.

Cook DJ, Crowther M. Thromboprophylaxis in the intensive care unit: focus on medical-surgical patients. *Crit Care Med.* 2010;38(2 suppl):S76-S82.

Cook D, Crowther M, Meade M, et al. Deep venous thrombosis in medical-surgical critically ill patients: prevalence, incidence, and risk factors. *Crit Care Med.* 2005;33(7):1565-1571.

Curtis JR, Cook DJ, Wall RJ, et al. Intensive care unit quality improvement: a "how-to" guide for the interdisciplinary team. *Crit Care Med.* 2006;34:211-218.

Gould CV, Umscheid CA, Agarwal RK, et al. Guideline for prevention of catheter-associated urinary tract infections 2009. *Infect Control Hosp Epidemiol.* 2010;31(4):319-326.

Hollenbeak CS, Schilling AL. The attributable cost of catheter-associated urinary tract infections in the United States: a systematic review. *Am J Infect Control.* 2018;46(7):751-757.

Langley GL, Moen R, Nolan KM, et al. *The Improvement Guide: A Practical Approach to Enhancing Organizational Performance.* 2nd ed. Jossey-Bass; 2009.

Marik PE, Vasu T, Hirani A, et al. Stress ulcer prophylaxis in the new millennium: a systematic review and meta-analysis. *Crit Care Med.* 2010;38:2222-2228.

Marwick C, Davay P. Care bundles: the holy grail of infectious risk management in hospital? *Curr Opin Infect Dis.* 2009;22:364-369.

Miller SE, Maragakis LL. Central line-associated bloodstream infection prevention. *Curr Opin Infect Dis.* 2012;25:412-422.

Mietto C, Pinciroli R, Patel N, et al. Ventilator associated pneumonia. Evolving definitions and preventive strategies. *Respir Care.* 2013;58(6):990-1003.

Morandi A, Brummel NE, Ely EW. Sedation, delirium and mechanical ventilation: the "ABCDE" approach. *Curr Opin Crit Care.* 2011;17:43-49.

O'Grady NP, Alexander M, Burns LA, et al. Guidelines for the prevention of intravascular catheter-related infections. *Am J Infect Control.* 2011;39(4 suppl 1):S1-S34.

Patel PK, Gupta A, Vaughn VM, et al. Review of strategies to reduce central line-associated bloodstream infection (CLABSI) and catheter-associated urinary tract infection (CAUTI) in adult ICUs. *J Hosp Med.* 2018;13(2):105-116.

Rossi PJ, Edmiston CE. Patient safety in the critical care environment. *Surg Clin N Am.* 2012;92:1369-1386.

Sagana R, Hyzy RC. Achieving zero central line-associated bloodstream infection rates in your intensive care unit. *Crit Care Clin.* 2013;29:1-9.

Siegel JD, Rhinehart E, Jackson M, et al. 2007 guideline for isolation precautions: preventing transmission of infectious agents in health care settings. *Am J Infect Control.* 2007;35(10 suppl 2):S65-S164.

Society of Critical Care Medicine. Critical Care Statistics. https://www.sccm.org/Communications/Critical-Care-Statistics

Tambyah PA, Oon J. Catheter-associated urinary tract infection. *Curr Opin Infect Dis.* 2012;25:365-370.

Wunsch H, Linde-Zwirble WT, Angus DC, Hartman ME, Milbrandt EB, Kahn JM. The epidemiology of mechanical ventilation use in the United States. *Crit Care Med.* 2010;38:1947-1953.

Young PJ, Bagshaw SM, Forbes AB, et al. Effect of stress ulcer prophylaxis with proton pump inhibitors vs histamine-2 receptor blockers on in-hospital mortality among ICU patients receiving invasive mechanical ventilation: the PEPTIC randomized clinical trial. *JAMA.* 2020;323(7):616-626.

Zimlichman MD, Henderson D, Tamir O, et al. Health care-associated infections: a meta-analysis of costs and financial impact on the US health care system. *JAMA Intern Med.* 2013;173(22):2039-2046.

Zimmerman JE, Kramer AA, Knaus WA. Changes in hospital mortality for United States intensive care unit admissions from 1988 to 2012. *Crit Care.* 2013;17:R81.

41 Ethical, Legal, and End-of-Life Issues in Intensive Care Unit Practice

Emmett Alexander Kistler, Sharon E. Brackett, and Michael J. Young

I. INTRODUCTION

In caring for patients who are critically ill, it is inevitable that ethical issues will arise. Critically ill patients often have complex medical conditions, multiple providers, and uncertain prognoses or treatment plans. This can lead to conflict and moral distress among patients, family, health care providers, and support staff. The COVID-19 pandemic with its higher mortality rates, need for unprecedented surge capacity, limited resources, and end-of-life care complexities exacerbated all these challenges.

Here, we describe a proactive approach to ethical issues in the intensive care unit (ICU). Adoption and adaptation of these measures may help minimize conflict and moral distress. Key ethical concepts and practical guidelines are provided to optimize care in a variety of circumstances. It is hoped that you will build trust and connect with your patients and their families through empathy, seeking to understand them, confronting (rather than avoiding) problems, managing expectations, and providing optimal clinical care.

II. PROACTIVE APPROACH

A. The Cost of Conflict: A proactive approach to ethical issues in the ICU can minimize conflict and moral distress. Conflict is common in the ICU and can lead to adverse patient experiences. Conflicts can arise within teams, between staff, and with families. Disagreements regarding value-laden clinical decisions and goals of care (GOC) may be aggravated by interpersonal tension within the team, breakdown or loss of usual communication channels, inability to establish trust, and challenging end-of-life care. The costs of unreconciled conflict are high and include misguided or goal-discordant treatment, poor health outcomes, moral distress, burnout, and increased staff turnover. Such poor outcomes should be prevented with proactive measures designed to enhance collaborative shared decision-making.

B. Proactive Measures: Modern critical care and education place a heightened focus on organ systems and specialty consultation, advanced treatment modalities, numbers, invasive monitoring, and computer-based documentation. Humanizing the ICU experience—for patients, family, and staff—can be challenging but remains a worthy endeavor and imperative that may reduce the chances that conflict arises. The essence of ethical care involves an engaged and person-focused attitude alongside an abundant concern for others including staff. The following measures comprise well-recognized strategies to promote patient-centered care (Table 41.1).

1. **Visiting and communication:** Guidelines for optimizing the visitor experience include inviting caregivers to rounds, facilitating introductions, minimizing medical jargon and offering to "translate" later, inviting corrections during staff presentations, and allowing a short period for questions at the end of rounds with the offer of more private time later. The opportunity to observe the "work" of rounds and the transparency of communication

TABLE 41.1 Proactive Measures to Minimize Moral Distress and ICU Conflict

ICU open visitation hours
Allowing family presence during rounds
Routine proactive family meetings
Process of informed consent
Relieving patients' distressing symptoms
Sensitivity to and respect for cultural norms
Provision of spiritual support
Interdisciplinary collaborative care
Team debriefings
Ethics rounds
ICU staff meetings
Ethics consultation
Integration of palliative care principles and practices into the ICU

ICU, intensive care unit.

can help build trust, mutual respect, and improve efficiency of family communication.

2. **Routine proactive family meetings:** Early (within 24-72 hours of ICU admission) and routine family meetings build trust between family and caregivers. They also elucidate patient values and establish agreed upon clinical goals and treatment options. Clinicians should be mindful of the range of potential cognitive biases that may bear on such discussions and aim to minimize self-fulfilling prophecy bias and disability bias in such meetings. A more detailed discussion can be found in **Section IV.**
3. **Interdisciplinary collaborative care:** The structure and function of an ICU team influences the prevalence of conflict and how it is handled. All members of the care team—nurses, physicians, students, social workers, chaplains, physical and respiratory therapists—should expect to interface with caregivers. Establishing this expectation and reviewing communication strategies can help normalize this idea for the unit.
4. **Team debriefings, daily huddles, clinical operations meetings, and unit-based ethics rounds** are a key mechanism for team collaboration and well-being. Debriefing with all staff after critical incidents allows for a retrospective review of what went well and what could be improved upon. Debriefings also provide opportunities to initiate discussions of larger topics: Are work rounds interdisciplinary and collaborative? What structured education would benefit staff? What are the overall mission and goals of the ICU?
5. **Get to Know Me Posters** offer another valuable mechanism to promote patient-centered care (Figure 41.1). These posters placed in the patient's room are completed by caregivers and allow the team to better know the patient as they were before admission. The information and photos provided by the family connect the team to the sometimes-voiceless patient. The interaction also helps the team develop rapport with the family. These posters were invaluable during mass causality events and the COVID-19 pandemic when visitor restrictions also limited the family's ability to "share the patient's story."

III. TREATMENT DECISIONS

A. **The Optimal Decision-Making Process** when there is conflict over value-laden clinical concerns is one that is fair, transparent, respectful, collaborative, and effective. Potential barriers to this level of care are numerous: within some

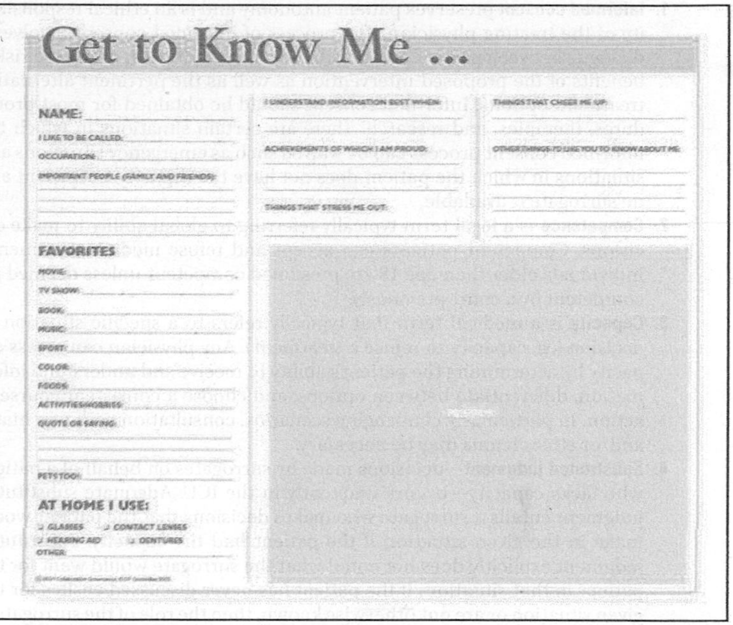

FIGURE 41.1 Get to Know Me Posters. These 20 × 24 inch posters in the intensive care unit (ICU) rooms are filled in by the patients' families as an opportunity for the team to get to know the patient better.

teams, there can be a diffusion of responsibility, whereas in others there might be a top-down authoritative approach in which some team or family members feel voiceless. Moral distress arises when individuals feel powerless to alter what they perceive to be suboptimal care. And yet, regardless of the team structure, each member of the team is a moral agent and should possess some degree of accountability for the decisions made and actions taken. A shared decision-making paradigm locates the responsibility between the patient (or surrogate) and the clinicians, thus aiming to respect patient autonomy and the beneficent intentions of caregivers.

B. Communication Is Key to the shared decision-making process. Effective communication enables clinicians to learn about the patient's values and goals and allows the patient/surrogate to learn about the clinical condition and which treatment paths are considered reasonable to pursue after review of the patient's values and goals. The process is dynamic and necessitates reassessment and adjustment of plans depending on the patient's evolving condition.

C. Key Ethical Tenets come into play daily in the ICU. These include the following:

1. Autonomy—the right of the patient to self-govern
2. Beneficence—the obligation to promote well-being and prevent/remove harm
3. Nonmaleficence—the need to refrain from inflicting harm
4. Justice—an allocation principle, striving for fair distribution of resources

D. Patient Autonomy, the respect for an individual patient's right to make decisions about own medical care, is a valued ethical principle. Autonomy is preserved by involving the patient in the decision-making process. Within autonomy, several terms warrant understanding:

1. **Informed consent** preserves patient autonomy and is an ethical responsibility of the treating physician. The process of informed consent involves a dialogue between patient and health care provider(s) describing the risks/benefits of the proposed intervention as well as the pertinent alternative treatment options. Informed consent should be obtained for most procedures, therapies, and research. There are certain situations in which the informed consent process can be waived such as emergency situations and situations in which the patient does not have the capacity to consent and no surrogate is available.
2. **Competence** is a legal term typically referring to global ability to make decisions. Competent patients can accept and refuse medical treatments. Individuals older than age 18 are presumed competent unless deemed incompetent by a court previously.
3. **Capacity** is a medical term that typically refers to a specific situation or decision (eg, capacity to refuse a treatment). Any physician can assess capacity by determining the patient's ability to receive and understand information, differentiate between options, and choose a consistent course of action. In particularly challenging scenarios, consultation with psychiatry and/or ethics teams may be necessary.
4. **Substituted judgment**—decisions made by surrogates on behalf of a patient who lacks capacity—occurs frequently in the ICU. Adequate substituted judgment entails a surrogate who makes decisions that the patient would make in the given situation if the patient had the capacity. Substituted judgment explicitly does not entail what the surrogate would want for the patient in that situation. If the patient has never discussed wishes for the given situation or are not otherwise known, then the role of the surrogate is to make the decision based on what is in the patient's best interests.

E. **Advanced Care Planning** encompasses the discussions and documentation of a patient's values and wishes regarding specific medical scenarios and interventions. These conversations are difficult, and the nature of certain medical conditions is unexpected such that the ICU team must frequently lead de novo advanced care planning. Ideally, however, discussions regarding advanced care planning should start in the outpatient setting, before ICU admission, because this allows more time to assess the patient's understanding of their illness, clarify goals and values over the illness trajectory, and discuss reasonable clinical goals. Here is a brief review of key documents that patients may have completed prior or during an ICU stay:

1. **Advanced directives** are statements specifying a patient's wishes that are designed to help guide decision-making in these situations. Advance directives vary from state to state and even from institution to institution. It has been recognized that advance directives may be verbal in nature and that conversations between the patient and their loved ones may provide an acceptable framework to guide decisions.
2. **A health care proxy** or **durable power of attorney for health care** is a legal document prepared by the patient appointing the person they wish to make health care decisions in their place in case they are unable to make decisions themselves.
3. **A living will** is a document describing therapies or interventions that the patient would wish to receive or refuse under specific circumstances. These documents often cover broad circumstances such as "persistent vegetative state" or "without meaningful recovery" and often do not apply to the nuanced situations that arise in the context of complex critical illness. Thus, these documents may only be marginally helpful and may overlap with other advanced directives. In some states, they are not legally binding and must be supplemented by communication with those close to the patient.

4. **Medical Order Forms:** Physician/Medical Orders for Life-Sustaining Treatment (POLST, MOLST) or Physician Order for Scope of Treatment (POST) forms are medical order forms that are completed by health care professionals after discussions with the patient regarding prognosis, treatments, and GOC. These forms provide a framework for patients to express their preferences about life-sustaining medical treatments and help relay this information between health care providers. Patients can update MOLST forms over time and verbally override preexisting wishes conveyed in a MOLST, although a change in GOC—particularly during an acute illness—should trigger additional discussion.

F. **Absence of a Surrogate:** In some cases, a surrogate decision-maker cannot be located. In these situations, as much information about the patient should be gathered from known contacts, other providers, and community supports. In some cases, such as those where conflict has arisen regarding surrogacy, a legal guardian may be appointed to serve as the decision-maker.

G. **Bundled Consent:** The need to perform life-saving procedures can often present suddenly in critical care and obtaining informed consent may delay potential life-saving interventions. For this reason, some ICUs have implemented a bundled or universal consent form. These forms include commonly performed procedures that may be urgent in nature such as intubation, central line placement, blood transfusion, and so on.

IV. THE FAMILY MEETING

A. **Rationale—for Patient and Provider:** Family meetings are one of the most effective means to achieve shared decision-making and can also help prevent or mitigate conflict. Think of the meeting as being like *a procedure* with its own set of skills to master. There are organizational, communication, and emotional skills needed to conduct an effective meeting. As with any procedure, preparation, performance, and follow-up are key components (Table 41.2).

1. **Family meetings within 72 hours** of ICU admission increase family satisfaction, reduce the length of ICU stay, and increase the likelihood of agreement between the providers and the family about the limitations of life-sustaining treatments. In addition, family satisfaction is higher if physicians spend a smaller proportion of time talking and more listening.
2. **Preparation:** Determine a time that both key stakeholders from the family and medical team can attend. Confirm there is space with adequate seating, comfort items (tissues, refreshments), and privacy with minimal interruptions. Hold a premeeting "huddle" to achieve consensus on facts, address areas of uncertainty, review an agenda and goals, and identify a suitable meeting leader before entering the room with the patient and/or family. Allow for adequate family/surrogate representation including via virtual attendance. In situations where consultant input may be informative (eg, neurology input regarding neurologic prognosis), create opportunities for the consultant to weigh in. In addition, ensure the bedside nurse is present because they spend the most time with the patient and visiting family members. The bedside nurse can speak most accurately to the patient's care requirements and day-to-day experience.

B. **Introduce Participants and the Purpose of Meeting:** Invite everyone to state their name and describe how they know the patient. Identify the patient's surrogate spokesperson. Politely establish a tone of courtesy and confidentiality. Clarify the purpose of the meeting (eg, to identify treatment options and goals that align with the patient's values, beliefs, and preferences).

C. **Obtain the Patient and/or Caregiver Perspective:** After introductions, a patient's caregivers should be asked to describe their understanding of the patient's

TABLE 41.2 Framework and Example Scripting for ICU Family Meetings

1. Prepare agenda and setting. Ensure team consensus on facts and plan. Decide who will be present and who will lead the discussion before seeing family.
2. Introduce participants and purpose of meeting. "Thank you all for coming today. We'd like to start with introductions. Can you share your name and how you know [patient's name]?" "The purpose of today's meeting is to provide a medical update and discuss next steps."
3. Assess patient/family perspective. "Can you tell us your understanding of (your/patient's name) medical condition?" "Tell us about [patient's name] outside of the hospital? What's important to her/him?"
4. Obtain an invitation. "Would it be ok for us to give you an update on how [patient's name] is doing?"
5. Summarize the patient's medical condition and key clinical decisions. "We obtained the test results, and unfortunately they did not show us what we hoped for." "[Patient's name] is doing worse. She/he has a new pneumonia. We're treating it, but he/she is requiring more support from the breathing machine."
6. Offer a recommendation if necessary. "God forbid his/her heart were to stop, at this time we would recommend against administering chest compressions and other invasive resuscitation efforts."
7. Process emotion and empathize. "I'm so sorry this is happening. I wish we didn't have to share this news." "I imagine this is overwhelming. Can you tell us more about what you're feeling?"
8. Summarize and strategize follow-up. "To summarize today's meeting, we discussed how [patient's name] is doing worse because of a new infection. We won't perform chest compressions if his heart stops, but we will keep treating the rest of his medical problems just like we have been." "Our next update will be tomorrow after the next set of tests, but you can call if you have questions before then."
9. Document the meeting and communicate content to team.

ICU, intensive care unit.

medical condition. Asking the family to speak first demonstrates respect and helps establish rapport. It is also diagnostic, allowing the team to discern what medical information and emotions will need to be addressed. We all have different communication styles—medical team and family members alike—and listening to the family first affords insight into how *this* family communicates.

D. Learn About the Patient: After the family describes the medical condition, there may be an opportunity to ask more about the patient in general: Who is this person outside of the hospital? What is important to them on a day-to-day basis? What would they say if they were present in the meeting? Before sharing the medical perspective, it can be invaluable to ask the caregiver about the patient's values, which subsequently inform the team's recommendations.

E. Acquire an Invitation: With this background in place, the staff member leading the meeting should then ask if the medical team's perspective and recommendations can be shared. Although small, this gesture provides caregivers with agency to accept this information. Most family members will want to know what is happening. For the few who decline to hear updates, explore the rationale and emotions underlying their desire not to hear what is happening.

F. Share Knowledge and Recommendations: After these steps have unfolded, the leading clinician can then concisely summarize the patient's medical condition, describe their trajectory, and ultimately frame recommendations based on the clinical details and the patient's values and goals. Treatment plans may be presented as time-limited trials with clearly stated duration and goals. If appropriate, this might also be the point in the meeting to address code status.

1. **Avoid "a la carte" recommendations** as much as possible. In general, it is unnecessary and burdensome to ask the family to decide about each diagnostic or treatment option. Rather, the medical team should propose a general plan consistent with the goals and values and then provide the family with an opportunity to respond.

G. Identify and Process Emotions: Providing critical updates, describing prognoses, and making recommendations can be an overwhelming experience. Helping caregivers identify and process emotions is as important as communicating accurate medical facts. Allowing periods of silence, asking caretakers about what they are experiencing, and offering reflective statements are all important strategies to help explore emotions. Exploring the patient's and family's fears and concerns uncovers opportunities to manage expectations and to provide psychosocial support for realistic hopes and fears—or to provide correction for unrealistic ones.

H. Summarize and Strategize: After recommendations have been shared and questions have been answered, the meeting leader should concisely summarize the content of the meeting before enumerating next steps and plans for future communication. It can be helpful to remind families that advanced care planning conversations are ongoing and will be revisited over time.

I. Document the meeting in the patient's record by writing a family meeting note—similar to writing a procedure note. Include who attended the meeting, what "the findings" were, what decisions and plans were made, justifications for those plans, what uncertainties or disagreements remained unreconciled, and plans for follow-up. Consider using a family meeting template to guide and document the meeting. Finally, verbally communicate salient points to pertinent team members (eg, supervising registered nurse [RN]) who were not present.

V. GOALS OF CARE

A. GOC and how medical providers address them vary depending on the patient's condition, clinical reasonableness of a given intervention, and the patient's values and expectations. For some patients, the goals are obvious, such as preventing imminent death, curing disease, and returning to their premorbid level of function. In other situations, the reality of a patient's condition warrants more tempered goals such as delay of a disease process (rather than its cure) or prolonging life to provide additional time with family and/or caregivers.

B. Code Status: Code status represents one of the main examples of GOC. The purpose of a code status is to clarify which therapies will be offered to the patient in the case of life-threatening instability. After discussing the disease process and prognosis (see **Section IV**), the patient, a surrogate, or physician may propose a "do not resuscitate" (DNR—sometimes referred to as "do not attempt resuscitation" or DNAR) or "do not intubate" (DNI) order. It is important to emphasize among staff and with the patient/family that DNR/DNI/DNAR orders do not signify that a patient's condition is hopeless or that the medical team's commitment to the patient has changed. Instead, the patient and family should be reassured that other interventions to evaluate and target underlying pathologies and manage symptoms will continue (if these efforts remain within the GOC).

1. **Transient reversals of code status:** It is not unusual for patients who are DNR/DNI to undergo diagnostic or therapeutic procedures that require reversal to a "full code." Typically, the rationale for periprocedural code status reversals is to allow the proceduralist and patient to endure possible complications of the procedure that could be reversed. These decisions should be decided on a case-by-case basis in the context of the patient's current health status, values, and goals. For patients undergoing elective surgical procedures requiring intubation or during which a reversible cause of cardiac arrest unrelated to their underlying illness may occur, it may still be reasonable to temporarily hold the DNR/DNI for a set period (eg, 72 hours post the procedure or extubation).
2. **Disagreements between patient/family and medical team:** Recommendations regarding code status and other GOC may not always be welcomed by the patient or caregivers. In these situations, the physician's first task is to explore the nature of the disagreement: What does "do everything" mean? Do the patient and family understand the nature of a specific intervention, its risks, and its benefits? Is there any common ground that can be identified ("I don't want to be kept alive by machines")? After gently interrogating the disagreement, offering education, and exploring emotions, the ICU physician can make the same recommendation, suggest a time-limited trial, or find other common ground to focus on before revisiting the recommendation later. It is important to remember that clinicians are not obligated to provide treatments that are not medically indicated.
3. **Futility:** There is no consensus on the precise definition of futility because it can entail value judgments when viewed through the differing lenses of the involved stakeholders. Clinicians often experience moral distress when they believe an intervention may be potentially inappropriate—ineffective, harmful, wasteful, or will not result in the patient's desired outcomes. If open communication does not resolve the situation, then the clinician may (i) attempt to transfer the patient to another caregiver, (ii) involve institutional ethics and legal consultation to discuss limitations of life-sustaining treatment despite the wishes of the patient and/or family, or (iii) seek adjudication to replace or override the surrogate. Certain decisions—withdrawing life-sustaining treatments, for example—require higher levels of ethical justification and support. They should not be made solely by individual physicians but rather with the backing of additional critical care opinion(s), formal ethics consultation, and, preferably, with institutional support.

C. Ethics Committees: Although varying between institutions, ethics committees usually comprise an interdisciplinary group of professionals and community members trained in clinical ethics consultation. Ethics consultation offers an objective analysis of the patient's care and, drawing upon ethical principles, employs a fair and transparent process to guide the patient, family, and medical team to a reasonable consensus or compromise. Ethics interventions have been shown to mitigate conflict and, for some, to reduce ICU length of stay, ventilator days, hospital stay, and cost without increasing mortality.

VI. PALLIATIVE CARE IN THE INTENSIVE CARE UNIT: IT IS NOT JUST FOR THE END OF LIFE

A. Symptoms—Frequent and Numerous: Patients in the ICU are at risk for suffering many unpleasant sensations during routine ICU care. Their underlying illnesses and the interventions imposed on them can lead to pain, dyspnea, anxiety, delirium, agitation, nausea, vomiting, secretions, pruritus, diarrhea, constipation, and other physical, psychosocial, or spiritual discomforts. For patients with neurocritical illness, management of neurologic symptoms such as dysautonomia, seizures, headache, dizziness, and spasticity require active management and may be also considered comfort focused. Preventing and palliating these distressing symptoms are goals shared by critical care and palliative care clinicians—whether the patient is receiving life-prolonging care or end-of-life care.

B. Primary Palliative Care entails symptom control, emotional support, and advanced care planning efforts led by the ICU team. ICU providers should develop a knowledge base and skillset for treating symptoms and discussing GOC because in the United States and elsewhere, the availability of subspecialty providers is inadequate relative to the demand.

C. Subspecialty Palliative Care: Common indications to involve palliative care specialists include uncontrolled symptoms recalcitrant to traditional interventions, complicated and often discordant GOC situations, and assistance formulating palliative ventilator withdrawal plans. Palliative care interventions reduce the length of stay and improve symptom control, communication, and the quality of dying in the ICU. Social service and chaplaincy interventions can be employed as part of or separately from palliative care consultation. Patients, families, and staff alike are often greatly supported by these services, especially under the stressful circumstances of ICU and end-of-life care.

VII. GUIDELINES FOR WITHDRAWING LIFE-SUSTAINING THERAPIES

A. The Goals for Limitation or Withdrawal of Life-Sustaining Therapies

1. Respecting the wishes of the patient
   - **a.** Withdrawing or withholding interventions that are not concordant with patient goals
   - **b.** Stopping or minimizing interventions that will no longer offer benefit
   - **c.** Continuing only those interventions that promote comfort
2. Supporting and respecting the caregivers
   - **a.** Physically, emotionally, and spiritually within their cultural norms
   - **b.** Offering expectations and education around the dying process
3. Allowing death to occur as peacefully and symptom-free as possible
   - **a.** Preventing or palliating distressing symptoms
   - **b.** Maintaining or achieving the patient's ability to communicate, if possible

B. Transitioning Focus: Although patients undergoing withdrawal of life-sustaining therapies (LSTs) may no longer be monitored invasively or administered high-intensity interventions, they nonetheless require equally as much—if not more—attention as any patient in the ICU. Providing this attention begins with communication: identifying what is important, offering clear expectations, and allowing the patient and caregivers the opportunity to explore their reactions.

1. **Elicit values:** If not already discussed, ask the patient and/or caregivers what they value and what is important to them now that time is short. Ask whether the patient would prefer specific religious, spiritual, or cultural practices or accommodations.
2. **Offer expectations:** The process of withdrawal should be clearly explained and the family educated about what to expect. Uncertainly should also be acknowledged because each patient is different and forecasting every aspect of the dying process is not possible.
   - **a.** Frame any clinical recommendations based on the patient's/family's values and your clinical expertise in end-of-life care. The anticipated rapidity of the dying process or realities of the patient's medical condition may determine specific choices concerning therapies to be withdrawn, the rate of withdrawal, and the ability to accommodate the requests of

families. Extubation, for example, may not be feasible in all situations; offer concise rationale if a request is not possible.

b. Provide education on what the dying process could entail: changes in skin color, noises due to airway secretions, and the irregular breathing pattern preceding death. Explain that these changes usually are not consciously felt by the patient.

3. Explore emotions: Transitioning focus in the ICU and the prospect of death can provoke a range of emotions. Emotions may be informed by prior experiences with in-hospital deaths or a complete lack thereof. Help identify emotions, recognize the difficulty of the situation, and allow space for them to continue processing.

4. Provide assurance that the patient will be comfortable throughout the process and invite family presence for as much as they would prefer and is medically allowable (a significant issue during the COVID-19 pandemic). Reaffirm that you will help them understand and cope with the end-of-life events as they unfold. Invite the family to ask questions at any point during the process.

C. Taking a Team-Based Approach: Once the decision has been made with the patient and/or caregivers to withdraw LSTs, the primary focus becomes the patient's comfort. Optimizing comfort at the end of life for patients in the ICU requires a significant reorientation of care in an environment otherwise designed for frequent, invasive care:

1. A huddle between clinicians, nurses, respiratory therapists, social work, spiritual care, and other members of the care team should occur before the transition to comfort measures to establish a plan for the transition, ensure all resources are available, and address any concerns. Discontinuation of LSTs may promptly lead to patient death—even when the patient is expected to live for a prolonged period—such that reviewing these details should be accomplished ahead of time to reduce the chances of an uncomfortable death.

2. Clinical orders should be reexamined and corrected with the primary nurse with a goal toward promoting palliative and comfort care. Anticipatory opioids, which decrease the chances of postextubation tachypnea, should be ordered.

3. Stop or minimize unnecessary interventions such as vital sign monitoring, alarms, and lab draws. If they are not providing significant relief, lines, tubes, drains, and indwelling catheters should also be discontinued, although at least one working intravenous (IV) line should be maintained for administration of IV pain and anxiety treatments. Reassess the equipment in the patient's room and remove unnecessary items to make room for comfortable seating for family members.

4. Stop life-prolonging interventions: Specific intervention modifications will be reviewed later, but in brief, therapies solely directed toward supporting physiologic homeostasis or treating the underlying disease processes are no longer indicated and should be discontinued. The benefit-to-burden ratio of each intervention should be used to determine which interventions should be eliminated. The precise order of discontinuation is tailored to the patient's situation and reasonable family preferences.

a. Avoid discussing with the family cessation of each individual therapy or asking for their input on a menu of options. Instead, provide a summary of what withdrawal of LSTs entails, providing additional details as questions arise.

b. Although a plan for each patient must be developed individually, we recommend that life-prolonging interventions be discontinued concurrently or within a short duration of time. A stepwise approach to withdrawal may be easier for caregivers to accept, but it is the patient who is the ICU team's main priority and whose life and potential suffering will be prolonged by serial discontinuation of therapies.

D. Withdrawal of Specific Interventions

1. **Nutrition, fluid resuscitation, blood replacement, and IV hydration** are considered forms of LSTs and are discontinued when prolonging life is no longer the goal. Case reports and controlled studies suggest that little, if any, discomfort accompanies the withdrawal of enteral nutrition and IV hydration. Continuation of artificially administered fluids and nutrition can lead to edema and distressing bowel symptoms in dying persons. Nevertheless, families can be quite upset if it is perceived that their loved one is being "starved." If so, it is key to review the natural slowing of metabolism during the dying process and the potential complications of artificial nutrition and hydration. An important exception is the patient who requests to eat and/or drink for comfort, religious, or cultural preferences—assuming all parties are aware and accepting of risks such as aspiration.
2. **Vasopressor and inotropic support** can be discontinued without weaning. The gradual withdrawal of circulatory support appears to offer no benefit for patient comfort.
3. **Antibiotics and other curative pharmacotherapy:** After the decision is made to terminate LSTs, therapies directed at cure are no longer consistent with the GOC. Such therapies include cancer chemotherapy, radiation therapy, steroids, and antimicrobials—unless the treatments play a significant palliative role (such as topical antifungal agents, oral hygiene, or antibiotics aimed at treating painful pathology).
4. **Neuromuscular blockade** must be discontinued, and adequate time must be allotted for residual paralytic to be metabolized, before withdrawing other LSTs. Paralysis limits the patient's ability to demonstrate signs/symptoms of discomfort, can generate significant distress for the conscious patient, and can directly precipitate death if other LSTs such as mechanical ventilation are removed before the paralytic has worn off. A train-of-four technique can evaluate for evidence of persistent muscle paralysis. If in doubt, allow additional time for the paralytic to be metabolized before withdrawing LSTs.
5. **Supplemental oxygen:** Supplemental oxygen is generally discontinued once the decision to withdraw LSTs is made because oxygen can prolong the dying process. Patients who cannot be extubated or utilize artificial airways should receive humidified air to avoid irritation and/or drying the airway. The more challenging situation entails the patient on a high-flow nasal cannula (HFNC) device, which can alleviate dyspnea through provision of high rates of flow projected through the nasal passages. In these situations, the clinician can discuss the timing of removal of the device with the patient, caregivers, nurse, and respiratory therapist versus reducing the oxygen supply to room air while maintaining a high flow rate.
6. **Mechanical ventilation:** Ventilatory support is the most common therapy withdrawn when LSTs are discontinued, and there are different approaches to its removal. We favor palliative extubation when medically feasible and when preferred by the family. Reasons to avoid extubation entail infectious contraindications (eg, for aerosolizing an infectious pathogen), high secretion burden, possibility for significant airway bleeding, and inability of the patient to protect the airway. Discuss with nursing, respiratory therapy, and caregivers to determine the best strategy for each patient.
   a. Mechanical ventilation may be gradually withdrawn over a short period by decreasing the inspired oxygen to room air, decreasing positive end-expiratory pressure, and then decreasing ventilatory rate. We

recommend that this be done over several minutes, not hours. The benefit of this strategy is that it allows time to titrate palliative medications to emerging symptoms as support is reduced. An overly slow "weaning" process should be avoided, however, because it may prolong the dying process and may provide the family with a misleading hope for survival.

b. Alternatively, mechanical ventilation may be discontinued abruptly, with the patient either extubated or the endotracheal tube left in place to provide humidified room air. Extubation may result in death more quickly compared with gradually decreasing the intensity of mechanical ventilation. It is important to anticipate, prevent, and be ready to treat dyspnea, obstruction, and air hunger.

c. The timing of death after the withdrawal of mechanical ventilation depends on the etiology and severity of respiratory failure. Death may occur within minutes for some, whereas in some studies, a small proportion of patients with chronic lung disease unexpectedly survived. This observation is humbling and a key reminder that our prognostication is imperfect.

7. Dialysis, including intermittent hemodialysis and the various forms of continuous hemodialysis, is generally discontinued when a decision to withdraw LSTs is made.

8. Anti-seizure medications for patients with seizure disorders may promote comfort and need not be discontinued.

9. Extracorporeal membrane oxygenation (ECMO), mechanical circulatory support devices, and other invasive novel therapies comprise an increasingly common set of interventions provided to some of the sickest patients. These devices require significant expertise and coordination of numerous resources and personnel. The main takeaway regarding withdrawal of LSTs for patients sustained by these devices is that significant planning between the patient, family, nurse, technician, primary ICU team, and subspecialty team managing the device must take place to ensure consensus is achieved around the decision to stop therapy and creation of a plan for how to support the patient thereafter.

E. Justification for Aggressive Symptom Control at the End of Life

1. Providing the standard of care: The administration of sedatives and analgesics during the withholding or withdrawal of life-sustaining treatments is consistent with the standard of care for the critically ill. Most patients in the ICU receive these medications during the withdrawal of support. Certainly, competent patients may refuse pharmacologic intervention to preserve lucidness. In addition, some medications may not be indicated for patients who will gain no benefit (eg, patients who are comatose).

2. Regarding concerns of "hastening death": Clinicians generally should not withhold measures necessary for comfort for fear of the double effect of hastening death.

a. Patients who are given large doses of opioids to treat discomfort during the withdrawal of life-sustaining treatments on average live as long as patients not given opioids, suggesting that it is the underlying disease process, not the use of palliative medications, that usually determines the time of death.

b. One is permitted to use medications to relieve suffering at the end of life—even if side effects of those medications might hasten death—if the intent of using the medications is to relieve suffering. For the terminally ill, risking the foreseen but unintended consequence of hastening death is justified under the "doctrine of double effect."

c. Cultural, philosophic, or religious objections to withdrawal of mechanical ventilation or other life-sustaining interventions should be explored and respected by clinicians, and unique approaches may be implemented to harmonize aims and preferences.

F. Common Symptoms at the End of Life and Associated Therapies

1. **Pain:** Pain is a common and treatable symptom at the end of life. When feasible, the patient's report of pain or discomfort is the best guide for treatment. However, as with many of the symptoms outlined later, patients undergoing withdrawal of LSTs are often unable to communicate their experiences. In these situations, other signs such as vocalization, grimacing, diaphoresis, tachypnea, and tachycardia must be used to guide treatment. Patients expressing or displaying symptoms should be provided both basal (standing extended release or infusion) and breakthrough (as needed) options for pain control. Opioids offer the mainstay of therapy; acetaminophen, nonsteroidal anti-inflammatory drugs (NSAIDs), topical therapies, and other adjunctives can also be employed. When increasing an infusion of an opioid, a bolus should be given simultaneously to ensure that immediate pain relief is provided because increases in infusions manifest slowly relative to the pace of symptoms.
2. **Air hunger, dyspnea, and irregular breathing patterns:** Dyspnea represents another common and treatable symptom at the end of life. Up to one-third of patients undergoing palliative extubation display postextubation tachypnea, a proxy for dyspnea. This percentage drops when anticipatory opioids are ordered before extubation. Anxiolytics such as benzodiazepines may also play a role in the management of dyspnea.
3. **Anxiety:** Alert patients may display varying levels of anxiety at the prospect of termination of life support. Although nonpharmacologic means of allaying anxiety can be extremely effective, sometimes patients request to be deeply sedated or unconscious before the discontinuation of LSTs such as mechanical ventilation. Although death might be hastened by deep sedation, such requests can be honored.
4. **Agitation or excessive motor activity:** Nonspecific motor activity may occur in some patients. Such activity is often interpreted as discomfort or distress by those attending the patient. It is reasonable that the level of sedation be increased in such situations. Neuromuscular blockade is rarely indicated.
5. **Death rattle:** Noisy, gargling breathing may occur in patients who are close to death. This is usually more distressing to family members who are present than to the patient. Treatment can include repositioning, gentle oropharyngeal suctioning, and anticholinergics. Preparation and reassurance of the family is also key.
6. **Avoidance of drug withdrawal:** Often, patients are already receiving high doses of opioids or sedatives during their illness and have developed drug tolerance. The patient's individual dose ranges should guide subsequent augmentation of opioids and sedatives during the discontinuation of support. Decreasing therapeutic doses of sedatives or opioids before the discontinuation of respiratory support is not advised.

VIII. PHARMACOLOGIC CHOICES (ALSO SEE CHAPTER 7)

A. Opioids are the first line of treatment for pain, dyspnea, or tachypnea during the discontinuation of life-sustaining measures. It is imperative that the route, dose, and schedule be individualized. IV administration is the most common route of administration, with bolus administration providing the fastest pain relief, followed by a continuous infusion and additional bolus doses available as needed. For patients lacking adequate IV access, subcutaneous, oral, or transdermal routes of administration are options. Opioids are cardiopulmonary depressants, but these risks may be tolerated because of the proportionately desirable antidyspneic, sedative, and analgesic effects justified under the principle of double effect. Gabapentin, lidocaine, and carbamazepine may be useful adjuncts for neuropathic pain.

B. Benzodiazepines are effective anxiolytics. However, because of the concern that benzodiazepines may be a risk factor for developing ICU delirium, critical care practice is leaning toward nonbenzodiazepines such as propofol or dexmedetomidine as preferable for routine sedation for adult patients who are mechanically ventilated. Nevertheless, in the end-of-life care setting, benzodiazepines still can play a role for their anxiolytic, hypnotic, sedative, and anticonvulsant properties. They can cause hypotension and respiratory depression—particularly when used in conjunction with opioids—but these risks are generally tolerated.

C. Dexmedetomidine or Haloperidol may be indicated in the presence of delirium (acute confusional states) or agitation. These medications do not affect the respiratory drive, but dexmedetomidine can cause hypotension, hypertension with bolus administration, bradycardia, and loss of airway stability resulting in obstruction if not intubated.

D. Propofol is a potent hypnotic agent that can be used for sedation or for rapid induction of unconsciousness. This may be helpful for procedures and to rapidly reach a desired level of sedation. It also has helpful hypnotic, anxiolytic, antiemetic, and anticonvulsant properties but provides no analgesia. Because dose-dependent decreases in arterial blood pressure and ventilatory drive are expected, some clinicians or institutions prefer not to use it for terminal ventilator withdrawal. The suppression of respiratory drive is enhanced by concomitant use of benzodiazepines and opioids.

E. Barbiturates are potent hypnotics that rapidly produce unconsciousness. Their pharmacodynamic effects are similar to those of propofol but their pharmacokinetic profile is much less favorable. Such agents might be reserved for patients who are refractory to other, more commonly used means of sedation.

F. Anticholinergic medications, such as glycopyrrolate, scopolamine, ipratropium bromide, and hyoscyamine, help diminish copious oral and respiratory secretions that can produce death rattle. Atropine should be avoided because of its potential central nervous system side effects.

G. Neuromuscular Blocking Agents are sometimes administered in the ICU to facilitate synchrony with mechanical ventilation in patients with severe acute respiratory failure. As discussed earlier, the indication for the use of neuromuscular blocking agents is lost once the decision to forgo LSTs is made.

H. Euthanasia Is Illegal in the United States; physician aid-in-dying (ie, assisted suicide, wherein a physician provides a lethal dose of a medication per the request of a competent patient with terminal illness) is legal in some states. Drugs should not be actively administered by physicians with the express purpose of causing death. Such interventions include physician administration of neuromuscular blocking agents to produce apnea or the administration of potassium chloride to produce asystole.

I. Palliative Sedation Is Legal in the United States and is not equivalent to active euthanasia. It is the monitored use of medications to relieve refractory and unendurable distressing symptoms. Protocols for this practice provide guidelines for the use of appropriate medications and the rationale for doing so. See, for example, the Palliative Sedation Protocol of the Hospice and Palliative Care Federation of Massachusetts.

IX. MEDICAL ERRORS IN THE INTENSIVE CARE UNIT

A. "To Err is Human" is the title of a seminal 2000 Institute of Medicine report that catalogs the high frequency of medical errors within health care, describes the significant impact these errors have on patients and providers, and emphasizes the need for a culture shift in medicine away from individual blame and toward a systems-level approach to prevention and management of medical errors. By nature of being human, physicians cannot be held to a standard of perfection, but we can be expected to identify and respond to errors when they occur for the benefit of the patient affected as well as for the sake of preventing future errors.

B. A Medical Error is omission, commission, or deviation from practice that results in harm to the patient. Harm can be categorized as physical, emotional, or financial. Errors typically result from an initial unsafe act progressing through a series of preexisting faults within the system before ultimately reaching the patient.

C. The Rate of Medical Errors Is High in the ICU—higher than in most other areas in the hospital—because of the high acuity of illness, the rapidity with which conditions develop and require management, and the massive amount of data collected on each patient. Although there are multiple lines of defense in place to prevent unsafe acts from reaching the patient, ICU providers must not only remain vigilant at the prospect of adverse events but also familiarize themselves with how to prevent and address medical errors.

D. Addressing Medical Errors With the Patient and Caregivers Begins With Disclosure: After an error has occurred, the first step is sharing that the error has occurred with the patient and family. There are often two stages to disclosure. First, the patient and/or caregivers should be notified of the medical error soon after it is recognized (within 24-72 hours). This initial conversation entails the nature of the error, the reason(s) why it occurred, the impact on the patient, and the steps being taken by the team to address the error. However, it is unlikely that all the details of how and why the error occurred will be understood this soon after it occurred. Unknowns should be acknowledged, and the patient and/or caregivers should be offered a second opportunity to discuss the error once a formal evaluation is complete. Depending on the complexity of the error and the individual institution, the error review process and root cause analysis can take weeks to be completed.

1. Error disclosure, when conveyed in an empathetic, nondefensive manner, can help patients undergo further treatment, address financial concerns, diminish distress about an otherwise unexplained problem, reestablish trust, and actually strengthen the doctor-patient relationship.
2. Compassionate and sensitive disclosure may reduce the risk of malpractice litigation, whereas failure to disclose errors has been linked to increased desire to file an insurance claim.
3. For particularly charged and/or complex scenarios, consider seeking advice from patient advocacy, risk management, legal services, and/or other experienced providers. There are preferred techniques for performing this difficult task.

E. Addressing Medical Errors for the ICU and Hospital System entails documenting an event or incident report. Incident reports are objective descriptions of a medical error, the contributory factors, and the impact on the patient, which are not part of the patient's medical record. These reports raise awareness that the medical error occurred to hospital administration and offer vital information for how to support staff and optimize the system which contributed to that error occurring. Incident reporting and review practices vary between institutions, but the importance of cataloging errors is ubiquitous.

F. Addressing Medical Errors for the Provider and/or others team members involved in the error represents the third key component to a comprehensive approach to medical errors. Medical errors and the broader issue of unintentionally harming a patient can significantly impact the well-being of those involved. An error review should be instructive, constructive, and nonpunitive.

Consolation, coaching, and education of those affected is ideally taken on by individuals trained in error management who are not direct members of the ICU team.

X. SUPPORTING PROVIDERS

A. The Intensive Care Unit Is a Challenging Place to Work: Multiple factors such as uncertain prognoses, high rates of mortality, high incidence of conflict, and challenging end-of-life issues can result in moral distress among providers, which can lead to impairment and burnout. The COVID-19 pandemic exacerbated many of these issues, casting the spotlight on provider well-being and the need for more investigation into the causes, effects, and approaches to reducing the emotional toll on health care providers.

1. **Impairment** is the inability or pending inability of a health care provider to practice according to accepted standards as a result of substance use, abuse, or dependency.
   a. It is estimated that approximately 10% to 15% of health care providers will misuse recreational drugs or alcohol at least once in their career. State, local, and some institutions provide affected clinician programs for rehabilitation and treatment. Recovery rates are higher for health care professionals than for the general population and many programs assist with reentry into practice.
2. **Physician burnout** as outlined by the World Health Organization entails fatigue or low energy, disassociation and pessimistic attitude from one's work, and reduced professional effectiveness.
   a. Conflict, poor communication, work hours, workplace organization, and involvement in end-of-life care increase the risk of burnout. Burnout among ICU providers is common and increased notably during the COVID-19 pandemic.
   b. There are multiple strategies to reduce risk of burnout. Improving overall health, increased personal/peer support, improved work conditions, and improving work satisfaction can help decrease burnout.

B. Ethics Debriefings in the ICU help mitigate moral distress and compassion fatigue related to challenging cases. Such discussions can allow providers to explore alternative strategies of addressing concerns, reach a team consensus, draw on the expertise of interdisciplinary team members, and help with consistent messaging to families. They can also provide awareness of moral distress and serve as educational opportunities for staff. Some ICUs schedule routine ethics rounds to discuss ethics topics, current troublesome cases, or recent past cases.

XI. SPECIAL POPULATIONS

A. The Pediatric Patient Deserves Special Consideration: Legally, end-of-life decisions are deferred to the parents. Ethically, however, the child may participate in these decisions, depending on developmental level and decision-making capacity. If the child is too immature to participate in decisions, parents are relied on to make decisions in the child's best interest by weighing the benefit versus burden of each therapy. Pediatric intensivists must be sensitive to individual family dynamics and parenting styles when approaching end-of-life discussions for the pediatric patient in the ICU.

B. Patients With Previous Disabilities: ICUs receive some patients from both the pediatric and adult populations who have been living with previous disabilities—whether physical or cognitive. Their home caregivers usually have expertise in their home-based complex care routines. Occasionally, tensions develop between home caregivers and ICU caregivers over various elements of care or over perceptions of quality of life. Proactive meetings among home and ICU caregivers early in the ICU course may help prevent or alleviate such tensions. Clinicians should avoid making assumptions about quality of life with disability. Patients with disability often consider their own quality of life to be significantly higher than external observers may assume it to be, a phenomenon known as the disability paradox. Clinicians should take care to avoid inappropriately imputing lower quality of life to patients solely based on actual or anticipated disability.

C. The Chronically Critically Ill: The term *chronically critically ill* refers to a group of patients who have survived an acute critical illness but continue to have persistent organ dysfunction requiring ongoing specialized care. Their course is usually characterized by fluctuations in care needs with slow progress and/or deterioration, which occurs over weeks to months, often interrupted by periodic acute events. These patients experience frequent changes in care venue, often traveling between ICU, step-down unit, short-term acute care, and long-term acute care facilities. One-year mortality is as high as 50%. In these situations, it can be difficult for patients, loved ones, and even health care providers to determine the optimum path. Continued conversations with patients and loved ones regarding prognosis, anticipated outcomes, future level of dependence, values, and goals are key because these can evolve as the state of chronic critical illness progresses. Palliative care involvement can be particularly helpful.

D. The Neurocritically Ill: Patients with acute severe neurologic illness, such as following brain injury, stroke, or status epilepticus, pose unique ethical challenges to clinicians and surrogates. Neurocritical illnesses are commonly accompanied by disorders of consciousness, rendering patients incapable of participating in medical decision-making and frequently carry high degrees of prognostic uncertainty. This confluence of neurologic acuity, decisional incapacity, and prognostic uncertainty can be challenging to navigate for clinicians who must craft time-sensitive, goal-concordant treatment plans in the context of significant uncertainty.

1. Recognizing these challenges and the importance of avoiding undue prognostic pessimism following brain injury, an American Academy of Neurology (AAN) 2018 guideline recommends that "when discussing prognosis with caregivers of patients with a disorder of consciousness during the first 28 days post injury, clinicians must avoid statements that suggest these patients have a universally poor prognosis."
2. The AAN guideline also notably recommends that "in situations where there is continued ambiguity regarding evidence of conscious awareness despite serial neurobehavioral assessments, or where confounders to a valid clinical diagnostic assessment are identified, clinicians may use multimodal evaluations incorporating specialized functional imaging or electrophysiologic studies to assess for evidence of awareness not identified on neurobehavioral assessment that might prompt consideration of an alternate diagnosis." The availability of advanced neuroimaging or electrophysiologic techniques to aid in the diagnosis or prognosis of consciousness may vary by location, and clinicians with expertise in the management of disorders of consciousness should be consulted.

E. Bridge to Nowhere: For some patients, a situation develops in which there is no hope for cure or improvement and yet, they seem "stranded" on a technologically complex and invasive intervention. The intervention may have been initially started as "a bridge" to some other, curative, treatment. An example of being on a "bridge to nowhere" is the continued use of ECMO for a patient who has lost candidacy for transplant or permanent ventricular assist device. In these situations, frank discussions establishing clear limits are necessary, as well as consultations with chaplaincy, palliative care, and ethics.

XII. ORGAN DONATION

A. Determination of Death Using Brain Criteria: Brain death is a clinical syndrome defined as the irreversible loss of clinical function of the entire brain, including the brain stem. Prerequisites include the following:

1. Proximate cause of brain injury is known and is permanently irreversible.
2. Exclusion of complicating medical conditions that may confound clinical assessment
3. Absence of drug intoxication or poisoning
4. Absent evidence of neuromuscular blockade
5. Core temperature greater than 36.5 °C (96.8 °F)
6. A period of 24 hours of observation without clinical change is necessary for comas of unknown etiology.
7. In the presence of confounding variables, brain death may be determined with the aid of ancillary testing.
   a. The three pivotal findings for brain death are irreversible **coma (absence of wakefulness and absence of awareness), absent brain stem reflexes, and apnea.**
   b. Confirmatory **ancillary tests** may be used when uncertainty about the reliability of the neurologic exam exists and apnea testing cannot be performed (such as patients on advanced circulatory support). In clinical practice, electroencephalogram (EEG), cerebral angiography, nuclear scan, transcranial Doppler, computed tomography (CT) angiography, and magnetic resonance imaging/magnetic resonance angiography (MRI/MRA) are used in adults.

B. Organ Donation After Brain Death: Patients who are declared brain dead may be considered for organ or tissue donation with premortem patient consent or postmortem surrogate consent.

1. Owing to a potential conflict of interest, conversations with the family regarding organ donation should not be conducted by the physician caring for the patient. Federal regulations require that these discussions be conducted by trained personnel for the regional organ procurement agency (OPA).
2. Early contact with the OPA by ICU clinicians is critical because OPAs generally have specific guidelines regarding medications, ventilator settings, and blood work to be performed before organ donation.

C. Organ Donation After Cardiac Death: The critically ill who depend on LSTs may be considered for organ donation after cardiac death (DCD). However, the decision to withdraw LSTs must be made before—and distinct from—the discussion and decision about organ donation. LSTs are not being removed *so that* the patient can become an organ donor. Rather, a decision is made to remove unwanted, burdensome, or ineffective LSTs, and the subsequent anticipated imminent death of the patient presents an opportunity for organ donation. Only if the patient is expected to die imminently upon withdrawal of LSTs can DCD be considered.

1. DCD organ procurement is challenging and demands adherence to guiding ethical principles. The institutional guidelines for DCD organ procurement should be followed. Care for the dying patient including analgesic and amnestic medications supersedes the goal of organ procurement. The institutional policy should clearly define the following:
   a. The separation of caregiving responsibilities for the donor and for the recipient to avoid conflict of interest
   b. The physician responsible for pronouncing cardiac death is a member of the patient's care team and not a member of the transplant team.
   c. Specify whether and what medications aimed at improving organ recovery may be administered before death.

d. The time interval after asystole at which death is declared (usually 2-5 minutes, to ensure no autoresuscitation but to minimize ischemic damage to organs)

e. The process for obtaining consent for and administering medications or procedures that are necessary for organ procurement, but are not otherwise of benefit to the patient (ie, heparin administration, femoral arterial line placement, etc)

f. The process for allowing family presence at the time of death

g. The time interval after which organ procurement will not be attempted in the case of unexpected patient survival after the withdrawal of LSTs

XIII. LIMITED RESOURCE ALLOCATION

A. Background and the Impact of COVID-19: With hundreds of thousands in the United States affected and tens of thousands requiring critical care, the COVID-19 pandemic led to an unprecedented demand for critical care staff, services, and provisions that outstripped the supply in some regions. This imbalance in supply and demand cast a spotlight on the triage of limited resources, also known as limited resource allocation. Limited resource allocation both before and during the COVID-19 pandemic was guided by several frameworks and expert opinions.

1. Although there is consensus on many issues within limited resource allocation, there is no single evidence-based gold standard. Across even the most well-recognized frameworks, small variations exist in the process (ie, how patients are prioritized) and principles (ie, who is prioritized or excluded) depending on the situations and populations for which they were designed. The New York State Guidelines for Ventilator Allocation, for example, were targeted toward a theoretical influenza pandemic and utilize the Sequential Organ Failure Assessment (SOFA) score as part of the priority calculation. These frameworks are subject to the limitations of our tools for evaluating mortality (eg, the SOFA score) and the situation they were designed for (eg, influenza instead of COVID-19).

B. Focusing on Survival: The primary goal of limited resource allocation is to maximize survival. "Survival" can be interpreted both with respect to short-term outcomes, such as maximizing the number of patients who live to hospital discharge, as well long-term outcomes, such as maximizing number of life-years. Some frameworks will focus on one interpretation more than the other. Defining the primary goal first is crucial because it influences the ethical obligations and eventual priority calculations. Maximizing survival translates to allocating limited resources to patients who are most likely to live by receiving them. Patients who are likely to survive without any intervention and the patients with the smallest likelihood of survival even with medical intervention therefore fall to a lower priority in the allocation framework.

C. Ethical Principles of Population Health: Providers grapple with medical ethics every day, especially in critical care. Medical ethics focus on the well-being of an individual patient. Allocation of a limited resource, however, requires maximizing its benefit to an entire population and approaching ethical issues at the population level. The following analogy can be drawn: Although the patient-focused ethical principles are intended to preserve the patient-provider relationship, the ethics of public health necessitate coordination of resources and policy at the regional level to uphold the relationship between the health care system and the public. Listed here are several key principles as well as the implication each has designing a resource allocation framework.

1. The duty to care comprises the fundamental obligation to tend to each individual patient. Physicians, nurses, and other members of frontline health care teams are responsible for the care of the individual patient regardless of the circumstances and should ideally be spared from responsibilities that would jeopardize the ability to provide direct care in an objective manner. During a pandemic, limited resource allocation requires approaching health care decisions from population- and systems-based mindsets that are difficult to reconcile with simultaneous bedside patient care. To respect the principle of the duty to care, then, the individual(s) charged with determining and carrying out the triage of limited resources should ideally not be directly caring for the patients for whom resources are being allocated. Furthermore, separating the roles reduces the amount of moral distress and bias introduced by a provider's relationship with a patient into the triage role.

2. **The duty to steward resources** encompasses the need for health care providers and governing institutions to responsibly manage limited resources. During a pandemic, the obligation to save as many patients as possible must be balanced with and will at times take precedence over the obligation to save one individual patient. The duty to steward resources necessitates that limited resources be triaged in an equitable way, and that the means of identifying who receives a resource and who does not is ethically sound and constructed in a way that is cognizant of possible sources of bias.
3. **Distributive justice** requires that an allocation protocol is applied broadly and consistently to ensure fairness and that vulnerable populations receive equal treatment. Implementing distributive justice, on one hand, requires a standardized process that can be implemented at the population level but, on the other hand, can account for regional variability in population and resource availability. Ideally, one triage system should be implemented by a local government in coordination with health care institutions to minimize discordance or worsen preexisting inequalities in health care access.
4. The principle of **transparency** necessitates that a system for allocating limited resources be constructed with the input and values of the public in mind. In addition, this principle calls for an ongoing dialogue between the health care system enacting the process and the public who are subject to its outcomes. More than simply educating the public on how the allocation process works, the idea of transparency also entails active review and updating of the allocation process based on public feedback to maintain public trust in that process.

D. Choosing a Framework: There are multiple strategies, each with its own benefits and pitfalls.

1. Common strategies with notable pitfalls include first-come first-serve (familiar to the public but will discriminate against already disadvantaged populations), randomization (ensures equal opportunity but random distribution of resources may not maximize the number of lives saved), and bedside physician clinical judgment (conflicts with duty to care, imposes large burden on provider, and prone to individual inconsistencies).
2. The allocation strategy recommended by prior guidelines entails triaging resources based on the likelihood of survival. Patients who are at the highest risk of mortality with or without the resource, as well as patients who are the most likely to survive without the resource, fall to a lower priority. When multiple patients are found to have an equivalent degree of priority, prior frameworks have employed clinical scores such as SOFA while others utilize randomization.

E. Operationalizing a Framework: A comprehensive description of how limited resource allocation occurs is out of the scope of this chapter, particularly because many details are determined by the nature of the crisis, the limited resource(s), and the capabilities of the health care system. Key takeaways from multiple models include determination of a clinical scoring system to determine priority, selection and coordination of triage officers (and sometimes committees of officers), and periodic assessment and reassessment of demand, availability, and allocation.

F. **Conclusion:** Reviewing the primary goal, identifying relevant public health ethical principles, and discussing how frameworks are implemented offer the first steps in grappling with a process as challenging as limited resource allocation. Even after the first waves of the COVID-19 pandemic, we still have much to learn about resource triage including the triggers for when crisis standards of care should be enacted, how to ensure equitable distribution of resources across multiple regions, and the optimal ways to discuss limited resource allocation with patients, families, and the public. Although the clear hope is that these frameworks will not have to be implemented again, the pandemic emphasized the need for further investigation and education around management of scarce resources in times of crisis.

Selected Readings

Azoulay E, Timsit JF, Sprung CL, et al. Prevalence and factors of intensive care unit conflicts: the conflicus study. *Am J Respir Crit Care Med.* 2009;180:853-860.

Baldisseri MR. Impaired healthcare professional. *Crit Care Med.* 2007;35(suppl 2):S106-S116.

Barr J, Fraser GL, Puntillo K, et al. Clinical practice guidelines for the management of pain, agitation, and delirium in adult patients in the intensive care unit. *Crit Care Med.* 2013;41:263-306.

Billings J, Keeley A, Bauman J, et al. Merging cultures: Palliative care specialists in the medical intensive care unit. *Crit Care Med.* 2006;34(11):S388-S393.

Boyle D, O'Connell D, Platt FW, et al. Disclosing errors and adverse events in the intensive care unit. *Crit Care Med.* 2006;34(5):1532-1537.

Bosslet GT, Pope TM, Rubenfeld GD, et al. An official ATS/AACN/ACCP/ESICM/SCCM policy statement: responding to requests for potentially inappropriate treatments in intensive care units. *Am J Respir Crit Care Med.* 2015;191(11):1318-1330.

Bülow H-H, Sprung CL, Reinhart K, et al. The world's major religions' points of view on end-of-life decisions in the intensive care unit. *Intensive Care Med.* 2008;34(3):423-430.

Chang DW, Neville TH, Parrish J, et al. Evaluation of time-limited trials among critically ill patients with advanced medical illnesses and reduction of nonbeneficial ICU treatments. *JAMA Intern Med.* 2021;181(6):786-794.

Christian MD, Sprung CL, King MA, et al. Triage: care of the critically ill and injured during pandemics and disasters: CHEST consensus statement. *Chest.* 2014;146(4 suppl): e61S-e74S.

Courtwright AM, Brackett, SE, Cadge W, et al. Experience with a hospital policy on not offering cardiopulmonary resuscitation when believed more harmful than beneficial. *J Crit Care.* 2015;30(1):173-177.

Emanuel EJ, Persad G, Upshur R, et al. Fair allocation of scarce medical resources in the time of COVID-19. *N Engl J Med.* 2020;382(21):2049-2055.

Fehnel CR, Armengol de la Hoz M, Celi LA, et al. Incidence and risk model development for severe tachypnea following terminal extubation. *Chest.* 2020;158(4):1456-1463.

Frontera J, Curtis JR, Nelson JE, et al. Integrating Palliative care into the care of neurocritically ill patients: a report from the improving palliative care in the ICU Project Advisory Board and the Center to Advance Palliative Care. *Crit Care Med.* 2015;43(9):1964-1977.

Greer DM, Shemie SD, Lewis A, et al. Determination of brain death/death by neurologic criteria: the World Brain Death Project. *JAMA.* 2020;324(11):1078-1097.

Hayes MM, Checkley W, Oakjones-Burgess K, et al. Use of a checklist for the withdrawal of ventilatory support to improve the quality of death and dying and nurse comfort with terminal extubation in a medical intensive care unit. Poster presentation. American Thoracic Society International Conference; Denver, Colorado, USA; May 19, 2015.

Institute of Medicine (US) Committee on Quality of Health Care in America. To err is human: building a safer health system. In: Kohn LT, Corrigan JM, Donaldson MS, eds. National Academies Press (US); 2000.

Luce JM, White DB. A history of ethics and law in the intensive care unit. *Crit Care Clin.* 2009;25: 221-237.

Macintyre NR. Chronic critical illness: the growing challenge to health care. *Respir Care.* 2012;57(6):1021-1027.
Miller DC, McSparron JI, Clardy PF, et al. Improving resident communication in the intensive care unit. The proceduralization of physician communication with patients and their surrogates. *Ann Am Thorac Soc.* 2016;13(9):1624-1628.
Morgantini LA, Naha U, Wang H, et al. Factors contributing to healthcare professional burnout during the COVID-19 pandemic: a rapid turnaround global survey. *PLoS One.* 2020;15(9):e0238217.
Netters S, Dekker N, van de Wetering, K, et al. Pandemic ICU triage challenge and medical ethics. *BMJ Support Palliat Care.* 2021;11(2):133-137.
New York State Task Force on Life and the Law, New York State Department of Health. Ventilator allocation guidelines. Published November 2015. Accessed July 27, 2021. https://www.health.ny.gov/regulations/task_force/reports_publications/docs/ventilator_guidelines.pdf
Ravitsky V. Timers on ventilators. *BMJ.* 2005;330(7488):415-417.
Ravitsky V, Steinberg A. Withholding and withdrawing: a religious-cultural path toward a practical resolution. *Am J Bioethics.* 2019;19(3):49-50.
Reich DJ, Mulligan DC, Abt PL, et al. ASTS recommended practice guidelines for controlled donation after cardiac death organ procurement and transplantation. *Am J Transplant.* 2009;9:2004-2011.
Robinson EM, Cadge W, Erler K, et al. Structure, operation, and experience of clinical ethics consultation 2007-2013: a report from the Massachusetts General Hospital Optimum Care Committee. *J Clin Ethics.* 2017;28(2):137-152.
Sprung CL, Zimmerman JL, Christian MD, et al. Recommendations for intensive care unit and hospital preparations for an influenza epidemic or mass disaster: summary report of the European Society of Intensive Care Medicine's Task Force for intensive care unit triage during an influenza epidemic or mass disaster. *Intensive Care Med.* 2010;36:428-443.
Truog RD, Campbell ML, Curtis JR, et al. Recommendations for end-of-life care in the intensive care unit: a consensus statement by the American Academy of Critical Care Medicine. *Crit Care Med.* 2008;36:953-963.
White DB, Lo B. Allocation of scarce critical care resources during a public health emergency. University of Pittsburgh Department of Critical Care Medicine. Published April 15, 2020. Accessed July 27, 2021. https://ccm.pitt.edu/sites/default/files/UnivPittsburgh_ModelHospitalResourcePolicy_2020_04_15.pdf
White DB, Lo B. Mitigating inequities and saving lives with ICU triage during the COVID-19 pandemic. *Am J Respir Crit Care Med.* 2021;203(3):287-295.
Wilmer A, Louie K, Dodek P, et al. Incidence of medication errors and adverse drug events in the ICU: a systematic review. *Qual Saf Health Care.* 2010;19(5):e7.
World Health Organization. Burn-out an "occupational phenomenon": International Classification of Diseases. Published May 28, 2019. Accessed July 25, 2021. https://www.who.int/news/item/28-05-2019-burn-out-an-occupational-phenomenon-international-classification-of-diseases
Young MJ, Bodien YG, Giacino JT, et al. The neuroethics of disorders of consciousness: a brief history of evolving ideas. *Brain.* 2021;144(11):3291-3310.

42 Intensive Care Unit Care After Organ Transplant

Amanda S. Xi

I. PRINCIPLES OF CARE FOR PATIENTS POST TRANSPLANT

A. Time Course: The complex clinical picture of patients post transplant may be simplified by considering time periods that emphasize different issues.

1. **First 7 days—donor and recipient surgery:** As a rule, the allograft is the organ most affected by hemodynamic changes. Proper allograft function will usually lead to swift overall clinical improvement. Allograft dysfunction, on the other hand, requires investigating the contribution of the recipient's preoperative status, intraoperative course, the quality of the donor organ, and the possibility of technical complications.
2. **After 1 week—acute rejection:** Because there are numerous steps in the complex cascade leading to full T-cell differentiation and activation, clinically detectable acute rejection does not usually occur until several days to weeks after transplantation. Assuming technical complications have been ruled out (eg, vascular thrombosis, biliary leak, and preservation injury), organ dysfunction at this time is usually attributed to rejection and can be treated with increased immunosuppression. At times, a liver biopsy in patients with hepatitis C may be helpful to distinguish acute rejection from disease recurrence. In renal transplantation, an early rejection episode may herald an antibody- or cellular-mediated mechanism, and the result of a biopsy may dictate different lines of therapy.
3. **After 6 months—chronic issues:** The risk of opportunistic infections increases with the degree of recipient immunosuppression. Thus, infections are more typical in the late postoperative period, especially if repeated bouts of rejection have required multiple courses of heightened immunosuppression. Late allograft dysfunction raises the possibility of disease recurrence or chronic rejection, both of which may lead to steadily worsening allograft failure and will be unresponsive to increased immunosuppression.

B. Immunosuppression: Administration of any immunosuppressive agent is limited by side effects. By combining different agents, it is possible to increase immunosuppression while limiting troublesome, unwanted effects. For this reason, in most whole-organ transplant cases, patients receive either double- or triple-drug immunosuppression (Table 42.1).

1. **Calcineurin inhibitors: Cyclosporine** and **tacrolimus** specifically target the activation of T lymphocytes (the immune cells principally responsible for rejection). **Calcineurin** inhibitors are the core of most current immunosuppressive protocols. Either one may be started perioperatively and taken orally as long-term maintenance. Both are nephrotoxic and require careful adjustment based on blood levels. Other side effects include hypertension, hyperkalemia, hyperglycemia (especially in patients on high-dose steroids), neurotoxicity (seizures and tremors), and hyperuricemia (gout).
2. **Antilymphocyte-depleting antibodies and interleukin-2 blocking antibodies: OKT3, antithymocyte globulin (ATG), basiliximab**, and **daclizumab** also target T cells, but can only be given via an intravenous (IV) line. The antibody-based agents are used for induction of immunosuppression, for treating steroid-resistant acute rejection, and as part of newer "tolerance"-inducing

TABLE 42.1 Immunosuppressive Medications

Medication name	Class/function
Cyclosporine (Neoral, Gengraf, Prograf)	Calcineurin inhibitor
Sirolimus (Rapamune)	Antiproliferative (mTOR inhibitor)
Mycophenolate mofetil (Cellcept)	Antiproliferative (IMPDH inhibitor)
Azathioprine (Imuran)	Antiproliferative (purine antimetabolite)
Methylprednisolone, prednisone	Corticosteroids
Basiliximab (Simulect), daclizumab (Zenapax)	IL-2 receptor antagonists
Muromonab-CD3 (Orthoclone OKT3)	CD3-specific monoclonal antibody
Antithymocyte globulin (Atgam, thymoglobulin)	Nonspecific polyclonal antibody

IL, interleukin; IMPDH, inosine-5′-monophosphate dehydrogenase; mTOR, mammalian target of rapamycin.

protocols. Multiple courses may have a decreased efficacy and can lead to infection and malignancy in the long term. In patients with postoperative renal failure, cyclosporine or tacrolimus may be discontinued, with OKT3 or thymoglobulin being substituted as equivalent, but non-nephrotoxic immunosuppression. This simplifies the early postoperative management but expends an important therapeutic option, which may be unavailable to treat subsequent resistant rejection later in the postoperative course.

3. **Antimetabolite agents: Mycophenolate** and **azathioprine** inhibit DNA or RNA synthesis and therefore block active lymphocyte proliferation. Dose reduction may be required if leukopenia, thrombocytopenia, or anemia occurs. Mycophenolate is also limited by gastrointestinal side effects that include mild ileus, gastritis, nausea, and vomiting.
4. **Corticosteroids** provide relatively nonspecific immunosuppression. High-dose IV **methylprednisolone** typically is initiated on the day of transplantation and tapered over the next 4 to 5 days to a maintenance level. **Prednisone** is substituted for methylprednisolone when feeding resumes. If rejection occurs, high-dose methylprednisolone boluses (500 mg IV every day for 2 days) are given as initial treatment. Patients may require stress dose supplementation for major procedures while receiving steroids. IV **hydrocortisone** (100 mg IV every 8 hours) is given on the day of surgery and tapered over 3 days. During this time, maintenance immunosuppression is continued with either oral prednisone or IV methylprednisolone. Patients on high-dose steroids are at risk for developing hyperglycemia and gastrointestinal bleeding, which may be mitigated by prophylactic histamine-2 (H_2) blockers.

C. **Efforts to Wean Immunosuppressive Agents:** There is ongoing research directed at the generation of true "transplantation tolerance" (specific immunologic nonreactivity toward the donor organ) and the development of clinical protocols for the reduction of traditional triple-drug immunosuppression down to monotherapy.

D. **Drug Interactions:** The patient's complex drug regimen post the transplant should constantly be reevaluated and simplified. This approach will improve compliance and avoid potentially catastrophic and sometimes unpredictable drug interactions. In particular, the addition of new medications to an immunosuppressive regimen should be carefully considered. For example, **allopurinol**, if administered in combination with azathioprine, may precipitate life-threatening leukopenia. Numerous medications (eg, **sucralfate**, **verapamil**, and **erythromycin**) may alter cyclosporine absorption and thus precipitate rejection or toxicity.

E. Infections

1. **Prophylactic strategies:** Between 60% and 80% of patients will develop some form of infection occurring days, weeks, or years after transplantation. However, different opportunistic infections occur within predictable time periods in the postoperative course, and prophylactic antibiotic regimens have been established. Long-term, low-dose **trimethoprim-sulfamethoxazole** effectively prevents *Pneumocystis* infections and may prevent urinary tract infections as well. During periods of heightened immunosuppression, **ganciclovir** or **acyclovir** (or their derivatives **valganciclovir** or **valacyclovir**) is added to lower the incidence of cytomegalovirus (CMV) and Epstein-Barr virus (EBV) infections. Because invasive procedures increase the risk of bacterial infections, systemic antibiotics are administered during the perioperative period and before cholangiograms or percutaneous biopsies.
2. **Preventative measures** include minimizing immunosuppression, avoiding endotracheal intubation and intravascular catheters, correcting malnutrition, and tight glycemic control. Evaluation of possible hematomas, abscesses, or fluid collections should be pursued by serial ultrasound or computed tomography (CT), and appropriate drainage should be expeditiously undertaken if there is a suspicion of active infection. Because immunosuppression blunts the usual signs of inflammation, an aggressive surveillance and diagnostic approach is crucial, with routine cultures (eg, biweekly cultures of sputum, urine, bile, and wound drainage) and daily chest radiographs while the recipient is receiving mechanical ventilation.

II. LIVER TRANSPLANTATION

A. Indications: Decompensated cirrhotic liver failure, acute fulminant hepatic failure, metabolic disorders, and liver failure with preserved hepatocyte function are all indications for liver transplantation and are discussed in detail in **Chapter 26**.

B. Donor allograft: The likelihood of early allograft failure is correlated with donor characteristics (obesity, prolonged intensive care unit [ICU] stay, malnutrition, terminal hypotension, and fatty liver changes). Although the characteristics of the "ideal donor" are well described, there has been increasing use of "extended criteria" donors (ECDs) in the United States. There is no precise definition of what constitutes an ECD liver; it may be from an older donor, may have steatosis, or have an increased risk of disease transmission (see Table 42.2). This practice is a response to the insufficient supply of needed donor organs. In many cases, recipients who are unlikely to receive organs because of severe illness may receive ECD grafts as an alternative to dying without a transplant. Careful selection of ECD livers can minimize poor postoperative and long-term recipient performance.

C. Efforts to Increase Organ Availability: In addition to the use of ECD livers, other efforts to increase the number of available organs include the use of **donors after cardiac death** (DCD), splitting cadaveric grafts for two recipients, and the use of living donors. DCD liver grafts may give inferior overall graft and patient survival, whereas grafts from living donors function well but place additional risk on a healthy donor. Quantitative algorithms using donor characteristics have been developed to better pair donor and recipient organ allocation to maximize utilization of donor organs. Splitting of well-chosen cadaveric organs for an adult-child recipient pair with one member critically ill has shown promising results. In addition, direct-acting antiviral therapy has made it possible to transplant **hepatitis C virus (HCV)–positive donor allografts** into recipients who are HCV negative. Preliminary data on medium-term outcomes suggest that the use of HCV-viremic donor organs does not impact patient or graft survival. Ongoing studies are needed to discern longer term impact of this strategy to expand the organ donor pool.

TABLE 42.2 Extended Donor Criteria for Liver Transplantation

Advanced age (age older than 60 in many institutions)
Macrovesicular steatosis
Organ dysfunction at procurement
- Prolonged ICU stay (5-7 d)
- Vasopressor use
- Elevated bilirubin (>3) or transaminases

Partial or split-donor liver
Donors with risk of disease transmission
- Hepatitis B
- Hepatitis C
- High-risk donors (eg, intravenous drug users)
- HIV
- Malignancy

Prolonged cold ischemia time
Donation after cardiac death

ICU, intensive care unit.

D. **Preservation:** Prolonged ischemia time is also correlated with allograft dysfunction. Allograft cold ischemia time is ideally limited to less than 12 hours and is less in marginal donor livers. During procurement, the donor allograft is flushed with the University of Wisconsin (UW) solution, which has been the gold standard in preservation solutions, and stored in ice until transplantation. Other preservation solutions such as histidine-tryptophan-ketoglutarate and Celsior, both of which lack starch, are currently being investigated as alternatives to the UW solution. Machine perfusion of the allograft from donors after circulatory death has led to a lower risk of nonanastomotic biliary strictures compared to conventional static cold storage.

E. **Recipient Operation**

1. **Native hepatectomy:** The coagulopathy of end-stage liver disease and the multiple venous collaterals of portal hypertension can lead to **massive blood loss**, which is directly correlated with postoperative morbidity and mortality. Therefore, this phase of the transplant procedure is often the most technically difficult. Once the liver is removed, patients frequently develop **metabolic acidosis**, requiring correction before reperfusion. Overcorrection with sodium bicarbonate, however, may lead to severe postoperative **metabolic alkalosis**. This phenomenon results from the metabolism of the **citrate** administered with transfused blood products to bicarbonate by the functioning allograft.
2. **Donor liver implantation** may be accomplished by different techniques with regard to the vena cava anastomosis. The traditional method utilizes anastomosis between the donor and recipient vena cava at the supra- and infrahepatic locations. Blood flow through the vena cava is typically disrupted, and a venovenous bypass circuit allows blood to shunt from the femoral and portal veins into the internal jugular or axillary vein. Alternately, the "piggyback" technique creates an end-to-side anastomosis between the donor suprahepatic vena cava and recipient vena cava, allowing for a continuous return of blood to the heart if a side-biting clamp is used while sewing the anastomosis. This is followed by portal vein, hepatic artery, and bile duct anastomosis (either a choledochocholedochostomy or Roux-en-Y choledochojejunostomy). A biliary stent or T-tube may be placed across the anastomosis and allowed to drain percutaneously. Peritoneal drains are also placed in the supra- and infrahepatic spaces.

3. **Reperfusion of the allograft,** usually within 60 minutes of warm ischemia time, returns a sudden bolus of cold, hyperkalemic, acidotic blood from the lower body and liver and may cause severe **pulmonary artery (PA) vasoconstriction** with resultant hypotension and possible dysrhythmia ("reperfusion phenomenon"). Reperfusion of the ischemic liver may also precipitate accelerated **fibrinolysis**. Aggressive replacement of coagulation factors and antifibrinolytic agent administration may be required to achieve hemostasis.

F. Posttransplant Management

1. **General care:** In addition to routine physical examination (checking mental status, abdomen, wound, and peritoneal and biliary drains) and invasive monitoring, evaluation includes serial laboratory studies, chest x-ray, and Doppler ultrasound examination in the first 48 hours to screen for hepatic artery thrombosis (HAT) (see later discussion). Neurologic complications are frequently attributable to encephalopathy, neurotoxicity due to immunosuppressants, cerebral hemorrhage, and stroke. Hypothermia must be avoided in the immediate postoperative setting and can be corrected by prewarming the ICU room, application of warm blankets, and the use of forced air warming machines. Maintenance IV fluids should always contain dextrose to avoid depletion of glycogen stores in the liver. Patients often tolerate sips by 24 to 48 hours after surgery, although feeding is resumed cautiously in patients with a Roux-en-Y choledochojejunostomy. On the fifth postoperative day, a cholangiogram is obtained if a biliary tube was placed. If no obstruction or leak is evident, the biliary stent or T-tube is clamped with removal planned for 3 to 6 months post the transplant.

2. **Cardiovascular**
   a. **Hemodynamics:** The high cardiac output and low peripheral vascular resistance typical of end-stage liver disease commonly persist into the early postoperative period, so inotropic agents are rarely required in recipients of liver transplants.
   b. **Hypotension:** The usual first therapeutic response is volume administration. Excessively high central venous pressures should be avoided because transmission back to the hepatic sinusoids may exacerbate allograft edema already present from reperfusion injury. If hypotension persists without detectable hypovolemia or cardiac dysfunction, sepsis should be suspected, blood cultures obtained, and empiric antibiotic therapy initiated. The use of prostaglandin E infusion to counter reperfusion injury may contribute iatrogenically to postoperative hypotension.
   c. **Hypertension:** Postoperative hypertension may be precipitated by pain, anxiety, fluid overload, and preexisting hypertension. Because of the increased risks of cerebral edema, hemorrhage, and seizures, sustained hypertension requires aggressive treatment.

3. **Respiratory:** In the presence of good graft function, successful endotracheal extubation usually can be accomplished within 12 to 48 hours, but it may be delayed by hepatic hydrothorax or right diaphragmatic paralysis from intraoperative placement of the suprahepatic vascular clamp or by metabolic alkalosis. "Fast-track" extubation of selected patients after an uneventful orthotopic liver transplantation may decrease the incidence of pulmonary complications and improve graft function and is becoming the norm at high-volume centers. Occasionally, diuresis is needed before extubation to reverse the effects of high-volume resuscitation. Judicious use of narcotics that are relatively unaffected by hepatic dysfunction (eg, fentanyl) may facilitate early extubation.

4. **Renal:** Many recipients of liver allografts develop mild postoperative renal dysfunction because of preexisting renal insufficiency, intraoperative caval occlusion, bleeding, hypotension, postimplantation hepatic allograft dysfunction, and nephrotoxic drugs such as cyclosporine and tacrolimus. Other nephrotoxic drugs, such as aminoglycosides, may cause intrinsic renal dysfunction and should be avoided. **Prostaglandin E_1** may have a beneficial effect on the recipient's renal function during the early postoperative period. Some patients whose preoperative renal dysfunction is a result of their liver failure (ie, those with the hepatorenal syndrome) will show posttransplant improvement. If postoperative oliguria persists despite optimized hemodynamics, a non-nephrotoxic antibody immunosuppressant can be substituted for tacrolimus or cyclosporine. With this approach, dialysis usually can be avoided. **Continuous venovenous hemofiltration** (CVVH) has less fluid shifts and electrolyte disturbances than does intermittent hemodialysis, and it is preferred if renal replacement therapy is indicated. Dialysis should be used with extreme caution because rapid osmotic shifts may worsen brain swelling already present in patients with hepatic failure. Mortality is high in patients whose renal dysfunction progresses to the need for dialysis.
5. **Hematology:** Leukopenia and thrombocytopenia secondary to hypersplenism typically persist into the early postoperative period, sometimes requiring a dose reduction of azathioprine. Should the white blood cell count fall below 1500/mm^3, **granulocyte colony-stimulating factor** can be administered to decrease the incidence of postoperative infections. The postoperative hematocrit is maintained in the range of 25% to 30%. In the absence of ongoing hemorrhage, an international normalized ratio between 1.5 and 2, a platelet count greater than 50 × 100/L, and a fibrinogen level greater than 100 mg/dL is generally permissible, yet specific benchmarks vary among institutions. The likelihood of significant postoperative bleeding is related directly to the degree of intraoperative bleeding and the quality of immediate allograft function. If major blood loss persists despite reversal of coagulopathy, surgical re-exploration is indicated. Even in patients whose early bleeding stops, re-exploration may be indicated to evacuate the clot. This may improve ventilation by reducing abdominal distension and prevent the development of secondarily infected hematomas of coagulated blood left in the abdomen.

G. Allograft Dysfunction

1. **Primary graft nonfunction (PGNF)**, defined as initial poor hepatic allograft function, occurs in approximately 2% to 10% of recipients and is a common cause of early retransplantation.
   a. PGNF must be differentiated from the reversible preservation injury that is frequently noted in the first 2 postoperative days. Preservation injury is typically associated with a serum glutamic-oxaloacetic transaminase (SGOT) peak less than 2000 U/L and rapid clinical improvement. Technical problems with any of the vascular anastomoses must be ruled out as well and is typically done with abdominal ultrasonography (see later discussion). In contrast, PGNF is associated with a marked elevation of bilirubin and transaminases (eg, SGOT >2000 U/L), persistent hepatic encephalopathy, minimal bile output (<30-60 mL/d, often colorless or white), uncorrectable coagulopathy, acidosis, hyperkalemia, worsening renal function, and profound hypoglycemia.
   b. **Treatment** consists of early prostaglandin E_1 infusion, intensive support, and retransplantation.
2. **Acute rejection:** Both acute rejection and acute viral hepatitis (B, C) or CMV may be heralded by a bilirubin and transaminase elevation. Acute rejection

is uncommon following liver transplantation but can occur during the first or second postoperative weeks, whereas recurrent hepatitis commonly occurs later. A percutaneous biopsy may be necessary to establish the correct diagnosis. Nearly half of recipients suffer some degree of acute rejection; of these, nearly 90% typically respond to steroid boluses. Retransplantation because of uncontrolled rejection is rarely required.

3. Technical complications

a. HAT is more common in pediatric recipients, especially those with small or multiple allograft arteries. Presentation varies: Approximately one-third demonstrate acute hepatic failure, with marked elevation of transaminases (SGOT 2000-10 000 U/L), or bile duct leak because the hepatic artery is the sole blood supply to the bile ducts; one-third have recurrent septic episodes with or without hepatic abscess; and one-third are asymptomatic, with the diagnosis found as an incidental finding. The late sequelae of HAT may include biliary dysfunction or ductal stricture. Doppler ultrasound is used liberally to screen for HAT, whereas an arteriogram may be required to confirm the diagnosis. Treatment options depend on the presentation and include retransplantation, reoperation, selective urokinase injection, and observation.

b. Bile duct complications may be detected by the appearance of bile in a drain or abdominal pain and an unexplained rise in serum bilirubin. Endoscopic retrograde cholangiopancreatography or re-exploration may be required.

c. Other complications, such as portal vein or vena cava thrombosis (manifested by ascites, variceal bleeding, or detected by radiographic studies), are exceedingly rare. Treatment options usually include medical support, radiologic intervention, and operative thrombectomy. Postoperative infections are the primary cause of death after liver transplantation and are a frequent cause of readmission to the ICU. Common sites of infection are the lungs and abdominal cavity.

III. RENAL TRANSPLANTATION

A. Indications: The most common indications for renal transplantation include **chronic glomerulonephritis, diabetic nephropathy, chronic pyelonephritis, malignant nephrosclerosis,** and **polycystic kidney disease.**

B. Recipients of Renal Transplants are at significant risk for cardiovascular complications. Diabetes is a leading indication for renal transplantation, and hypertension and hypercholesterolemia often complicate renal failure. Cardiovascular complications are nevertheless relatively rare in the immediate postoperative period because of aggressive pretransplant screening and preoperative treatment of occult coronary artery disease.

C. Donor Allograft: Adverse donor characteristics, such as advanced age, terminal or prolonged hypotension, and the need for vasopressors, are highly correlated with posttransplant acute tubular necrosis (ATN). Nevertheless, if the allograft has reasonable underlying parenchyma (established by biopsy), recovery may be expected. Prolonged cold ischemia time, associated with shipping renal grafts long distances and the use of DCD donors, can also contribute to poor intra- and postoperative graft function. Delayed allograft function is much easier to manage in kidney recipients than in liver recipients because of the availability of dialysis. ATN is extremely rare in living donor recipients. Although efforts at human leukocyte antigen (HLA) matching have proved successful in lengthening the half-life of well-matched renal allografts, no difference in perioperative immunosuppression or performance is expected.

D. Recipient Operation: The allograft is implanted in the pelvis, with the renal artery and vein sewn into the corresponding iliac vessels. If the ureter is implanted into the bladder, a Foley catheter is left in place for 5 days to prevent bladder distension and strain on the ureter-bladder anastomosis. If a ureteroureterostomy is constructed (after a native nephrectomy), prolonged bladder catheter drainage is not required, although it may be useful to monitor urine output. In either case, a Jackson-Pratt drain is left in place at the site of the ureteral anastomoses.

E. Immediate Postoperative Course

1. Immediate allograft function is heralded by a massive diuresis necessitating aggressive fluid replacement (eg, replace fluid equal to the previous hour's urine output in milliliters plus 30 mL every hour, limited to 400 mL/h) and diligent electrolyte monitoring.
2. Oliguria in the early postoperative course is usually due to reversible ATN but technical complications must be excluded.

F. Late Course: Elevated creatinine could be due to nephrotoxins or rejection, resulting in a decision about whether to reduce the dose of a nephrotoxic immunosuppressant (cyclosporine or tacrolimus) or to increase immunosuppression to treat rejection. A biopsy often is required to determine the cause of graft dysfunction.

G. Complications: The most common vascular complication following kidney transplant is renal artery stenosis, which often manifests as severe hypertension. Treatment may be surgical or via percutaneous balloon-based techniques. Urologic complications include leak from the bladder closure or ureteral anastomosis, and ureteral obstruction. Lymphocele of the transplant bed can be avoided with careful ligation of the surrounding lymphatics during recipient preparation.

IV. LUNG TRANSPLANTATION

A. Indications include end-stage chronic obstructive pulmonary disease (**COPD**), **cystic fibrosis, pulmonary fibrosis, α-1-antitrypsin deficiency, sarcoidosis, bronchiectasis, lymphangioleiomyomatosis, occupational lung diseases**, and **pulmonary hypertension**. Candidates with end-stage pulmonary disease have an estimated survival of 2 to 3 years without transplantation.

B. Donor Organs: Improved organ preservation and perioperative management have expanded the pool of potential donor organs, but **the lung remains more susceptible to ischemic injury than does any other transplanted organ.** Ischemic time for lung transplantation should be limited to 6 to 8 hours; lungs from older donors are less tolerant of long ischemic times than are those from younger donors. **Living related lung donation** (with two donors each donating a lung lobe) is an option exercised with increasing frequency in experienced centers. DCD has also been performed for lung transplantation.

C. Recipient characteristics affect the postoperative course. For example, patients with systemic disease such as cystic fibrosis may suffer from other organ involvement. Similarly, years of tobacco abuse may be associated with peripheral vascular disease and pulmonary disease in single-lung recipients postoperatively.

D. Recipient Operation

1. **Monitoring:** Patients undergoing single- or double-lung transplantation are usually monitored with pulmonary and systemic arterial catheters and possibly with transesophageal echocardiography. The procedure necessitates endotracheal intubation with a technique that allows for selective lung ventilation, usually with double-lumen tracheal tube.
2. **The recipient surgical operation** consists of a posterior lateral thoracotomy for single-lung transplantation or a bilateral anterothoracosternotomy for bilateral lobe transplantation. Double-lung transplantation with a single tracheal anastomosis is rarely performed because of anastomotic complications.

E. Postoperative Management

1. **General:** Postoperative issues in lung transplants generally involve management of respiratory status, hemodynamics, prevention and treatment of infection, continuation of immunosuppressive regimen, and pain control.
2. **Respiratory management:** The goal of postoperative respiratory management in lung transplants is to achieve adequate oxygenation and ventilation while avoiding oxygen toxicity and barotrauma. Positive end-expiratory pressure (PEEP) is generally added to a level of 5 to 10 cm H_2O. Limiting tidal volume and peak airway pressures to less than 40 cm H_2O is thought to decrease barotrauma and bronchial anastomotic complication. **Pulmonary reimplantation response** is a phenomenon of noncardiogenic pulmonary edema lasting up to 3 weeks and requiring ventilatory support but is generally associated with a good prognosis. Following extubation, patients demonstrate a hypoventilatory response to hypercapnia, although the etiology is not fully delineated.
3. **Hemodynamic management:** Postoperative hemodynamic management after a lung transplant is a fine balance between adequate volume for vital organ function and prevention of pulmonary edema, and, thus, monitoring the patient with a PA catheter may facilitate management. Hemorrhage is more common following transplantation in which cardiopulmonary bypass (CPB) has been utilized. CPB may also increase postoperative transfusion requirement, intubation duration, and overall hospital stay. Pulmonary hypertension is common in the immediate postoperative period; patients may benefit from treatment with inhaled nitric oxide to decrease PA pressures without systemic hypotension.
4. **Pain management** generally involves either systemic opioids or epidural analgesia. Those with chronic respiratory failure due to either COPD or cystic fibrosis may be particularly susceptible to the development of hypercapnia when treated with systemic opioids. Although epidural opioids may also cause hypercapnia, equivalent analgesia can generally be achieved with a significantly lower opioid dose. Epidural analgesia may decrease times to extubation and discharge from the ICU. However, their use is institution dependent and may be contraindicated in the setting of anticoagulation when CPB is used.

F. Immunosuppression: Most centers initiate immunosuppression in the operating room. Almost all protocols include a nonspecific anti-inflammatory corticosteroid. Side effects of corticosteroids such as hyperglycemia and myopathy must be considered. A calcineurin inhibitor such as **cyclosporine** is generally initiated as well. Side effects include nephrotoxicity, hypertension, and neurotoxicity. **Tacrolimus** has essentially the same mechanism of action as cyclosporine but is more effective in preventing acute rejection. Tacrolimus does have higher rates of neurotoxicity, nephrotoxicity, and new-onset diabetes. **Azathioprine** or **mycophenolate**, both of which inhibit lymphocyte proliferation, may be adjunct immunosuppressant agents. Toxicities include leukopenia, hepatitis, and cholestasis. Finally, antilymphocyte preparations such as polyclonal **antilymphocyte globulin, ATG**, and **OKT3** may be initiated.

G. Infections: Immunosuppression increases the recipient's incidence of both bacterial and viral infection. Early infections tend to be bacterial, with gram-negative organisms predominating. **CMV** is the most common early viral infection and may be due to reactivation of an infection in a seropositive recipient (secondary) or, more commonly, new infection in a seronegative recipient from the seropositive donor organ (primary). The most serious manifestation of CMV is pneumonitis or pneumonia; treatment is with **ganciclovir**, which, when given prophylactically, may decrease the incidence. *Aspergillus fumigatus* is the most common fungal infection, with a peak incidence within the first 2 months. Manifestations include ulcerations, pseudomembranes, and tracheobronchitis.

H. Rejection: Hyperacute, acute, and chronic rejection may be encountered in the ICU. Hyperacute rejection is extremely uncommon, occurring within the first minutes to hours after transplantation, and is almost universally fatal. It is due to preformed antibodies against HLA and ABO antigens and may be confused with ischemia-reperfusion injury. Acute rejection occurs within the first 3 to 6 months. Symptoms of acute rejection include fever, cough, dyspnea, and anorexia. Decreases in pulmonary spirometry or diffusion capacity may aid the diagnosis, which requires biopsy for confirmation. Treatment of acute rejection consists of a course of high-dose steroids and elimination of other causes of symptoms. Chronic rejection occurs generally between 6 and 12 months and is typically manifested as bronchiolitis obliterans (BO). The pathophysiology of BO is poorly understood, but the syndrome is typically characterized by airflow limitation due to fibroproliferation in the small airways. Treatment includes corticosteroids and immunosuppressants, but mortality remains high despite treatment.

Selected Readings

Abt PL, Desai NM, Crawford MD, et al. Survival following liver transplantation from non-heart-beating donors. *Ann Surg.* 2004;239:87-92.

Allan JS. Immunosuppression for lung transplantation. *Semin Thorac Cardiovasc Surg.* 2004;16:333-341.

Arcasoy SM, Kotloff RM. Lung transplantation. *N Engl J Med.* 1999;340:1081-1091.

Busuttill RW, Klintmaim GB. *Transplantation of the Liver.* 2nd ed. Elsevier Saunders; 2005.

Busuttil RW, Shaked A, Millis JM, et al. One thousand liver transplants. The lessons learned. *Ann Surg.* 1994;219:490-497.

Cotter TG, Aronsohn A, Reddy KG, Charlton M. Liver transplantation of HCV-viremic donors into HCV-negative recipients in the United States: increasing frequency with profound geographic variation. *Transplantation.* 2021;105(6):1285-1290.

DeMeo DL, Ginns LC. Clinical status of lung transplantation. *Transplantation.* 2001;72:1713-1724.

Feng S, Goodrich NP, Bragg-Gresham JL, et al. Characteristics associated with liver graft failure: the concept of a donor risk index. *Am J Transplant.* 2006;6:783-790.

Findlay JY, Jankowski CJ, Vasdeve GM, et al. Fast track anesthesia for liver transplantation reduces postoperative ventilation time but not intensive care unit stay. *Liver Transpl.* 2002;8:670-675.

Ghobrial RM, Busuttil RW. Future of adult living donor liver transplantation. *Liver Transpl.* 2003;9:S73-S79.

Kawai T, Cosimi AB, Spitzer TR, et al. HLA-mismatched renal transplantation without maintenance immunosuppression. *N Engl J Med.* 2008;358:353-361.

Miller LW, Kasiske BL, Gaston RS, et al. Consensus conference on standardized listing criteria for renal transplant candidates. *Transplantation.* 1998;66:962-967.

Ng CY, Madsen JC, Rosengard BR, Allan JS. Immunosuppression for lung transplantation. *Front Biosci.* 2009;14:1627-1641.

Organ Procurement and Transplantation Network. https://optn.transplant.hrsa.gov/

Ploeg RJ, D'Alessandro AM, Knechtle SJ, et al. Risk factors for primary dysfunction after liver transplantation—a multivariate analysis. *Transplantation.* 1993;55:807-813.

Renz JF, Emond JC, Yersiz H, et al. Split-liver transplantation in the United States: outcomes of a national survey. *Ann Surg.* 2004;239:172-181.

Singh H, Bossard FR. Perioperative anaesthetic considerations for patients undergoing lung transplantation. *Can J Anaesth.* 1997;44:284-299.

Sleiman C, Mal H, Fournier M, et al. Pulmonary reimplantation response in single-lung transplantation. *Eur Respir J.* 1995;8:5-9.

Sollinger HW, Knechtl SJ, Reed A, et al. Experience with 100 consecutive simultaneous kidney-pancreas transplants with bladder drainage. *Ann Surg.* 1991;214:703-711.

Starzl TE, Murase N, Abu-Elmagd K, et al. Tolerogenic immunosuppression for organ transplantation. *Lancet.* 2003;361:1502-1510.

Tolkoff RN, Rubin RH. The infectious disease problems of the diabetic renal transplant recipient. *Infect Dis Clin North Am.* 1995;9:117-130.

Tzakis AG, Gordon RD, Shaw BW Jr, et al. Clinical presentation of hepatic artery thrombosis after liver transplantation in the cyclosporin era. *Transplantation.* 1985;40:667-671.

Zhang T, Dunson J, Kanwal F, et al. Trends in outcomes for marginal allografts in liver transplant. *JAMA Surg.* 2020;155:926-932.

43 Disaster Management

Ed George

The more you sweat in peace, ... the less you bleed in war.
—General Patton

I. BACKGROUND

A. The past several years has unfortunately raised our awareness of the nature and scope of disasters and society's vulnerabilities. All health care institutions have now faced the challenges associated with responding to a disaster in the context of the recent disaster. The etiology of such events may be varied—a natural disaster such as an earthquake, the challenges imposed by a pandemic, or a man-made event as a result of an accident or an act of terrorism. Regardless of the nature, one of the most significant concerns that affect all involved is that the *assets may be overwhelmed by demand.* And assets range from personnel to equipment, to space, to support services; essentially everything and anything that allows an institution to function may be constrained because of the effects of a disaster.

B. One of the most vulnerable components of an institution's ability to provide patient care, in the setting of a disaster, is its ability to provide critical care services. Although such events levy an extraordinary burden on emergency department (ED) resources, the most grievously injured/ill require care in the institutions' intensive care units (ICUs).

C. The specialized clinical capabilities in ICUs, coupled with the limitation of available individuals trained to provide critical care, and the availability of physical resources to support these requirements, position ICUs as one of the most vital "choke points" in the response to any disaster. The experiences of the COVID-19 pandemic, having extended over several years, can offer a common and valuable example of the challenges associated with disaster management. Although these experiences have been most often described by focusing on the management of clinical challenges associated with severe respiratory illness, the volume of patients resulted in clinicians managing multiple morbidities, often with worsening of the disease process leading to sepsis, multi-organ system failure, and death.

D. The intent of this chapter is not to specifically address a unique type of disaster. The focus is to offer to provide insight and guidance regarding common factors known to arise in the setting of institutional disaster management to allow institutions and ICUs the opportunity to anticipate key areas of concern and establish guidelines and policies that best position the ICU to face the demands of a disaster, regardless of the nature. Experience gained during the COVID-19 pandemic is vital in predicting the challenges of other types of disasters. Examining the common elements in a reflective manner will help frame overall disaster management policies.

E. Clinical care during a disaster always presents challenges. However, the development and execution of a care plan for a patient is similar, if not identical to the same plan effected under routine operational conditions. The challenges of disaster management are predominantly tied to insufficient preparation and limited resources. Significant elements of concern have been reported over the experiences during the response(s) to the COVID-19 pandemic; significant findings are noted in Table 43.1.

II. MANAGEMENT

The most critical component of disaster management is planning/preparation. The development and promulgation of effective policies for response implementation are the foundations of the process. Recognition that regular and comprehensive training exercises must be a priority, from the level of institutional leadership to activities directly impacting delivery of bedside care, is key to disaster management.

A. Prioritization/Approach

Institutional leadership must have an approach to establish control over a potentially chaotic event. Prioritizing clear lines of responsibility and interactions, as well as communication, will help all plans for disaster management.

To facilitate disaster planning and management in the ICU, it is important that ICU leadership appreciate institutional-level plans and policies. The Hospital Incident Command System (HICS) provides a framework to understand organization in clinically challenging times and offers distinct means for managing an institutional challenge, as well as the ability to interact with municipalities and other government agencies to obtain support as required.

B. Hospital Incident Command System

Initially, the Incident Command System (ICS) was developed as an approach for emergency response units in the setting of forest fires and mining disasters experienced in the 1960s and 1970s. At the national level, the Federal Emergency Management Agency (FEMA) evolved to offer a hierarchy of coordination from the highest level of government. And Health and Human Services (HHS), along with its precedent agencies, and others such as the Department of Homeland Security (DHS) continue efforts to refine response capabilities to assist states and municipalities confronted by emergency situations requiring resources in excess of organic assets.

The HICS structure is an ICS structure specifically designed for hospitals. The HICS, a standardized approach to disaster management in clinical settings, has evolved from these efforts and has been vital in institutions dealing with the COVID-19 pandemic. Familiarization with institutional HICS plans and procedures is key to development of training and vital in times of disaster. Figure 43.1 provides a structural overview of the basic elements of the HICS design.

TABLE 43.1 Global Planning Shortfalls[a]

Resource Shortfalls
- Equipment
- Medications
- PPE

Inadequate staff[b]
Preparation/education

PPE, personal protective equipment.

[a]Primary shortfalls experienced in the earliest phases of response to the COVID-19 pandemic. Deficiencies regarding the anticipation of strains on intensive care unit (ICU) operations during a disaster demonstrate key shortfalls. Advance preparation and training remain an area that may best limit operations limitations during a disaster.

[b]Academic centers fare better than community hospitals.

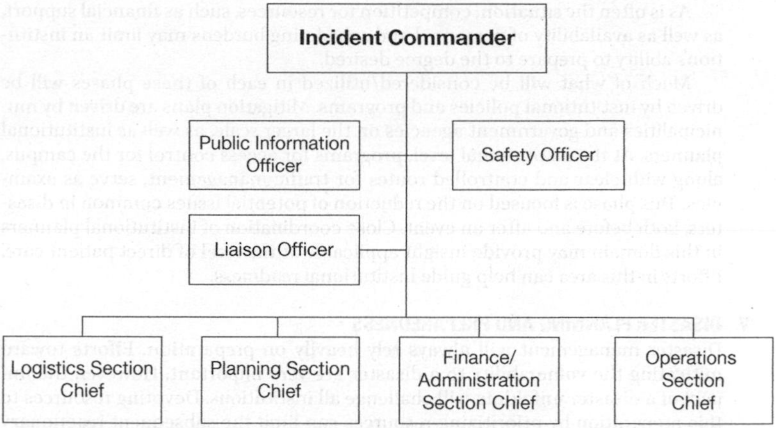

FIGURE 43.1 The Incident Command System structure offers a simple mechanism to facilitate command and control during a disaster. Limiting spans of control and offering latitude in design, the structure can be established by an institution and adjusted for any unique elements of a given setting.

It represents a standardized means for command, control, and communications for emergency situations that can be task organized to address the needs of a specific incident. Adopted by health care institutions, HICS uses principles that have been proved to improve efficiency and effectiveness in a business setting and applies these principles to emergency response.

Although the system is designed to ensure that all personnel appreciate the chain of command, it also provides the incident commander with the ability to design/adjust the structure to best represent the challenges of a particular situation. It serves to help establish reasonable spans of control at all levels and offers the ability to have individuals serving in multiple roles as needed.

The command element typically provides the incident commander with staff specialists to facilitate coordination with external agencies and oversee institutional policies. Typically, this cadre of staff can include a public information officer, a safety officer, an external liaison officer, and a safety officer, as well as clinical and technical specialists.

A team of section chiefs comprise the leadership directly overseeing clinical operations, logistics, planning, and finance. Subserved by personnel engaged in overseeing/providing/supporting direct patient care, these individuals or section teams, must provide timely input to the incident commander to permit ongoing care and anticipate future requirements.

A key component of the HICS concept remains the inherent flexibility for adjustment. The incident commander may choose to reassign individuals and/or functions to best address the needs of the disaster. For example, the finance section can be set up as an operational section or as an element of the command staff, as needed.

III. OVERVIEW OF DISASTER MANAGEMENT

Disaster management commonly comprises four distinct and related phases:

- Mitigation: ongoing effort; minimize impact
- Preparedness: evaluate, equip, and train
- Response: handle the threat
- Recovery: debrief, learn, restore

As is often the situation, competition for resources, such as financial support, as well as availability of personnel and scheduling burdens may limit an institution's ability to prepare to the degree desired.

Much of what will be considered/utilized in each of these phases will be driven by institutional policies and programs. Mitigation plans are driven by municipalities and government agencies on the larger scale, as well as institutional planners. At the institutional level, programs for access control for the campus, along with clear and controlled routes for traffic management, serve as examples. This phase is focused on the reduction of potential issues common in disasters, both before and after an event. Close coordination of institutional planners in this domain may provide insight applicable at the level of direct patient care. Efforts in this area can help guide institutional readiness.

IV. DISASTER PLANNING AND PREPAREDNESS

Disaster management will always rely heavily on preparation. Efforts toward mitigating the vulnerability to a disaster are very important. However, the impact of a disaster unfolding will challenge all institutions. Devoting resources to this preparation by prioritizing resources can limit the subsequent reactionary efforts with the arrival of a disaster. Table 43.2 outlines basic steps in planning that may be undertaken in advance of any disaster.

Planning and preparation for disaster mandate both generic (all hazards) and specific designs. It is important to appreciate that disasters present unique demands related to the nature of the disaster encountered, as well as generic requirements tied to the overall demand, on an institution/unit when urgent/emergent challenges exceed organic assets. Planners at every level are confronted by common challenges ranging from personnel and equipment shortfalls to space and event duration.

Organizing efforts for disaster preparedness and response mandate a coordinated effort utilizing resources organic to the ICU, as well as support services and assets not resident in the ICU. Exercises and tabletop drills can help identify areas requiring support.

Table 43.3 provides an outline that can be used as a checklist in guiding leadership in analysis and preparation. By mapping out a strategy from the level

TABLE 43.2 Elements of Disaster Preparation[a]

- Develop a disaster team/review existing unit-institutional plans
- Assess current capabilities and liabilities
- Coordinated triage plan(s)
- Internal/external patient flow
- Infection control issues
- Surge capacity
- Logistics plans
- Data maintenance
- Team training/simulation
- Communication plans
- Staff well-being
- Care for family members
- Ethics training
- Behavioral health resources
- Conflict resolution

[a]Key elements of disaster management. Institutional emphasis for critical care is primarily focused on preparation. However, knowledge of efforts regarding mitigation can facilitate the intensive care unit (ICU) leadership's planning efforts.

of the ICU can quickly identify areas that will require additional support and areas that may remain dynamic in requirements as a disaster evolves.

Advance preparation is, to a degree, limited by the uncertainty associated with the varied nature of a future disaster. Investing heavily in purchasing/stockpiling extra ventilators in anticipation of a respiratory pandemic can limit obtaining other types of equipment that may be vital in addressing a different type of disaster that may present primarily with trauma patients. Equipping and training

TABLE 43.3 Preparation for Disaster Management

Form a disaster team (unit-based)

- Medical and nursing leadership
  - Critical support/vested groups (organic and otherwise)
  - Respiratory care
  - Pharmacy
  - ID
  - Trauma, OR, and ED
  - Imaging/laboratory
  - Mental health providers

Review existing plans/protocols

- Staff
  - Availability
  - Emergency recall/platooning
  - Protection (PPE, immunization, isolation, negative pressure)
  - Cross-training additional staff
- Space
  - Expansion/surge capabilities
  - Family members
- Supplies
  - Medications, gases, monitors, disposables
- Standard of care (conventional—contingency—crisis)
  - Staff-to-patient ratio
  - Ventilators
  - Infection control

Coordinate with Institutional Disaster Planning leadership for threat assessment

Exercise and revise

- Tabletop
- Unit-based
- Institutional
- Simulation/VR training

Formulate a unit-based plan

- Coordinate with other ICUs.
- Vette with institutional agenda(s).

Establishing a focus on basic elements, such as personnel and equipment, can help position an intensive care unit (ICU) to manage a future disaster. Developing a plan of action and designing exercises to familiarize personnel can best position an ICU to effectively react to an evolving disaster. ED, emergency department; ICU, intensive care unit; ID, infectious diseases; OR, operating room; PPE, personal protective equipment.

in anticipation of a known type of disaster affords specific targets of opportunity. However, the same efforts framed against nonspecific disaster situations place leadership in the position of looking to common features, such as increased patient volume and operational tempo, with the requirements of a specific disaster being addressed as part of the evolution of a disaster.

Figure 43.2 illustrates some of the differences associated with planning/preparing for a known disaster (ie, COVID-19) versus the nonspecific nature of designing the more generic/nonspecific disaster plan, capable of being adjusted to a described threat. Preparedness occurs before the direct challenge of a disaster. Planning for generic (all hazards) and specific challenges (pandemic, mass casualty, etc) shares common goals. Obtaining necessary supplies such as personal protective equipment (PPE), gloves, and cleaning equipment, as well as more specific equipment such as monitors and ventilators, and processes such as recall plans for personnel and evacuation plans for patients all demonstrate various considerations typically undertaken during the preparedness phase. It is important that ICUs are engaged in all phases of higher level discussions. The specific requirements by units can vary, tied as they are to the unit's primary roles (ie, surgical versus medical), as well as potential requirements for a unit to be utilized/transitioned to provide critical care of a nature different from that typically encountered in a specialized patient population.

Commonly developed and reviewed in institutional committees charged with, for example, emergency planning or disaster preparation, these discussions are often led by ED leadership, in conjunction with senior management. During a disaster, emergency services are often the initial source for information, as well as for clinical demands. In the response to a disaster, programs and policies instituted in the ICU should be closely coordinated with operations in the ED. Critical care personnel are often called upon to assist with the care of patients in the ED and may serve as a vital liaison to the ICU. These roles should be specified in the institution's HICS design.

The specific requirements for individual units can vary as a function of the particular role of an ICU (ie, surgical vs medical; burn units, etc), as well as potential requirements for a unit to be utilized to provide critical care of a nature different (overflow or repurposing) from that typically encountered in a specialized patient population. As such, education/exercises should consider elements

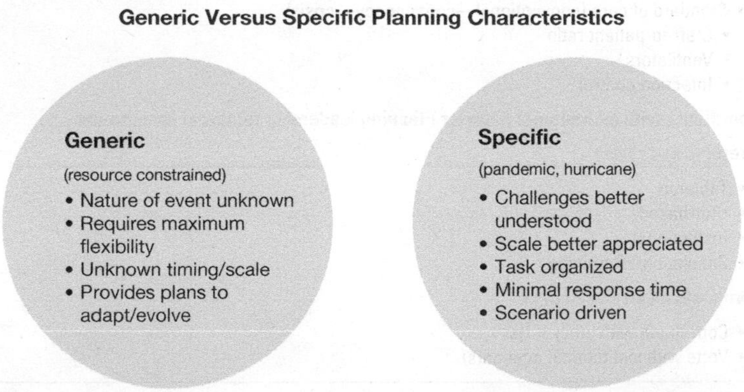

Generic Versus Specific Planning Characteristics
Generic
(resource constrained)
• Nature of event unknown
• Requires maximum flexibility
• Unknown timing/scale
• Provides plans to adapt/evolve
Specific
(pandemic, hurricane)
• Challenges better understood
• Scale better appreciated
• Task organized
• Minimal response time
• Scenario driven

FIGURE 43.2 The challenge of uncertainty regarding potential disaster limits "complete" efforts regarding anticipatory planning. Adjusting planning to consider the probabilities suggested in an institution's HVA and help guide the efficiency of planning.

of clinical cross-training to better prepare personnel to work in areas other than their primary roles. A post-anesthesia care unit (PACU) can quickly be repurposed to an ICU role in critical capacity management situations. Meeting rooms may be utilized as family waiting areas. The element of flexibility must be reinforced in all operational planning and exercises.

Many experiences during the COVID-19 pandemic can serve as examples for determination of requirements. With acute respiratory failure presenting as the most common condition requiring management, many institutions were challenged to provide adequate resources to intensive care sites, both in the domain of space and physical resources as well as personnel and clinical expertise. Examination of challenges anticipated/encountered can categorize limitations into broad areas that can be applied to all phases.

Some elements/functions outlined in the HICS are subdivided to a degree not necessarily applicable to units engaged in direct patient care. For example, a particular ICU may not be directly involved in fiscal management issues or in the framing of public affairs announcements. However, resources and policies from institutional leadership will often impact the processes associated with direct patient care. Therefore, clear understanding, by all personnel, of the institution's expectations of ICUs in the setting a disaster response is vital.

Organizing an ICU's abilities and requirements into a few basic domains can help examine assets/liabilities and provide the ability to communicate to leadership overall capabilities and shortfalls. Dividing unit functionality into three or four generic categories can help anticipate challenges, as well as identify resources/capabilities that can assist in meeting institutional challenges. Most activities in an ICU could be viewed in the context administrative, operational, or a logistic function.

Typically, these elements will have subordinate areas, tied to the nature of the unit as well as the diverse requirements tied to the nature of a specific disaster. And limiting to fewer domains may help unit personnel address key issues and relay requirements in a more concise and efficient manner.

Disaster planning may not be the focus of day-to-day activities for an institution. Competing costs and resource availability can limit the focus to more of a weekly or monthly time scale. However, as more recent experiences have demonstrated, prioritizing disaster planning and preparation must be an institutional focus.

Most often performed at the institutional and regional levels, a hazard vulnerability assessment (HVA) can assist in envisioning the nature and likelihood of various types of disasters. A pandemic may be estimated to occur every decade, whereas a mass casualty event, such as a shooting, may be a more likely occurrence. Guided by the potential for events of each type to occur and the anticipation of the types of patients likely to present for treatment, the ICU can strategize and develop plans that can establish immediate actions and identify areas that may be vulnerable to early exhaustion, or be markedly limited from the outset.

V. INTENSIVE CARE UNIT DISASTER TEAM

Organizing an ICU's abilities and needs along a few simple domains can help examine assets/liabilities and provide the ability to communicate to leadership overall capabilities and shortfalls. Creating an ICU disaster plan, for a single ICU or for multiple ICUs in an institution, requires a coordinated effort engaging subject matter experts (SMEs) in the domain, as well as the appreciation of plans at higher levels of the institution.

A. Unit-Based Disaster Team

A unit-based disaster team is a group dedicated to the evaluation and planning processes and can serve as a framework for guiding operations during a disaster. The team should comprise senior individuals/stakeholders from all disciplines involved in the ICU. A team leader must be designated. Figure 43.3 outlines the key participants in an ICU's disaster team. Both personnel working as primary ICU staff (intensivists, nurses, respiratory therapists [RTs], etc) and individuals supporting multiple ICUs are important members of the team.

B. Intensive Care Unit Surge Team

A subset of the disaster team may be designated as the ICU surge team. This group would, as required, develop contingency plans for increased tempo of operations (ie, higher acuity) as well as increased patient volume necessitating

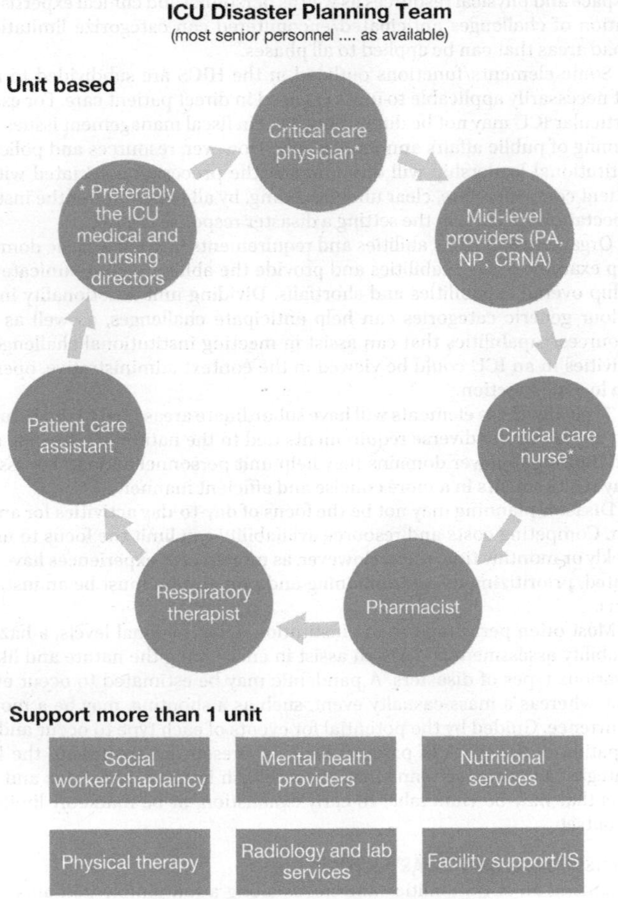

FIGURE 43.3 A planning team for an ICU can provide direction to specific efforts for planning and preparation. Comprising personnel assigned to a given ICU, as well as those specialties supporting multiple ICUs, this team can offer insight to leadership and can be tasked with developing training scenarios and exercises. CRNA, certified registered nurse anesthetist; ED, emergency department; ICU, intensive care unit; IS, information services; OR, operating room; NP, nurse practitioner; PA, physician assistant.

expansion of available beds. Planning is important because such actions will often be institution-wide and directed by the HICS team. Having discussed and rehearsed such contingencies in advance would greatly facilitate execution during a disaster.

C. Critical Care Disaster Committee

Discussions must be open and all input is encouraged. The team leader will serve both as an arbitrator and as a resource to bring any concerns to the institutional leadership. Hospitals with multiple ICUs may establish a critical care disaster committee that can serve as a representative to the HICS to better reflect the overall posture of institutional critical care capabilities and requirements.

VI. UNIT ANALYSIS

This most critical stage of planning offers some flexibility to unit leadership regarding the evaluation of unit capabilities. ICU operations can be divided into a few basic categories to help evaluate unit functions needing support. This may be performed in the context of an identified challenge, such as a mass casualty, or in a less specific manner, simply anticipating a more generic increase in operational tempo associated with larger scale emergencies.

A. Architecture of the Hospital Incident Command System Command Elements

There are multiple approaches to the evaluation, planning, implementation, and execution of disaster management in the ICU. An ICU can choose to approach disaster planning along the architecture of the HICS command elements using basic component categories. Evaluating functionalities in the context of planning, administrative, operational, and logistic domains may be helpful to smaller institutions.

B. Systems-Oriented Process

A systems-oriented process can be employed to parallel functionally within a unit, as well as resources designated to support unit requirements. This view may offer a more global approach to assessment. Such analysis can be of use in larger units faced with diverse populations and more strongly integrated with developing institutional-level programs. Here, the planners may become engaged in discussions addressing data management and epidemiologic registries, as well as formulating plans for cross-training staff to assist in other units.

Categorizing unit functionality into three or four basic areas can simplify and help clarify unit readiness, as well as convey capabilities and shortfalls to the institutional leadership via HICS reporting pathways, facilitating leaderships meeting institutional challenges. Smaller ICUs may find that limiting the domains for the purpose of evaluation may help unit personnel address key issues and relay requirements in a more efficient manner.

C. Role-Based Approach

However, a role-based approach to the analysis can offer all personnel the chance to provide insight into every phase of disaster management. Led by the disaster team, the various "stakeholders" in the function of the ICU(s), both from the staff working in the ICU and those providing clinical or support services to many sites in the hospital, have the opportunity to contribute to the assessment process and provide insight from a perspective perhaps not resident in staff solely assigned to a particular ICU.

D. Stakeholder-Based Approach

A stakeholder-based approach may be the most efficient manner of performing a unit-based needs analysis, particularly during an initial evaluation. This can be conducted along role groups in the ICU, with those groups/disciplines external (imaging, laboratory, etc) to the ICU engaged as the analysis/planning progresses.

VII. KEY ROLES AND STAKEHOLDERS

A. Intensivists

Critical care physicians offer specialized insight and experience in the care of the severely ill patient. Specialization along the disciplines of surgical, pulmonary, cardiac, pediatric, and burn domains positions these physicians in ICUs, most often directing the care of a unique subset of critically ill/injured patients. However, the common elements of critical care do place these physicians in a position to assist in the care of patients not typically placed in a specialized ICU. And it also offers the intensivist as a resource that could be employed in a different ICU, supplementing existing staff and serving as an institutional resource.

Intensivists may be called upon to manage emergency airway and resuscitation teams in the hospital, as well as affording an institution-wide service for obtaining access in patients requiring central lines and arterial access/invasive monitoring. Critical care physicians can also work with other specialties, such as anesthesia and emergency medicine physicians, to design and implement a cross-training plan for education that would permit non-critical illness–trained physicians to help in overseeing the care of critically ill patients as patient volume increases.

With critical care nursing, intensivists can offer insight and oversight in training and using specialized nurses, such as nurse practitioners (NPs) and certified registered nurse anesthetists (CRNAs), as well as physician assistants (PAs), to augment direct patient care during personnel constraints. In addition to directing the clinical care provided by trainees (fellows, residents, medical students), the intensivist must help plan a mechanism to anticipate personnel shortfalls and make sure that the incident command staff is kept aware in a timely manner. Protecting clinical staff from exhaustion is vital, particularly so in a protracted disaster, such as the COVID-19 pandemic.

The critical care physicians and nursing leadership can identify personnel with experience in other areas of care, in either other areas of critical care or in different specialty areas. As the patient population increases, the ICUs may admit patients not commonly received in a specialized unit. Identifying, in advance, personnel with additional specialty experience/training (ie, pediatric, neonate, obstetrics, cardiac, neurosurgery) may facilitate assigning these individuals to a direct care function, or as taking on a role to oversee less experienced staff.

B. Critical Care Nurses

ICUs are completely dependent on the many roles served by the ICU nursing staff in the operation of the unit. Ranging from direct delivery of bedside care to the management of teaching programs, every aspect of day-to-day operations is influenced by the nursing staff. An additional consideration involves the administrative functioning of the ICU. The nursing director/manager of an ICU most often oversees multiple domains of staff/functions in the ICU. Personnel for administrative support and patient care, as well as clinical support subspecialties, such as diet, nutrition, and others are most often overseen by the nursing leadership of the ICU. Equipment calibration, triage and evacuation planning, visitation policies, and issues pertaining to the needs of the patient's family members all require the attention of nursing leadership.

On a day-to-day basis, staff shortages owing to illness/emergencies, equipment and supply challenges, and the ever-present competition for limited resources are most often resolved at the level of nursing leadership. Adding the demands/constraints of either acute or protracted disasters will almost certainly exceed the resources immediately available to the unit. Nursing and physician leadership must work closely to make sure requirements are met and must inform the HICS group of any requirement for assistance.

C. Respiratory Therapists

Resources can vary as a function of institutional size, as well as specialization. However, the availability of RTs and the associated capabilities remain in the forefront of disaster planning and management. As highlighted in the COVID-19 pandemic, the need for RTs was paramount. Managing ventilators and providing inhalational therapies, as well as maintenance of oxygen and specialized gases, required that the RT had intimate knowledge of the patient's care plan, and the ability to coordinate with logistic elements in the institution to obtain necessary equipment. And these demands became more challenging in the setting of surge operations and the expansion of ICU care into non-ICU spaces (PACUs, operating rooms [ORs], wards, etc). The RT is also vital in planning and implementing care strategies not often used in the ICU—specialized beds, ventilator sharing, prone ventilation, ventilator turnover, and so on. Scope of practice may also permit the RT to have a primary role in intubations, intravenous (IV) insertion, and in initiating noninvasive mechanical ventilation (NIMV). In mass casualty events, the RT can be used as a key element of monitoring and triage strategies.

D. Infectious Disease

Not commonly part of the staff based in the ICU, the infectious disease (ID) and infection control personnel are vital components of any disaster management plan. The critical roles played by these services were one of the primary points of focus during the COVID-19 pandemic. Both disease containment and the interpretation of the newest guidelines of care were essential as the pandemic evolved. The guidance for protection of staff personnel was provided by the infection control group: This was particularly challenging because guidelines provided by regulatory agencies evolved/changed over the earlier days of the pandemic.

Although a pandemic may highlight the role of the ID team, other types of disasters also require specific expertise. Injuries associated with mass casualties often present medical challenges associated with infections. Contaminated wounds, hospital- and ventilator-associated pneumonias, and other types of comorbidities often require the assistance of ID services. And during a disaster, where ICU staff ratios may be impacted, the ID personnel can augment a care team and alleviate some of the requirements of care normally provided by the ICU team.

E. Emergency Department, Trauma Team, and Perioperative Services

1. Emergency Department

The ED is most often the portal of entry to the hospital during times of disaster. Often, the ED serves as the source of early warning, as well as the gatekeeper to the institution in performing the earliest and perhaps most critical function of triage. The ED typically has a close relationship with the municipality's emergency medical and law enforcement resources. This relationship can afford important information regarding a disaster that can provide the institution valuable lead time to initiate emergency protocols and forewarn all departments.

The ED is often required to initiate critical care for patients arriving because of a disaster. As the number of patients increase, and the institution begins to experience capacity challenges, there will almost certainly be a delay in transferring patients to ICUs. In this setting, critical care personnel from the ICUs may be required to oversee care of these patients in the ED for extended periods, thereby freeing ED staff to continue primary services.

2. Trauma Team

Trauma teams, with specialized surgical and nursing staff, work closely with the ED, the ICU, and perioperative services, and are usually involved early on in any disaster where injuries may require surgical intervention. Trauma teams are often involved with providing care during a disaster. And trauma has become increasingly viewed as a disease process and it is clear that the earliest of interventions may have a dramatic impact on morbidity and mortality. The ability to help direct care in the ED, communicate with the OR, and to provide additional triage to assist in patient disposition is essential to efficient patient movement. And in coordination with the ICU, trauma teams may choose to send a patient to imaging, with subsequent transfer to the ICU for resuscitation, before undergoing surgery. This can contribute to improved patient care and help relieve overburdened sites of care, such as the ED.

In addition, the team can help communicate with surgical colleagues and OR leadership to evaluate processes for postponing elective cases. This may facilitate scheduling urgent and emergent cases, as well as clearing a pathway to use OR facilities and personnel in nonsurgical roles, that is, additional ICU space.

3. Perioperative Services

Perioperative services can be engaged in several manners. In addition to the management of the ORs and support services and recovery of surgical patients, these facilities can be utilized as auxiliary triage areas. Perioperative resources may be used for additional supplies and additional ICU space for surge capacity. Staff, such as OR nurses, can be used in the ICU to perform dressing changes and other specialized patient care, freeing critical care nurses to attend to other issues requiring special skills (administration of vasoactive agents, delivery of analgesics, ventilator management, etc). These services may also be utilized in the process of initiating emergency recall of personnel to assist in providing needed services. Serving as a coordination center, perioperative services can provide briefings and direct personnel arriving from outside the hospital to areas of need. Likely a hub of activity during a crisis such as a mass casualty, perioperative services also have a vital role in keeping the leadership and the HICS staff informed.

F. Specialty Services

1. Pediatrics, Neonate, and Obstetrics

These services are closely related, can offer experience as consultants, and may be able to assist in staffing other ICUs. The specialized monitoring required of a pregnant patient and a fetus may challenge some ICUs in terms of equipment, supplies, and experience. The ability to confer with personnel experienced with maternal-fetal medicine will enhance the ICU's ability to care for such patients during a disaster.

2. Dietary, Nutritional, Physical, and Occupational Therapy

The nature of these services, routinely involved in the day-to-day care provided in the ICU, affords insight into patient requirements and capabilities. The demands associated with a disaster can markedly impact these important services. And, compromise in the delivery can impact patient care and disposition. During a pandemic, patients can require prolonged ICU care. Both from the extended time required for recovery and commonly associated comorbidities that require treatment, the expertise offered by nutritional and dietary services can help avoid unnecessary deterioration in patient progress. And if unit expansion is required during surge activities, these services must be involved as early as possible to make sure that appropriate resources are available, despite new and perhaps more austere physical settings.

G. Mental Health

Psychologists, psychiatrists, and specifically trained providers must be engaged in every phase of disaster management. During the World Trade Center disaster in 2001, the devastation was incomprehensible to the survivors, as well as to many of the personnel working to rescue/recover survivors. Individuals, including health care and rescue workers, were often overcome by the magnitude of the event to the point of requiring relief from duty, consoling, and counseling both in the moment and longitudinally. Mental health providers were in the forefront of providing on-site care, as well as assisting in the subsequent needs of survivors and rescuers.

In a protracted disaster, such as a pandemic, staff are required to work longer hours, with more frequent shifts, often caring for severely ill/injured patients. Subjected to such stress, to include the challenges experienced in assisting family members and friends levies an emotional burden on staff that must not be overlooked. Psychiatrists, psychologists, and other specialized personnel can offer assistance to those staff impacted by these stressors. These providers can also monitor staff for early signs of stress associated with the increased tempo of operations and severity of encountered illness, thereby offering immediate assistance and educational sessions. Keeping leadership informed regarding the overall emotional burden on unit personnel is also another vital function of these specialized providers. These same insights are also very helpful in gauging the impact of the situation on friends and family of survivors.

H. Ethicists

Ethicists are often closely integrated with the mental health services needed during disaster management. Although the cannons of care during a disaster should never be compromised, resource allocation may impart a different urgency.

During routine operations, providers in the ICU may encounter situations where a terminal patient, sustained on multiple modalities of life support, has reached the stage where continued care is futile. The ability to help family members through the decisions involved in the limitation of life-sustaining therapies or limiting escalation of care can be demanding on all involved. It may require significant time to help those family and friends close to the patient understand these issues. Here, members of the care team must often proceed slowly in providing guidance to help family members.

In the setting of the increased operational tempo experienced during a disaster, the prolonged course required for these same decisions may impact the ability to admit other patients needing critical care. And in both settings, the assistance of the ethicist may help provide comfort and guidance to family members and caregivers not accustomed to what may feel as an accelerated process.

Not offering mechanical ventilation or hemodialysis to a patient where there is no benefit may be more challenging in the setting of heightened emotions experienced in a disaster. Here also the ethicist can offer to provide insight and support, both in the moment and later, to the family and the staff.

I. Chaplaincy and Social Services

Caring for patients located throughout the hospital, chaplains and social service personnel are a vital component of ICU care during a disaster. Chaplains can provide valuable assistance to family, friends, and patients, as well as staff. Offering spiritual support, chaplains may learn information during interactions with family and friends that can assist the care team; and it is often a member(s) of the social services team who initially obtains important details.

Information appreciated in this setting can help the social worker in developing appropriate plans for the patient and the family. Certain constraints, such as financial or geographic, may not be obvious to other members of the team, yet can have a large impact in the design of a discharge plan.

J. Clinical Support Services

These vital elements in any hospital may feel the impact of a disaster to an extent and manner on parallel to that experienced in the ICU. These services are involved in helping with almost all patients admitted to the hospital, as well as those going through the ED for discharge home. The tempo of operations may rapidly escalate and the ability to adapt is clearly tied to advance planning.

1. **Imaging/Interventional Services**
   The requirements placed on imaging/interventional services may be the most demanding of any services during a disaster. ICU patients routinely transported to undergo studies may be too unstable for transport and may require studies performed with portable equipment. It is important to appreciate this potential chokepoint and make sure training focuses on developing portable ultrasound capabilities in the ICU to be utilized where appropriate to provide information needed to treat the patient. In addition, the interventional service may be called upon to assist in the care of disaster patients, further burdening physical resources. Contingency planning with members of these support services can help establish a process to maximize utilization, while minimizing service obligations.
2. **Laboratory Testing**
   Laboratory and testing capabilities experience an increase in demand during a disaster. Emphasizing point-of-care testing can help limit the burden on these services. These services can provide education regarding the conservative limitation of requests, both in type and frequency, to what is necessary for clinical decision-making. This can contribute to efficiency and help limit service burdens.
3. **Patient Transport**
   Patient transport resources may be overlooked but remain essential. Institutional plans likely address the ability to augment this service, perhaps by assigning personnel from other services to patient transport. However, the ICU leadership must always consider the potential for patient transport to be a rate-limiting factor. And plans to utilize ICU personnel to help in transport should be established.
4. **Police and Security**
   Police and security will likely be one of the busiest support services. Not only providing for the safety of staff, patients, and visitors, they also have a close relationship with ED and municipal functions. This can offer important information to ICU leadership that can provide insight, not only in preparing for an ongoing disaster but also in providing "real-time" information as the disaster evolves. The ability for security and safety personnel to communicate when other resources may be limited can afford ICU leadership key information in a timely manner. And the presence of security can be very helpful in managing/limiting the movement of family members during acute phases of response.

VIII. EVALUATION BY FUNCTIONAL DOMAINS

Preparing an evaluation of ICU capabilities for disaster management can also be performed by examining a few functional areas, rather than the detailed, role by role, evaluations used as planning matures. Analyzing requirements along the lines of a few component categories is often helpful as an initial approach to disaster management/planning. This method of categorization during initial planning stages may be of merit in smaller intuitions with limited ICU capabilities.

Staff members are asked to examine needs relative to providing a service and assigning the function to one (or more) of the main categories. This can help all members appreciate the dependence and interdependence of unit functions on multiple personnel in the unit, as well as those providing externally based services.

IX. COMPONENT CATEGORIES

Using fewer, basic divisions of elements, along parallel and often interrelated lines, can help planning activities and provide staff with an understanding about potential areas of overlapping responsibilities. HICS employs such an approach, broadened to address both the needs of the care units and institutional requirements that may require outside assistance. A simple stratification using the categories mentioned can offer a basic scheme of attack; a training program along these lines can be modified as necessary. Table 43.4 details some of the significant activities in day-to-day ICU function.

Logistic, operational, and administrative areas are examined in detail and may reflect key areas of focus within the HICS. This review can also facilitate effective communication with institutional leadership. Considering each of these areas in the context of the various phases of disaster planning earlier mentioned can provide anticipatory and reactionary insights.

Categorization is not rigid. And there is often overlap regarding the impact of a particular challenge. For example, a disaster that produces personnel shortfalls will almost certainly provide constraints regarding operational capabilities. However, examining the impact of challenges over these domains can help simplify solutions.

Examining unit functions in this manner can also serve to provoke discussions across the various members of the ICU staff. A simple request for a patient to undergo an imaging procedure, scheduled by the administrative group, illustrates the complexity of the requirement. The scheduling may require communication with resources not usually part of the ICU's cadre of resources. The process requires coordination with logistics for transport and respiratory therapy if such services are required. A nurse and/or a physician may be required to accompany the patient out of the unit, thereby impacting available staff resources in the ICU. And the care team may be required to identify a window of opportunity in the day's activities best suited to permit the patient leaving the ICU. Many of these requirements rely on the administrative staff to coordinate efforts.

A. Logistics

Traditionally, the rate-limiting element in any major undertaking, personnel involved in logistical support of an ICU must be involved in any consideration for disaster planning/management. In close coordination with operational and administrative components, the logistic support team may be resident in the ICU or function as an external resource supporting several clinical activities.

In addition to providing needed equipment, supplies, and a myriad of additional services, a key role played by logistics personnel during planning phases is to offer feasibility assessments when plans are being developed or care is being proposed. Requiring 20 additional ventilators for an ICU may appear to the clinicians as a reasonable request. However, storage space may not be available, institutional availability may be limited, external resources may

TABLE 43.4 Component Categories[a]

Logistics	Operations	Administrative
• Supplies	• Direct care	• Patient records
• Communications	• Provide consults	• Consult requests
• Transport	• Code team	• Family/visitors
• Food	• Training	• Order admin
• Coordinate (with admin and ops)	• Coordinate (with log and admin)	• Coordinate (with log and ops)

Admin, administrative; log, logistics; ops, operations.[a]

Functional categories can assist planners in understanding specific actions and the interdependence of elements within the ICU. Operational efforts remain the focus of all functions.

not be available, and support personnel for testing, calibration, and operation may already be overwhelmed. Such situations mandate coordination with the logistics team to arrive at practical and supportable solutions.

This role of assessing the feasibility of a plan may be the most important element of personnel involved in logistic support. Where it is human nature to ask for everything possible, the logistician may address many requirements along the just-in-time concept of resupply.

Communication support may also be assigned to logistic elements. A communication plan, established by the ICU leadership, is often dependent on institutional assets and HICS guidance. The logistician, in coordination with both the ICU leadership and HICS personnel, may be required to oversee communications. This process illustrates the interdependence of the other major components within the ICU, administrative and operational, on logistics support.

Technical requirements for equipment in the ICU are often overseen by logistics personnel. In close coordination with nursing leadership, monitors, ventilators, defibrillators, and other equipment requiring regular maintenance and calibration are managed by the logistician, often in collaboration with institutional biomedical resources. Any planning is only as effective as is the logistician's ability to support it. Involving the logistics elements in all phases of disaster management is essential to success.

Employing component categories of function to develop a plan for disaster management can assist leadership in developing an initial assessment. Rather than list every action taken by every individual associated with the ICU, framing a functional view can be particularly helpful to smaller ICUs, as well as ICUs with little previous experience in disaster management.

B. Operational

Delivery of direct patient care in an ICU can range from the more routine activities of obtaining vital signs and conducting examinations to performing emergent procedures and managing resuscitations. In the setting of operations during a disaster, many elements can potentially be compromised. Staffing ratios may increase, supplies may not be immediately available, and resource personnel may be limited as the duration of a disaster may be prolonged and personnel may be reassigned to provide help elsewhere. Longer shifts and hours worked per week will, to some degree, erode staff productivity and morale.

Although a key element of clinical training emphasizes the necessity of anticipation, the challenges encountered in disaster management may place staff and institutions in a reactionary mode of operation. This can be tied to sheer volumes of patients needing care or the heterogeneous nature of the clinical challenges that may place staff in situations where primary expertise/experience may be limited.

Direct patient care and elements tied to providing urgent and emergent responses are the hallmarks of disaster care. ICUs, although most often specialized, provide care to the most grievously injured and ill patients in the institution.

The challenges of a disaster will likely impact ICU operations in both qualitative and quantitative aspects. The scope of care may change to require providing care to more heterogeneous clinical requirements. A neurosurgical ICU may be required to provide care to general trauma or medical patients. It is important to appreciate the common elements of critical care between various types of ICUs, as well as identifying areas where additional expertise may be required.

Familiarity with staff capabilities and expertise in other clinical domains should be noted by unit leadership because previous experience may (and should) be leveraged as clinical demands broaden.

Individuals may be asked to fill clinical roles for which specific experience may be limited. During the initial responses to the World Trade Center bombing, medical and surgical ICU nurses were used in burn ICUs to fill in staffing shortfalls. As the COVID pandemic escalated, most ICUs did not have enough critical care nurses experienced in managing mechanically ventilated patients. And the high volume of ventilated patients often exceeded the number of available RTs. Many institutions utilized anesthesiologists and CRNAs to help bridge this gap. The Department of Defense's experiences during the Gulf War demonstrated shortfalls in available orthopedic trauma surgeons. Programs were implemented to train general trauma surgeons in forward areas to place external fixation devices to treat fractures.

There are many additional examples of individuals being called upon to help in areas where background may be less than robust. The point is to emphasize the necessity of developing and rehearsing contingency plans. It is important that staff, from unit leadership to caregivers at the bedside, as well as support personnel, appreciate that in constrained situations flexibility is vital.

A pandemic requires specialists in ID and infection control to be integrated into ICU care teams. Special precautions, such as the use of PPE and other specialized equipment, can levy burdens, not only on caregivers but also on staff involved in obtaining these items. Training in procurement, use, and disposal places additional burdens on administrative and logistic elements.

Operational requirements can incorporate every activity in the ICU. However, examining the key components of care delivery to the patient can help planners, in the earliest stage, appreciate the hierarchy and prioritize requirements that can then be addressed more specifically.

C. Administrative

Commonly considered the "paperwork" end of the clinical activities, administrative functions can incorporate several key activities. Before the promulgation of the electronic medical record, most record keeping was done on paper. Alarm systems for vital signs and central station monitoring were rudimentary. And communications between colleagues in a unit relied on telephones, pagers, or face-to-face interactions.

1. Electronic Systems

A disaster compromising electronic systems could markedly impact the administrative elements of patient care. An internet failure may eliminate data recording and informational exchange in a timely manner. Given present-day dependence on electronic systems, emergency use of paper records may be the only alternative during a disaster. However, newer, recently trained personnel may be unfamiliar with completing the somewhat complicated and archaic ICU paper records and may require assistance from more senior/experienced personnel. Burdening senior staff with basic training requirements for record keeping during the evolution of a disaster could compromise the ability to respond to the disaster and deliver patient care. An administrative plan to familiarize all staff with paper records would be helpful in avoiding unnecessary delays due to record keeping.

2. Personnel

Personnel-associated issues are an additional area that is often addressed by administrative elements. Administrative staff often assist unit leadership in coordination with human resources. Challenges may range from determining that all shifts have adequate personnel, to include specialized providers, as well as identifying shortfalls to institutional leadership in a manner commonly outlined in HICS procedural guidelines. Activating recall of staff may also be assigned to the administrative personnel.

Administrative functions most likely have a role in logistic support. For example, ordering additional/specialized equipment, reordering medication and supplies, helping coordinate pastoral care, and working with dietary resources to obtain additional meals for patients and family, as well as the potential to provide meals to staff in a high-tempo setting where leaving the unit may not be practical. One of the major challenges encountered during the earlier phases of response to the COVID epidemic involved obtaining adequate supplies of PPE. Again, the burden of requesting/finding/tracking appropriate supplies often fell to the administrative staff of the unit, working closely with the logistic staff.

In the event of a mass casualty event, patients may require emergent disposition/treatment before being identified. EDs and perioperative services maintain systems to provide a mechanism to provide each patient, yet an unknown identity, with an event-specific, synthetic, and individualized identity specifically tied to a set of records. This permits appropriate tracking of a patient and all information until a positive identification is made. This process relies heavily on administrative personnel to make sure these records are maintained and, upon identification of a given patient, the information is flawlessly transferred to the patient's permanent record. Administrative personnel can also help in coordinating family visits and interaction with emergency response personnel.

X. RECOVERY

As the management of any disaster approaches its end, the challenge(s) of recovery begins. This phase is not simply repair and resupply but also brings a significant educational approach to disaster management in the ICU.

As in the case of managing a patient's resuscitation, when the efforts are complete regarding the patient, the care team should immediately debrief. This affords a nonjudgmental review of the recent event, permits all involved to offer perspective, and, most importantly, offers an excellent forum for providing recommendations for improvement. These suggestions can address protocols, equipment, performance, or any other issues germane to the effort. The initial debriefing may be abbreviated because patient care requirements may require additional clinical efforts. However, when possible, a meeting should occur to facilitate a more formal review.

This concept of debriefing is every bit as vital in the success of the recovery phase of disaster management. More complex/detailed, leadership must organize formal sessions to review overall performance and solicit feedback from all members of the ICU personnel.

These sessions can be supported by the development of tools/questionnaires by leadership to make sure all key areas are addressed. The process must make sure that all comments/criticisms are confidential and maintain an appropriate level of professionalism.

The review process may be dictated by elements of the HICS. However, the degree of resolution offered by those directly involved in providing/supporting bedside care offers invaluable insight to all levels of leadership.

From both the level of the individual ICU to the HICS group, information must be analyzed, both in the face of the given disaster and in the elements applicable to general disaster management. This information can be incorporated into action plans for improving unit function as well as for the support of unit function from institutional leadership.

A recovery phase can also take on a longitudinal approach. In the case of a more prolonged disaster, such as the recent pandemic, leadership can direct certain personnel to regularly review unit performance. This value-added approach facilitates corrections/adjustments to unit function while facing an ongoing challenge.

Selected Readings

Harris G, Adalja A. ICU preparedness in pandemics: lessons learned from the coronavirus disease-2019 outbreak. *Curr Opin Pulm Med.* 2012;27(2):73-78.

Minnesota Department of Health. Patient care strategies for scarce resource situations. Published August 2021. https://www.health.state.mn.us/communities/ep/surge/crisis/standards.pdf

Troug RD, Mitchel C, Daley RD. The toughest triage—allocating ventilators in a pandemic. *N Engl J Med.* 2019;382:1973-1975.

Wax RS. Preparing the intensive care unit for disaster. *Crit Care Clin.* 2019;35551–562.

Wilcox ME, Rowen KM, Harrison DM, Dodge JM. Does unprecedented ICU capacity strain, as experienced during the COVID-19 pandemic, impact patient outcome? *Crit Care Med.* 2022;50:e548-e556.

INDEX

Note: Page numbers followed by *f* denotes figure; those followed by *t* denote tables

D

E

J

K

L

M

Q

R